IMMUNOLOGY

A Short Course

Icons used in this book

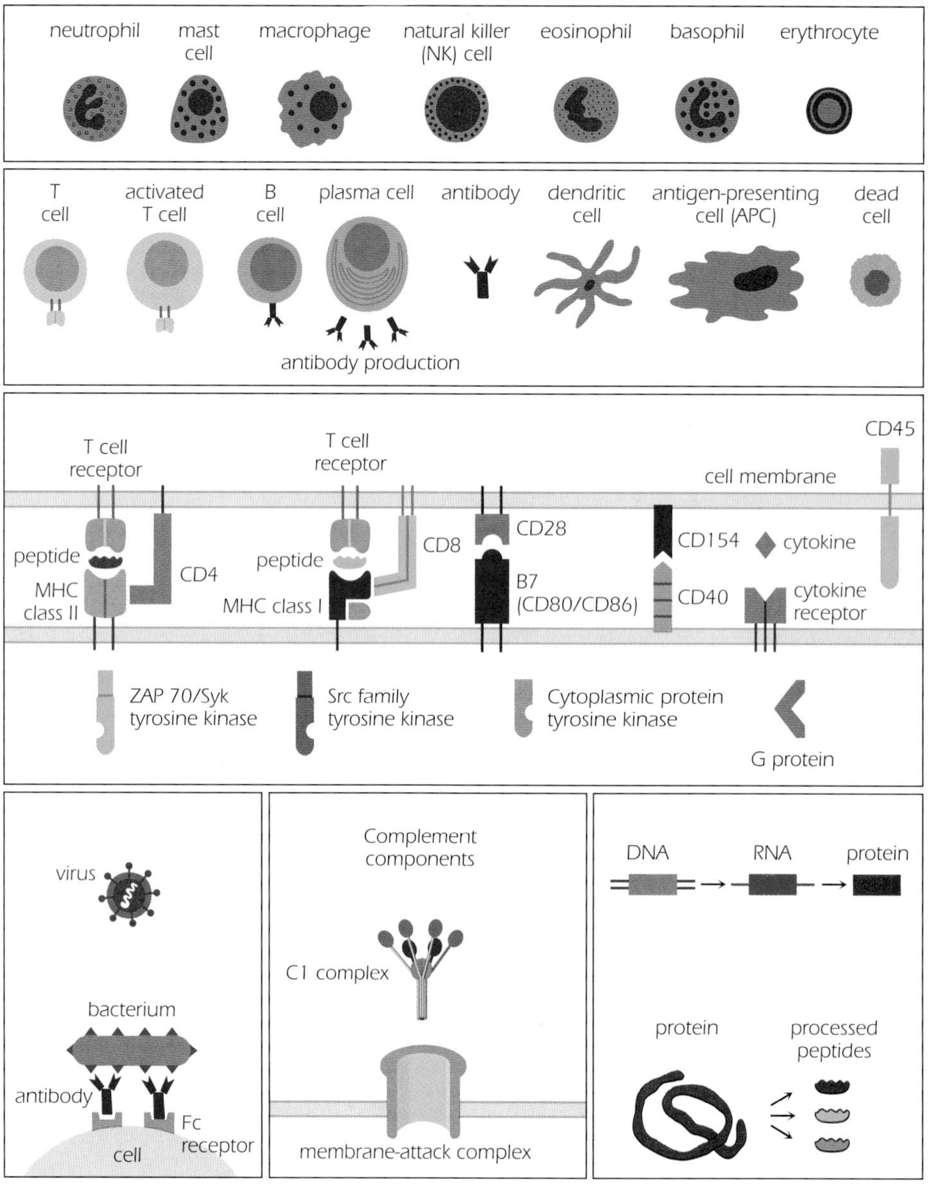

neutrophil
mast cell
macrophage
natural killer (NK) cell
eosinophil
basophil
erythrocyte
T cell
activated T cell
B cell
plasma cell
antibody
dendritic cell
antigen-presenting cell (APC)
dead cell
antibody production
T cell receptor
peptide
MHC class II
CD4
T cell receptor
peptide
MHC class I
CD8
CD28
B7 (CD80/CD86)
CD154
CD40
cytokine
cytokine receptor
cell membrane
CD45
ZAP 70/Syk tyrosine kinase
Src family tyrosine kinase
Cytoplasmic protein tyrosine kinase
G protein
virus
bacterium
antibody
Fc receptor
cell
Complement components
C1 complex
membrane-attack complex
DNA
RNA
protein
protein
processed peptides

IMMUNOLOGY
A Short Course

FIFTH EDITION

Richard Coico
Professor and Chairman
Department of Microbiology and Immunology
City University of New York Medical School
New York, New York

Geoffrey Sunshine
Senior Scientist
Health Effects Institute
Boston, Massachusetts
and
Lecturer, Department of Pathology
Tufts University School of Medicine
Boston, Massachusetts

Eli Benjamini
Professor Emeritus
Department of Medical Microbiology and Immunology
University of California School of Medicine
Davis, California

WILEY-LISS
A JOHN WILEY & SONS, INC., PUBLICATION

Published by John Wiley & Sons, Inc., Hoboken, New Jersey.

Published simultaneously in Canada.

Library of Congress Cataloging-in-Publication Data:

Coico, Richard.
Immunology : a short course / Richard Coico, Geoffrey Sunshine, Eliezer Benjamini.—5th ed.
p. cm.
Previous ed. cataloged under: Benjamini, Eli.
Includes bibliographical references and index.
ISBN 0-471-22689-0 (alk. paper)
1. Immunology. I. Sunshine, Geoffrey. II. Benjamini, Eli. III. Title.
QR181.B395 2003
616.07′9—dc21 2002156133

Printed in the United States of America

10 9 8 7 6 5 4

To
Lisa, Jonathan, and Jennifer
R.C.

To
Ilene, Caroline, Alex, and Pearl
G.S.

To
Joshua and Matthew, my grandsons
E.B.

CONTENTS IN BRIEF

CONTENTS

4 ANTIBODY STRUCTURE AND FUNCTION, 39

5 ANTIGEN–ANTIBODY INTERACTIONS, IMMUNE ASSAYS, AND EXPERIMENTAL SYSTEMS, 59

6 THE GENETIC BASIS OF ANTIBODY STRUCTURE, 79

ABOUT THE AUTHORS

Richard Coico is a professor and chairman of the Department of Microbiology and Immunology at the City University of New York Medical School. For the past eight years, he has directed the Microbiology and Immunology course taught to medical students, and also participates in the teaching of immunology to graduate students and physician assistant students at CUNY. He is a currently President of the Association of Medical School Microbiology and Immunology Chairs (AMSMIC) and he chairs the AMSMIC Education Committee. His research interests include genomic and proteomic studies aimed at defining epitopes expressed by several human pathogens that bind promiscuously to a variety of class I MHC alleles. His laboratory uses computational immunology (bioinformatic) approaches and database-building to investigate candidate epitopes and to create shared knowledgebases.

Geoffrey Sunshine is a Senior Scientist at the Health Effects Institute in Cambridge, Massachusetts, where he reviews research on the biologic effects of air pollutants. He is also a lecturer in the Department of Pathology at Tufts University School of Medicine. For several years, he has directed a course in immunology for graduate dental students at Tufts University Dental School and previously directed a course for veterinary students at Tufts University Veterinary School. He was also a member of the Sackler School of Graduate Biomedical Sciences at Tufts University, doing research in antigen presentation and teaching immunology to medical, graduate, and undergraduate students.

Eli Benjamini is a professor emeritus of immunology in the Department of Medical Microbiology and Immunology at the School of Medicine of the University of California at Davis. Dr. Benjamini has taught immunology to undergraduate, graduate, and medical students, as well as having served for 10 years as Chairman of the Graduate Program of Immunology on the Davis campus—a program that he was instrumental in forming. His research interests include the immunobiology of protein antigens, mechanisms of immune regulation, and principles of synthetic vaccine.

CONTRIBUTORS

Arturo Casadevall, M.D., Ph.D.
Department of Medicine
Albert Einstein College of Medicine
Bronx, New York

Betty Diamond, M.D.
Department of Microbiology and Immunology
Albert Einstein College of Medicine
Bronx, New York

Susan R. S. Gottesman, M.D., Ph.D.
Department of Pathology
State University of New York
Health Science Center at Brooklyn
Brooklyn, New York

Linda Spatz, Ph.D.
Department of Microbiology and Immunology
City University of New York Medical School
New York, New York

PREFACE AND ACKNOWLEDGMENTS TO THE FIFTH EDITION

The Fifth Edition of *Immunology: A Short Course* preserves our commitment to the motto "less is more," which has been our guiding principle in all the previous editions. Given the historic scientific events that have occurred since the publication of the Fourth Edition–including the sequencing of the human genome and the development of new areas such as genomics, proteomics, and bioinformatics–maintaining this tradition has been a formidable challenge for the authors. Despite this explosion of information, we have tried to include only what we think is essential *need to know* material in immunology for those new to the field.

In addition, since the publication of the Fourth Edition, our knowledge of how the immune system develops and functions and ways in which these physiological phenomena can fail or be compromised and thereby cause disease has significantly expanded. To reflect this new knowledge, every chapter in the Fifth Edition has been either updated, rewritten to incorporate new findings, or has had information deleted that no longer reflects current thinking. One major example is that the topics of tolerance and autoimmunity in the current edition are now discussed in a unified approach in a single chapter. We are very grateful to Drs. Linda Spatz and Betty Diamond who contributed Chapter 12, "Tolerance and Autoimmunity." We would also like to thank Drs. Susan Gottesman and Arturo Casadevall, who updated the chapters entitled "Immunodeficiency Disorders and Neoplasias of the Lymphoid System" and "Resistance and Immunization to Infectious Diseases," respectively. In addition, we would like to thank Dr. John P. Atkinson, Washington University School of Medicine, St. Louis, Missouri, for reviewing the completely revised chapter on complement in the current edition.

Richard Coico would like to acknowledge the loving, enduring support of his family during the writing of this book: Lisa, for her encouragement and inspiration, Jonathan (a budding writer himself) and Jennifer, for their patience and good humor. Special thanks are extended to the following list of colleagues who generously provided their insightful scientific expertise and many helpful suggestions for the Fifth Edition: Drs. Ethan Shevach (NIH), David Margulies (NIH), Lloyd Mayer (Mount Sinai School of Medicine), and Viera Lima (CUNY Medical School). Finally, he would like to posthumously acknowledge his mentors, Dr. Robert A. Good, the founder of modern immunology who introduced him to immunologic research and the experiments of nature that offer biological insights to host defense, and Dr. G. Jeanette Thorbecke, who greatly influenced his commitment and passion to the science of immunology.

Geoffrey Sunshine would like to thank Peter Brodeur (Tufts University Medical School) for his unstinting help during the preparation of his section of the current edition. He is also grateful to the many friends and colleagues who answered questions about their areas of expertise, especially Mark Exley, Antonio da Silva, and Paula Hochman. In addition, he would like to thank his wife, Ilene, and children, Caroline and Alex, for their continued support and understanding during the writing. He too acknowledges the role that the late Robert Good played in his development as a scientist. As a postdoctoral fellow in Dr. Good's institute in New York, Geoffrey was immersed for the first time in the exciting world of immunology.

The authors wish to express their appreciation to the staff members of John Wiley and Sons, Inc., who helped with the publication of the Fifth Edition. Special thanks also go to our co-workers, including secretaries, office assistants, and other staff members, who helped with the preparation of the manuscript.

IMMUNOLOGY: A SHORT COURSE ON THE WEB

The Web site is designed as an additional resource for students and educators who adopt the book for use in their courses (http://www.wiley.com/immuno-shortcourse.com). The site uses a versatile online course management tool—namely, WebCT. The following features are included in the Web site:

- Table of contents
- Information about the authors
- Sample chapter
- All figures and tables published in the 4th edition
- Icon page with downloadable clip art images
- Embellished and regularly updated CD Antigens and Cytokine tables
- Embellished and regularly updated Glossary
- Embellished and regularly updated Review Questions and Answers section
- Links to other useful Web sites

The authors chose to use the WebCT course management tool because it is the undisputed e-learning leader in higher education. The Web site and its WebCT backbone allow those who adopt the Fifth Edition of Immunology: A Short Course to teach *their* courses *their* way.

We are committed to updating the Web site regularly with the goal of facilitating the teaching efforts of instructors and, of course, student e-learning. First and foremost, our commitment in maintaining this Web site will be to provide an immunology-related educational resource that presents appropriate current information in a clear, concise, and student-friendly manner.

PREFACE AND ACKNOWLEDGMENTS TO THE FOURTH EDITION

Since the last edition, significant developments in biomedical research have helped to refine and, in some cases, redefine our understanding of many aspects of the immune system. As a result, every chapter published in the fourth edition has been either updated or rewritten to incorporate new findings and to delete information that no longer reflects current thinking. In addition, several new chapters have been added to the book, including one on cytokines and another on resistance and immunization to infectious diseases. Finally, a new section on experimental systems has been added to Chapter 5. Describing how and why biomedical scientists utilize various experimental tools to investigate the complexities of the immune system is essential to a student's understanding of the subject of immunology.

As in the first three editions, we remain committed to the motto "less is more." Therefore, our objective in creating this edition has been to present what we consider to be the most pertinent material in a concise, palatable, and easily digestible fashion to the introductory student of immunology. Additional supportive material for students and course instructors can also now be found on a Web site (see below).

We are deeply indebted to Dr. Susan Gottesman, who contributed the chapter entitled, "Immunodeficiency and Other Disorders of the Immune System." We also thank Dr. Karen Yamaga, who updated the autoimmunity chapter. The important contributions of Dr. Patricia Giclas, who updated the complement chapter, and Dr. Arturo Casadevall, who added the new final chapter on resistance and immunization to infectious diseases, are also gratefully acknowledged.

Richard Coico would like to acknowledge the loving support of his family during the writing of this book. Their fortitude, inspiration, and enduring patience helped make the job an enjoyable adventure. Special thanks is extended to the following list of colleagues who generously provided their insightful scientific expertise and many helpful suggestions for the Fourth Edition: Drs. Ethan Shevach (NIH), David Margulies (NIH), Lloyd Mayer (Mount Sinai School of Medicine), Lakshmi Tamma (CUNY Medical School), Linda Spatz (CUNY Medical School), Laurel Eckhardt (Hunter College), Kathleen Barnes (Johns Hopkins School of Medicine), Soldano Ferrone (Roswell Park Memorial Institute), and Harriet Robinson (Emory University). Finally, he would like to thank his mentors, Drs. Ronald Curley, Susan Krown, Robert A. Good, and G. Jeanette Thorbecke, each of whom has greatly influenced his commitment and passion to the road taken.

Geoffrey Sunshine would like to thank Peter Brodeur (Tufts University Medical School) and Cindy Theodos (Tufts University Veterinary School) for their unstinting help during the preparation of his section of the current edition; they reviewed chapters in both the Third and Fourth Editions, and offered suggestions for making the material relevant and accessible to introductory readers. He is also grateful to the many friends and colleagues who answered questions about their areas of expertise, especially Mark Exley, Susan Kalled, and Paula Hochman. In addition, he would like to thank his family for their continued support and understanding during the writing.

The authors wish to express their appreciation to the staff members of John Wiley and Sons, Inc., who helped to bring the Fourth Edition to publication and did so with skill, patience, and good humor. Special thanks to our co-workers, including secretaries, office assistants, and other staff members, who helped with the preparation of the manuscript.

Finally, we wish to acknowledge the important contributions made by Dr. Sidney Leskowitz to the earlier editions of this book. The Hypersensitivity chapters are dedicated to his memory.

SPECIAL DEDICATION

In the 1980s, Dr. Sidney Leskowitz, one of the two original authors of *Immunology: A Short Course,* was convinced of the need for a textbook that would provide the bare essentials of immunology in a palatable form. As a result, *Immunology: A Short Course* was conceived and written along the lines of the dictum attributed to the noted architect Mies van der Rohe: "Less is more." Indeed, the book's clear presentation of the basics of immunology continues to strike a responsive chord with readers, and is a testament to the success of Dr. Leskowitz's approach.

The field of immunology has evolved significantly since the publication of the first edition, and this text has kept up with these changes through extensive revision and expansion. At the same time, the present authors have made every effort to remain true to Dr. Leskowitz's philosophy. It is to the bright memory of Dr. Sidney Leskowitz, who contributed immeasurably to the ongoing success of *Immunology: A Short Course,* that this fifth edition is dedicated.

PREFACE AND ACKNOWLEDGMENTS TO THE THIRD EDITION

Since the last edition, the intense efforts of research scientists around the world have produced significant new findings that have reshaped our understanding of many aspects of the immune system. As a result, every chapter in the current edition has been either updated or rewritten to incorporate new findings and to delete information that no longer reflects current thinking.

As in the first and second editions, we remain committed to the motto "less is more." Our task has been to present what we consider the most relevant material in a concise, palatable, and easily digestible fashion to the introductory student. That reader will be the best judge of whether we have succeeded.

We are deeply indebted to Dr. Demosthenes Pappagianis, who contributed the chapter on immunoprophylaxis and immunotherapy, and Dr. Karen Yamaga, who contributed the chapter on control mechanisms in the immune response and on autoimmunity. We wish to thank the many co-workers and students who contributed to the first and second editions and those who were helpful in the preparation of the third edition, in particular, Dr. Robert J. Scibienski of the School of Medicine, University of California at Davis, and Dr. Donna M. Rennick, DNA Research Institute, Palo Alto, California. Geoffrey Sunshine would like to thank the many friends who patiently answered his questions during the writing of the third edition, in particular, Peter Brodeur, Mark Exley, and Paula Hochman. He would also like to thank his family for their continued support: Ilene, for her encouragement and dedication to the cause, and Alex and Caroline, for their optimism. His sections are dedicated to his father Harry, who did not live to see the new edition.

PREFACE TO THE SECOND EDITION

An anxiety common to authors of textbooks in rapidly developing fields is the necessity of relatively frequent revisions to include material that, in the previous edition, was in the "twilight zone," between fact and fancy but that since has gained the status of important fact. Indeed, the rapidly developing field of immunology requires continuous revisions; hence, the present edition.

In this second edition, various concepts and findings have been updated and expanded; new information has been added on such diverse topics as the molecular biology and genes controlling antibody synthesis and isotype switch, T-cell differentiation and the T-cell receptor, antigen processing and presentation, cytokines and lymphokines, new therapeutic approaches for immunodeficiency disorders and tumors, and new aspects of prophylaxis and immunotherapy of infectious diseases. In addition, we have added a section on AIDS and several techniques such as Western blots and fluorescence-activated cell sorting. We have also expanded the glossary and added review questions as well as several clinical correlates.

Although we have deleted and shortened some sections, the expanded and added material increased somewhat the size of the book. We can, however, assure the readers that with this second edition, as with the first edition, we remain committed to the motto "less is more" and have attempted to present the principles of immunology in a concise, palatable, and easily digestible form.

Revision and change is the constant burden that authors writing about a dynamically changing field have to carry. Students, too, have to partake of that burden and must prepare themselves with the realization that science is not static and they must continually move on to new levels of understanding. Good luck to us both.

PREFACE TO THE FIRST EDITION

Why was this book written? At a time when so many excellent, extensive, and beautifully illustrated texts flood the bookstores, why offer another one? The reasons are fairly simple and rather unsophisticated. In our collective 40 some-odd years of teaching all kinds of students, we have become convinced that most texts fail their purpose because they overshoot the mark.

Anyone coming into contact with these students year after year cannot fail to appreciate the burden under which they operate. If they are to graduate, they must learn an enormous amount of material on an exceptionally diverse series of subjects, each increasing in scope yearly. As any student can tell you, every faculty lecturer considers his/her particular topic absolutely essential for future graduates, and so the pile of required "essentials" grows and grows. This is a manifestly untenable approach to curriculum.

A second cruel observation arises from long years of questioning students: many of them are not really that interested in immunology! As exciting, dynamic, and all-encompassing in its passion that we practitioners of immunology find it to be, the students have many other interests and concerns, one of which is to pass the five or six other subjects usually taken simultaneously with immunology.

This book was therefore conceived along the lines of the noted architect Mies van der Rohe's dictum, "less is more." We have devised this text to present the bare essentials of immunology in a palatable form that will enable most students to grasp the essential principles of immunology sufficiently to pass their course. For those developing a deeper interest in the field, numerous advanced and more complete texts exist to further their interests.

The book follows the outlines of most immunology courses and is divided into chapters that mostly approximate the length of an average lecture reading assignment. A short introduction setting the stage precedes the main text of each chapter, the end of each chapter contains a summary, and a series of study questions appears at the very end. The questions are designed to enable students to evaluate their own progress and comprehension; the appended answers are meant as a further learning experience. As new terms or concepts are introduced, they are highlighted in italics and boldface and defined for easy recognition and recall.

It is our hope that students using this text will avoid that choking sensation so common in a course in immunology and even conceive a curiosity about the subject that will lead to further study.

1

INTRODUCTION AND OVERVIEW

INTRODUCTION

Anyone who has had the good fortune to hear an orchestra brilliantly perform a symphony composed by one of the great masters knows that each of the carefully tuned musical instruments contributes to the collective, harmonious sound produced by the musicians. In many ways, the normally *tuned* immune system continuously plays an orchestrated symphony to maintain homeostasis in the context of host defenses. However, as William Shakespeare noted "untune that string, and, hark, what discord follows!" (*Troilus and Cressida*). Similarly, an *untuned* immune system can cause discord, which manifests as autoimmunity, cancer, or chronic inflammation. Fortunately, for most of us, our immune system is steadfastly vigilant in regard to tuning (regulating) itself to ensure that its cellular components behave and interact symbiotically to generate protective immune responses that ensure good health.

In his penetrating essays, scientist–author Lewis Thomas, discussing symbiosis and parasitism, described the forces that would drive all living matter into one huge ball of protoplasm were it not for regulatory and recognition mechanisms that allow us to distinguish ***self*** from ***nonself.*** The origins of these mechanisms go far back in evolutionary history, and many, in fact, originated as markers for allowing cells to recognize and interact with each other to set up symbiotic households. Genetically related sponge colonies that are placed close to each other, for example, will tend to grow toward each other and fuse into one large colony. Unrelated colonies, however, will react in a different way, destroying cells that come in contact and leaving a zone of rejection between the colonies.

In the plant kingdom, similar types of recognition occur. In self-pollinating species, a pollen grain landing on the stigma of a genetically related flower will send a pollen tubule down the style to the ovary for fertilization. A pollen grain from a genetically distinct plant either will not germinate or the pollen tubule, once formed, will disintegrate in the style. The opposite occurs in cross-pollinating species: self-marked pollen grains disintegrate, whereas nonself grains germinate and fertilize.

The nature of these primitive recognition mechanisms has not been completely worked out, but almost certainly it involves cell surface molecules that are able to specifically bind and adhere to other molecules on opposing cell surfaces. This simple method of molecular recognition has evolved over time into the very complex immune system that retains, as its essential feature, the ability of a protein molecule to recognize and bind specifically to a particular shaped structure on another molecule. Such molecular recognition is the underlying principle involved in the discrimination between self and nonself during an immune response. It is the purpose of this book to describe how the fully mature immune system—which has evolved from this simple beginning—makes use of this principle of recognition in increasingly complex and sophisticated ways.

The study of immunology as a science has gone through several periods of quiescence and active development,

Immunology: A Short Course, Fifth Edition, By Richard Coico, Geoffrey Sunshine, and Eli Benjamini
ISBN 0-471-22689-0

TABLE 1.1. Major Properties of the Innate and Adaptive Immune Systems

Property	Innate	Adaptive
Characteristics	Antigen nonspecific Rapid response (minutes) No memory	Antigen specific Slow response (days) Memory
Immune components	Natural barriers (e.g., skin) Phagocytes Soluble mediators (e.g., complement) Pattern-recognition molecules	Lymphocytes Antigen-recognition molecules (B cell and T cell receptors) Secreted molecules (e.g., antibody)

usually succeeding the introduction of a new technique or a changed paradigm for thinking about the subject. Perhaps the biggest catalyst for progress in this and many other biomedical areas has been the advent of molecular biologic techniques. It is important to acknowledge, however, that certain technological advances in the field of molecular biology were made possible by earlier progress in the field of immunology. For example, the importance of immunologic methods (Chapter 5) used to purify proteins as well as identify specific cDNA clones cannot be understated. These advances were greatly facilitated by the pioneering studies of Kohler and Milstein (1975), who developed a method for producing monoclonal antibodies. Their achievement was rewarded with the Nobel Prize in Medicine. It revolutionized research efforts in virtually all areas of biomedical science. Some monoclonal antibodies produced against so-called tumor-specific antigens have now been approved by the U.S. Food and Drug Administration for use in patients to treat certain malignancies. Monoclonal antibody technology is, perhaps, an excellent example of how the science of immunology has transformed not only the field of medicine but also fields ranging from agriculture to the food science industry.

Given the rapid advances occurring in immunology and the many other biomedical sciences and, perhaps most important, the sequencing of the human genome, every contemporary biomedical science textbook runs a considerable risk of being outdated before it appears in print. Nevertheless, we take solace from the observation that new formulations generally build on and expand the old rather than replacing or negating them completely.

OVERVIEW

Innate and Acquired Immunity

The Latin term *immunis,* meaning "exempt," gave rise to the English word ***immunity,*** which refers to all the mechanisms used by the body as protection against environmental agents that are foreign to the body. These agents may be microorganisms or their products, foods, chemicals, drugs, pollen, or animal hair and dander. Immunity may be innate or acquired.

Innate Immunity. Innate immunity is conferred by all those elements with which an individual is born and that are always present and available at very short notice to protect the individual from challenges by foreign invaders. Most of these elements are discussed in detail in Chapter 2. Table 1.1 summarizes and compares some of the features of the innate and adaptive immune systems. Elements of the innate system include body surfaces and internal components, such as the skin, the mucous membranes, and the cough reflex, which present effective barriers to environmental agents. Chemical influences, such as pH and secreted fatty acids, constitute effective barriers against invasion by many microorganisms. Another noncellular element of the innate immune system is the complement system. As in the previous editions of this book, we cover the subject of complement in a separate chapter (Chapter 13).

Numerous other components are also features of innate immunity: fever, interferons (Chapter 11), other substances released by leukocytes, and pattern-recognition molecules, which can bind to various microorganisms (Toll-like receptors or TLRs; Chapter 2), as well as serum proteins such as β-lysin, the enzyme lysozyme, polyamines, and the kinins, among others. All of these elements either affect pathogenic invaders directly or enhance the effectiveness of host reactions to them. Other internal elements of innate immunity include phagocytic cells such as granulocytes, macrophages, and microglial cells of the central nervous system, which participate in the destruction and elimination of foreign material that has penetrated the physical and chemical barriers.

Acquired Immunity. Acquired immunity is more specialized than innate immunity, and it supplements the protection provided by innate immunity. Acquired immunity came into play relatively late, in evolutionary terms, and is present only in vertebrates.

Although an individual is born with the capacity to mount an immune response to a foreign invader, immunity is acquired by contact with the invader and is specific to that invader only, hence the term *acquired immunity.* The initial contact with the foreign agent (***immunization***) triggers a chain of events that leads to the activation of ***lymphocytes*** and other cells and the synthesis of proteins, some of which exhibit specific reactivity against the foreign agent. By this process, the individual acquires the immunity to withstand and resist a subsequent attack by, or exposure to, the same offending agent.

The discovery of acquired immunity predates many of the concepts of modern medicine. It has been recognized for centuries that people who did not die from such life-threatening diseases as bubonic plague and smallpox were subsequently more resistant to the disease than were people who had never been exposed to it. The rediscovery of acquired immunity is credited to the English physician Edward Jenner, who, in the late eighteenth century, experimentally induced immunity to smallpox. If Jenner performed his experiment today, his medical license would be revoked, and he would be the defendant in a sensational malpractice lawsuit: He inoculated a young boy with pus from a lesion of a dairy maid who had cowpox, a relatively benign disease that is related to smallpox. He then deliberately exposed the boy to smallpox. This exposure failed to cause disease! Because of the protective effect of inoculation with cowpox (*vaccinia,* from the Latin word *vacca,* meaning "cow"), the process of inducing acquired immunity has been termed ***vaccination.***

The concept of vaccination or immunization was expanded by Louis Pasteur and Paul Ehrlich almost 100 years after Jenner's experiment. By 1900, it had become apparent that immunity could be induced against not only microorganisms but also their products. We now know that immunity can be induced against enumerable natural and synthetic compounds, including metals, chemicals of relatively low molecular weight, carbohydrates, proteins, and nucleotides.

The compound to which the acquired immune response is induced is termed an ***antigen,*** a term initially coined due to the ability of these compounds to cause ***anti***body responses to be ***gen***erated. Of course, we now know that antigens can generate antibody-mediated and T cell–mediated responses.

Active, Passive, and Adoptive Immunization

Acquired immunity is induced by immunization, which can be achieved in several ways:

- **Active immunization** refers to immunization of an individual by administration of an antigen.
- **Passive immunization** refers to immunization through the transfer of specific antibody from an immunized individual to a nonimmunized individual.
- **Adoptive immunization** refers to the transfer of immunity by the transfer of immune cells.

Characteristics of the Acquired Immune Response

The acquired immune response has several generalized features that characterize it and distinguish it from other physiologic systems, such as circulation, respiration, and reproduction. These features are as follows:

- **Specificity** is the ability to discriminate among different molecular entities and to respond only to those uniquely required, rather than making a random, undifferentiated response.
- **Adaptiveness** is the ability to respond to previously unseen molecules that may in fact never have naturally existed before on earth.
- **Discrimination between self and nonself** is a cardinal feature of the specificity of the immune response; it is the ability to recognize and respond to molecules that are foreign (nonself) and to avoid making a response to those molecules that are self. This distinction, and the recognition of antigen, is conferred by specialized cells (lymphocytes) that bear on their surface antigen-specific receptors.
- **Memory** a property shared with the nervous system, is the ability to recall previous contact with a foreign molecule and respond to it in a learned manner—that is, with a more rapid and larger response. The term used to describe immunologic memory is ***anamnestic response.***

When you reach the end of this book, you should understand the cellular and molecular bases of these features of the immune response.

Cells Involved in the Acquired Immune Response

For many years, immunology remained an empirical subject in which the effects of injecting various substances into hosts were studied primarily in terms of the products elicited. Most progress came in the form of more quantitative methods for detecting these products of the immune response. A major change in emphasis came in the 1950s with the recognition that lymphocytes were the major cellular players in the immune response, and the field of cellular immunology came to life.

It is now firmly established that there are three major cell types involved in acquired immunity and that complex interactions among these cell types are required for the expression of the full range of immune responses. Two of these cell types come from a common lymphoid precursor cell but differentiate along different developmental lines. One line matures in the thymus and is referred to as ***T cells;*** the other matures in the bone marrow and is referred to as ***B cells.*** Cells of the B and T lymphocyte series differ in many functional aspects but share one of the important properties of the immune response—namely, they exhibit specificity toward an antigen. Thus the major recognition and reaction functions of the immune response are contained within the lymphocytes.

Antigen-Presenting cells (APCs), such as macrophages and dendritic cells, constitute the third cell type that

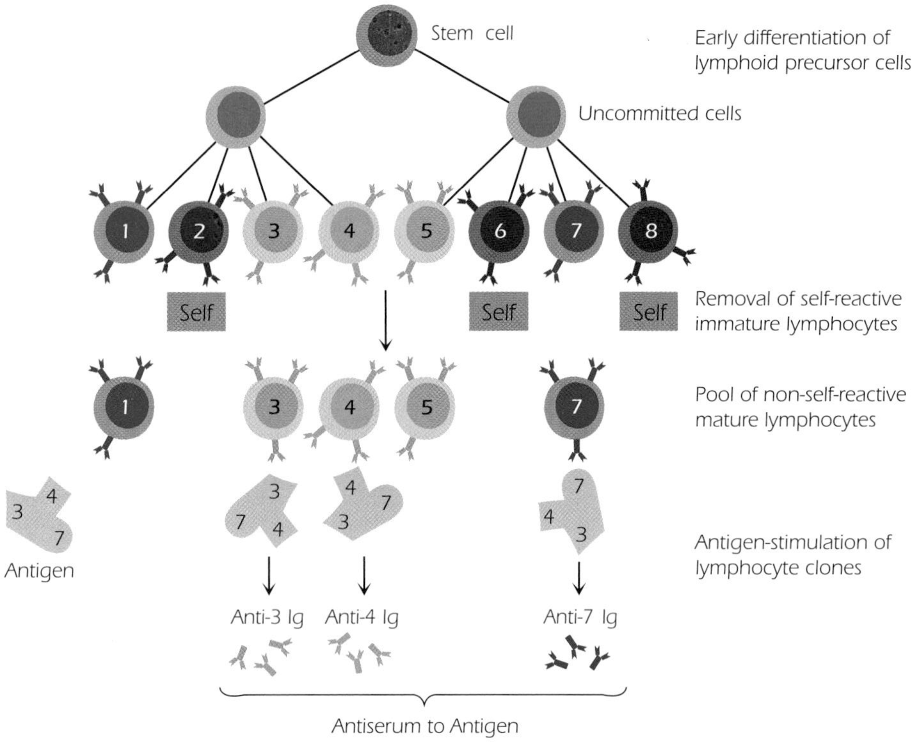

Figure 1.1. The clonal selection theory of B cells leading to antibody production.

participates in the acquired immune response. Although these cells do not have antigen-specific receptors as do the lymphocytes, their important function is to ***process and present antigen*** to the specific receptors (T cell receptors) on T lymphocytes. The APCs have on their surface two types of special molecules that function in antigen presentation. These molecules, called ***major histocompatibility complex*** (MHC) ***class I*** and ***MHC class II molecules,*** are encoded by a set of genes that is also responsible for the rejection or acceptance of transplanted tissue. The processed antigen is noncovalently bound to MHC class I or class II molecules (or both). Antigen presented on MHC class I molecules is presented to and participates in activation of one T cell subpopulation (cytotoxic T cells), whereas antigen processed and expressed on APCs in the context of MHC class II molecules results in activation of another subpopulation (helper T cells). This is discussed in more detail in Chapter 9.

In addition, other cell types, such as neutrophils and mast cells, participate in immune responses. In fact, they participate in both innate and acquired immunity. They are involved primarily in the effector phases of the response. These cells have no specific antigen recognition properties and are activated by various substances, collectively termed cytokines, which are released by various cells, including activated antigen-specific lymphocytes.

Clonal Selection Theory

A turning point in immunology came in the 1950s with the introduction of a Darwinian view of the cellular basis of specificity in the immune response. This was the now universally accepted ***clonal selection theory*** proposed and developed by Jerne and Burnet (both Nobel Prize winners) and by Talmage. The essential postulates of this theory are summarized below.

The specificity of the immune response is based on the ability of its components (namely, antigen-specific T and B lymphocytes) to recognize particular foreign molecules (antigens) and respond to them in order to eliminate them. Inherent in this theory is the need to clonally delete lymphocytes that may be self-reactive, or autoreactive. If such a mechanism were absent, autoimmune responses might occur routinely. Fortunately, lymphocytes with receptors that bind to self-antigens are eliminated during the early phases of lymphocyte development, thus ensuring tolerance of self (Fig. 1.1).

Since, as we have already stated, the immune system is capable of recognizing enumerable foreign antigens, how is a response to any one antigen accomplished? In addition to the now-proven postulate that self-reactive clones of lymphocytes are functionally inactive, the clonal selection theory proposed that

- T and B lymphocytes of myriad specificities exist before there is any contact with the foreign antigen.
- The lymphocytes participating in the immune response have antigen-specific receptors on their surface membranes. As a consequence of antigen binding to the lymphocyte, the cell is activated and releases various products. In the case of B lymphocytes, the receptors are molecules (antibodies) bearing the same specificity as

the antibody that the cell will subsequently produce and secrete. T cells have receptors denoted as ***T cell receptors*** (TCRs). Unlike the B cell, the T cell products are not the same as their surface receptors but are other protein molecules, called cytokines, that participate in elimination of the antigen by regulating the many cells needed to mount an effective immune response.

- Each lymphocyte carries on its surface receptor molecules of only a single specificity as demonstrated in Figure 1.1 for B cells, and holds true also for T cells.

These three postulates describe the existence of a large repertoire of possible specificities formed by cellular multiplication and differentiation *before* there is any contact with the foreign substance to which the response is to be made.

The introduction of the foreign antigen then selects from among all the available specificities those with specificity for the antigen, enabling binding to occur. The scheme shown in Figure 1.1 for B cells also applies to T cells; however, T cells have receptors that are not antibodies and secrete molecules other than antibodies.

The remaining postulates of the clonal selection theory account for this process of selection by the antigen from among all the available cells in the repertoire.

- Immunocompetent lymphocytes combine with the foreign antigen, or a portion of it, termed the ***epitope,*** by virtue of their surface receptors. They are stimulated under appropriate conditions to proliferate and differentiate into clones of cells with the corresponding identical receptors to the particular portion of the antigen, termed antigenic determinant, or epitope. With B cell clones, this will lead to the synthesis of antibodies having precisely the same specificity. Collectively, the clonally secreted antibodies constitute the polyclonal antiserum, which is capable of interacting with the multiple epitopes expressed by the antigen. T cells will be similarly selected by appropriate antigens or portions thereof. Each selected T cell will be activated to divide and produce clones of the same specificity. Thus the clonal response to the antigen will be amplified, the cells will release various cytokines, and subsequent exposure to the same antigen will now result in the activation of many cells or clones of that specificity. Instead of synthesizing and releasing antibodies like the B cells, the T cells synthesize and release cytokines. These cytokines, which are soluble mediators, exert their effect on other cells to grow or become activated facilitating elimination of the antigen. Several distinct regions of an antigen (epitopes) can be recognized: Several different clones of B cells will be stimulated to produce antibody, whose sum total is an antigen-specific antiserum that is made up of antibodies of differing specificity (Fig. 1.1); all the T cell clones that recognize various epitopes on the same antigen will be activated to perform their function.

A final postulate was added to account for the ability to recognize self-antigens without making a response:

- Circulating self-antigens that reach the developing lymphoid system before some undesignated maturational step will serve to shut off those cells that recognize it specifically, and no subsequent immune response will be induced.

This formulation of the clonal selection theory had a truly revolutionary effect on the field and changed forever our way of looking at and studying the immune system.

Humoral and Cellular Immunity

There are two arms (branches) of acquired immunity, which have different sets of participants and different purposes but one common aim: to eliminate the antigen. As we shall see later, these two arms interact with each other and collaborate to achieve the final goal of eliminating the antigen. Of these two arms of the acquired immune response, one is mediated mainly by B cells and circulating antibodies, a form of immunity referred to as ***humoral*** (the word *humors* was formerly used to define body fluids). The other is mediated by T cells, which, as we stated before, do not synthesize antibodies but instead synthesize and release various cytokines that affect other cells. Hence this arm of the acquired immune response is termed ***cellular*** or ***cell-mediated immunity.***

Humoral Immunity. Humoral immunity is mediated by serum antibodies, which are the proteins secreted by the B cell compartment of the immune response (see Chapter 7). B cells are initially activated to secrete antibodies after the binding of antigens to specific membrane ***immunoglobulin*** (Ig) molecules (B cell receptors [BCRs]), which are expressed by these cells. It has been estimated that each B cell expresses $\sim 10^5$ BCRs of exactly the same specificity. Once ligated, the B cell receives signals to begin making the secreted form of this immunoglobulin, a process that initiates the full-blown antibody response whose purpose is to eliminate the antigen from the host. Antibodies are a heterogeneous mixture of serum globulins, all of which share the ability to bind individually to specific antigens. All serum globulins with antibody activity are referred to as immunoglobulins.

All immunoglobulin molecules have common structural features, which enable them to do two things: (1) recognize and bind specifically to a unique structural entity on an antigen (namely, the ***epitope***), and (2) perform a common biologic function after combining with the antigen. Basically, each immunoglobulin molecule consists of two identical light (L) chains and two identical heavy (H) chains, linked by disulfide bridges. The resultant structure is shown in Figure 1.2.

The portion of the molecule that binds antigen consists of an area composed of the amino-terminal regions of both H and L chains. Thus each immunoglobulin molecule is symmetric

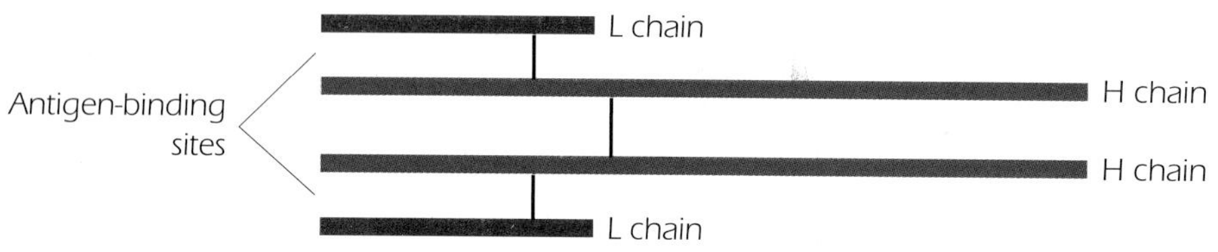

Figure 1.2. Typical antibody molecule composed of two heavy (H) and two light (L) chains. Antigen-binding sites are noted.

and is capable of binding two identical eptitopes present on the same antigen molecule or on different molecules.

In addition to differences in the antigen-binding portion of different immunoglobulin molecules, there are other differences, the most important of which are those in the H chains. There are five major classes of H chains (termed γ, μ, α, ε, and δ). On the basis of differences in their H chains, immunoglobulin molecules are divided into five major classes IgG, IgM, IgA, IgE, and IgD each of which has several unique biologic properties. For example, IgG is the only class of immunoglobulin that crosses the placenta, conferring the mother's immunity on the fetus, and IgA is the major antibody found in secretions such as tears and saliva. It is important to remember that antibodies in all five classes may possess precisely the same specificity against an antigen (antigen-combining regions), while at the same time having different functional (biologic effector) properties.

The binding between antigen and antibody is not covalent but depends on many relatively weak forces, such as hydrogen bonds, van der Waals forces, and hydrophobic interactions. Since these forces are weak, successful binding between antigen and antibody depends on a very close fit over a sizable area, much like the contacts between a lock and a key.

Another important element involved in humoral immunity is the complement system (Chapter 13). The reaction between antigen and antibody serves to activate this system, which consists of a series of serum enzymes, the end result of which is lysis of the target or enhanced ***phagocytosis*** (ingestion of the antigen) by phagocytic cells. The activation of complement also results in the recruitment of highly phagocytic polymorphonuclear (PMN) cells, which constitute part of the innate immune system. These activities maximize the effective response made by the humoral arm of immunity against invading agents.

Cell-Mediated Immunity. The antigen-specific arm of cell-mediated immunity consists of the T lymphocytes (Fig. 1.3). Unlike B cells, which produce soluble antibody that circulates to bind its specific antigens, each T cell, bearing many identical antigen receptors called TCRs ($\sim 10^5$ /cell) circulates directly to the site of antigen expressed on APCs and interacts with the APCs in a cognate (cell-to-cell) fashion (Chapter 10).

There are several phenotypically distinct subpopulations of T cells, each of which may have the same specificity for an antigenic determinant (epitope), although each subpopulation may perform different functions. This is analogous to the different classes of immunoglobulin molecules, which may have identical specificity but different biologic functions. Two major subsets of T cells exist: helper T cells (***T_H cells***) which express molecules called ***CD4,*** and cytotoxic T cells (***T_C cells***) which express ***CD8*** molecules on their surface.

The functions ascribed to the various subsets of T_H cells include the following:

- **Cooperation with B cells to enhance the production of antibodies.** Such T cells function by releasing cytokines, which provide various activation signals for the B cells. As mentioned earlier, cytokines are soluble substances, or mediators, released by cells; such mediators released by lymphocytes are also termed *lymphokines.* A group of low molecular weight cytokines has been given the name *chemokines.* These play a role in inflammatory

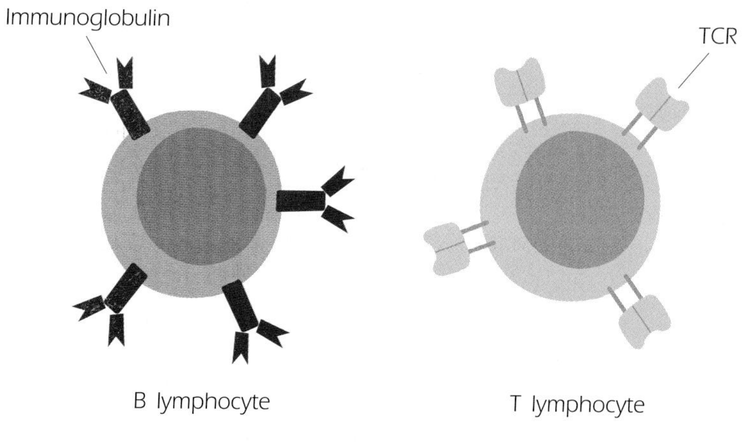

Figure 1.3. Antigen receptors expressed as transmembrane molecules on B and T lymphocytes.

responses, as discussed below. Additional information about cytokines is presented in Chapter 11.

- **Inflammatory effects.** On activation, a certain T cell subpopulation releases cytokines, which induce the migration and activation of monocytes and macrophages, leading to the so-called delayed-type hypersensitivity inflammatory reactions (Chapter 16). This subpopulation is sometimes called T_{DTH}, for T cells participating in delayed-type hypersensitivity, and others term this subpopulation simply T_H.
- **Cytotoxic effects.** The T cells in this subset become cytotoxic killer cells that, on contact with their target, are able to deliver a lethal hit, leading to the death of the target cells. These T cells are termed T cytotoxic (T_C) cells. In contrast with T_H cells, they express molecules called CD8 on their membranes and are, therefore, $CD8^+$ cells.
- **Regulatory effects.** Helper T cells can be divided into different functional subsets, which are defined by the cytokines they release. As you will learn in subsequent chapters, these subsets (T_H1, T_H2) have distinct regulatory properties that are mediated by the cytokines they release (Chapter 11). Moreover, T_H1 cells can negatively cross-regulate T_H2 cells and vice versa. Another population of regulatory or suppressor T cells co-expresses CD4 and CD25 (CD25 is the interleukin 2 receptor α chain; Chapter 11). The regulatory activity of these $CD4^+/CD25^+$cells and their role in actively suppressing autoimmunity are discussed in Chapter 12.
- **Cytokine effects.** T cells and other cells within the immune system (e.g., macrophages) exert numerous effects on many cells, lymphoid and nonlymphoid, through many different cytokines that they release. Thus, directly or indirectly, T cells communicate and collaborate with many cell types.

For many years, immunologists have recognized that cells activated by antigen manifest a variety of effector phenomena. It is only in the last few decades that they began to appreciate the complexity of events that take place in activation by antigen and communication with other cells. We know today that just mere contact of the T cell receptor with antigen is not sufficient to activate the cell. In fact, at least two signals must be delivered to the antigen-specific T cell for activation to occur: Signal 1 involves the binding of the TCR to antigen, which must be presented in the appropriate manner by antigen-presenting cells. Signal 2 involves costimulators that include certain cytokines such as interleukin 1 (IL-1), IL-4, and IL-6 (Chapter 11) as well as cell-surface molecules expressed on APCs, such as CD40 and CD86 (Chapter 10). Recently, the term ***costimulator*** has been broadened to include stimuli such as microbial products (infectious nonself) and damaged tissue (Matzinger's "danger hypothesis") that will enhance signal 1 when that signal is relatively weak. Once T cells are optimally signaled for activation, a series of events take place and the activated cell synthesizes and releases cytokines. In turn, these cytokines come in contact with appropriate receptors on different cells and exert their effect on these cells.

Although both the humoral and cellular arms of the immune response have been considered as separate and distinct components, it is important to understand that the response to any particular pathogen may involve a complex interaction between both, as well as the components of innate immunity. All this with the purpose of ensuring a maximal survival advantage for the host by eliminating the antigen and, as we shall see, by protecting the host from mounting an immune response against self.

Generation of Diversity in the Immune Response

The most recent tidal surge in immunologic research represents a triumph of the marriage of molecular biology and immunology. While cellular immunology had delineated the cellular basis for the existence of a large and diverse repertoire of responses, as well as the nature of the exquisite specificity that could be achieved, arguments abounded on the exact genetic mechanisms that enabled all these specificities to become part of the repertoire in every individual of the species.

Briefly, the arguments were as follows:

- By various calculations, the number of antigenic specificities toward which an immune response can be generated could range upward of 10^6–10^7.
- If every specific response, in the form of either antibodies or T cell receptors, were to be encoded by a single gene, did this mean that $>10^7$ genes (one for each specific antibody) would be required in every individual? How was this massive amount of DNA carried intact from individual to individual?

The pioneering studies of Tonegawa (a Nobel laureate) and Leder, using molecular biologic techniques, finally addressed these issues by describing a unique genetic mechanism by which immunologic receptors expressed on B cells (BCRs) of enormous diversity could be produced with a modest amount of DNA reserved for this purpose.

The technique evolved by nature was one of genetic recombination in which a protein could be encoded by a DNA molecule composed of a set of recombined minigenes that made up a complete gene. Given small sets of these minigenes, which could be randomly combined to make the complete gene, it was possible to produce an enormous repertoire of specificities from a limited number of gene fragments. (This is discussed in detail in Chapter 6.)

Although this mechanism was first elucidated to explain the enormous diversity of antibodies that are not only released by B cells but that in fact constitute the antigen- or epitope-specific receptors on B cells (BCR), it was subsequently established that the same mechanisms operate in generating diversity of the antigen-specific T cell receptor (TCR). Mechanisms operating in generating diversity of B cell receptors and antibodies are discussed in Chapter 6. Those operating in generating diversity of TCR are discussed in Chapter 8. Suffice it to say at this point that various techniques of molecular biology that permit genes not only to be analyzed but also to be moved around at will from one cell to another have continued to provide impetus to the on-rushing tide of immunologic progress.

Benefits of Immunology

While we have thus far discussed the theoretical aspects of immunology, its practical applications are of paramount importance for survival and must be part of the education of students.

The field of immunology has been in the public limelight since the successful use of polio vaccines in the mid-twentieth century. More recently, the spectacular transplantation of the human heart and other major organs, such as the liver, has been the focus of much publicity. Public interest in immunology was intensified by the potential application of the immune response to the detection and management of cancer; and in the 1980s, the general public became familiar with some aspects of immunology because of the alarming spread of acquired immune deficiency syndrome (AIDS).

The innate and acquired immune systems play an integral role in the prevention of and recovery from infectious diseases and are, without question, essential to the survival of the individual. Metchnikoff was the first to propose in the 1800s that phagocytic cells formed the first line of defense against infection and that the inflammatory response could actually serve a protective function for the host. Indeed, innate immune responses are responsible for the detection and rapid destruction of most infectious agents that are encountered in the daily life of most individuals. We now know that innate immune responses operate in concert with adaptive immune responses to generate antigen-specific effector mechanisms that lead to the death and elimination of the invading pathogen. Chapter 20 presents information concerning how our immune systems respond to microorganisms and how methods developed to exploit these mechanisms are used as ***immunoprophylaxis.*** Vaccination against infectious diseases has been an effective form of prophylaxis. Immunoprophylaxis against the virus that causes poliomyelitis has reduced this dreadful disease to relative insignificance in many parts of the world and, for the first time, a transmission of a previously widespread disease, smallpox, has been eliminated from the face of the earth. The last documented case of natural transmission of smallpox virus was in 1972. Unfortunately, the threat of biologic weapons has prompted new concerns regarding the reemergence of certain infectious diseases, including smallpox. Fortunately, public health vaccination initiatives can be applied to prevent or significantly curtail the threat of weaponized microbiological agents, including smallpox.

Recent developments in immunology also hold the promise of immunoprophylaxis against malaria and several other parasitic diseases that plague many parts of the world and affect billions of people. Vaccination against diseases of domestic animals promises to increase the production of meat in developing countries, while vaccination against various substances that play roles in the reproductive processes in mammals offers the possibility of long-term contraception in humans and companion animals such as cats and dogs.

Damaging Effects of the Immune Response

The enormous survival value of the immune response is self-evident. Acquired immunity directed against a foreign material has as its ultimate goal the elimination of the invading substance. In the process, some tissue damage may occur as the result of the accumulation of components with nonspecific effects. This damage is generally temporary. As soon as the invader is eliminated, the situation at that site reverts to normal.

There are instances in which the power of the immune response, although directed against innocuous foreign substances—such as some medications, inhaled pollen particles, or substances deposited by insect bites—produces a response that may result in severe pathologic consequences and even death. These responses are known collectively as hypersensitivity reactions or allergic reactions. An understanding of the basic mechanisms underlying these disease processes has been fundamental in their treatment and control but, in addition, has contributed much to our knowledge of the normal immune response. The latter is true because both use essentially identical mechanisms; however, in hypersensitivity, these mechanisms are misdirected or out of control.

Hypersensitivity reactions are categorized in accordance with the effectors involved in these reactions. One category is antibody-mediated and may be passively transferred to another individual by the appropriate amount and type of antibody in serum. This group is, in turn, divided into three classes, depending on the specific underlying mechanisms involving either mast cells or complement and neutrophils. These reactions have in common a rapidity of response that can range from minutes to a few hours following the exposure to antigen and are, therefore, generally grouped as immediate hypersensitivity reactions (hypersensitivity reactions are discussed in Chapters 14–16).

The second major category of hypersensitivity reactions is mediated largely by T cells with consequent involvement of monocytes and is appropriately termed cell-mediated immunity (CMI). These responses are much more delayed in appearance, generally taking 18–24 h to reach their full expression, and have been traditionally referred to as delayed-type hypersensitivity (DTH). Unlike antibody-mediated hypersensitivity, which can be transferred from a sensitive individual to a nonsensitive individual via serum, DTH may only be transferred by T cells.

It should be reemphasized that all these hypersensitivity reactions have a normal counterpart in that the same mechanisms may operate to protect the host from invading organisms. It is only when the consequences of these responses are misplaced or exaggerated that deleterious effects to the host occur, and we call them hypersensitivity reactions.

Regulation of the Immune Response

Given the complexity of the immune response and its potential for inducing damage, it is self-evident that it must operate under carefully regulated conditions, as does any other physiologic system. These controls are multiple and include feedback inhibition by soluble products as well as cell–cell interactions of many types, which may either heighten or reduce the response. The net result is to maintain a state of homeostasis so that, when the system is perturbed by a foreign invader, enough response is generated to control the invader, and then the system returns to equilibrium—in other words, the immune response is shut down. However, its memory of that particular invader is retained so that a more rapid and heightened response will occur should the invader return.

Disturbances in these regulatory mechanisms may be caused by conditions such as congenital defects, hormonal imbalance, or infection, any of which may have disastrous consequences. AIDS may serve as a timely example; it is associated with an infection of T lymphocytes that participate in regulating the immune response. As a result of infection with the human immunodeficiency virus (HIV), which causes AIDS, there is a decrease in occurrence and function of one vital subpopulation of T cells, which leads to immunologic deficiency and renders the patient powerless to resist infections by microorganisms that are normally benign.

An important form of regulation concerns the prevention of immune responses against self-antigens. For various reasons, this regulation may be defective, thus causing an immune response against self to be mounted. This type of immune response is termed ***autoimmunity*** and is the cause of diseases such as some forms of arthritis, thyroiditis, and diabetes, which are very difficult to treat.

The Future of Immunology

For the student, a peek into the world of the future of immunology suggests many exciting areas in which the application of molecular and computational techniques promises significant dividends. To cite just a few examples, let's focus on vaccine development and control of the immune response. In the former, rather than the laborious, empirical search for an attenuated virus or bacterium for use in immunization, it is now possible to use pathogen-specific protein sequence data and sophisticated computational methods (bioinformatics) to identify candidate immunogenic peptides that can be tested as vaccines. Alternatively, DNA vaccines involving the injection of DNA vectors that encode immunizing proteins may revolutionize vaccination protocols in the not-too-distant future. The identification of various genes and the proteins or portions thereof (peptides) that they are encoding makes it possible to design vaccines against a wide spectrum of biologically important compounds.

Another area of great promise is the characterization and synthesis of various cytokines that enhance and control the activation of various cells associated with the immune response as well as with other functions of the body. Techniques of gene isolation, clonal reproduction, the polymerase chain reaction, and biosynthesis have contributed to rapid progress. Powerful and important modulators have been synthesized by the methods of recombinant DNA technology and are being tested for their therapeutic efficacy in a variety of diseases, including many different cancers. In some cases, cytokine research efforts have already moved from the bench to the bedside with the development of therapeutic agents used to treat patients.

Finally, and probably one of the most exciting areas, is the technology to genetically engineer various cells and even whole animals, such as mice, that lack one or more specific traits (gene knockout) or that carry a specific trait (transgenic). These and other immune-based experimental systems are the subject of Chapter 5. They allow the immunologist to study the effects of such traits on the immune system and on the body as a whole with the aim of understanding the intricate regulation, expression, and function of the immune response and with the ultimate aim of controlling the trait to the benefit of the individual. Thus our burgeoning understanding of the functioning of the immune system, combined with the recently acquired ability to alter and manipulate its components, carries enormous implications for the future of humankind.

In the remaining chapters we provide a more detailed account of the workings of the immune system, beginning with its cellular components, followed by a description of the structure of the reactants and the general methodology for measuring their reactions. This is followed by chapters describing the formation and activation of the cellular and molecular components of the immune apparatus required to generate a response. A discussion of the control mechanisms that regulate the scope and intensity of immune responses completes the description of the basic nature of immunity. Included in this section of the book is a chapter on cytokines, the soluble mediators that regulate immune responses and play a significant role in hematopoiesis. Next are chapters that deal with the great variety of diseases involving immunologic components. These vary from ineffective or absent immune response (immunodeficiency) to those produced by aberrant immune responses (hypersensitivity) to responses to self-antigens (autoimmunity). This is followed by chapters that describe the role of the immune response in transplantation and discuss antitumor reactions. A final chapter focuses on the spectrum of microorganisms that challenge the immune system and how immune responses are mounted in a vigilant, orchestrated fashion to protect the host from infectious diseases. Included is a discussion of immunoprophylaxis using vaccines that protect us from variety of pathogenic organisms. Without question, the successful use of vaccines helped revolutionize the field of medicine in the twentieth century. What lies ahead in the twenty-first century are research efforts related to the development of crucial new vaccines to protect humankind from naturally occurring pathogenic viruses and microorganisms that have just begun to plague us (most notably, HIV), have been engineered as potential biologic weapons, or have yet to be identified.

With the enormous scope of the subject and the extraordinary richness of detail available, we have made every effort to adhere to fundamental elements and basic concepts required to achieve an integrated, if not extensive, understanding of the immune response. If the reader's interest has been aroused, many current books, articles, and reviews, and growing numbers of educational Internet sites, including the one that supports this textbook (see the Preface), are available to flesh out the details on the scaffolding provided by this book.

REFERENCES

Baxter AG, Hodgkin PD (2002): Activation rules: the two-signal theories of immune activation. *Nature Rev Immunology* 2:439.

Shevach EM (2002): $CD4^+$, $CD25^+$ suppressor T cells: More questions than answers. *Nature Rev Immunol* 2:389.

Matzinger P (1994): Tolerance, danger and the extended family. *Ann Rev Immunol* 12:991.

2

ELEMENTS OF INNATE AND ACQUIRED IMMUNITY

INTRODUCTION

Every living organism is confronted by continual intrusions from its environment. Our immune systems are equipped with a network of mechanisms to safeguard us from infectious microorganisms that would otherwise take advantage of our bodies for their own survival. In short, the immune system has evolved as a surveillance system poised to initiate and maintain protective responses against virtually any harmful foreign element we might encounter. These defenses range from physical barriers, such as our skin, to highly sophisticated systems, such as the acquired immune response. This chapter describes the defense systems: the elements that constitute the defense, the participating cells and organs, and the action of the participants in the immune response to foreign substances that invade the body.

In vertebrates, immunity against microorganisms and their products or against other foreign substances that may invade the body is divided into two major categories: ***innate,*** or ***nonspecific immunity*** and ***acquired,*** or ***adaptive immunity.*** These two types of immunities and their origins, components, and interrelationships are discussed in this chapter. Here, and in the chapters that follow, it will become apparent that innate immune responses are important not only because they are an independent arm of the immune system but also because they profoundly influence the nature of adaptive immune responses.

INNATE IMMUNITY

Innate immunity is present from birth and consists of many factors that are relatively nonspecific—that is, it operates against almost any substance that threatens the body. Its principle role is to provide an early, nonspecific, first line of defense against ***pathogens.*** Most ***microorganisms*** encountered daily in the life of a healthy individual are detected and destroyed within minutes to hours by innate defense mechanisms.

Innate immunity is related to many attributes of the individual that are determined genetically. Differences in innate immunity among various people may, in addition, be attributed to age, race, and the hormonal and metabolic conditions of the individual. This section describes the major cellular, noncellular, and receptor components of innate immunity. It serves as an important backdrop for subsequent discussions of the links between innate and adaptive immunity.

Physical and Chemical Barriers

Most organisms and foreign substances cannot penetrate intact ***skin*** but can enter the body if the skin is damaged. Some microorganisms can enter through sebaceous glands and hair follicles. However, the ***acid pH*** of sweat and sebaceous secretions and the presence of various ***fatty acids*** and ***hydrolytic enzymes*** (e.g., ***lysozymes***) all have some antimicrobial

Immunology: A Short Course, Fifth Edition, By Richard Coico, Geoffrey Sunshine, and Eli Benjamini
ISBN 0-471-22689-0 © 2003 John Wiley & Sons, Inc.

effects, therefore minimizing the importance of this route of infection. In addition, soluble proteins, including the ***interferons*** and certain members of the ***complement system*** found in the serum (see Chapter 13), contribute to nonspecific immunity. Interferons are a group of proteins made by cells in response to virus infection, which essentially induce a generalized antiviral state in surrounding cells (see Chapter 11). Activation of complement components in response to certain microorganisms results in a controlled enzymatic cascade, which targets the membrane of pathogenic organisms and leads to their destruction.

An important innate immune mechanism involved in the protection of many areas of the body, including the respiratory and gastrointestinal tracks, involves the simple fact that surfaces in these areas are covered with mucous. In these areas, the mucous membrane barrier traps microorganisms, which are then swept away, by ciliated epithelial cells, toward the external openings. The hairs in the nostrils and the cough reflex are also helpful in preventing organisms from infecting the respiratory tract. Alcohol consumption, cigarette smoking, and narcotics suppress this entire defense system.

The elimination of microorganisms from the respiratory tract is aided by pulmonary or alveolar macrophages, which, as we shall see later, are phagocytic cells able to engulf and destroy some microorganisms. Other microorganisms that have penetrated the mucous membrane barrier can be picked up by macrophages or otherwise transported to lymph nodes, where many are destroyed.

The environment of the gastrointestinal tract is made hostile to many microorganisms by other innate mechanisms, including the hydrolytic enzymes in saliva, the low pH of the stomach, and the proteolytic enzymes and bile in the small intestine. The low pH of the vagina serves a similar function.

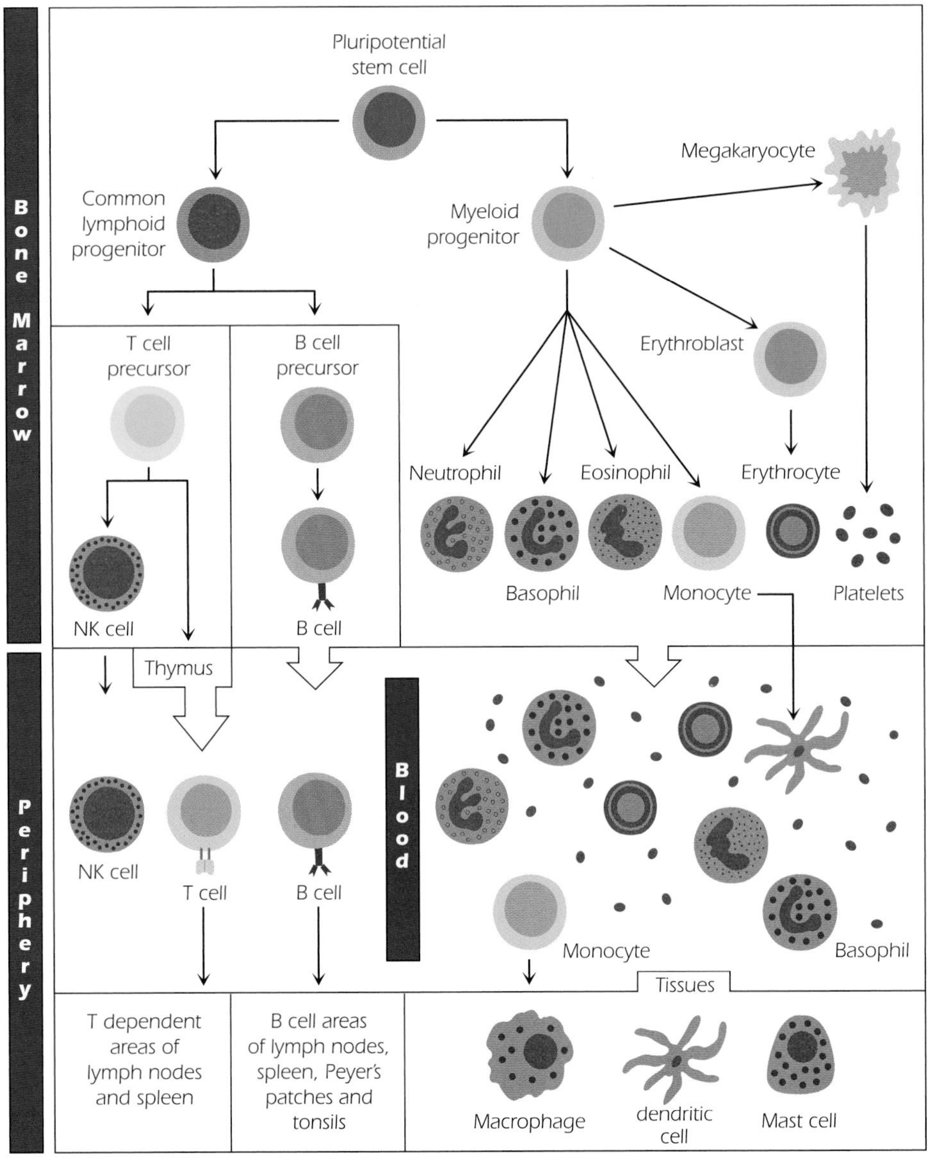

Figure 2.1. The developmental pathway of various cell types from pluripotential bone marrow stem cells.

Cellular Defenses

Once an invading microorganism has penetrated the various physical and chemical barriers, the next line of defense consists of various specialized cells whose purpose is to destroy the invader. There are several cell types that fulfill this function. The developmental pathways of hematopoietic cells and the interrelationships among the various cell types, which will be discussed in this and subsequent chapters, are shown in Figure 2.1.

Phagocytosis and Extracellular Killing

As part of its innate immunity, the body has developed defenses mediated by specialized cells that destroy the invading microorganism by first ingesting and then destroying it (phagocytosis) or by killing it extracellularly (without ingesting it).

Endocytosis and Phagocytosis. Two innate immune mechanisms result in the internalization of foreign macromolecules and cells and can lead to their intracellular destruction and elimination. These involve processes called endocytosis and phagocytosis.

Endocytosis. ***Endocytosis*** is the process whereby macromolecules present in extracellular tissue fluid are ingested by cells. This can occur either by pinocytosis, which involves nonspecific membrane invagination, or by receptor-mediated endocytosis, a process involving the selective binding of macromolecules to specific membrane receptors. In both cases, ingestion of the foreign macromolecules generates endocytic vesicles filled with the foreign material, which then fuse with acidic compartments called endosomes. Edosomes then fuse with lysosomes containing degradative enzymes (e.g., nucleases, lipases, proteases) to reduce the ingested macromolecules to small breakdown products, including nucleotides, sugars, and peptides (Fig. 2.2).

Phagocytosis. ***Phagocytosis*** is the ingestion by individual cells of invading foreign particles, such as bacteria. It is a critical protective mechanism of the immune system. Many microorganisms release substances that attract phagocytic cells. Phagocytosis may be enhanced by a variety of factors that make the foreign particle an easier target. These factors, collectively referred to as ***opsonins*** (Greek word meaning "prepare food for"), consist of antibodies and various serum components of complement (see Chapter 13). After ingestion, the foreign particle is entrapped in a phagocytic vacuole (***phagosome***), which fuses with ***lysosomes*** forming the ***phagolysosome*** (Fig. 2.2). The latter release their powerful enzymes, which digest the particle.

Phagocytes can also damage invading pathogens through the generation of toxic products in a process known as the

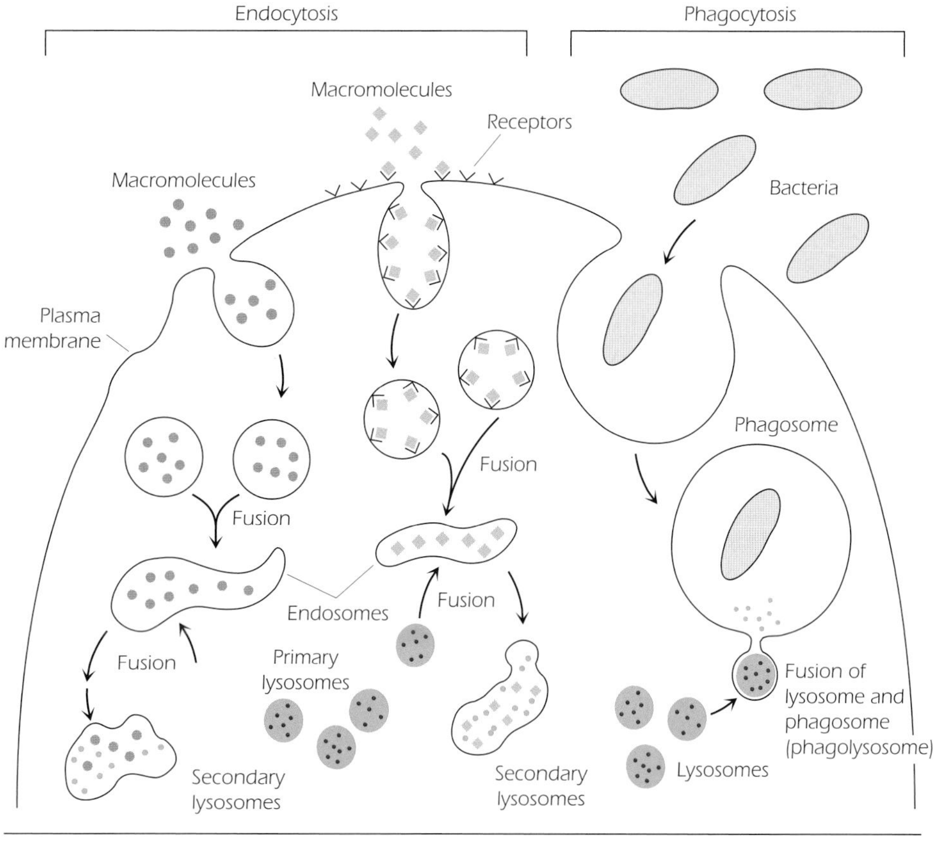

Figure 2.2. Endocytosis and phagocytosis by macrophages.

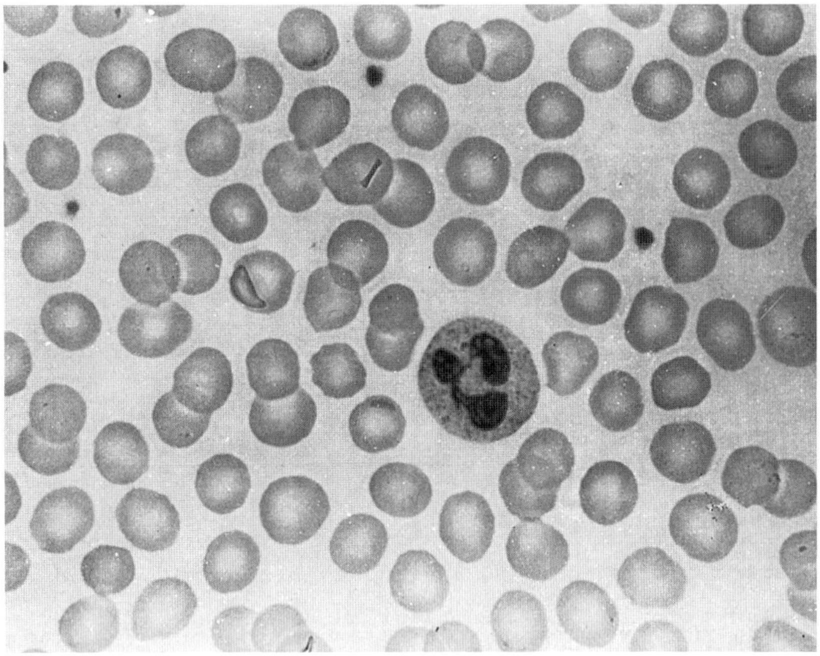

Figure 2.3. A polymorphonuclear leukocyte (surrounded by erythrocytes in a blood smear) with a trilobed nucleus and cytoplasmic granules. ×950. (Courtesy of Dr. AC Enders, School of Medicine, University of California at Davis.)

respiratory burst. Production of these toxic metabolites is induced during phagocytosis of pathogens such as bacteria and catalyzed by a set of interrelated enzyme pathways. The most important of these are nitric oxide (inducible nitric oxidase synthase), hydrogen peroxide and superoxide anion (phagocyte NADPH oxidase), and hypochlorous acid (myeloperoxidase), each of which is toxic to bacteria. These microbicidal products can also damage host cells. Fortunately, a series of protective enzymes produced by phagocytes controls the action of these products so that their microbicidal activity is primarily limited to the phagolysosome (i.e., fused phagosomes and lysosomes – see Figure 2.2), thereby focusing their toxicity on ingested pathogens. These protective enzymes include catalase, which degrades hydrogen peroxide, and superoxide dismutase, which converts the superoxide anion into hydrogen peroxide and oxygen. The absence of, or an abnormality in, any one of the respiratory burst components from phagocytic cells results in a form of immunodeficiency that predisposes individuals to repeated infections (Chapter 17).

Cells Involved in the Innate Immune System

Many cell types participate in innate host defense mechanisms. As noted above, phagocytosis is a fundamental protective mechanism and is carried out by several cell types, including the polymorphonuclear leukocytes, phagocytic monocytes (e.g., macrophages), and fixed macrophages of the reticuloendothelial system. On activation, all these cells release soluble substances called cytokines, which have different effects on various cells (see Chapter 11). Many of these and other cells that participate in innate immunity are also involved in key steps required for induction of adaptive immunity, including antigen presentation.

Polymorphonuclear Leukocytes. ***Polymorphonuclear*** (PMN) ***leukocytes*** are a population of cells also referred to as granulocytes. These include the basophils, mast cells, eosinophils, and neutrophils. Granulocytes are short-lived phagocytic cells that contain the enzyme-rich lysosomes, which can facilitate destruction of infectious microorganisms (Fig. 2.3). They also produce peroxide and superoxide radicals, which are toxic to many microorganisms. Some lysosomes also contain bactericidal proteins, such as lactoferrin. PMN leukocytes play a major role in protection against infection. Defects in PMN cell function are accompanied by chronic or recurrent infection.

Macrophages. ***Macrophages*** are phagocytes derived from blood ***monocytes*** (Fig. 2.4). The monocyte itself is a small, spherical cell with few projections, abundant cytoplasm, little endoplasmic reticulum, and many granules. Following migration of monocytes from the blood to various tissues, they undergo further differentiation into a variety of histologic forms, all of which play a role in phagocytosis, including the following:

- ***Kupffer cells,*** in the liver; large cells with many cytoplasmic projections.
- ***Alveolar macrophages,*** in the lung.
- ***Splenic macrophages,*** in the white pulp.
- ***Peritoneal macrophages,*** free-floating in peritoneal fluid.
- ***Microglial cells,*** in the central nervous tissue.

Each of these macrophage populations is included in the ***reticuloendothelial system*** (RES), which is widely distributed throughout the body. The major function of the RES is to

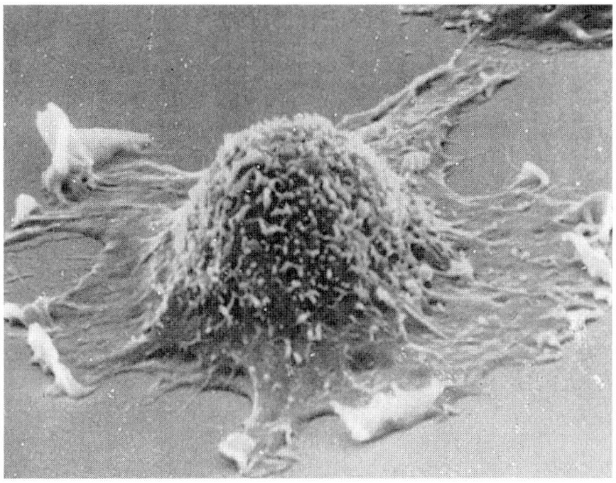

Figure 2.4. A scanning electron micrograph of a macrophage with ruffled membranes and a surface covered with microvilli. ×5200. (Courtesy of Dr. KL Erickson, School of Medicine, University of California at Davis; reproduced with permission from Lippincott/Harper & Row.)

phagocytize microorganisms and foreign substances that are in the bloodstream and in various tissues. The RES also functions in the destruction of aged and imperfect cells, such as erythrocytes.

Although associated with diverse names and locations, many of these cells share common features, such as the ability to bind and engulf particulate materials and antigens. Because of their location along capillaries, these cells are most likely to make first contact with invading pathogens and antigens and, as we shall see later, play a large part in the success of innate as well as acquired immunity.

In general, cells of the macrophage series have two major functions. One, as their name ("large eater") implies, is to engulf and, with the aid of all the degradative enzymes in their lysosomal granules, break down trapped materials into simple amino acids, sugars, and other substances for excretion or reuse. Thus these cells play a key role in the removal of bacteria and parasites from the body. As discussed in later chapters, the second major function of the macrophages is to take up antigens, process them by denaturation or partial digestion, and present them, on their surfaces, to specific T cells. Thus macrophages also function as antigen-presenting cells (see Chapter 9).

Dendritic cells are long-lived and reside in an immature state in most tissues, where they recognize and phagocytize pathogens and other antigens. They are found as ***interdigitating cells of the thymus,*** and ***Langerhans cells*** in the skin are derived from the same hematopoietic precursor cells as monocytes. Direct contact with many pathogens leads to the maturation of dendritic cells, leading to a significant increase in their antigen-presentation capacity. In fact, such maturation allows them to activate naive antigen-specific T cells. Thus they are important in both innate immunity and the initiation of adaptive immune responses.

From this outline, it can be seen that each of these cellular components of the innate immune system has diverse roles within the nonspecific limb of the immune system. They also play a key role in the afferent or induction limb of the acquired immune response (by initiating T cell responses). Finally, the macrophages play a role in the efferent or effector limb of the acquired immune response as the end cells that become activated by cytokines produced largely by T cells, which enhance their killing of pathogens.

Natural-Killer Cells. Altered features of the membranes of abnormal cells, such as those found on virus-infected or cancer cells, are recognized by cytotoxic or killer cells that destroy the target cell not by phagocytosis but by releasing biologically potent molecules that, within a very short time, kill the target cell. Such killer cells include the antigen-specific cytotoxic T lymphocytes, which are members of the adaptive or acquired immune system (discussed in more detail in Chapter 10), and the ***natural-killer*** (***NK***) cells, which are members of the innate immune system.

NK cells probably play a role in the early stages of viral infection or tumorogenesis, before the cytotoxic T lymphocytes of the acquired immune response increase in numbers. NK cells are large granular lymphocytes that are able to lyse certain virus-infected cells and tumor cells without prior stimulation. Unlike cytotoxic T lymphocytes, which recognize antigen-bearing target cells via their T cell receptors (TCRs), NK cells lack antigen-specific TCRs. How, then, do they seek and destroy their targets? They do this by using a mechanism involving cell–cell contact, which allows them to determine whether a potential target cell has lost a particular self-antigen—major histocompatibility complex (MHC) class I. MHC class I is expressed on virtually all nucleated cells. NK cells express non-TCR-related receptors, called ***killer-cell inhibitory receptors (KIR),*** which bind to MHC class I molecules. When ligated, KIRs protect the target from being killed by NK cells. Virus-infected or transformed (tumor) cells have reduced MHC class I on their surfaces. Thus, when such cells encounter NK cells, they fail to effectively engage these killer cell inhibitory receptors and therefore become susceptible to NK cell–mediated cytotoxicity (Fig. 2.5)

Killing is achieved by the release of various cytotoxic molecules. Some of these molecules cause the formation of pores in the membrane of the target cell, leading to its lysis. Other molecules enter the target cell and cause apoptosis (programmed cell death) of the target cell by enhanced fragmentation of its nuclear DNA. The activity of NK cells is highly increased by soluble mediators, such as interleukin-2 (IL-2), IL-12, and interferons. As discussed in Chapter 11, interferons-α and -β are antiviral proteins synthesized and released by leukocytes, fibroblasts, and virally infected cells; IL-2 and interferon-γ are released by activated T lymphocytes.

NK T Cells. Another population of cells with phenotypic and functional properties that are similar to NK cells is the thymus-derived ***NK T cell***. Like other T cells, these

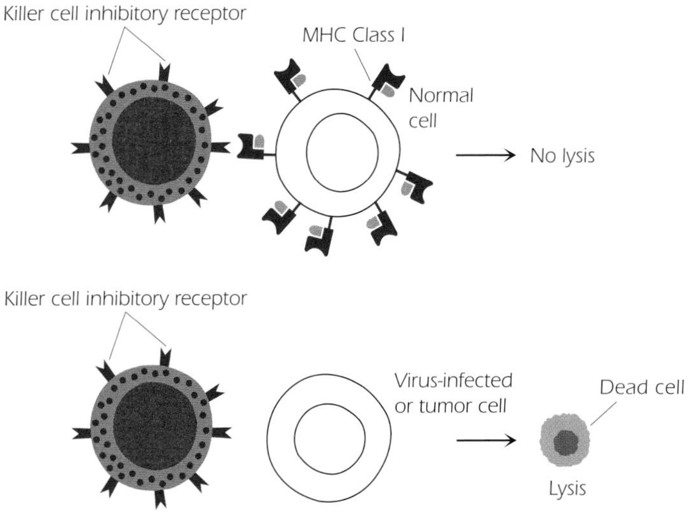

Figure 2.5. NK cell inhibitory receptors and killing.

cells express TCRs, although with restricted variability. Unlike other T cells, these cells express a marker called NK1.1, which recognizes an MHC-associated CD1 receptor expressed on antigen-presenting cells. NK1.1 T cells are unusual in terms of their functional status because they fall somewhere between the innate and the adaptive immune systems. Following activation, they secrete several cytokines, including IL-4 and interferon-γ (thus they play an immunoregulatory role) and kill target cells via Fas–Fas ligand interactions which cause apoptosis (Chapter 10).

Inflammation

An important function of phagocytic cells is their participation in inflammation, a major component of the body's defense mechanisms. The important aspects of inflammation are summarized below.

Inflammation is a complex process initiated by tissue damage caused by endogenous factors (such as tissue necrosis or bone fracture) and by exogenous factors. These include various types of damage, such as mechanical injury (e.g., cut), physical injury (e.g., burn), chemical injury (e.g., exposure to a corrosive chemical), biologic injury (e.g., infection by microorganisms; see Chapter 20), and immunologic injury (e.g., hypersensitivity reactions; see Chapters 14–16). The inflammatory response constitutes an important part of both innate and acquired immunity. It has evolved as a protective response against injury and infection. Although in certain cases, such as hypersensitivity, inflammation becomes the problem rather than the solution to a problem, by and large the inflammatory response is protective; it is one of the major responses to injury and constitutes a process aimed at bringing the injured tissue back to its normal state.

The hallmark signs of inflammation are ***pain, redness,*** and ***heat.*** Each of these is the result of specific changes in the local blood vessels. Pain is caused by ***increased vascular diameter,*** which leads to ***increased blood flow,*** thereby causing heat and redness in the area. A subsequent ***reduction in blood velocity*** and concomitant cytokine- and kinin-induced increased expression of so-called ***adhesion molecules*** on the endothelial cells lining the blood vessel promote the ***binding of circulating leukocytes.*** These events facilitate the attachment and entry of leukocytes into tissues and the ***recruitment of neutrophils and monocytes*** to the site of inflammation. Another major change in the local blood vessels is ***increased vascular permeability.*** This results from the separation of previously tightly joined endothelial cells lining the blood vessels leading to the exit of fluid and proteins from the blood and their accumulation in the tissue. These events account for the ***swelling*** (***edema***) associated with inflammation, which contributes significantly to the pain.

Within minutes after injury, the inflammatory process begins with the activation and increased concentration of pharmacologically powerful substances, such as a group of proteins known as ***acute-phase proteins.*** The ***acute-phase response*** induces both localized and systemic responses. Localized inflammatory responses are generated, in part, as a result of the activation of the ***kinins*** and the ***coagulation system*** (***clotting***).

The ***kinins*** have several important effects:

- They act directly on local smooth muscle and cause muscle contraction.
- They act on axons to block nervous impulses, leading to a distal muscle relaxation.
- Most important, they act on vascular endothelial cells (e.g., the vasoactive peptide ***bradykinin***), causing them to contract and leading to increase in vascular permeability, and to express ***endothelial cell adhesion molecules*** (ECAMs), leading to leukocyte adhesion and ***extravasation.***
- Kinins are very potent nerve stimulators and are the molecules most responsible for pain (and itching) associated with inflammation.

Kinins are rapidly inactivated after their activation by proteases, which are generated during these localized responses.

The ***coagulation pathway*** consists of plasma enzymes that are activated in a cascading manner following damage to blood vessels. Its role in the inflammatory response is to form a physical barrier (***clot***) that prevents microorganisms from entering the bloodstream.

The ***systemic inflammatory response*** includes the induction of ***fever*** (discussed below), increased white blood cell production, increased synthesis of hydrocortisone and adrenocorticotropic hormone (ACTH), and production of the acute-phase proteins (see Chapter 11). An important member of the acute-phase proteins is ***C-reactive protein.*** This protein binds to the membrane of certain microorganisms and activates the complement system (Chapter 13). This results in the lysis of the microorganism or its enhanced phagocytosis by phagocytic cells, as well as other important biologic functions, as we shall see later.

Cytokines play a key role in the inflammatory response. IL-1, IL-6, and tumor necrosis factor-α (TNFα) are among the most important cytokines involved (Chapter 11). These cytokines, released by activated macrophages, induce adhesion molecules on the walls of vascular endothelial cells to which neutrophils, monocytes, and lymphocytes adhere before moving out of the vessel—through a process called extravasation—to the affected tissue. These cytokines also induce coagulation and increased vascular permeability. Other cytokines, including IL-8 and interferon-γ, exert additional effects, such as increased chemotaxis for leukocytes and increased phagocytosis. All these effects result in the accumulation of fluid (edema) and leukocytic cells in the injured areas. These, in turn, amplify the response, since additional biologically active compounds are transported in the fluid and are released from the accumulated cells, attracting and activating still more cells.

Most of the cells involved in the inflammatory response are phagocytic cells, first consisting mainly of the polymorphonuclear leukocytes, which accumulate within 30–60 min, phagocytize the intruder or damaged tissue, and release their lysosomal enzymes in an attempt to destroy the intruder. If the cause of the inflammatory response persists beyond this point, within 4-6 h the area will be infiltrated by mononuclear cells, which include macrophages and lymphocytes. The macrophages supplement the phagocytic activity of the polymorphonuclear cells, thus adding to the defense of the area. Moreover, the macrophages participate in the processing and presentation of antigen to lymphocytes, which respond to the foreign antigens of the invader by inducing the acquired immune response specific to those antigens.

If the injury or the invasion by microorganisms continues, the inflammatory response will be supplemented and augmented by elements of acquired immunity, including antibodies and cell-mediated immunity. The antibody response initiates the complement cascade in which pharmacologically active compounds are activated and released. These include substances that increase vascular permeability and capillary dilatation as well as chemotactic substances that attract and activate additional polymorphonuclear cells and antigen-specific lymphocytes. The lymphocytes themselves are capable of destroying some foreign invaders. More important, they release cytokines that activate macrophages and other cells to participate in destroying and removing the invaders.

Many substances activated during the inflammatory process participate in repairing the injury. During this remarkable process, many cells, including leukocytes, are being destroyed. The macrophages present in the area phagocytize the debris, and the inflammation subsides; the tissue may be restored to its normal state, or scar tissue may be formed.

Sometimes it is difficult or impossible to remove the causes of inflammation. This results in chronic inflammation, which occurs in situations of chronic infection (e.g., tuberculosis) or chronic activation of the immune response (e.g., rheumatoid arthritis and glomerulonephritis). In these cases, the inflammatory response continues and can be only temporarily modified by the administration of an anti-inflammatory agents, such as aspirin, ibuprofen, and cortisone. These and other drugs act on several of the metabolic pathways involved in the elaboration and activation of some of the pharmacologic mediators of inflammation. However, they do not affect the root cause of the inflammation; so when they are withdrawn, the symptoms may return.

Fever

Although fever is one of the most common manifestations of infection and inflammation, there is still limited information about the significance of fever in the course of infection in mammals. Fever is caused by many bacterial products, most notably the ***endotoxins*** of gram-negative bacteria, generally as the result of the release of endogenous ***pyrogens,*** which derive from monocytes and macrophages and include IL-1 and certain interferons.

Biologically Active Substances

Many tissues synthesize substances that are harmful to microorganisms. Examples are ***degradative enzymes, toxic free radicals, acids, inhibitors of growth, acute-phase proteins,*** and ***interferons.*** Thus, depending on their ability to synthesize these substances, certain tissues may have a heightened resistance to infection by some microorganisms.

Receptors Involved in the Innate Immune System

Unlike the adaptive immune system, which uses antigen-specific receptors to allow effector B and T cells to target antigens, the innate immune system lacks such specificity. These receptors are not clonally distributed, whereas antigen-specific receptors are. Thus a given set of receptors will be present on all the cells of the same cell type. The diversity of innate immune cell receptors also includes those involved in phagocytosis. For example, neutrophils express the ***f-Met-Leu-Phe receptor,*** a chemotactic receptor that binds the N-formylated peptides expressed by certain bacteria and guides neutrophils to the site of infection.

Certain families of ***pattern recognition receptors*** are also expressed on many cell types involved in the innate immune system. These receptors recognize conserved microbial structures directly as signatures of certain classes of pathogens. In doing so, they contribute to the specific detection of pathogens. One pattern recognition receptor type is the ***mannan-binding*** (MB) ***lectin,*** which enables phagocytes to recognize pathogenic microbe-expressed polysaccharides that have a sugar composition and residue spacing not found on host cells. Ligation of the phagocyte MB lectin (receptor) with these sugars initiates and activates the MB lectin pathway of complement. This results in the generation of complement components that coat the microorganism (opsonization), making them more susceptible to phagocytosis (see Chapter 13). A second set of phagocytic receptors are the ***scavenger receptors,*** which recognize specific anionic polymers and acetylated low-density lipoproteins expressed by certain pathogens as well as old dying red blood cells, leading to the removal of these cells.

Recently, a family of ***Toll-like receptors*** (TLRs) have been discovered to be essential for the recognition of pathogen-specific components shared by microorganisms. The Toll gene family was originally discovered for its contribution to dorsoventral patterning in *Drosophila melanogaster* embryos. Later, studies showed that Toll genes encode proteins that play a critical role in the fly's innate immune response to microbial infection. Further investigation then confirmed the existence of homologous proteins in mammals (TLR) that can activate phagocytes and tissue dendritic cells to respond to pathogens. TLRs make up a large family of receptors and each recognizes specific microbial components. Activation of TLRs by microbial components leads not only to activation of the innate immune system but also to development of adaptive immunity through production of proinflammatory cytokines and expression of costimulatory molecules.

ADAPTIVE (ACQUIRED) IMMUNITY

Under circumstances in which an infectious organism is not eliminated by nonspecific innate immune mechanisms, adaptive immune responses ensue, with the generation of ***antigen-specific lymphocytes*** (effector cells) and ***memory cells*** that can prevent reinfection with the same organism. These adaptive responses (sometimes called acquired responses) take more time to develop (> 96 h) because the rare B and T cells specific for the invading microorganism must undergo clonal expansion before they can differentiate into effector cells to help eliminate the infection. In contrast to innate immunity, which is an attribute of every living organism, adaptive immunity is a more specialized form of immunity. It developed late in evolution and is found only in vertebrates. The various elements that participate in innate immunity do not exhibit specificity against the foreign agents they encounter; by contrast, acquired immunity always exhibits such specificity. As its name implies, acquired immunity is a consequence of an encounter with a foreign substance. The first encounter with a particular foreign substance that has penetrated the body triggers a chain of events that induces an immune response with specificity against that foreign substance.

CELLS AND ORGANS INVOLVED IN THE ADAPTIVE IMMUNE RESPONSE

Acquired immunity is usually exhibited only after an initial encounter with the substance. Thus acquired immunity develops only after exposure to or immunization with a given substance.There are two major lymphocyte populations that participate in acquired immunity: B lymphocytes (so named because they originate in the bone marrow), and T lymphocytes (named for their differentiation in the thymus). B and T lymphocytes are responsible for the specificity exhibited by the acquired immune response. B lymphocytes synthesize and secrete into the bloodstream antibodies with specificity against the foreign substance. This is termed ***humoral immunity***. The T lymphocytes, which also exhibit specificity against the foreign substance by virtue of their receptors (TCRs), do not make antibodies but perform various effector functions when antigen-presenting cells (APCs) bring antigens into the secondary lymphoid organs. T lymphocytes also interact with B cells and help the latter make antibodies; they activate macrophages and have a central role in the development and regulation of acquired immunity (see Chapter 10). Acquired immunity mediated by T lymphocytes is termed ***cellular immunity*** or ***cell-mediated immunity*** (CMI). As we have seen, macrophages are phagocytic cells; they do not exhibit specificity against a given substance but are involved in the processing and presentation of foreign substances to T lymphocytes and activation of T lymphocytes (see Chapters 9 and 10).

In mammalian species, circulating blood cells have their common origin in a small cluster of cells that move from the primitive yolk sac to the fetal liver and finally to the bone marrow, where they take up permanent residence. These cells are the ***hematopoietic stem cells,*** so called because they are the undifferentiated cells from which all the other specialized cells in the blood develop (Fig. 2.1).

The undifferentiated stem cells are characterized by an ability to proliferate throughout life as a self-renewing reservoir, replenishing the pool of more mature cells as they are used up during normal activity. These early stem cells are considered to be ***pluripotent***—that is, they are capable of developing into any of the more differentiated lines of cells,

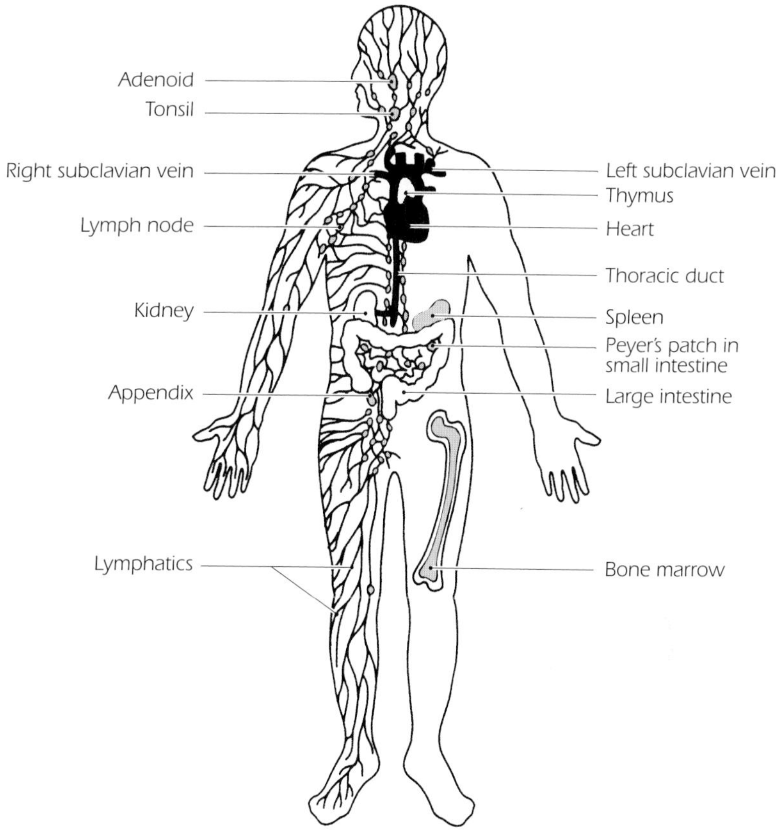

Figure 2.6. The distribution of lymphoid tissues in the body. (Reproduced with permission from FS Rosen and RS Geha, *Case Studies in Immunology,* Garland Publishing.)

under the influence of a variety of soluble factors that control both the extent and the direction of maturation. Isolation and characterization of these earliest hematopoietic and pluripotent stem cells have been facilitated by the recent identification on their surface of a molecule referred to as CD34. (The CD nomenclature is discussed in Chapter 5.) Expression of CD34 is quite specific for early progenitor cells (as well as for endothelial cells). Once differentiation in any direction has occurred, the cells become committed to make only a single type of cell lineage—that is, they become unipotent, and CD34 expression decreases. One pathway of differentiation (***myeloid differentiation***) starts from a bone marrow stem cell that gives rise to differentiated precursors and culminates with erythrocytes, thrombocytes (platelets), and the various granule-containing cells of the granulocyte–monocyte series. The other pathway of differentiation (***lymphocytic differentiation***) leads to two distinct cell types called B and T lymphocytes.

Lymphatic Organs

The lymphatic organs are those organs in which lymphocyte maturation, differentiation, and proliferation take place. They are generally divided into two categories. The ***primary (central) lymphoid organs*** are those in which the maturation of T and B lymphocytes into antigen-recognizing lymphocytes occurs. As we shall see in subsequent chapters, developing T and B cells acquire their antigen-specific receptors in primary lymphoid organs. Mature B and T lymphocytes migrate from the ***bone marrow*** and ***thymus,*** respectively, through the bloodstream to the peripheral lymphoid tissues, including the lymph nodes, spleen, and gut-associated lymphoid tissues such as the tonsils. These ***secondary (peripheral) lymphoid organs*** are those organs in which antigen-driven proliferation and differentiation take place (Fig. 2.6).

Primary Lymphoid Organs. There are two major primary lymphoid organs, one in which the T cells develop and the other in which the B cells develop.

Thymus Gland. Progenitor cells from the bone marrow migrate to the primary lymphoid organ, the thymus gland, where they differentiate into T lymphocytes. The thymus gland is a bilobed structure, derived from the endoderm of the third and fourth pharyngeal pouches (Fig. 2.7). During fetal development, the size of the thymus increases. The growth continues until puberty. Thereafter, the thymus undergoes atrophy with aging.

The thymus is a ***lymphoepithelial*** organ and consists of epithelial cells organized into cortical (outer) and medullary (central) areas that are infiltrated with lymphoid cells (***thymocytes***). The cortex is densely populated with lymphocytes of various sizes, most of which are immature, and scattered macrophages involved in clearing apoptotic thymocytes.

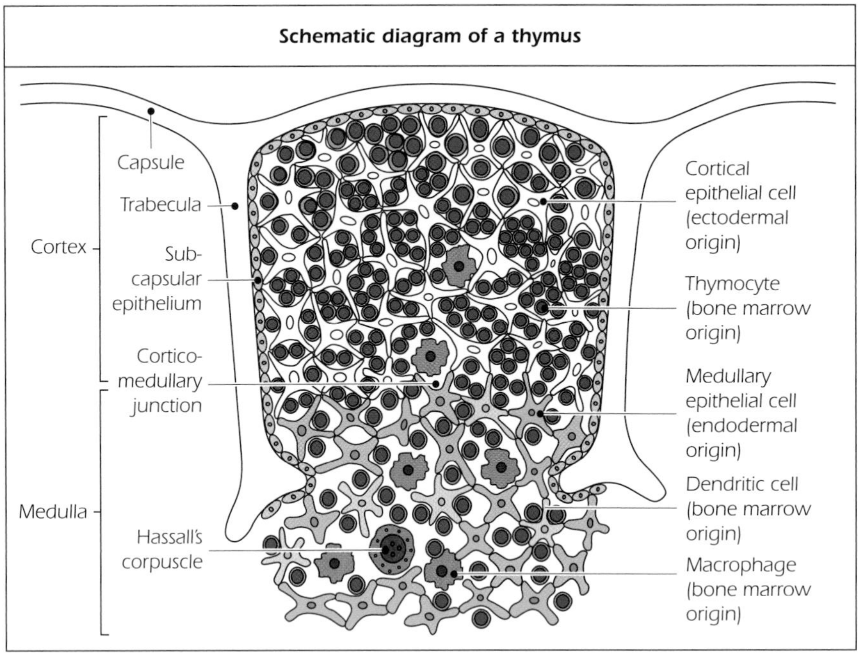

Figure 2.7. The cellular organization of the thymus. (Reproduced with permission from FS Rosen and RS Geha, *Case Studies in Immunology,* Garland Publishing.)

T lymphocytes mature in the cortex and migrate to the medulla, where they encounter macrophages and dendritic cells. Here, they undergo thymic selection, which results in the development of mature, functional T cells, which then leave to enter the peripheral blood circulation, through which they are transported to the secondary lymphoid organs. (T-cell development is discussed in detail in Chapter 8.) It is in these secondary lymphoid organs that the T cells encounter and respond to foreign antigens.

Maturation of the T lymphocyte involves the commitment of a given T cell to recognize and respond to a given determinant or epitope of a foreign antigen. This recognition is achieved by a specific receptor on the T cell (TCR), which is acquired during differentiation in the thymus (Chapter 8). Mature T lymphocytes in the medulla are capable of responding to foreign antigens in the same way that they would respond in the secondary lymphoid organs. However, the thymus is considered to be a primary lymphoid organ, because it is the site where T cells differentiate to express TCRs.

The maturation of T lymphocytes occurs mainly during fetal development and for a short time after birth. In mice, removal of the thymus gland from a neonate results in a severe reduction in the quantity and quality of T lymphocytes and produces a potentially lethal wasting disease. Removal of the thymus from an adult generally has little effect on the quantity and quality of the T lymphocytes, which have already matured and populated the secondary lymphoid organs. However, adult thymectomy could, in time, result in a deficiency of T cells if there is acute death of the T cells that originally populated the secondary lymphoid organs (such as following whole-body irradiation). Without the thymus, there would be no mechanism for repopulation of the secondary organs with new T lymphocytes.

Only 5–10% of maturing lymphocytes survive and eventually leave the thymus; 90–95% of all thymocytes die in the thymus. It is clear that the lymphocytes that die have developed specificity to self-structures or have failed to make functional receptors and, therefore, are eliminated. The lymphocytes that survive develop specificity against foreign antigens. This is discussed in detail in Chapter 9.

Bursa of Fabricius and Bone Marrow. In birds, B cells undergo maturation in the bursa of Fabricius. This organ, situated near the cloaca, consists of lymphoid centers that contain epithelial cells and lymphocytes. Unlike the lymphocytes in the thymus, these lymphocytes consist solely of antibody-producing B cells (see Chapter 7).

Mammals do not have a bursa of Fabricius. Consequently, much work has been directed toward the identification of a mammalian equivalent of the primary lymphoid organ in which B cells develop and mature. It is now clear that in embryonic life, B cells differentiate from hematopoietic stem cells in the fetal liver. After birth and for the life of the individual, this function moves to the bone marrow, a structure that is considered to be a primary lymphoid organ with functions equivalent to that of the avian bursa. Each mature B lymphocyte bears antigen-specific receptors that have a structure and specificity identical to the antibody later synthesized by that B cell. The mature B cells are transported by the circulating blood to the secondary lymphoid organs, where they encounter and respond to foreign antigens.

Secondary Lymphoid Organs. The ***secondary lymphoid organs*** consist of certain structures in which mature, antigen-committed lymphocytes are stimulated by antigen to undergo further division and differentiation. The major secondary lymphoid organs are the ***spleen*** and the ***lymph nodes.*** In addition, tonsils, appendix, clusters of lymphocytes distributed in the lining of the small intestine (***Peyer's patches***), and lymphoid aggregates spread throughout mucosal tissue are considered secondary lymphoid organs. These secondary lymphoid organs are found in various areas of the body, such as the linings of the digestive tract, in the respiratory and genitourinary tracts, in the conjunctiva, and in the salivary glands, where mature lymphocytes interact with antigen and undergo activation. These mucosal secondary lymphoid organs have been given the name ***mucosa-associated lymphoid tissue*** (MALT). Those lymphoid tissues associated with the gut are ***gut-associated lymphoid tissue*** (GALT); those associated with the bronchial tree are termed ***bronchus-associated lymphoid tissue*** (BALT).

The secondary lymphoid organs have two major functions: They are highly efficient in trapping and concentrating foreign substances, and they are the main sites of production of antibodies and the induction of antigen-specific T lymphocytes.

The Spleen. The spleen is the largest of the secondary lymphoid organs (Fig. 2.8). It is highly efficient in trapping and concentrating foreign substances carried in the blood. It is the major organ in the body in which antibodies are synthesized and from which they are released into the circulation. The spleen is composed of ***white pulp,*** rich in lymphoid cells,

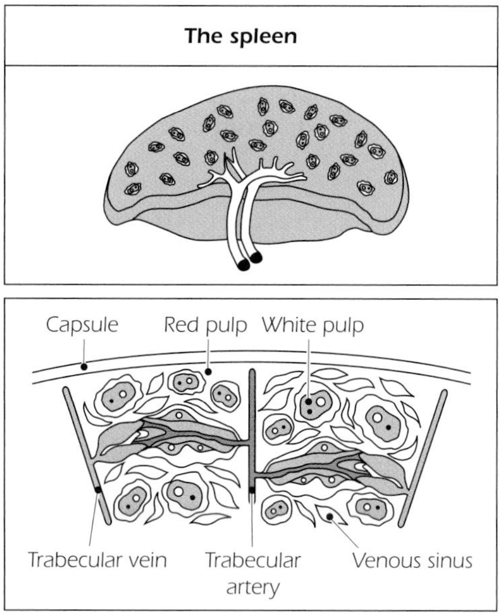

Figure 2.8. Overall and section views of the spleen. (Reproduced with permission from FS Rosen and RS Geha, *Case Studies in Immunology,* Garland Publishing.)

and ***red pulp,*** which contains many sinuses as well as large quantities of erythrocytes and macrophages, some lymphocytes, and a few other cell types.

The areas of white pulp are located mainly around small arterioles, the peripheral regions of which are rich in T cells; B cells are present mainly in germinal centers. Approximately 50% of spleen cells are B lymphocytes; 30–40% are T lymphocytes. After antigenic stimulation, the germinal centers contain large numbers of B cells and plasma cells. These cells synthesize and release antibodies.

Lymph Nodes. Lymph nodes are small ovoid structures (normally < 1 cm in diameter) found in various regions throughout the body (Fig. 2.9). They are close to major junctions of the lymphatic channels, which are connected to the thoracic duct. The thoracic duct transports lymph and lymphocytes to the vena cava, the vessel that carries blood to the right side of the heart (Fig. 2.10), from where it is redistributed throughout the body.

The lymph nodes are composed of a medulla with many sinuses and a cortex, which is surrounded by a capsule of connective tissue (Fig. 2.9A). The cortical region contains primary lymphoid follicles. After antigenic stimulation, these structures enlarge to form secondary lymphoid follicles with germinal centers containing dense populations of lymphocytes (mostly B cells) that are undergoing mitosis. In response to antigen stimulation, antigen-specific B cells proliferating within these germinal centers also undergo a process known as affinity maturation to generate clones of cells with higher affinity receptors (antibody) for the antigenic epitope that triggered the initial response (see Chapter 7). The remaining antigen-nonspecific B cells are pushed to the outside to form the mantle zone. The deep cortical area or paracortical region contains T cells and dendritic cells. Antigens are brought into these areas by dendritic cells, which present antigen fragments to T cells, events that result in activation of the T cells. The medullary area of the lymph node contains antibody-secreting plasma cells that have traveled from the cortex to the medulla via lymphatic vessels.

Lymph nodes are highly efficient in trapping antigen that enters through the afferent lymphatic vessels. In the node, the antigen interacts with macrophages, T cells, and B cells, and that interaction brings about an immune response, manifested by the generation of antibodies and antigen-specific T cells. Lymph, antibodies, and cells leave the lymph node through the efferent lymphatic vessel, which is just below the medullary region.

LYMPHOCYTE RECIRCULATION

Blood lymphocytes enter the lymph nodes through ***postcapillary venules*** and leave the lymph nodes through ***efferent lymphatic vessels,*** which eventually converge in the ***thoracic duct.*** This duct empties into the ***vena cava,*** the vessel that

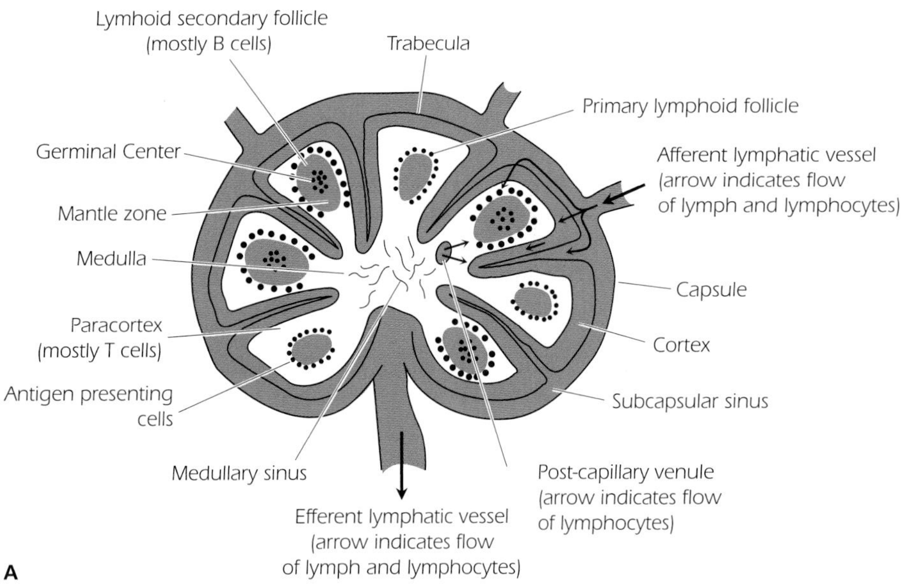

A

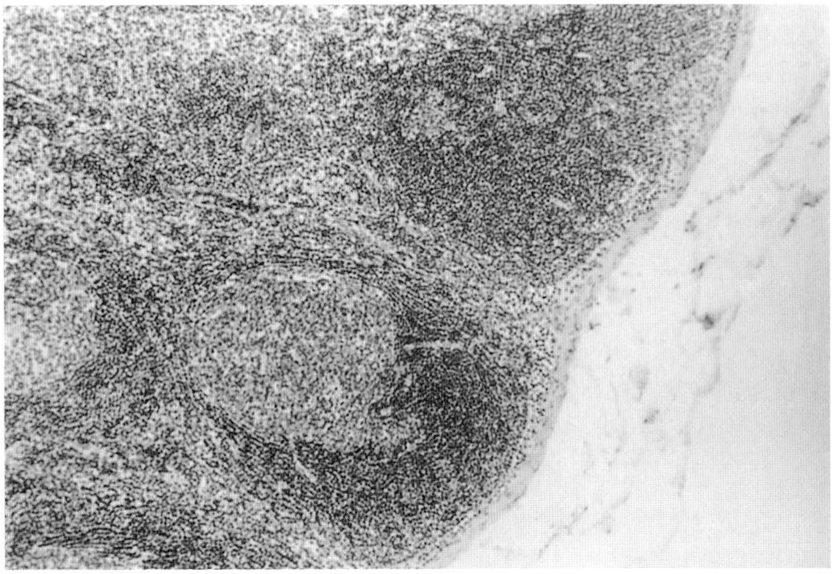

B

Figure 2.9. **(A)** A section of a lymph node. *Arrows,* flow of lymph and lymphocytes. **(B)** A section through a lymph node showing the capsule, the subcapsular sinus, the medulla (**upper left**), and the cortex with secondary follicles containing germinal centers. Also shown (**upper right**) is a follicle without a germinal center. ×140. (Panel B courtesy of Dr. AC Ender, School of Medicine, University of California at Davis.)

returns the blood to the ***heart,*** thus providing for the continual recirculation of lymphocytes.

The spleen functions in a similar manner. Arterial blood lymphocytes enter the spleen through the hilus and pass into the trabecular artery, which along its course becomes narrow and branched. At the farthest branches of the trabecular artery, capillaries lead to lymphoid nodules. Ultimately, the lymphocytes return to the venous circulation through the trabecular vein. Like lymph nodes, the spleen contains efferent lymphatic vessels through which lymph empties into the lymphatics from which the cells continue their recirculation through the body and back to the afferent vessels.

The migration of lymphocytes between various lymphoid and nonlymphoid tissue and their homing to a particular site is highly regulated by means of various ***cell-surface adhesion molecules*** (CAMs) and receptors to these molecules. Thus, except in the spleen where small arterioles end in the parenchyma, allowing access to blood lymphocytes, blood lymphocytes must generally cross the endothelial vascular lining of postcapillary vascular sites, termed ***high endothelial venules*** (HEVs). This process is called ***extravasation***. Recirculating lymphocytes selectively bind to specific receptors on the HEV of lymphoid tissue or inflammatory tissue spaces and appear to completely ignore other vascular endothelium. Moreover, it appears that a selective binding of finer specificity operates between the HEV and various distinct subsets of lymphocytes, further regulating the migration of lymphocytes into the various lymphoid and nonlymphoid tissue. Recirculating monocytes and granulocytes also express adhesion molecule receptors and migrate to tissue sites using a similar mechanism.

The traffic of lymphocytes between lymphoid and nonlymphoid tissue ensures that on exposure to an antigen, the antigen and the lymphocytes specific to that antigen are

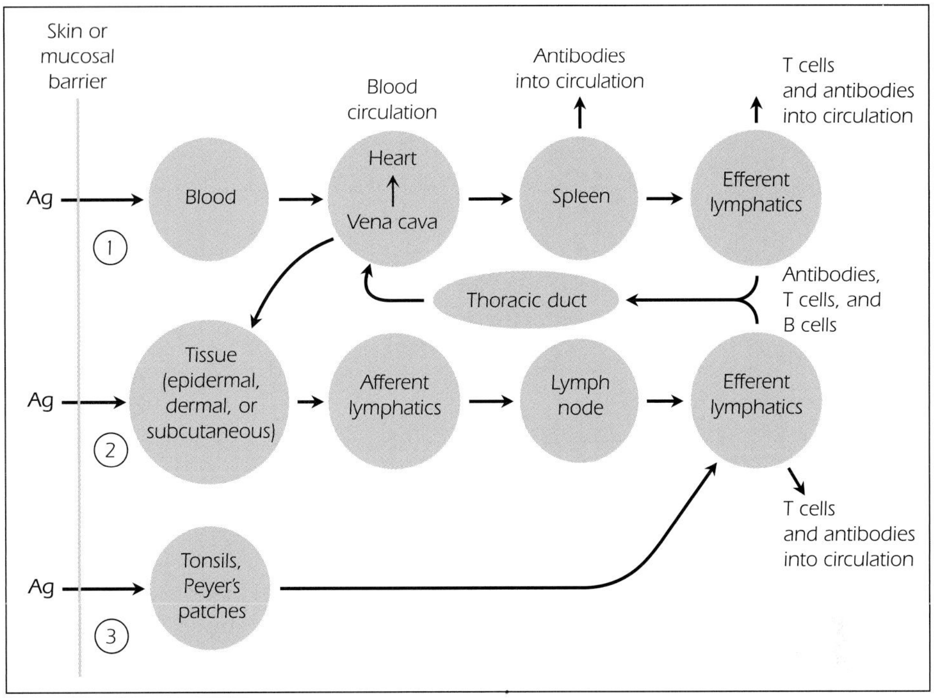

Figure 2.10. Circulation of lymph and fate of antigen following penetration through *(1)* the bloodstream, *(2)* the skin, and *(3)* the gastrointestinal or respiratory track.

sequestered in the lymphoid tissue, where the lymphocytes undergo proliferation and differentiation. The differentiated cells (memory cells) leave the lymphoid organ and are disseminated in the body to reconcentrate at the site where antigen persists and, at that place, exert their protective function.

THE FATE OF ANTIGEN AFTER PENETRATION

The ***reticuloendothelial system*** is designed to trap foreign antigens that have penetrated the body and to subject them to ingestion and degradation by the phagocytic cells of the system. Also, there is constant movement of lymphocytes throughout the body, and this movement permits deposition of lymphocytes in strategic places along the lymphatic vessels. The system not only traps antigens but also provides loci (the secondary lymphoid organs) where antigen, macrophages, T cells, and B cells can interact within a very small area to initiate an immune response.

The fate of an antigen that has penetrated the physical barriers and the cellular and antibody components of the ensuing immune response are shown in Figure 2.10. Three major routes may be followed by an antigen after it has penetrated the interior of the body:

- The antigen may enter the body through the bloodstream. In this case, it is carried to the spleen, where it interacts with APCs, such as dendritic cells and macrophages. B cells also serve as APCs, although their major role is to produce antibodies in response to the antigenic stimulus. APCs are essential in the activation of antigen-specific T cells. The interactions between APCs and T cells ultimately leads to activation of B and T cells and hence the immune response. The spleen then releases the antibodies directly into the circulation. Lymphocytes also leave the spleen through the efferent lymphatics, to reenter the circulation via the thoracic duct.
- The antigen may lodge in the epidermal, dermal, or subcutaneous tissue, where it may cause an inflammatory response. From these tissues, the antigen, either free or trapped by APCs, is transported through the afferent lymphatic channels into the regional draining lymph node. In the lymph node, the antigen, macrophages, dendritic cells, T cells, and B cells interact to generate the immune response. Eventually, antigen-specific T cells and antibodies, which have been synthesized in the lymph node, enter the circulation and are transported to the various tissues. Antigen-specific T cells, B cells, and antibodies also enter the circulation via the thoracic duct.
- The antigen may enter the gastrointestinal or respiratory tract, where it lodges in the MALT. There it will interact with macrophages and lymphocytes. Antibodies synthesized in these organs are deposited in the local tissue. In addition, lymphocytes entering the efferent lymphatics are carried through the thoracic duct to the circulation and are thereby redistributed to various tissue.

The induction of an acquired immune response necessitates the interaction of the foreign antigen with lymphocytes that recognize that specific antigen. It has been estimated that in a naive (nonimmunized) animal, only one in every 10^3–10^5 lymphocytes is capable of recognizing a typical antigen. Therefore, the probability that an antigen will

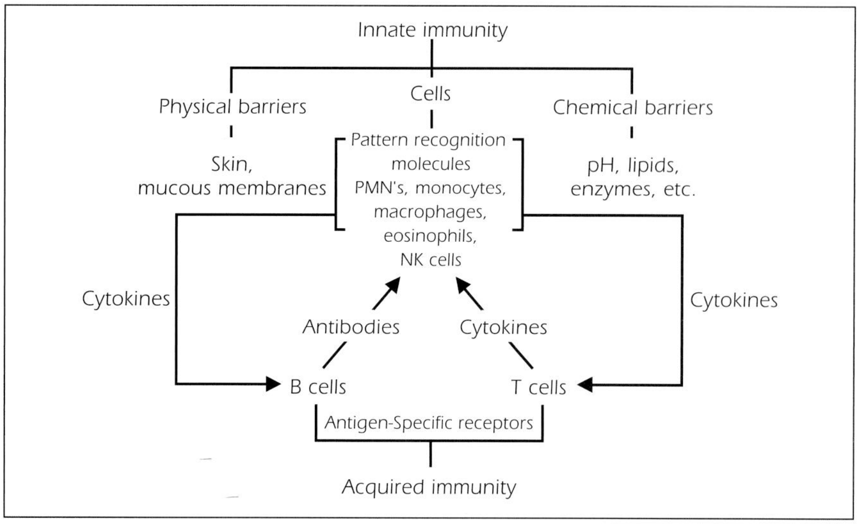

Figure 2.11. The interrelationship between innate and acquired immunity.

encounter these cells is very low. The problem is compounded by the fact that, for synthesis of antibody to ensue, two different kinds of lymphocytes, the T lymphocyte and B lymphocyte, each with specificity against this particular antigen, must interact.

Statistically, the chances for the interaction of specific T lymphocytes with their particular antigen, and then with B lymphocytes specific for the same antigen, are very low. However, nature has devised an ingenious mechanism for bringing these cells into contact with antigen: The antigen is carried via the draining lymphatics to the secondary lymphoid organs. In these organs, the antigen is exposed on the surface of fixed specialized cells. Because both T and B lymphocytes circulate at a rather rapid rate, making the rounds every several days, some circulating lymphocytes with specificity for the particular antigen should pass by the antigen within a relatively short time. When these lymphocytes encounter the antigen for which they are specific, the lymphocytes become activated, and the acquired immune response, with specificity against this antigen, is triggered.

INTERRELATIONSHIP BETWEEN INNATE AND ACQUIRED IMMUNITY

The innate and acquired arms of the immune system have developed a beautiful interrelationship. The intricate and ingenious communication system through the various cytokines and cell adhesion molecules allows components of innate and acquired immunity to interact, send each other signals, activate each other, and work in concert toward the final goal of destroying and eliminating the invading microorganism and its products. The interrelationship between innate and acquired immunity is shown in Figure 2.11.

SUMMARY

1. There are two forms of immunity: (a) innate, or nonspecific, and (b) acquired, or adaptive.
2. Many elements participate in innate immunity, including various physical barriers (e.g., skin), chemical barriers (e.g., low pH in stomach), cellular components (e.g., phagocytes), and pattern recognition receptors (e.g., TLRs).
3. Two major types of cells participate in acquired immunity and clonally express antigen-specific receptors: (a) B lymphocytes and (b) T lymphocytes.
4. Macrophages constitute an essential part of the reticuloendothelial system and function to trap, process, and present antigen to T lymphocytes, thus assuming an important function in both innate and acquired immunity.
5. B and T lymphocytes have receptors that are specific for particular antigens and thus constitute the components of acquired immunity that are responsible for antigenic specificity.
6. B and T lymphocytes develop in primary lymphoid organs. B cells are derived from lymphoid progenitor cells and differentiate within the bone marrow; T cells are derived from the same lymphoid progenitor cells as B cells and differentiate in the thymus to become functional cells before migrating to the peripheral lymphoid organs.

7. Mature B and T lymphocytes differentiate and proliferate in response to antigenic stimulation. These events generally take place in secondary lymphoid organs.

8. B lymphocytes synthesize and secrete antibodies. T lymphocytes participate in cell-mediated immunity; they help B cells make antibodies by providing them with soluble growth and differentiation factors (cytokines) needed for B cell activation. They also participate in various other regulatory aspects of the immune response by releasing cytokines.

9. Lymphocytes continuously recirculate between the blood, lymph, lymphoid organs, and tissues. Receptors on lymphocytes interact with CAMs located on specialized HEVs, facilitating extravasation to tissue sites where immune-cell activation occurs.

REFERENCES

Aderem A, Underhill DM (1999): Mechanisms of phagocytosis in macrophages. *Ann Rev Immunol* 17:593.

Akira S, Takeda K, Kaiso T (2001): Toll-like receptors: critical proteins linking innate and acquired immunity. *Nature Immunol* 2:675.

Bowie A, O'Neill LA (2000): The interleukin-1 receptor/Toll-like receptor superfamily: signal generators for pro-inflammatory interleukins and microbial products. *J Leukocyte Biol* 67: 508.

Gallatin M, St John TP, Siegelman M, Reichert R, Butcher CE, Weissman I (1986): Lymphocyte homing receptors. *Cell* 44:673.

Lanier, LL (1998): NK cell receptors. *Annu Rev Immunol* 16:359.

Stekel DJ, Parker CE, Nowak MA (1997): A model for lymphocyte recirculation. *Immunol Today* 18:216.

REVIEW QUESTIONS

For each question, choose the ONE BEST answer or completion.

1. Which of the following generally does not apply to bone marrow (a primary lymphoid organ)?
   A) cellular proliferation
   B) differentiation of lymphocytes
   C) cellular interaction
   D) antigen-dependent response

2. Which of the following apply uniquely to secondary lymphoid organs?
   A) presence of precursor B and T cells
   B) circulation of lymphocytes
   C) terminal differentiation
   D) cellular proliferation

3. Which of the following does not apply to innate immune mechanisms?
   A) absence of specificity
   B) activation by a stimulus
   C) involvement of multiple cell types
   D) a memory component

4. Which of the following is the major function of the lymphoid system?
   A) innate immunity
   B) inflammation
   C) phagocytosis
   D) acquired immunity

5. Removal of the bursa of Fabricius from a chicken results in
   A) a markedly decreased number of circulating T lymphocytes.
   B) anemia.
   C) a delayed rejection of skin grafts.
   D) low serum levels of antibodies.
   E) a deficient innate immunity.

6. The germinal centers found in the cortical region of lymph nodes and the peripheral region of splenic periarteriolar lymphatic tissue
   A) support the development of immature B and T cells.
   B) function in the removal of damaged erythrocytes from the circulation.
   C) act as the major source of stem cells and thus help maintain hematopoiesis.
   D) provide an infrastructure that on antigenic stimulation contains large populations of B lymphocytes and plasma cells.
   E) are the sites of NK cell differentiation.

7. Which of the following is a correct statement about NK cells?
   A) They proliferate in response to antigen.
   B) They kill target cells by phagocytosis and intracellular digestion.

C) They are a subset of polymorphonuclear cells.
D) They kill target cells in an extracellular fashion.
E) They are particularly effective against certain bacteria.

8. Mature dendritic cells are capable of which of the following?

A) activating naive antigen-specific T cells
B) removing red blood cells
C) producing bradykinin
D) extracellular killing of target cells

ANSWERS TO REVIEW QUESTIONS

1. *D* Cellular proliferation, differentiation of lymphocytes, and cellular interactions can take place in bone marrow (or bursa of Fabricius). However, antigen-dependent responses occur in the secondary lymphoid organs, such as the spleen and lymph nodes.

2. *C* Terminal differentiation of B cells into plasma cells occurs only in secondary lymphoid organs, such as the spleen and lymph nodes. Circulation of lymphocytes and cellular proliferation (but not antigen-dependent responses of terminal differentiation) also take place in the primary lymphoid organs, such as the bursa of Fabricius, or its equivalent, and the thymus. The bone marrow is the site where pluripotential stem cells differentiate into precursor B and T cells.

3. *D* Innate immunity has none of the antigenic specificity exhibited by acquired immunity. It is activated by such stimuli as the invasion of the foreign particles into the body. Innate immunity involves multiple cell types, such as those of the monocytic series (macrophages) and those of the granulocytic series (neutrophils, eosinophils, etc.).

4. *D* The major function of the lymphoid system is the recognition of foreign antigen by lymphocytes, which leads to the acquired immune response. Functions such as phagocytosis and inflammation do not necessarily require the lymphoid system, and they constitute part of innate immunity.

5. *D* Removal of the bursa of Fabricius from a chicken results in low levels of antibodies in serum, since this organ serves as a primary lymphoid organ in which B lymphocytes (which eventually synthesize and secrete antibodies) undergo maturation. The removal of the organ will not result in a marked decrease in the number of circulating T lymphocytes, nor will it result in anemia, characterized by a marked decrease in erythrocyte count, since erythrocytes undergo maturation outside the bursa. Bursectomy has no effect on rejection of skin grafts.

6. *D* On antigenic stimulation, the germinal centers contain large populations of B lymphocytes undergoing mitosis and plasma cells secreting antibodies. Virgin immunocompetent lymphocytes are developed in the primary lymphoid organs, not in the secondary lymphoid organs, such as the spleen and lymph nodes. Germinal centers do not participate in the removal of damaged erythrocytes, nor are they a source of stem cells; the latter are found in the bone marrow.

7. *D* NK cells are large granular lymphocytes. Their number does not increase in response to antigen. Their killing is extracellular, and their target cells are virus-infected cells or tumor cells. They are not particularly effective against bacterial cells.

8. *A* When immature dendritic cells are activated following their engulfment of pathogens (phagocytosis), they mature and become more efficient at antigen presentation and, in fact, can activate antigen-specific naive T cells.

3

IMMUNOGENS AND ANTIGENS

INTRODUCTION

Immune responses arise as a result of exposure to foreign stimuli. The compound that evokes the response is referred to either as ***antigen*** or as ***immunogen.*** The distinction between these terms is functional. An antigen is any agent capable of binding specifically to components of the immune system, such as the B cell receptor (BCR) on B lymphocytes and soluble antibodies. By contrast, an immunogen is any agent capable of inducing an immune response and is therefore ***immunogenic.*** The distinction between the terms is necessary because there are many compounds that are incapable of inducing an immune response, yet they are capable of binding with components of the immune system that have been induced specifically against them. Thus all immunogens are antigens, but not all antigens are immunogens. This difference becomes obvious in the case of low molecular weight compounds, a group of substances that includes many antibiotics and drugs. By themselves, these compounds are incapable of inducing an immune response, but when they are coupled with much larger entities, such as proteins, the resultant conjugate induces an immune response that is directed against various parts of the conjugate, including the low molecular weight compound. When manipulated in this manner, the low molecular weight compound is referred to as a ***hapten*** (from the Greek *hapten,* which means "to grasp"); the high molecular weight compound to which the hapten is conjugated is referred to as a ***carrier.*** Thus a hapten is a compound that, by itself, is incapable of inducing an immune response but against which an immune response can be induced by immunization with the hapten conjugated to a carrier.

Immune responses have been demonstrated against all the known biochemical families of compounds, including carbohydrates, lipids, proteins, and nucleic acids. Similarly, immune responses to drugs, antibiotics, food additives, cosmetics, and small synthetic peptides can also be induced, but only when these are coupled to a carrier. In this chapter, we discuss the major attributes of compounds that render them antigenic and immunogenic.

REQUIREMENTS FOR IMMUNOGENICITY

A substance must possess the following characteristics to be immunogenic: (1) foreignness; (2) high molecular weight; (3) chemical complexity; and, in most cases, (4) degradability and interaction with host major histocompatibility complex (MHC).

Foreignness

Animals normally do not respond immunologically to self. Thus, for example, if a rabbit is injected with its own serum albumin, it will not mount an immune response; it recognizes

Immunology: A Short Course, Fifth Edition, By Richard Coico, Geoffrey Sunshine, and Eli Benjamini
ISBN 0-471-22689-0

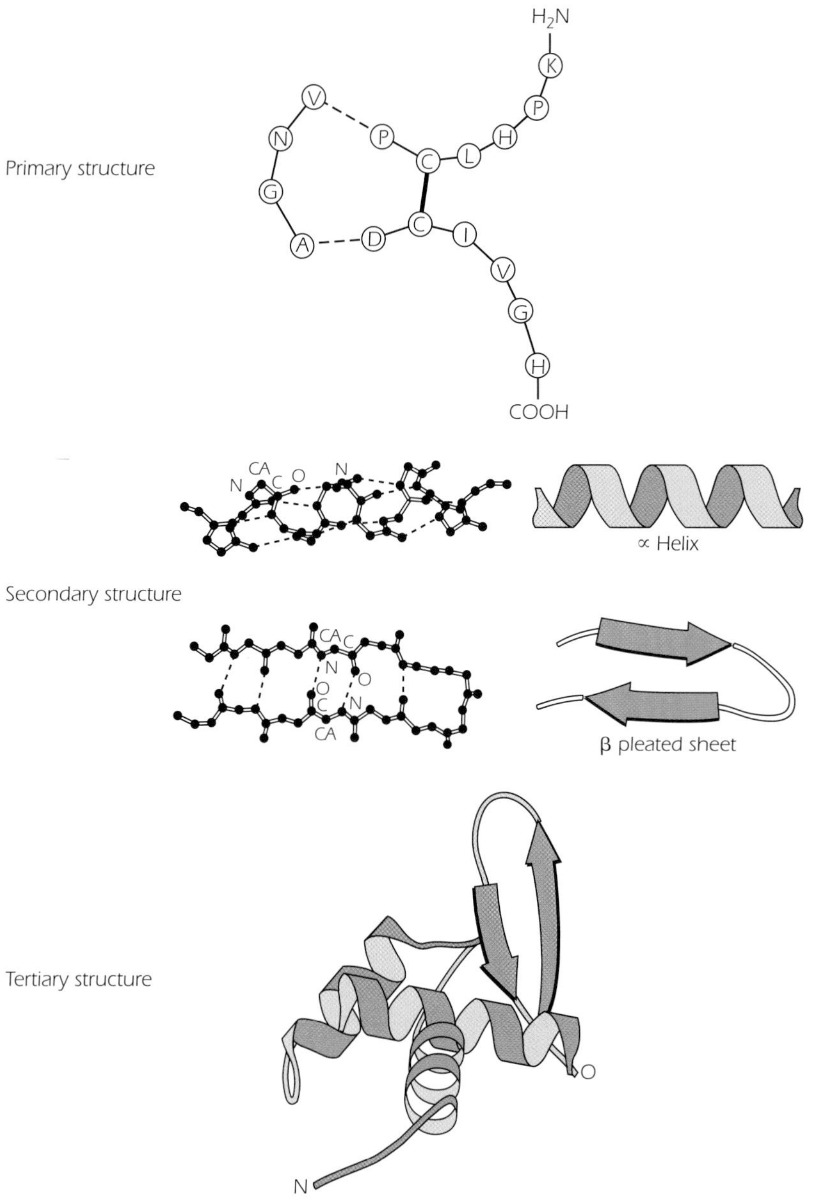

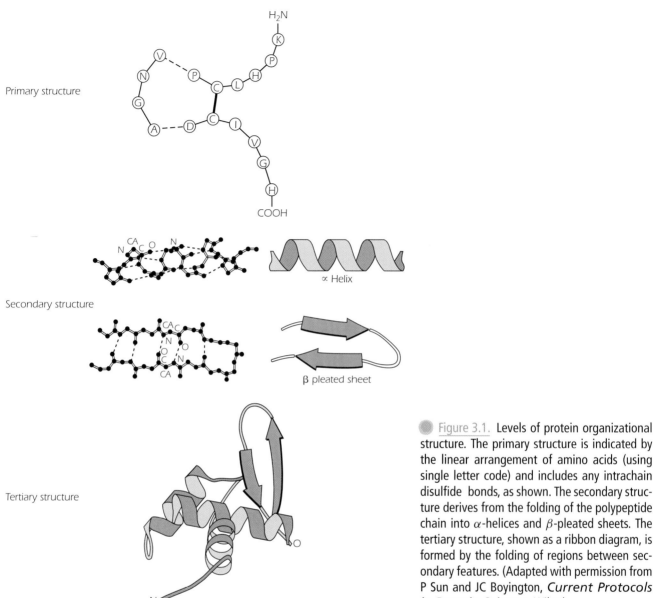

Figure 3.1. Levels of protein organizational structure. The primary structure is indicated by the linear arrangement of amino acids (using single letter code) and includes any intrachain disulfide bonds, as shown. The secondary structure derives from the folding of the polypeptide chain into α-helices and β-pleated sheets. The tertiary structure, shown as a ribbon diagram, is formed by the folding of regions between secondary features. (Adapted with permission from P Sun and JC Boyington, *Current Protocols in Protein Science*, Wiley.)

the albumin as self. By contrast, if rabbit serum albumin is injected into a guinea pig, the guinea pig recognizes the rabbit serum albumin as foreign and mounts an immune response against it. To prove that the rabbit, which did not respond to its own serum albumin, is immunologically competent, it can be injected with guinea pig albumin. The competent rabbit will mount an immune response to guinea pig serum albumin, because it recognizes the substance as foreign. Thus the first requirement for a compound to be immunogenic is foreignness. The more foreign the substance, the more immunogenic it is.

In general, compounds that are part of self are not immunogenic to the individual. However, there are exceptional cases in which an individual mounts an immune response against his or her own tissues. This condition is termed ***autoimmunity*** (see Chapter 12).

High Molecular Weight

The second requirement for being immunogenic is that the compound must have a certain minimal molecular weight. In general, small compounds with a molecular weight <1000 Da (e.g., penicillin, progesterone, aspirin) are not immunogenic; those of molecular weight between 1000 and 6000 Da (e.g., insulin, adrenocorticotropic hormone) may or may not be immunogenic; and those of molecular weight >6000 Da (e.g., albumin, tetanus toxin) are generally immunogenic. In short, relatively small substances have decreased immunogenicity, whereas large substances have increased immunogenicity.

Chemical Complexity

The third characteristic necessary for a compound to be immunogenic is a certain degree of physicochemical complexity. Thus, for example, simple molecules such as homopolymers of amino acids (e.g., a polymer of lysine with a molecular weight of 30,000 Da) are seldom good immunogens. Similarly, a homopolymer of poly-γ-D-glutamic acid (the capsular material of *Bacillus anthracis*) with a molecular weight of 50,000 Da is not immunogenic. The absence of immunogenicity is because these compounds, although of high molecular weight, are not sufficiently chemically complex. However, if the complexity is increased by attaching various moieties—such as dinitrophenol or other low molecular weight compounds—that, by themselves, are not immunogenic, to the epsilon amino group of polylysine, the entire macromolecule becomes immunogenic. The resulting immune response is directed not only against the coupled low molecular weight compounds but also against the high molecular weight homopolymer. In general, an increase in the chemical complexity of a compound is accompanied by an increase in its immunogenicity. Thus copolymers of several amino acids, such as polyglutamic, alanine, and lysine (poly-GAT), tend to be highly immunogenic.

Because many immunogens are proteins, it is important to understand the structural features of these molecules. Each of the four levels of protein contributes to the molecule's immunogenicity. The acquired immune response recognizes many structural features and chemical properties of compounds. For example, antibodies can recognize various structural features of a protein, such as its primary structure (the amino acid sequence), secondary structures (the structure of the backbone of the polypeptide chain, such as an α-helix or β-pleated sheet), and tertiary structures (formed by the three-dimensional configuration of the protein, which is conferred by the folding of the polypeptide chain and held by disulfide bridges, hydrogen bonds, hydrophobic interactions, etc.) (Fig. 3.1). They can also recognize quaternary structures (formed by the juxtaposition of separate parts, if the molecule is composed of more than one protein subunit) (Fig. 3.2).

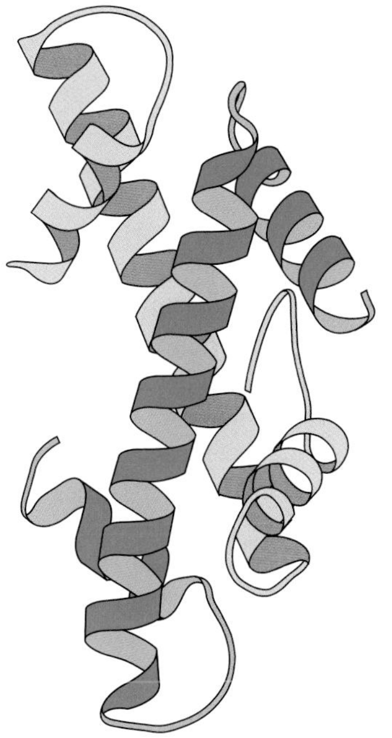

Figure 3.2. The quaternary structure of proteins results from the association of two or more polypeptide chains, which form a polymeric protein. (Adapted with permission from P Sun and JC Boyington, *Current Protocols in Protein Science,* Wiley.)

Degradability

For antigens that activate T cells to stimulate immune responses, interactions with MHC molecules expressed on antigen-presenting cells (APCs) must occur (see Chapter 9). APCs must first degrade the antigen through a process known as antigen processing (enzymatic degradation of antigen) before they can express antigenic epitopes (small fragments of the immunogen) on their surface. Once degraded and noncovalently bound to MHC, these epitopes stimulate the activation and clonal expansion of antigen-specific effector T cells. A protein antigen's susceptibility to enzymatic degradation largely depends on two properties: (1) It has to be sufficiently stable so that it can reach the site of interaction with B cells or T cells necessary for the immune response and (2) the substance must be susceptible to partial enzymatic degradation that takes place during antigen processing by APCs. Peptides composed of D-amino acids, which are resistant to enzymatic degradation, are not immunogenic, whereas their L-isomers are susceptible to enzymes and are immunogenic. By contrast, carbohydrates are not processed or presented and are thus unable to activate T cells, although they can activate B cells.

In general, a substance must have all four of these characteristics to be immunogenic; it must be foreign to the individual in whom it is administered, have a relatively high molecular weight, possess a certain degree of chemical complexity, and be degradable.

Haptens

As noted earlier, substances called ***haptens*** fail to induce immune responses in their native form because of their low molecular weight and their chemical simplicity. These compounds are not immunogenic, unless they are conjugated to high molecular weight, physiochemically complex ***carriers.*** Thus an immune response can be evoked to thousands of chemical compounds—those of high molecular weight and those of low molecular weight, provided the latter is conjugated to high molecular weight complex carriers.

Further Requirements for Immunogenicity

Several other factors play roles in determining whether a substance is immunogenic. The genetic makeup (genotype) of the immunized individual plays an important role in determining whether a given substance will stimulate an immune response. Genetic control of immune responsiveness is largely controlled by genes mapping within the MHC. Another factor that plays a crucial role in the immunogenicity of substances relates to the B and T cell repertoires of an individual. Acquired immune responses are triggered following the binding of antigenic epitopes to antigen-specific receptors on B and T lymphocytes. If an individual lacks a particular clone of lymphocytes consisting of cells bearing the identical antigen-specific receptor needed to respond to the stimulus, an immune response to that antigenic epitope will not take place. Finally, practical issues such as the ***dosage*** and ***route*** of administration of antigens play a role in determining whether the substance is immunogenic.

Insufficient doses of antigen may not stimulate an immune response either because the amount administered fails to activate enough lymphocytes or because such a dose renders the responding cells unresponsive. The latter phenomenon induces a state of tolerance to that antigen (discussed further in Chapter 12). Besides the need to administer a threshold amount of antigen to induce an immune response, the number of doses administered also affects the outcome of the immune response generated. As discussed below, repeated administration of antigen is required to stimulate a strong immune response.

Finally, the route of administration can affect the outcome of the immunization strategy, because this determines which organs and cell populations will be involved in the response. Antigens administered via the most common route—namely, ***subcutaneously,*** generally elicit the strongest immune responses. This is due to their uptake, processing, and presentation to effector cells by Langerhans cells present in the skin, which are among the most potent APCs. Responses to subcutaneously administered antigens take place in the lymph nodes draining the injection site. ***Intravenously*** administered antigens are carried first to the spleen, where they can either induce immune unresponsiveness or tolerance or, if presented by APCs, generate an immune response. Orally administered antigens (***gastrointestinal route***) elicit local antibody responses within the intestinal lamina propria but often produce a systemic state of tolerance (antigen unresponsiveness) (see Chapter 12 for a detailed discussion about tolerance). Finally, administration of antigens via the respiratory track (***intranasal route***) often elicits allergic responses (see Chapter 14).

Since immune responses depend on multiple cellular interactions, the type and extent of the immune response is affected by the cells populating the organ in which the antigen is ultimately delivered. The stringent requirements given above constitute a portion of the delicate control mechanisms, expanded and elaborated in subsequent chapters, which, on one hand, trigger the acquired immune response and, on the other hand, protect the individual from responding to substances in cases where such responses are detrimental.

PRIMARY AND SECONDARY RESPONSES

The first exposure of an individual to an immunogen is referred to as the primary immunization, which generates a ***primary response.*** As we shall see in subsequent chapters, many events take place during this primary immunization—cells process antigen, triggering antigen-specific lymphocytes to proliferate and differentiate. T lymphocyte subsets interact with other subsets and induce the latter to differentiate into T lymphocytes with specialized function. T lymphocytes also interact with B lymphocytes, inducing them to synthesize and secrete antibodies.

A second exposure to the same immunogen results in a ***secondary response.*** This second exposure may occur after the response to the first immune event has leveled off or has totally subsided (within weeks or even years). The secondary response differs from the primary response in many respects. Most notably and biologically relevant is the much quicker onset and the much higher magnitude of the response. In a sense, this secondary (and subsequent) exposure behaves as if the body remembered that it had been previously exposed to that same immunogen. In fact, secondary and subsequent responses exploit the expanded number of antigen-specific lymphocytes generated in response to the primary immune response. Thus the increased arsenal of responding lymphocytes accounts, in part, for the magnitude of the response observed. The secondary response is also called the memory or anamnestic response, and the B and T lymphocytes that participate in the memory response are termed ***memory cells.*** The kinetics of antibody production after immunization are given in detail in Chapter 4 and Figure 4.12.

ANTIGENICITY AND ANTIGEN-BINDING SITE

An immune response induced by an antigen generates antibodies or lymphocytes that react specifically with the antigen. The antigen-binding site of an antibody or a receptor on a lymphocyte has a unique structure that allows a complementary fit to some structural aspect of the specific antigen. The portion of the immunoglobulin that specifically binds to the antigenic determinant or epitope is concentrated in several hypervariable regions of the molecule, which form the ***complementarity-determining region*** (CDR). Additional structural features of the immunoglobulin molecule are described in Chapter 4.

Various studies indicate that the size of an epitope that combines with the CDR on a given antibody is approximately equivalent to 5–7 amino acids. These dimensions were calculated from experiments that involved the binding of antibodies to polysaccharides and to peptide epitopes. Such dimensions would also be expected to correspond roughly to the size of the complementary antibody-combining site,

TABLE 3.1. Antigen Recognition by B and T Cells

Characteristic	B Cells[a]	T Cells
Antigen interaction	B cell receptor (membrane Ig) binds Ag	T cell receptor binds Ag and MHC
Nature of antigens	Protein, polysaccharide, lipid	Peptide
Binding soluble antigens	Yes	No
Epitopes recognized	Accessible, sequential, or nonsequential	Internal linear peptides produced by antigen processing (proteolytic degradation)

[a] *Ig*, immunoglobulin; *Ag*, antigen.

termed *paratope,* and indeed this expectation has been confirmed by X-ray crystallography. The small size of an epitope (peptide) that binds to a specific T cell receptor (TCR) (peptides with 8–12 amino acids) is made functionally larger, since it is noncovalently associated with MHC proteins of the antigen-presenting cell. This bimolecular epitope–MHC complex then binds to the TCR, forming a ***trimolecular complex*** (TCR–epitope–MHC).

EPITOPES RECOGNIZED BY B CELLS AND T CELLS

There is a large body of evidence pointing out that the properties of many epitopes recognized by B cells differ from those recognized by T cells (Table 3.1). In general, membrane-bound antibody present on B cells recognizes and binds free antigen in solution. Thus these epitopes are typically on the outside of the molecule, accessible for interaction with the B cell receptor. Terminal side chains of polysaccharides and hydrophilic portions on protein molecules generally constitute B cell epitopes. An example of an antigen with five ***linear*** B cell epitopes located on the exposed surface of myoglobulin is shown in Figure 3.3. B cell epitopes may also form as a result of the folded conformation of molecules, as shown in Figure 3.4. Such epitopes are called ***conformational (discontinuous) epitopes,*** in which nonsequential residues along a polypeptide chain are brought together by the folded conformation of the protein, as shown in Figure 3.3.

In contrast to B cells, T cells are unable to bind soluble antigen. The interaction of an epitope with the T-cell receptor requires APC processing of the antigen in which enzymatic degradation takes place to yield small peptides, which then associate with MHC. Thus T cell epitopes can be only ***continuous*** or ***linear*** since they are composed of a single segment of a polypeptide chain. Figure 3.5 illustrates the structural organization of a MHC class I molecule bound to an antigenic peptide. Generally, such processed epitopes are internal denatured linear hydrophobic areas of proteins. Polysaccharides do not yield such areas and indeed are not known to bind or activate T cells. Thus polysaccharides contain solely B cell–recognizable epitopes, whereas proteins contain both B and T cell–recognizable epitopes (Table 3.1). Antigenic epitopes may have the characteristics shown in Figure 3.6. Therefore, they may consist of a single epitope (hapten) or have varying numbers of the same epitope on the same molecule (e.g., polysaccharides). The most common antigens (proteins) have varying numbers of different epitopes on the same molecule.

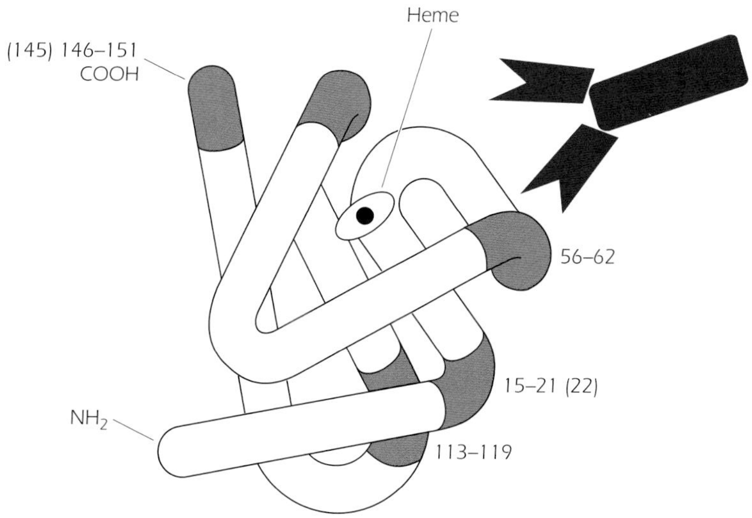

Figure 3.3. An example of an antigen (sperm whale myoglobin) containing five linear B cell epitopes (*red*), one of which is bound to the antibody-binding site of an antibody specific for amino acid residues 56–62.

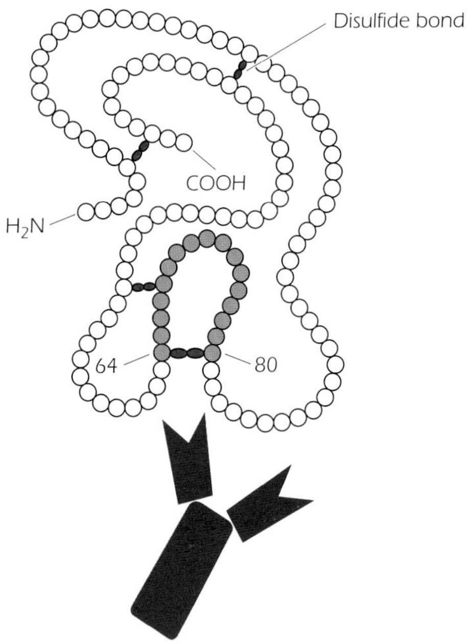

Figure 3.4. An antigen showing amino acid residues (*circles*), which form a nonsequential epitope "loop" (*blue*) resulting from a disulfide bond between residues 64 and 80. Note the binding of an epitope-specific antibody to the nonsequential amino acids that constitute the epitope.

MAJOR CLASSES OF ANTIGENS

The following major chemical families may be antigenic:

- **Carbohydrates (polysaccharides).** Polysaccharides are immunogenic only when associated with protein carriers. For example, polysaccharides that form part of more complex molecules (glycoproteins) will elicit an immune response, part of which is directed specifically against the polysaccharide moiety of the molecule. An immune response, consisting primarily of antibodies, can be induced against many kinds of polysaccharide molecules, such as components of microorganisms and of eukaryotic cells. An excellent example of antigenicity of polysaccharides is the immune response associated with the ABO blood groups, which are polysaccharides on the surface of the red blood cells.
- **Lipids.** Lipids are rarely immunogenic, but an immune response to lipids may be induced if the lipids are conjugated to protein carriers. Thus, in a sense, lipids may be regarded as haptens. Immune responses to glycolipids and to sphingolipids have also been demonstrated.
- **Nucleic acids.** Nucleic acids are poor immunogens by themselves, but they become immunogenic when they are conjugated to protein carriers. DNA, in its native

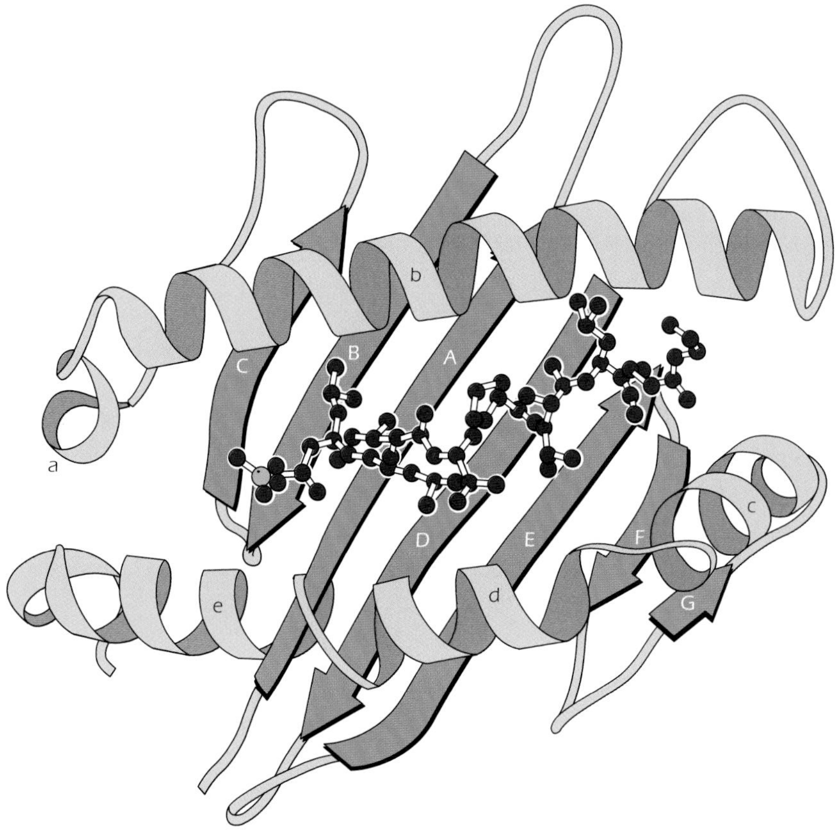

Figure 3.5. Structure of MHC class I molecule (*ribbon diagram*) with an antigenic peptide (*ball-and-stick model*).

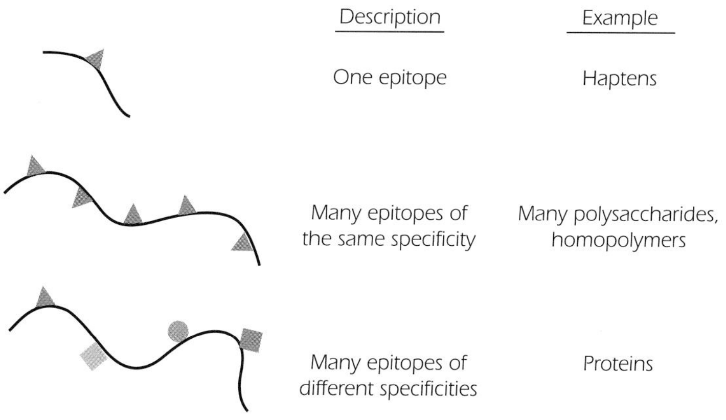

Figure 3.6. Some possible antigenic structures containing single and multiple epitopes.

helical state, is usually nonimmunogenic in normal animals. However, immune responses to nucleic acids have been reported in many instances. One important example in clinical medicine is the appearance of anti-DNA antibodies in patients with systemic lupus erythematosus (discussed in detail in Chapter 12).

- **Proteins.** Virtually all proteins are immunogenic. Thus the most common immune responses are those to proteins. Furthermore, the greater the degree of complexity of the protein, the more vigorous will be the immune response to that protein. Because of their size and complexity, proteins contain multiple epitopes.

BINDING OF ANTIGEN WITH ANTIGEN-SPECIFIC ANTIBODIES OR T CELLS

The binding between antigen and antibodies is discussed in detail in Chapters 4 and 5. The interactions of antigen with both B and T cells and subsequent activation events are discussed in Chapter 10. At this point, it is important to emphasize only that the binding of antigen with antibodies or T cell receptors does not involve covalent bonds. The ***noncovalent binding*** may involve ***electrostatic interactions, hydrophobic interactions, hydrogen bonds,*** and ***van der Waals forces.*** Since these interactive forces are relatively weak, the fit between antigen and its complementary site on the antigen receptor must occur over an area large enough to allow the summation of all the possible available interactions. This requirement is the basis for the exquisite specificity observed in immunologic interactions.

CROSS-REACTIVITY

Since macromolecular antigens contain several distinct epitopes, some of these macromolecules can be altered without totally changing the immunogenic and antigenic structure of the entire molecule. This concept is important in relation to immunization against highly pathogenic microorganisms or highly toxic compounds. Obviously, immunization with the pathogenic toxin is unwise. However, it is possible to destroy the biologic activity of this and a broad variety of other toxins (e.g., bacterial toxins and snake venoms) without appreciably affecting their immunogenicity. A toxin that has been modified to the extent that it is no longer toxic but still maintains some of its immunochemical characteristics is called a ***toxoid.*** Thus we can say that a toxoid ***cross-reacts*** immunologically with the toxin. Accordingly, it is possible to immunize individuals with the toxoid and thereby induce immune responses to some of the epitopes that the toxoid still shares with the native toxin because these epitopes have not been destroyed by the modification. Although the molecules of toxin and toxoid differ in many physicochemical and biologic respects, they nevertheless cross-react immunologically. They share enough epitopes to allow the immune response to the toxoid to mount an effective defense against the toxin itself. An immunologic reaction in which the immune components, either cells or antibodies, react with two molecules that share epitopes but are otherwise dissimilar is called a ***cross-reaction.*** When two compounds cross-react immunologically, the compounds will have one or more epitopes in common, and the immune response to one of the compounds will recognize one or more of the same epitope(s) on the other compound and react with it. Another form of cross-reactivity is seen when antibodies or cells with specificity to one epitope bind, usually more weakly, to another epitope that is not quite identical but has a structural resemblance to the first epitope.

To denote that the antigen used for immunization is different from the one with which the induced immune components are then allowed to react, the terms ***homologous*** and ***heterologous*** are used. *Homologous* denotes that the antigen and the immunogen are the same; *heterologous* denotes that the substance used to induce the immune response is different from the substance that is then used to react with the products of the induced response. In the latter case, the heterologous antigen may or may not react with the immune components. If reaction does take place, it may be concluded that the heterologous and homologous antigens exhibit immunologic cross-reactivity.

Although the hallmark of immunology is specificity, immunologic cross-reactivity has been observed on many levels. This does not mean that the immunologic specificity has been diminished but rather that the cross-reacting compounds share ***antigenic determinants.*** In cases of cross-reactivity, the antigenic determinants of the cross-reacting substances may have identical chemical structures or they may be composed of similar but not identical physicochemical configurations. In the example described above, a toxin and its corresponding toxoid represent two molecules, the toxin being the native molecule and the toxoid being a modified molecule that cross-reacts with the native molecule.

There are other examples of immunologic cross-reactivity, wherein the two cross-reacting substances are unrelated to each other, except that they have one or more epitopes in common, specifically, one or more areas that have similar three-dimensional characteristics. These substances are referred to as ***heterophile antigens.*** For example, human blood group A antigen reacts with antiserum raised against pneumococcal capsular polysaccharide (type XIV). Similarly, human blood group B antigen reacts with antibodies to certain strains of *Escherichia coli.* In these examples of cross-reactivity, the antigens of the microorganisms are referred to as the heterophile antigens (with respect to the blood group antigen).

ADJUVANTS

To enhance the immune response to a given immunogen, various additives or vehicles are often used. An ***adjuvant*** (from the Latin, *adjuvare,* "to help") is a substance that, when mixed with an immunogen, enhances the immune response against the immunogen. It is important to distinguish between a carrier for a hapten and an adjuvant. A hapten will become immunogenic when conjugated covalently to a carrier; it will not become immunogenic if mixed with an adjuvant. Thus an adjuvant enhances the immune response to immunogens but does not confer immunogenicity on haptens.

Adjuvants have been used to augment immune responses to antigens for >70 years. Interest in the identification of adjuvants for use with vaccines is growing because many new vaccine candidates lack sufficient immunogenicity. This is particularly true of peptide-based vaccines. Adjuvant mechanisms include (1) increasing the biological or immunological half-life of vaccine antigens; (2) increasing the production of local inflammatory cytokines; and (3) improving antigen delivery and antigen processing and presentation by APCs, especially the dendritic cells. Empirically, it has been found that adjuvants containing microbial components (e.g., mycobacterial extracts) are the best adjuvants. Pathogen components induce macrophages and dendritic cells to express co-stimulatory molecules and to secrete cytokines. More recently, it has been shown that such induction by microbial components involves pattern recognition molecules (e.g., Toll-like receptor 2) expressed by these cells. Thus binding of microbial components to Toll-like receptors (TLRs) signals the cells to express co-stimulatory molecules and to release cytokines.

While many adjuvants have been developed in animal models (Table 3.2) and tested experimentally in humans, only one has been accepted for routine vaccination. Currently, aluminum hydroxide and aluminum phosphate (alum) are the only adjuvants used for licensed human vaccines in

TABLE 3.2. Common Adjuvants and Their Mechanism of Action

Adjuvant	Composition	Mechanism of Action
Aluminum hydroxide or aluminum phosphate (alum)	Aluminum hydroxide gel	Enhanced uptake of antigen by APCs; delayed release of antigen
Alum with a mycobacterial-derived dipeptide	Aluminum hydroxide gel with muramyl dipeptide	Enhanced uptake of antigen by APCs; delayed release of antigen; induction of costimulatory molecules on APCs
Alum with *Bordetella pertusis*	Aluminum hydroxide gel with killed *Bordetella pertusis*	Enhanced uptake of antigen by APCs; delayed release of antigen; induction of costimulatory molecules on APCs
Freund's complete adjuvant	Oil in water with killed mycobacteria	Enhanced uptake of antigen by APCs; delayed release of antigen; induction of costimulatory molecules on APCs
Freund's incomplete adjuvant	Oil in water	Enhanced uptake of antigen by APCs; delayed release of antigen
Immune stimulatory complexes	Open cagelike structures containing cholesterol and a mixture of saponins	Delivery of antigen to cytosol, allowing induction of cytotoxic T cell responses

the United States. As an inorganic salt, alum binds to proteins, causing them to precipitate, and elicits an inflammatory response that nonspecifically increases the immunogenicity of antigen. When injected, the precipitated antigen is released more slowly than antigen alone at the injection site. Moreover, the increased size of the antigen, which occurs as a consequence of precipitation, increases the probability that the macromolecule will be phagocytized.

Many adjuvants have been used in experimental animals. One commonly used adjuvant is ***Freund's complete adjuvant*** (FCA), consisting of killed *Mycobacterium tuberculosis* or *M. butyricum* suspended in oil, which is then emulsified with an aqueous antigen solution. The oil-emulsified state of the adjuvant–antigen mixture, allows the antigen to be released slowly and continuously, helping sustain the recipient's exposure to the immunogen. Other microorganisms used as adjuvants are bacille Calmette-Guerin (BCG) (an attenuated *Mycobacterium*), *Corynebacterium parvum,* and *Bordetella pertussis.* In reality, many of these adjuvants exploit the immune cell activation properties of microbe-expressed molecules, including lipopolysaccharide (LPS), bacterial DNA containing unmethylated CpG dinucleotide motifs, and bacterial heat-shock proteins. Many of these microbial cell adjuvants bind to pattern recognition signaling receptors, such as TLRs. Ligation of TLRs expressed by many cell types within the innate immune system, facilitates the stimulation of adaptive B and T cell responses. For example, dendritic cells are important APCs involved in the activity of microbial adjuvants. They respond by secreting cytokines and expressing costimulatory molecules, which, in turn, stimulate the activation and differentiation of antigen-specific T cells.

SUMMARY

1. Immunogenicity is the capacity of a compound to induce an immune response. Immunogenicity requires that a compound (a) be foreign to the immunized individual, (b) possesses a certain minimal molecular weight, (c) possesses a certain degree of chemical complexity, and (d) be degradable or susceptible to antigen processing and presentation through its interaction with MHC.

2. Antigenicity refers to the ability of a compound to bind with antibodies or with cells of the immune system. This binding is highly specific; the immune components are capable of recognizing various physicochemical aspects of the compound. The binding between antigen and immune components involves several weak forces operating over short distances (van der Waals forces, electrostatic interactions, hydrophobic interactions, and hydrogen bonds); it does not involve covalent bonds.

3. The smallest unit of antigen that is capable of binding with antibodies is called an antigenic determinant or epitope. Compounds may have one or more epitopes capable of reacting with immune components. The immune response against these compounds involves the production of antibodies or the generation of cells with specificities directed against most or all of the epitopes.

4. B cell membrane immunoglobulin or secreted antibody tends to recognize amino acid sequences that are accessible, usually hydrophobic and mobile. These can be contiguous or noncontiguous amino acids (conformational determinants), which are brought into proximity by the three-dimensional folding of the protein. B cell membrane immunoglobulins and antibody are capable of recognizing polysaccharides and lipids.

5. T cells recognize internal amino acid sequences of proteins in the context of MHC class I or class II molecules. Peptide fragments of protein antigens are generated by antigen processing may associate with MHC molecules and be presented to T cells.

6. Immunologic cross-reactivity denotes a situation in which two or more substances, which may have various degrees of dissimilarity, share epitopes and would, therefore, react with the immune components induced against any one of these substances. Thus a toxoid, which is a modified form of toxin, may have one or more epitopes in common with the toxin. Immunization with the toxoid leads to an immune response capable of reacting not only with the toxoid but also with the native toxin.

7. Adjuvants are substances that can accelerate, prolong, and enhance the quality of specific immune responses. When administered with antigens, adjuvants facilitate immune responses that are specific for the antigen (not for adjuvant itself) since the adjuvant nonspecifically amplifies the response. The principle mechanisms or adjuvants activity include increased antigen presentation by APCs (especially dendritic cells), induction of costimulatory molecules, and induction of local inflammatory cytokine responses.

REFERENCES

Atassi MZ (1977): Immunochemistry of Proteins, Vols 1 and 2. New York: Plenum.

Benjamin DC, Berzofsky JA, East IJ, Gurd FRN, Hannum C, Leach SJ, Margoliash E, Michael JG, Miller A, Prager EM, Reichlin M, Sercarz EE, Smith-Gill SJ, Todd PE, Wilson AC (1984): The antigenic structure of proteins: a reappraisal. *Annu Rev Immunol* 2:67.

Berzofsky JA, Berkower IJ (1998): Immunogenicity and antigen structure. In Paul WE (ed): Fundamental Immunology, 4th ed. New York: Lippincott-Raven. Berzofsky JA, Cease KB, Cornette JL, Spouge JL, Margalit H, Berkower IJ, Good FM, Miller LH, DeLisi C (1987): Protein antigenic structures recognized by T cells: potential applications to vaccine design. *Immunol Rev* 98:9.

Davis DR, Cohen GH (1996): Interactions of protein antigens with antibodies. *Proc Natl Acad Sci USA* 93:7.

Davis, MM, Boniface, JJ, Reich, Z, Lyons, D, Hampl, J, Arden, B, Chien, Y. (1998): Ligand recognition by $\alpha\beta$ T cell receptors. *Annu Rev Immunol* 16:523.

Freund J, Calals J, Hosmer EP (1937): Sensitization and antibody formation after injection of tubercle bacilli and paraffin oil. *Proc Soc Exp Biol Med* 37:509.

Novotny J, Handschumacher H, Bruccoleri RE (1987): Protein antigenicity: a static surface property. *Immunol Today* 8:26.

Rothbard JB, Gefter ML (1991): Interactions between immunogenic peptides and MHC proteins. *Annu Rev Immunol* 9:527.

Watts C (1997): Capture and processing of exogenous antigens for presentation on MHC molecules. *Annu Rev Immunol* 15:821.

REVIEW QUESTIONS

For each question, choose the ONE BEST answer or completion.

1. A large protein has been enzymatically digested in the laboratory to yield a mixture of peptides ranging in size from 4 to 10 amino acids in length. Which of the following would be expected if the peptide mixture were administered to an experimental animal?
A) Peptide-specific antibodies would be generated using the peptide mixture alone.
B) Peptide-specific antibodies would be generated only if an adjuvant were administered with the peptide mixture.
C) Peptide-specific antibodies would be generated if they were first coupled to a protein carrier.
D) Peptide-specific antibody and T cell responses would be generated using the peptide mixture alone.
E) Peptide-specific antibodies and T cell responses would be generated only if an adjuvant were administered with the peptide mixture.

2. The protection against smallpox virus infection afforded by prior infection with cowpox virus represents
A) antigenic specificity.
B) antigenic cross-reactivity.
C) enhanced viral uptake by macrophages.
D) innate immunity.
E) passive protection.

3. Converting a toxin to a toxoid
A) makes the toxin more immunogenic.
B) reduces the pharmacologic activity of the toxin.
C) enhances binding with antitoxin.
D) induces only innate immunity.
E) increases phagocytosis.

4. Haptens
A) require carrier molecules to be immunogenic.
B) react with specific antibodies when homologous carriers are not employed.
C) interact with specific antibody, even if the haptens are monovalent.
D) cannot stimulate secondary antibody responses without carriers.
E) all of the above

5. An adjuvant is a substance that
A) increases the size of the immunogen.
B) enhances the immunogenicity of haptens.
C) increases the chemical complexity of the immunogen.
D) enhances the immune response to the immunogen.
E) enhances immunologic cross-reactivity.

6. An antibody made against the antigen tetanus toxoid (TT) reacts with it even when the TT is denatured by disrupting all disulfide bonds. Another antibody against TT fails to react when the TT is similarly denatured. The most likely explanation can be stated as follows:
A) The first antibody is specific for several epitopes expressed by TT.
B) The first antibody is specific for the primary amino acid sequence of TT, whereas the second is specific for conformational determinants.
C) The second antibody is specific for disulfide bonds.
D) The first antibody has a higher affinity for TT.

ANSWERS TO REVIEW QUESTIONS

1. **C** Peptides (4–10 amino acids in length) are low molecular weight molecules that are unable to generate antibody responses owing to their small size. When coupled or bound to a protein carrier, they can be immunogenic.

2. **B** The protection against smallpox provided by prior infection with cowpox is an example of antigenic cross-reactivity. Immunization with cowpox leads to an immune response capable of reacting with smallpox because the two viruses share several identical, or structurally similar, determinants.

3. **B** Conversion of a toxin to a toxoid is performed to reduce the pharmacologic activity of the toxin, so that sufficient toxoid can be injected to induce an immune response.

4. **E** Haptens are substances, usually of low molecular weight and univalent, that, by themselves, cannot induce immune responses (primary or secondary) but can do so if conjugated to high molecular weight carriers. The haptens can and do interact with the induced antibodies, without it being necessary that they be conjugated to the carrier.

5. **D** An immunologic adjuvant is a substance that, when mixed with an immunogen, enhances the immune response against that immunogen by mechanisms that depend on the specific adjuvant used (e.g., enhanced antigen presentation, delayed release of antigen). It does not increase its size or chemical complexity. In addition, it does not enhance the immune response against a hapten, which requires its conjugation to an immunogenic carrier to induce a response against the hapten. The adjuvant has no relevance to possible toxicity of an immunogen.

6. **B** Antibodies can recognize single epitopes formed by primary sequence structures or secondary, tertiary, and quaternary conformational structures. Denaturing a protein by disrupting disulfide bonds generally destroys conformational determinants. Therefore it is likely that the first antibody reacts with a primary amino acid sequence determinant that is present on both native and denatured TT, while the second antibody sees a conformational determinant only on native TT.

4

ANTIBODY STRUCTURE AND FUNCTION

INTRODUCTION

One of the major functions of the immune system is the production of soluble proteins that circulate freely and exhibit properties that contribute specifically to immunity and protection against foreign material. These soluble proteins are the ***antibodies,*** which belong to the class of proteins called *globulins* because of their globular structure. Initially, owing to their migratory properties in an electrophoretic field, they were called γ-globulins (in relation to the more rapidly migrating albumin, α-globulin, and β-globulin); today they are known collectively as ***immunoglobulins*** (Igs).

Immunoglobulins are expressed as secreted and membrane-bound forms. Secreted antibodies are produced by plasma cells—the terminally differentiated B cells that serve as antibody factories housed largely within the bone marrow. Membrane-bound antibody is present on the surface of B cells, where it serves as the antigen-specific receptor. The membrane-bound form of antibody is associated with a heterodimer called Igα/Igβ to form the ***B cell receptor*** (BCR). As will be discussed in Chapter 7, the Igα/Igβ heterodimer mediates the intracellular signaling mechanisms associated with B cell activation.

The structure of immunoglobulins incorporates several features essential for their participation in the immune response. The two most important of these features are specificity and biologic activity. As discussed later in this chapter, ***specificity*** is attributed to a defined region of the antibody molecule that contains the hypervariable or ***complementarity-determining region*** (CDR). This restricts the antibody to combine only with those substances that contain one particular antigenic structure. The existence of a vast array of potential antigenic determinants or epitopes (see Chapter 3) has necessitated the evolution of a system for producing a repertoire of antibody molecules, each of which is capable of combining with a particular antigenic structure. Thus antibodies collectively exhibit great diversity, in terms of the types of molecular structures with which they are capable of reacting, but individually they exhibit a high degree of specificity, since each is able to react with only one particular antigenic structure.

Despite the large numbers of different specific individual antibodies capable of reacting with many different structural entities, the biologic effects of such reactions are rather few in number. These include neutralization of toxins, immobilization of microorganisms, neutralization of viral activity, agglutination (clumping together) of microorganisms or of antigenic particles (see Chapter 5), binding with soluble antigen leading to the formation of precipitates (which are readily phagocytized and destroyed by phagocytic cells; see Chapter 2), and activating serum complement to facilitate the lysis of microorganisms (see Chapter 13) or their phagocytosis and destruction either by phagocytic cells or by killer lymphocytes. Still another important biologic function of antibodies is their ability to cross the placenta from the mother to the fetus. Not all antibody molecules are equal in the performance of all of these biologic tasks.

Immunology: A Short Course, Fifth Edition, By Richard Coico, Geoffrey Sunshine, and Eli Benjamini
ISBN 0-471-22689-0

The differences in the various biologic activities of antibodies are attributed to their ***isotypic (class)*** structure. While one part of the antibody molecule must be adaptable to allow the accommodation of a large number of epitopes, another part of the antibody molecule must be adaptable to allow the antibody molecule to participate in biologic activities common to many antibodies. The determination of the structure of antibody, the establishment of the relationship between this structure and function, and the elucidation of the genetic organization of the immunoglobulin molecule have contributed to our understanding of the evolution of the immune system. It exists as a sophisticated, highly specialized system in which diverse structures (immunoglobulins) all recognize the same antigen, but in which the combination of immunoglobulin with antigen leads to an array of diverse biologic effects. This chapter deals with the structural and biologic properties of immunoglobulins.

ISOLATION AND CHARACTERIZATION

Serum is the antibody-containing component of blood left when it has clotted and the clot, which contains cells and clotting factors, is removed. When serum is subjected to ***electrophoresis*** (separation in an electrical field) in slightly alkaline pH (8.2) conditions, five major components can normally be visualized (Fig. 4.1). The slowest, in terms of migration toward the anode, called γ-globulin, has been shown to contain antibody. The demonstration entailed a simple comparison of the electrophoretic pattern of antiserum from a hyperimmune rabbit (one that had received multiple immunizations with a test antigen) before and after the test antigen-specific antibody had been removed by precipitation with the antigen. Only the size of the γ-globulin fraction was diminished by this procedure. Analysis showed that when this fraction was collected separately, all measurable antibodies were contained within it. Later, it was shown that antibody activity is present not only in the γ-globulin fraction but also in a slightly more anodic area. Consequently, all globular proteins with antibody activity are generically referred to as immunoglobulins, as exemplified by the γ-peak (Figure 4.1).

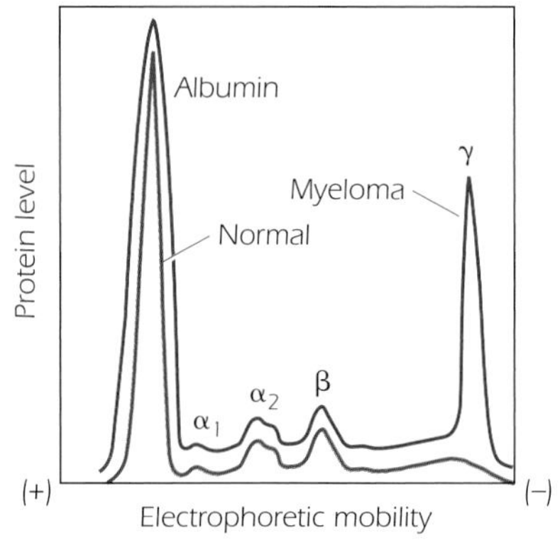

Figure 4.1. Electrophoretic mobility of serum proteins obtained from a normal individual (*blue*) and from a patient with IgG myeloma (*red*). (Courtesy of Dr. C Miller, School of Medicine, University of California at Davis.)

From the broad electrophoretic peaks, it is clear that a heterogeneous collection of immunoglobulin molecules with slightly different charges is present. This heterogeneity was one of the early obstacles in attempts to determine the structure of antibodies, since analytical chemistry requires homogeneous, crystallizable compounds as starting material. This problem was solved, in part, by the discovery of ***myeloma proteins,*** which are homogeneous immunoglobulins produced by the progeny of a single plasma cell that has become neoplastic in the malignant disease called ***multiple myeloma.*** This is clearly demonstrated by the γ-globulin spike in the electrophoretic pattern of serum proteins of a patient with multiple myeloma (Fig. 4.1). When it became clear that some myeloma proteins bound antigen, it also became apparent that they could be dealt with as typical immunoglobulin molecules.

Another aid to structural studies of antibodies was the discovery of ***Bence Jones proteins*** in the urine. These homogeneous proteins, produced in large quantities by some patients with multiple myeloma, are ***dimers of immunoglobulin*** κ ***or*** λ ***light chains.*** They were very useful in the determination of the structure of this portion of the immunoglobulin molecule. Today, the powerful technique of cell–cell hybridization (hybridomas) permits the production of large quantities of homogeneous preparations of monoclonal antibody of virtually any specificity (see Chapter 5).

STRUCTURE OF LIGHT AND HEAVY CHAINS

Analysis of the structural characteristics of antibody molecules really began in 1959 with two discoveries revealing that the molecule could be separated into analyzable parts suitable for further study. In England, Porter found that proteolytic treatment with the enzyme ***papain*** split the immunoglobulin molecule (molecular weight, 150,000 Da) into three fragments of about equal size (Fig. 4.2). Two of these fragments were found to retain the antibody's ability to bind antigen specifically, although, unlike the intact molecule, they could no longer precipitate the antigen from solution. These two fragments are referred to as ***Fab*** (fragment antigen binding) regions and are considered to be univalent, possessing one binding site each and being in every way identical to each other. The third fragment could be crystallized out of solution, a property indicative of its apparent homogeneity. This fragment is called ***Fc*** (crystallizable fragment). It cannot bind antigen, but, as was subsequently shown, it is responsible for the biologic functions of the antibody molecule after antigen has been bound to the Fab part of the intact molecule.

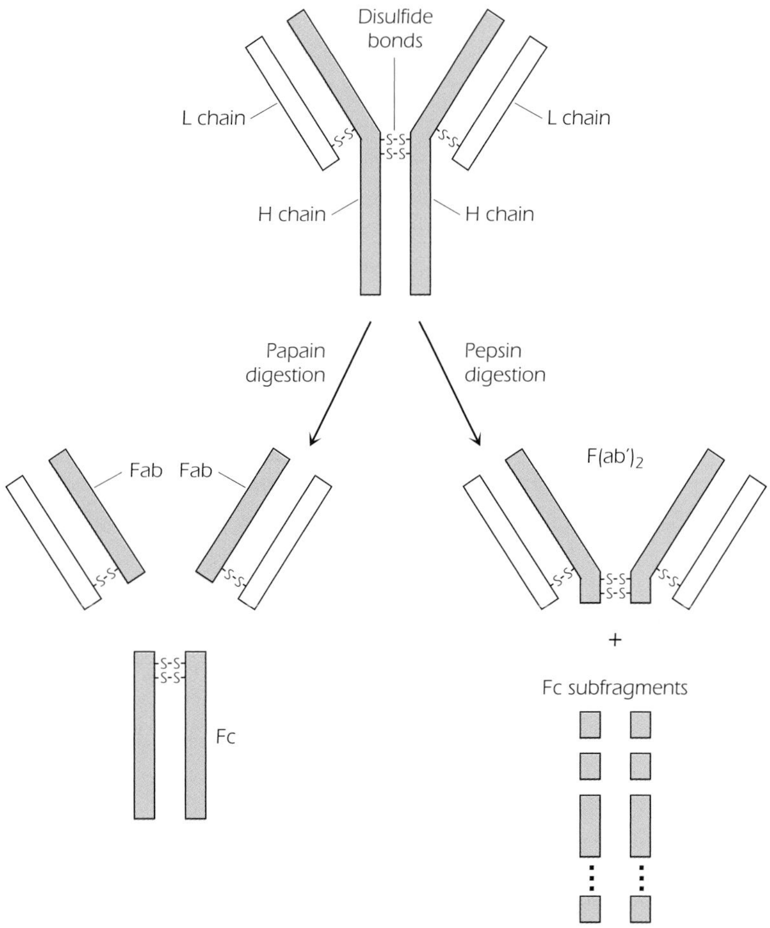

Figure 4.2. Proteolytic digestion of immunoglobulin using papain and pepsin.

At about the same time, Edelman in the United States discovered that when γ-globulin was extensively reduced by treatment with mercaptoethanol (a reagent that breaks SS bonds), the molecule fell apart into four chains: two identical chains with a molecular weight of about 53,000 Da each and two others of about 22,000 Da each. The larger molecules were designated ***heavy*** (H) ***chains*** and the smaller ones, ***light*** (L) ***chains.*** On the basis of these results, the structure of immunoglobulin molecules, as depicted in Figure 4.2, was proposed. This model was subsequently shown to be essentially correct, and Porter and Edelman shared the Nobel Prize for the elucidation of antibody structure. Thus all immunoglobulin molecules consist of a basic unit of four polypeptide chains, two identical heavy chains and two identical light chains, held together by a number of disulfide bonds. It should be noted that papain digestion of the immunoglobulin molecule results in cleavage N-terminally to the disulfide bridge between the heavy chains at the hinge region, yielding two monovalent Fab fragments and an Fc fragment. On the other hand, ***pepsin*** digestion results in cleavage C-terminally to the disulfide bridge, resulting in a divalent fragment referred to as ***F(ab')₂***, consisting of two ***Fab regions*** joined by the disulfide bond and several Fc subfragments (Figure 4.2). A more detailed view of a generic immunoglobulin molecule, consisting of two glycosylated heavy chains and two light chains, is shown in Figure 4.3. Note that in addition to the interchain disulfide bonds that hold the chains together, the heavy and light chains each contain intrachain disulfide bonds, creating the ***immunoglobulin fold domains,*** which form the antiparallel β-pleated sheet structure characteristic of antibody molecules. As discussed later in this chapter, other molecules belonging to the so-called ***immunoglobulin superfamily*** share this structural feature.

As is the case with other proteins, immunoglobulins of one species are immunogenic in another species. The use of immunoglobulins of a given species as immunogens in another species allowed the production of a variety of antisera that could distinguish between features of different immunoglobulin chains. By a combination of biochemical and serologic (using serum antibodies) techniques, it was shown that almost all species studied have two major classes of light chains: κ and λ. Any one individual of a species produces both types of light chain, but the ratio of κ chains to λ chains varies with the species (mouse: 95% κ; human: 60% κ). However, in any one immunoglobulin molecule, the light chains are always either both κ or both λ, never one of each. While there are two types of light chains, the immunoglobulins of virtually all species have been shown to consist

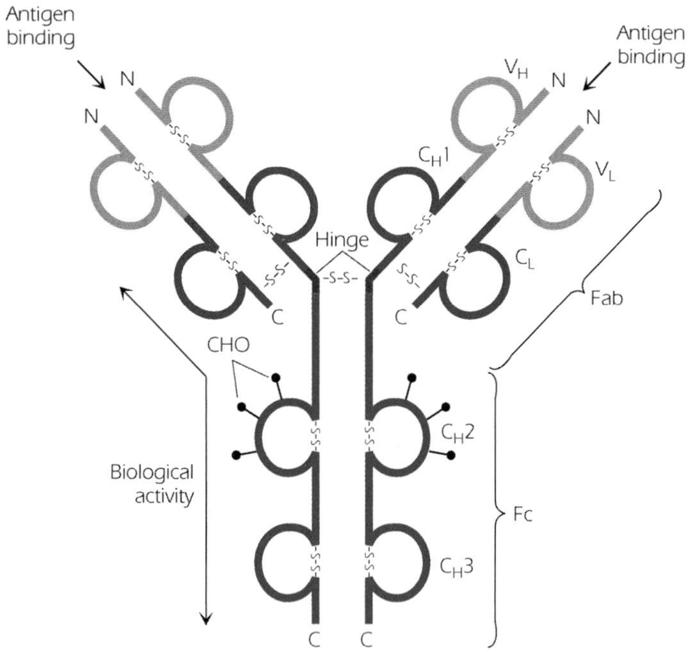

Figure 4.3. An immunoglobulin molecule showing immunoglobulin fold domains formed by intrachain disulfide bonds.

of five different classes (isotypes) that differ in the structure of the heavy chains. These heavy chains differ as antigens (serologically), in carbohydrate content, and in size. Most important, they confer different biologic functions on each isotype. The heavy chains, whose constant regions are derived from immunoglobulin heavy chain genes (discussed in detail in Chapter 6) are designated with Greek letters as shown in Table 4.1.

The genes encoding the constant regions of the heavy chains are similarly designated (see Chapter 6). Therefore, the genes encoding these constant (C) regions responsible for the μ, δ, γ, α, and ε heavy chains are called $C\mu$, $C\delta$, $C\gamma$, $C\alpha$, and Cgεs respectively.

Any individual of a species makes all heavy chains, in proportions characteristic of the species; but in any one antibody molecule, both heavy chains are identical (e.g., 2γ or 2ε). Thus an antibody molecule of the IgG class could have the structure $\kappa_2\gamma_2$ with two identical κ light chains and two identical γ heavy chains. Alternatively, it could have the structure $\lambda_2\gamma_2$ with two identical λ light chains and two identical γ heavy chains. In contrast, an antibody of the IgE class could have the structure $\kappa_2\varepsilon_2$ or $\lambda_2\varepsilon_2$. In each case, it is the nature of the heavy chains that confers on the molecule its unique biologic properties, such as its half-life in the circulation, its ability to bind to certain receptors, and its ability to activate enzymes (see Chapter 13) on combination with antigen.

TABLE 4.1. Immunoglobulin Heavy Chain Isotypes

Isotype	Heavy Chain
IgM	μ
IgD	δ
IgG	γ
IgA	α
IgE	ϵ

Further characterization of these isotypes by specific antisera has led to the designation of several subclasses based on more subtle differences. Thus the major class of human IgG can be subdivided into the ***subclasses*** IgG_1, IgG_2, IgG_3, and IgG_4. IgA has been divided similarly into two subclasses, IgA_1 and IgA_2. The subclasses differ from one another in numbers and arrangement of interchain disulfide bonds as well as by alterations in other structural features. These alterations, in turn, produce some changes in functional properties, discussed later.

DOMAINS

Early in the study of the structure of immunoglobulins, it became apparent that, in addition to interchain disulfide bonds that hold together light and heavy chains and the two heavy chains, intrachain disulfide bonds exist that form loops within the chain. The ***globular structure*** of immunoglobulins and the ability of enzymes to cleave these molecules at restricted positions into large entities instead of degrading them to oligopeptides and amino acids indicate a very compact structure. Furthermore, the presence of intrachain disulfide bonds at regular and approximately equal intervals of 100–110 amino acids leads to the prediction that each loop in the peptide chains should form a compactly folded ***globular domain.*** In fact, light chains have two domains each, and heavy chains have four or five domains, separated by a short unfolded stretch (Fig. 4.3). These configurations have been confirmed by direct observation and by genetic analysis (see Chapter 6).

Immunoglobulin molecules are assemblies of separate domains, each centered on a disulfide bond and each having so much homology with the others as to suggest that they evolved from a single ancestral gene that duplicated itself several times and then changed its amino acid sequence to enable the resultant different domains to fulfill different functions. Each domain is designated by a letter, indicating whether it is on a light chain or a heavy chain, and a number, indicating its position. As we shall soon discuss in more detail, the first domain on light and heavy chains is highly variable, in terms of amino acid sequence, from one antibody to the next; it is designated V_L or V_H, accordingly (Fig. 4.3). The second and subsequent domains on both heavy chains are much more constant in amino acid sequence and are designated C_L or C_H1, C_H2, and C_H3 (Fig. 4.3). In addition to their interchain disulfide bonding, the globular domains bind to each other in homologous pairs, largely by hydrophobic interactions, as follows: V_HV_L, C_H1C_L, C_H2C_H2, and C_H3C_H3.

HINGE REGION

In the immunoglobulins (with the possible exception of IgM and IgE), the hinge region is composed of a short segment of amino acids and is found between the C_H1 and C_H2 regions of the heavy chains (Fig. 4.3). This segment is made up predominantly of cysteine and proline residues. The cysteines are involved in formation of interchain disulfide bonds, and the proline residues prevent folding in a globular structure. This region of the heavy chain provides an important structural characteristic of immunoglobulins. It permits ***flexibility between the two Fab arms*** of the Y-shaped antibody molecule. It allows the two Fab arms to open and close to accommodate binding to two identical epitopes, separated by a fixed distance, as might be found on the surface of a bacterium. In addition, since this stretch of amino acids is open and as accessible as any other nonfolded peptide, it can be cleaved by proteases, such as papain, to generate the Fab and Fc regions described above (Fig. 4.2).

VARIABLE REGION

The biologic functions of the antibody molecule derive from the properties of a constant region, which is identical for antibodies of all specificities within a particular class. It is the variable region that constitutes the part of the molecule that binds to the epitope. A major problem for immunologists was to determine how so many individual specificities, which are required to meet the enormous variety of antigenic challenges, are generated from the variable region. As we shall see in Chapter 6, this issue has been largely resolved.

When the amino acid sequences of proteins of sufficient homogeneity (e.g., myeloma proteins, Bence Jones proteins) were determined, it was found that the greatest variability in sequence existed in the N-terminal 110 amino acids of both the light and heavy chains. Kabat and Wu compared the amino acid sequences of many different V_L and V_H regions. They plotted the variability in the amino acids at each position in the chain and showed that the greatest amount of variability (defined as the ratio of the number of different amino acids at a given position to the frequency of the most common amino acid at that position) occurred in three regions of the light and heavy chains. These regions are called ***hypervariable regions.*** The less variable stretches, which occur between these hypervariable regions, are called framework regions. It is now clear that the hypervariable regions participate in the binding with antigen and form the region complementary in structure to the antigen epitope. Consequently, hypervariability regions are termed ***complementarity-determining regions*** of the light and heavy chains: CDR1, CDR2, and CDR3 (Fig. 4.4).

The hypervariable regions, although separated in the linear, two-dimensional model of the peptide chains, are actually brought together in the folded form of the intact antibody molecule. Together, they constitute the combining site,

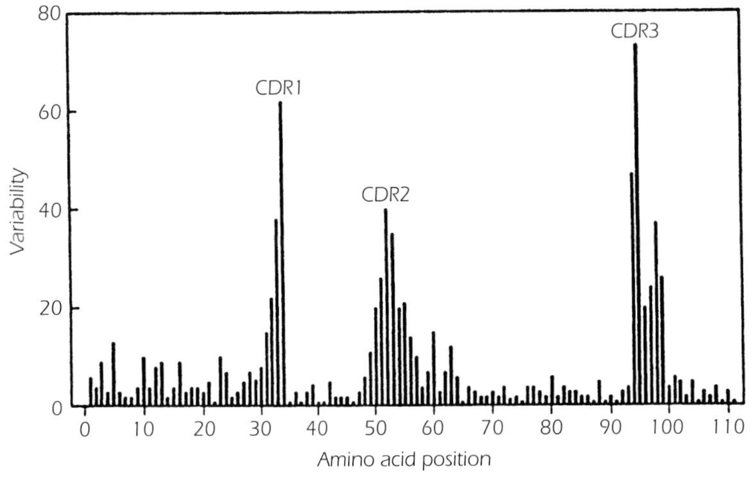

Figure 4.4. Variability of amino acids representing the N-terminal residues of V_H in a representative immunoglobulin molecule.

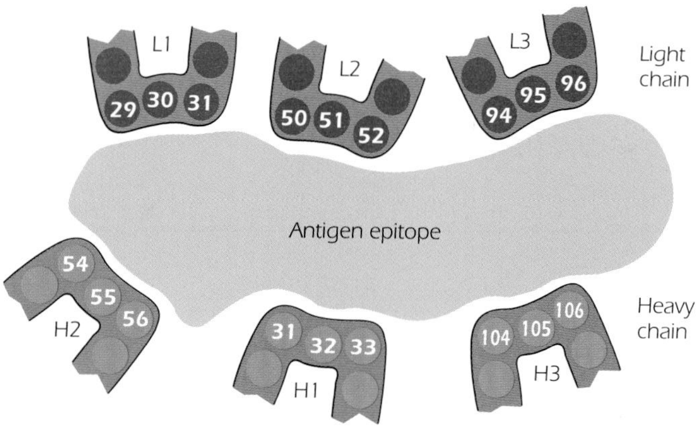

Figure 4.5. The complementarity between an epitope and the antibody-combining site, consisting of the hypervariable areas of the L and H chains. *Numbered letters,* CDRs of H and L chains; *circled numbers,* the number of the amino acid residue in the CDRs.

which is complementary to the epitope (Fig. 4.5). The variability in these CDRs provides the diversity in the shape of the combining site that is required for the function of antibodies of different specificities. All the known ***forces involved in antigen–antibody interactions are weak, noncovalent interactions*** (e.g., ionic, hydrogen bonding, van der Waals forces, and hydrophobic interactions). It is, therefore, necessary that there be a close fit between antigen and antibody over a sufficiently large region to allow a total binding force that is adequate for stable interaction. Contributions to this binding interaction by both heavy and light chains are involved in the overall association between epitope and antibody.

It should now be apparent that two antibody molecules with different antigenic specificities must have different amino acid sequences in their hypervariable regions and that those with similar sequences will generally have similar specificities. However, it is possible for two antibodies with different amino acid sequences to have specificity to the same epitope. In this case, the ***binding affinities*** of the antibodies with the epitope will probably be different, because there will be differences in the number and types of binding forces available to bind identical antigens to the different binding sites of the two antibodies.

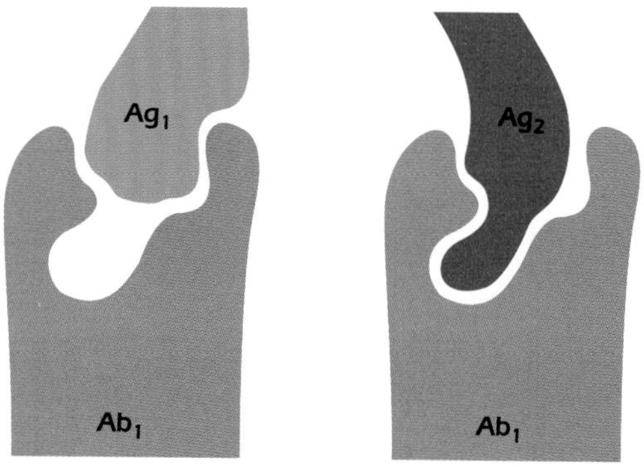

Figure 4.6. How an antibody (*Ab*) of a given specificity can exhibit binding with two different epitopes (Ag_1 and Ag_2).

An additional source of variability involves the size of the combining site on the antibody, which is usually (but not always) considered to take the form of a depression or cleft. In some instances, especially when small hydrophobic haptens are involved, the epitopes do not occupy the entire combining site, yet they achieve sufficient affinity of binding. It has been shown that antibodies specific for such a small hapten may, in fact, react with other antigens that have no obvious similarity to the hapten (e.g., dinitrophenol and sheep red cells). These large, dissimilar antigens bind either to a larger area or to a different area of the combining site on the antibody (Fig. 4.6). Thus a particular antibody-combining site may have the ability to combine with two (or more) apparently diverse epitopes, a property called *redundancy.* The ability of a single antibody molecule to cross-react with an unknown number of epitopes may reduce the number of different antibodies needed to defend an individual against the range of antigenic challenges.

IMMUNOGLOBULIN VARIANTS

Isotypes

Thus far we have described the features common to all immunoglobulin molecules, such as the four-chain unit and the structural domains. In its defense against invading foreign substances, the body has evolved a variety of mechanisms, each dependent on a somewhat different property or function of an immunoglobulin molecule. Thus when a specific antibody molecule combines with a specific antigen or a pathogen, several different effector mechanisms come into play. These different mechanisms derive from the different classes of immunoglobulin (isotypes), each of which may combine with the same epitope, but each of which triggers a different response. These differences result from structural variations in heavy chains, which have generated domains that mediate a variety of functions. The structural features are discussed here. A summary of the properties of the immunoglobulin classes is given in Tables 4.2 and 4.3.

TABLE 4.2. The Most Important Features of Immunoglobulin Isotopes

Feature	Isotype				
	IgG	IgA	IgM	IgD	IgE
Molecular weight	150,000	160,000 for monomer	900,000	180,000	200,000
Additional protein subunits	—	J and S	J	—	—
Approximate concentration in serum (mg/mL)	12	1.8	1	0–0.04	0.00002
Percent of total Ig	80	13	6	0.2	0.002
Distribution	~Equal: intravascular and extravascular	Intravascular and secretions	Mostly intravascular	Present on lymphocyte surface	On basophils and mast cells present in saliva and nasal secretions
Half-life (days)	23	5.5	5	2.8	2.0
Placental passage	++	—	—	—	—
Presence in secretion	—	++	—	—	—
Presence in milk	+	+	0 to trace	—	—
Activation of complement	+	—	+++	—	—
Binding to Fc receptors on macrophages, polymorphonuclear cells, and NK[a] cells	++	—	—	—	—
Relative agglutinating capacity	+	++	+++	—	—
Antiviral activity	+++	+++	+	—	—
Antibacterial activity (gram negative)	+++	++ (with lysozyme)	+++ (with complement)	—	—
Antitoxin activity	+++	—	—	—	—
Allergic activity	—	—	—	—	++

[a] Natural killer

ALLOTYPES

Another form of variation in the structure of immunoglobulins is allotypy. It is based on ***genetic differences among individuals.*** It depends on the existence of ***allelic forms*** (allotypes) of the same protein, as a result of the presence of different forms of the same gene at a given locus. As a result of allotypy, a heavy or light chain constituent of any immunoglobulin can be present in some members of a species and absent in others. This situation contrasts with that of immunoglobulin classes or subclasses, which are present in all members of a species.

Allotypic differences at known loci usually involve changes in only one or two amino acids in the constant region of a chain. With a few exceptions, the presence of allotypic differences in two identical immunoglobulin molecules does not generally affect binding with antigen, but it serves as an important marker for analysis of Mendelian inheritance.

Some known allotype markers constitute a group on the γ-chain of human IgG (called ***Gm*** for IgG markers), a group on the κ chain (called ***Km***), and a group on the α chain (called ***Am***).

Allotypic markers have been found in the immunoglobulins of several species, usually by the use of antisera generated by immunization of one member of a species with antibody from another member of the same species. As with other allelic systems, allotypes are inherited as dominant Mendelian traits. The genes encoding the markers are expressed

TABLE 4.3. Important Differences among Human IgG Subclasses

Characteristic	IgG_1	IgG_2	IgG_3	IgG_4
Occurrence (% of total IgG)	70	20	7	3
Half-life	23	23	7	23
Complement binding	+	+	+++	—
Placental passage	++	±	++	++
Binding of monocytes	+++	+	+++	±

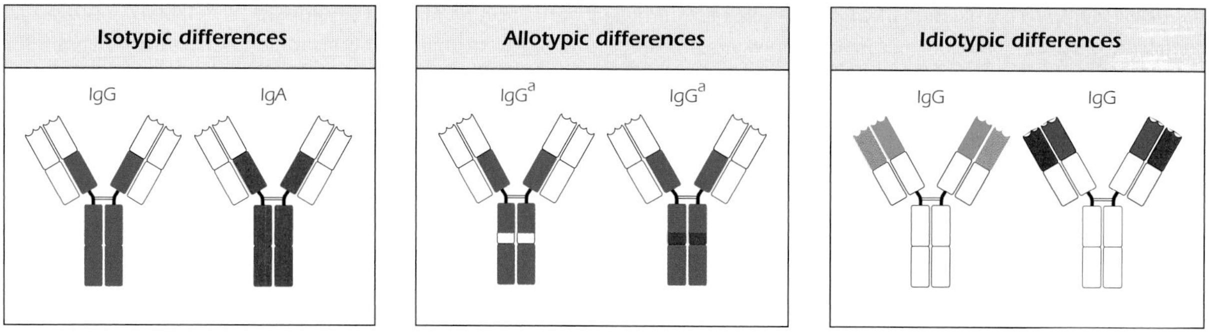

Figure 4.7. Different types of immunoglobulin variation.

codominantly, so that an individual may be homozygous or heterozygous for a given marker.

Idiotypes

As we have seen, the combining site of a specific antibody molecule is made up of a unique combination of amino acids in the variable regions of the light and heavy chains. Since this combination is not present in other antibody molecules, it should be immunogenic and capable of stimulating an immunologic response against itself in an animal of the same species. Such was actually found to be the case by Oudin and Kunkel, who, in the early 1960s, showed that experimental immunization with a particular antibody or myeloma protein could produce an antiserum specific only for the antibody that was used to induce the response and for no other immunoglobulin of the species. These antisera contain populations of antibodies specific for several epitopes, called ***idiotopes,*** which are present in the variable (heavy and light) region of the antibody used for inoculation. The collection of all idiotopes on the inoculated antibody molecule is called the ***idiotype*** (Id). In some cases, anti-idiotypic sera prevent binding of the antibody with its antigen, in which event the idiotypic determinant is considered to be in or very near the combining site itself. Anti-idiotypic sera, which do not block binding of antibody with antigen, are probably directed against variable determinants of the framework area, outside the combining site (Fig. 4.8). On theoretical grounds, it is possible to visualize that an anti-idiotypic antibody with a combining site complementary to that of the idiotype resembles the epitope, which is also complementary to the idiotype's combining site. Thus the anti-idiotype may represent a facsimile or an internal image of the nominal epitope. Indeed, there are examples of immunization of experimental animals using anti-idiotypic internal images as immunogens. Such immunogens induce antibodies capable of reacting with the antigen that carries the epitope to which the original idiotype is directed. Such antibodies are induced without the immunized animal ever having seen the original antigen.

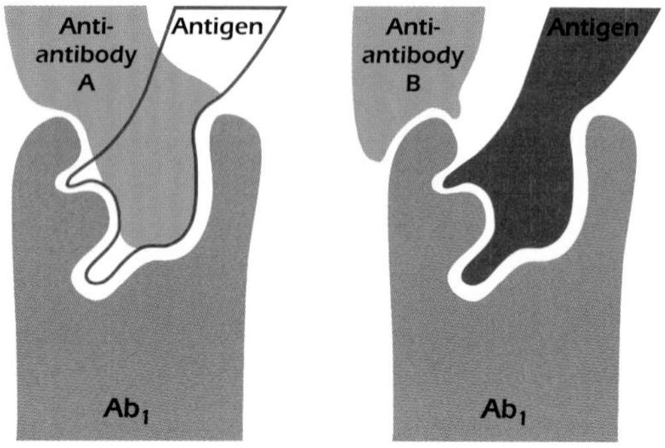

Figure 4.8. Two anti-idiotypic antibodies to Ab_1. **(A)** The anti-idiotypic antibody is directed to the combining site of Ab_1, preventing binding of Ab_1 with the antigen. **(B)** The anti-idiotypic antibody binds with framework areas of Ab_1 and does not prevent its binding with antigen.

In some instances, especially with inbred animals, anti-idiotypic antibodies react with several different antibodies that are directed against the same epitope and share idiotypes. These idiotypes are called public or ***cross-reacting idiotypes,*** and this term frequently defines families of antibody molecules. By contrast, sera that react with only one particular antibody molecule define a private idiotype. As we discuss in Chapter 10, the presence of idiotypic determinants on immunoglobulin molecules may have a role in the control and modulation of the immune response, as envisioned in the Jerne network theory, although this remains controversial.

Figure 4.9 summarizes the different types of variation seen among immuoglobulins. Differences between constant regions as a result of the use of different heavy and light chain constant region genes are called isotypes. Differences owing to different alleles of the same constant region gene are called allotypes. Finally, within a given isotype (e.g., IgG), differences in particular rearranged V_H and V_L genes are called idiotypes.

STRUCTURAL FEATURES OF IgG

IgG is the predominant immunoglobulin in blood, lymph fluid, cerebrospinal fluid, and peritoneal fluid. The IgG

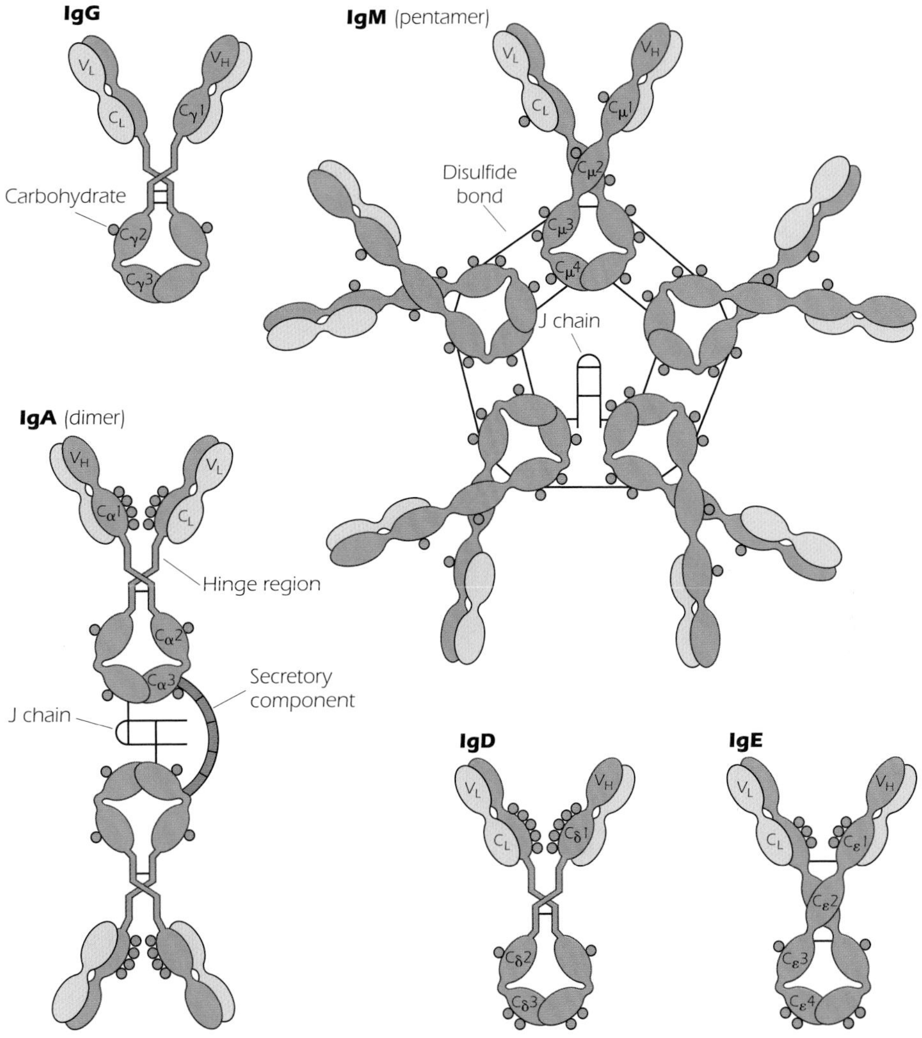

Figure 4.9. Structures of the five major classes of secreted antibody. Light chains are shown in *green;* heavy chains are shown in *blue. Orange circles* denote areas of glycosylation. The polymeric IgM and IgA molecules contain a polypeptide known as the J chain. The dimeric IgA molecule shown includes the secretory component (*red*).

molecule consists of two γ heavy chains of molecular weight ~50,000 Da each and two light chains (either κ or λ) of molecular weight ~ 25,000 Da each, held together by disulfide bonds (Fig. 4.9). Thus the IgG molecule has a molecular weight of ~ 150,000 Da and a sedimentation coefficient of 7S. Electrophoretically, the IgG molecule is the least anodic of all serum proteins, and it migrates to the γ range of serum globulins; hence its earlier designation as γ-globulin or 7S immunoglobulin.

The IgG class of immunoglobulins ***in humans contains four subclasses designated IgG_1, IgG_2, IgG_3, and IgG_4,*** named in order of their abundance in serum (IgG_1 being the most abundant). Except for their variable regions, all the immunoglobulins within a class have about 90% homology in their amino acid sequences, but only 60% homology exists between classes (e.g., IgG and IgA). This degree of homology means that an antiserum to IgG may be produced against a determinant that is common to, and specific for, all members of a given class (e.g., all members of the IgG class) while other antisera may be raised that are specific for determinants found in only one of the subclasses (e.g., in IgG_2). This variation was first detected antigenically by the use of antibodies against various γ chains. The IgG subclasses differ in their chemical properties and, more important, in their biologic properties, which are discussed below.

BIOLOGIC PROPERTIES OF IgG

IgG present in the serum of human adults represents about 15% of the total protein (other proteins include albumins, globulins, and enzymes). IgG is distributed approximately equally between the intravascular and extravascular spaces.

Except for the IgG_3 subclass, which has a rapid turnover, with a half-life of 7 days, ***the half-life of IgG is approximately 23 days,*** which is the longest half-life of all immunoglobulin isotypes. This persistence in the serum makes IgG the most suitable for passive immunization by transfer of antibodies. Interestingly, as the concentration of IgG in the serum increases (as in cases of multiple myeloma or after the transfer

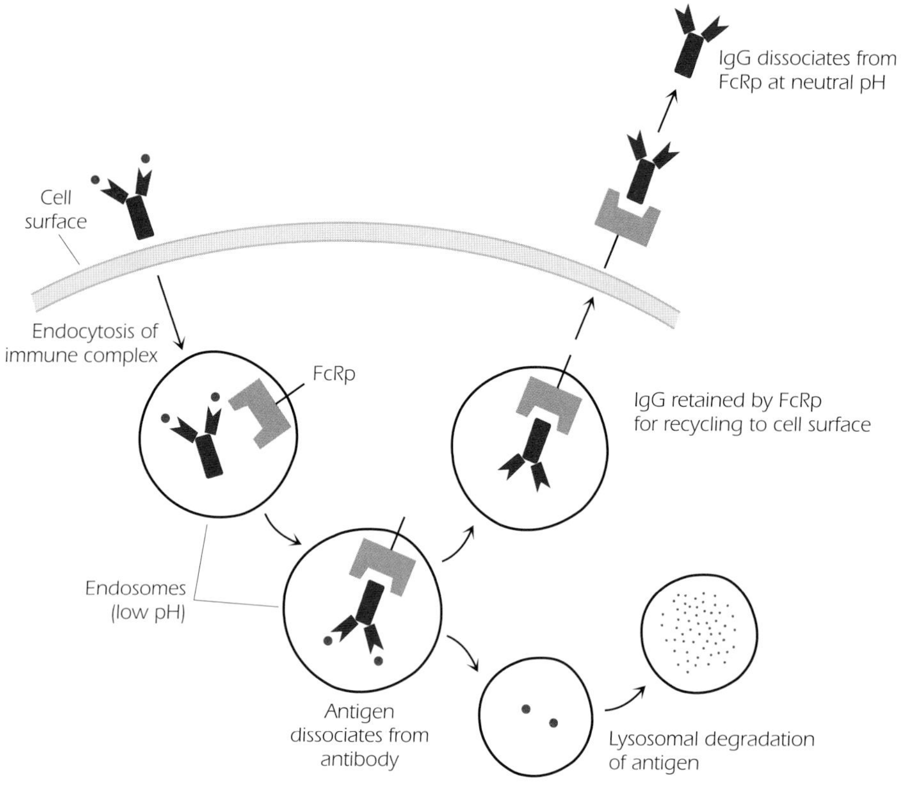

Figure 4.10. Recycling of IgG using the protector receptor (FcRp). Circulating monomeric IgG plus antigen (immune complex) enters an antigen-presenting cell through the process of endocytosis. Within the endosome, the complex binds FcRp; IgG and antigen dissociate, allowing the IgG to be directed to the cell surface for recycling. The antigen undergoes lysosomal degradation (antigen processing), and its proteolytic fragments are ultimately expressed on the cell surface in the context of MHC class II molecules.

of very high concentrations of IgG), the rate of catabolism of IgG increases, and the half-life of IgG decreases to 15–20 days or even less. Recent studies have provided a clear explanation for the prolonged survival of IgG relative to other serum proteins and why its half-life decreases at high concentrations. A saturable IgG protection receptor (FcRp, also called the Brambell receptor) has been identified and shown to bind to the Fc region of this isotype. This receptor is found in cellular endosomes and selectively recycles endocytized IgG (e.g., following endocytosis of antigen–antibody immune complexes) back to the circulation. Figure 4.10 illustrates how this mechanism operates to cleanse IgG antibody of antigen and harvest antigen for presentation without antibody destruction. Conditions associated with high IgG levels saturate the FcRp receptors, rendering the catabolism of excess IgG indistinguishable from albumin or other Ig isotypes.

Agglutination and Formation of Precipitate

IgG molecules can cause the ***agglutination*** or clumping of particulate (insoluble) antigens such as microorganisms. The reaction of IgG with soluble, multivalent antigens can generate ***precipitates*** (see Chapter 5). This property of IgG is undoubtedly of considerable survival value since insoluble antigen–antibody complexes are easily phagocytized and destroyed by phagocytic cells. IgG molecules may be made to aggregate by a variety of procedures. For example, precipitation with alcohol, a method employed in the purification of IgG, and heating at 56° C for 10 min, a method used to inactivate complement (see Chapter 13), cause aggregation. Aggregated IgG can still combine with antigen.

Many of the properties that are attributed to antigen–antibody complexes are exhibited by aggregated IgG (without antigen), for example, attachment to phagocytic cells as well as the activation of complement and other biologically active substances that may be harmful to the body. Such activation is attributable to the juxtaposition of Fc domains by the aggregation process in a way analogous to that produced by antigen-induced immune complex formation. It is, therefore, imperative that no aggregated IgG be present in passively administered IgG.

Passage through the Placenta and Absorption in Neonates

The IgG isotype (except for subclass IgG_2) is the only class of immunoglobulin that can pass through the placenta, enabling the mother to transfer her immunity to the fetus. Placental transfer is facilitated by expression of an IgG protection receptor (FcRn) expressed on placental cells. FcRn was recently shown to be identical to the IgG protection receptor (FcRp) found in the cellular endosomes. Analysis of fetal immunoglobulins shows that, at the 3rd or 4th month of pregnancy, there is a rapid increase in the concentration of IgG. This IgG must be of maternal origin, since the fetus is unable to synthesize immunoglobulins at this age. Then, during the 5th month of pregnancy, the fetus begins to synthesize IgM and trace amounts of IgA. It is not until 3 or 4 months after birth, when the level of inherited maternal IgG drops as a result of catabolism (the half-life of IgG is 23 days), that the infant begins to synthesize its own IgG antibodies. Thus the resistance of the fetus and the neonate to infection is conferred almost entirely by the mother's IgG, which passes across the placenta. It has been established that passage across the placenta is mediated by the Fc portion of the IgG molecule; $F(ab')_2$ or Fab regions of IgG do not pass through the placenta. It is of interest to note that the IgG protection receptor (FcRn) expressed on placental cells is transiently superexpressed in the intestinal tissue of neonates. Absorption of maternal IgG contained in the colostrum of nursing mothers is achieved by its binding to these high density receptors in intestinal tissue. FcRn is downregulated in intestinal tissue at 2 weeks of age.

While passage of IgG molecules across the placenta confers immunity to infection on the fetus, it may also be responsible for hemolytic disease of the newborn (erythroblastosis fetalis) (see Chapter 15). This is caused by maternal antibodies to fetal red blood cells. The maternal IgG antibodies to Rh antigen produced by an Rh^- mother, pass across the placenta and attack the fetal red blood cells that express Rh antigens (Rh^+).

Opsonization

IgG is an opsonizing antibody (from the Greek ***opsonin,*** which means "to prepare for eating") thereby facilitating phagocytosis. It reacts with epitopes (e.g., those expressed on microorganisms) via its Fab portions, but it is the Fc portion that confers the opsonizing property. Many phagocytic cells, including macrophages and polymorphonuclear phagocytes, express membrane receptors for the Fc portion of the IgG molecule. These cells adhere to the antibody-coated bacteria by virtue of their Fc receptors. The net effect is a zipper-like closure of the surface membrane of the phagocytic cell around the organism, as receptors for Fc and the Fc regions on the antibodies continue to combine, leading to the final engulfing and destruction of the microorganism (Fig. 4.11).

Antibody-Dependent, Cell-Mediated Cytotoxicity

The IgG molecule plays an important role in ***antibody-dependent, cell-mediated cytotoxicity*** (ADCC). In this form of cytotoxicity, the Fab portion binds with the target cell, whether it is a microorganism or a tumor cell, and the Fc portion binds with specific receptors for Fc that are found on certain large granular lymphocytic cells called natural killer (NK) cells (see Chapter 2). By this mechanism, the IgG molecule focuses the killer cells on their target, and the killer cells destroy the target, not by phagocytosis but with the various substances that they release.

Activation of Complement

In Chapter 13, we discuss the major properties of the complement system. In brief, complement is a set of plasma proteins that can be activated either by binding to certain pathogens or by binding to antibody (e.g., pathogen-specific antibodies). Complement activation is often described as a series of ***cascading enzymatic events,*** leading to the generation specific complement components that cause ***opsonization*** and ***phagocytosis*** of infectious agents as well as direct ***lysis of the invading organism*** among other important immunologic phenomena. Structural features of the early complement components involved in the activation cascade in which antibodies are involved dictate the antibody classes to which complement will bind.

The IgG molecule can activate the complement system (see Chapter 13). Activation of complement results in the release of several important biologically active molecules and leads to lysis if the antibody is bound to antigen on the surface of a cell. Some of the complement components are also opsonins; they bind to the target antigen and thereby direct phagocytes, which carry receptors specific for these opsonins, to focus their phagocytic activity on the target antigen. Other components from the activation of complement are chemotactic; specifically, they attract phagocytic cells. All in all, the activation of complement by IgG has profound biologic effects on the host and on the target antigen, whether it is a live cell, a microorganism, or a tumor cell.

Neutralization of Toxin

The IgG molecule is an excellent antibody for the ***neutralization*** of toxins, such as ***tetanus and botulinus,*** or for the inactivation of, for example, snake and scorpion venoms. Because of its ability to neutralize such poisons (mostly by blocking their active sites) and because of its relatively long half-life, the IgG molecule is the isotype of choice for ***passive immunization*** (i.e., the transfer of antibodies) against toxins and venoms.

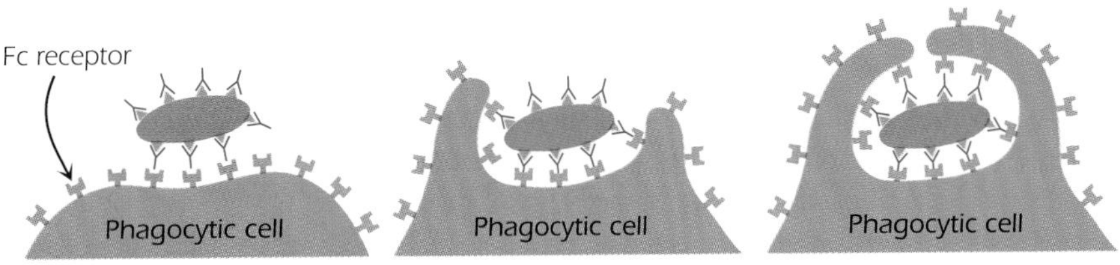

Figure 4.11. Phagocytosis of a particle coated with antibodies.

Immobilization of Bacteria

IgG molecules are efficient in immobilizing various motile bacteria. Reaction of antibodies specific for the flagella and cilia of certain microorganisms causes them to clump, thereby arresting their movement and preventing their ability to spread or invade tissue.

Neutralization of Viruses

IgG antibody is an efficient virus-neutralizing antibody. One mechanism of neutralization is that in which the antibody binds with antigenic determinants present on various portions of the virus coat, among which is the region used by the virus for attachment to the target cell. Inhibition of viral attachment effectively arrests infection. Other antibodies are thought to inhibit viral penetration or shedding of the viral coat required for release of the viral DNA or RNA needed to induce infection.

The versatility in function of the IgG molecule makes it a very important molecule in the immune response. Its importance is underscored in those immune deficiency disorders in which an individual is unable to synthesize IgG molecules (see Chapter 17). Such individuals are prone to infections that may result in toxemias and death.

STRUCTURAL FEATURES OF IgM

As we shall see later in this chapter, ***IgM is the first immunoglobulin produced following immunization.*** Its name derives from its initial description as a macroglobulin (M) of high molecular weight (900,000 Da). It has a sedimentation coefficient of 19S, and it has an extra C_H domain. In comparison to the IgG molecule, which consists of one four-chain structure, ***IgM is a pentameric molecule*** composed of five such units, each of which consists of two light and two heavy chains, all joined together by additional disulfide bonds between their Fc portions and by a polypeptide chain termed the J chain (Fig. 4.9). The J chain, which, like light and heavy chains, is synthesized in the B cell or plasma cell, has a molecular weight of 15,000 Da. This pentameric ensemble of IgM, which is held together by disulfide bonds, comes apart after mild treatment with reducing agents, such as mercaptoethanol.

Surprisingly, each pentameric IgM molecule appears to have a valence of 5 (i.e., five antigen combining sites), instead of the expected valence of 10 predicted by the 10 Fab segments contained in the pentamer. This apparent reduction in valence is probably the result of conformational constraints imposed by the polymerization. It is known that pentameric IgM has a planar configuration, such that each of its 10 Fab portions cannot open fully with respect to the adjacent Fab, when it combines with antigen, as is possible in the case of IgG. Thus any large antigen bound to one Fab may block a neighboring site from binding with antigen, making the molecule appear pentavalent (or of even lesser valence).

BIOLOGIC PROPERTIES OF IgM

IgM present in adult human serum is found predominantly in the intravascular spaces. The half-life of the IgM molecule is approximately 5 days. In contrast to IgG, IgM antibodies are not very versatile; they are poor toxin-neutralizing antibodies, and they are not efficient in the neutralization of viruses. IgM is also found on the surface of mature B cells together with IgD (see below), where it serves as an antigen-specific BCR. Once the B cell is activated by antigen following ligation of the BCR, it may undergo class switching (see Chapter 6) and begins to secrete and express other membrane immunoglobulin isotypes (e.g., IgG).

Because of its pentameric form, ***IgM is an excellent complement-fixing or complement-activating antibody.*** Unlike other classes of immunoglobulins, a single molecule of IgM, on binding to antigen with at least two of its Fab arms, can initiate the complement sequence, making it the most efficient immunoglobulin as an initiator of the complement-mediated lysis of microorganisms and other cells. This ability, taken together with the appearance of IgM as the first class of antibodies generated after immunization or infection, makes IgM antibodies very important as providers of an early line of immunologic defense against bacterial infections.

IgM antibodies do not pass through the placenta; however, since this is the only class of immunoglobulins that is synthesized by the fetus, beginning at approximately 5 months of gestation, elevated levels of IgM in the fetus indicate congenital or perinatal infection.

IgM is the isotype synthesized by children and adults in appreciable amounts after immunization or exposure to T-independent antigens, and it is the first isotype that is synthesized after immunization (Fig. 4.12). Thus ***elevated levels of IgM usually indicate either recent infection or recent exposure to antigen.***

Agglutination

IgM molecules are efficient agglutinating antibodies. Because of their pentameric form, IgM antibodies can form macromolecular bridges between epitopes on molecules that may be too distant from each other to be bridged by the smaller IgG antibodies. Furthermore, because of their pentameric form and multiple valence, the IgM antibodies are particularly well suited to combine with antigens that contain repeated patterns of the same antigenic determinant, as

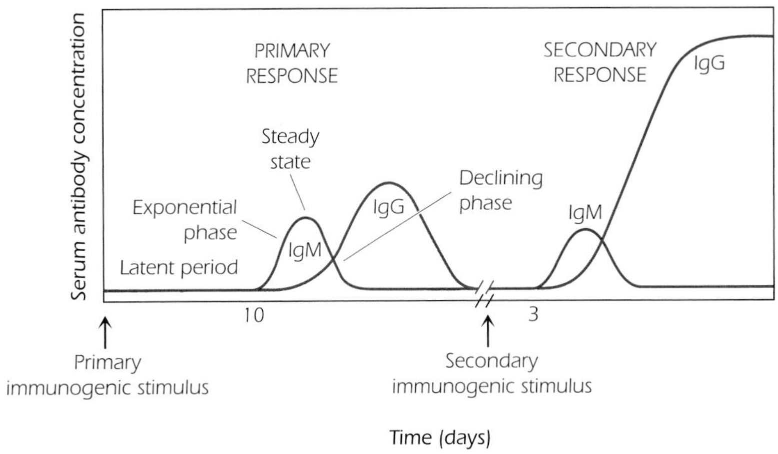

Figure 4.12. The kinetics of an antibody response.

in the case of polysaccharide antigens or cellular antigens, which are multiply expressed on cell surfaces.

Isohemagglutinins

The IgM antibodies include the ***isohemagglutinins***—the naturally occurring antibodies against the red blood cell antigens of the ABO blood groups. These antibodies are presumed to arise as a result of immunization by bacteria in the gastrointestinal and respiratory tracts, which bear determinants similar to the oligosaccharides of the ABO blood groups. Thus, without known prior immunization, people with the type O blood group have isohemagglutinins to the A and B antigens; those with the type A blood group have antibodies to the B antigen; and those with the B antigen have antibodies to the A antigen. An individual of the AB group has neither anti-A nor anti-B antibodies. Fortunately, the ***IgM isohemagglutinins do not pass through the placenta,*** so incompatibility of the ABO groups between mother and fetus poses no danger to the fetus. However, transfusion reactions, which arise as a result of ABO incompatibility, and in which the recipient's isohemagglutinins react with the donor's red blood cells, may have disastrous consequences.

STRUCTURAL AND BIOLOGIC PROPERTIES OF IgA

IgA is the major immunoglobulin in external secretions such as ***saliva, mucus, sweat, gastric fluid,*** and ***tears.*** It is, moreover, the major immunoglobulin found in the ***colostrum*** of milk in nursing mothers, and it may provide the neonate with a major source of intestinal protection against pathogens during the first few weeks after birth. The IgA molecule consists of either two κ light chains or two λ light chains and two α heavy chains. The α-chain is somewhat larger than the γ-chain. The molecular weight of monomeric IgA is ~165,000 Da, and its sedimentation coefficient is 7S. Electrophoretically, it migrates to the slow β- or fast γ-region of serum globulins. Dimeric IgA has a molecular weight of 400,000 Da.

The IgA class of immunoglobulins contains two subclasses: IgA_1 (93%) and IgA_2(7%). It is interesting to note that if all production of IgA on mucosal surfaces (respiratory, gastrointestinal, and urinary tracts) is taken into account, IgA would be the major immunoglobulin in terms of quantity.

Serum IgA has a ***half-life of 5.5 days.*** The ***IgA present in serum is predominantly monomeric*** (one four-chain unit) and has presumably been released before dimerization so that it fails to bind to the secretory component. Secretory IgA is very important biologically, but little is known of any function for serum IgA.

Most IgA is present not in the serum, but in secretions such as tears, saliva, sweat, and mucus, where it serves an important biologic function such as being part of the mucosa-associated lymphoid tissue (MALT), as mentioned in Chapter 2. ***Within mucous secretions, IgA exists as a dimer*** consisting of two four-chain units linked by the same joining (J) chain found in IgM molecules (Fig. 4.9). IgA-secreting plasma cells synthesize the IgA molecules and the J chains, which form the dimers. Such plasma cells are located predominantly in the connective tissue called ***lamina propria,*** which lies immediately below the basement membrane of many surface epithelia (e.g., in the parotid gland, along the gastrointestinal tract in the intestinal villi, in tear glands, in the lactating breast, or beneath bronchial mucosa). When these dimeric molecules are released from plasma cells, they bind to the poly-Ig receptor expressed on the basal membranes of adjacent epithelial cells. This receptor transports the molecules through the epithelial cells and releases them into extracellular fluids (e.g., in the gut or bronchi). Release is facilitated by enzymatic cleavage of the poly-Ig receptor, leaving a large 70,000 Da fragment (i.e., the secretory component) of the receptor still attached to the Fc piece of the dimeric IgA molecule (Fig. 4.13). The secretory component may help protect the dimeric IgA from proteolytic cleavage. It should be noted that the secretory component also binds

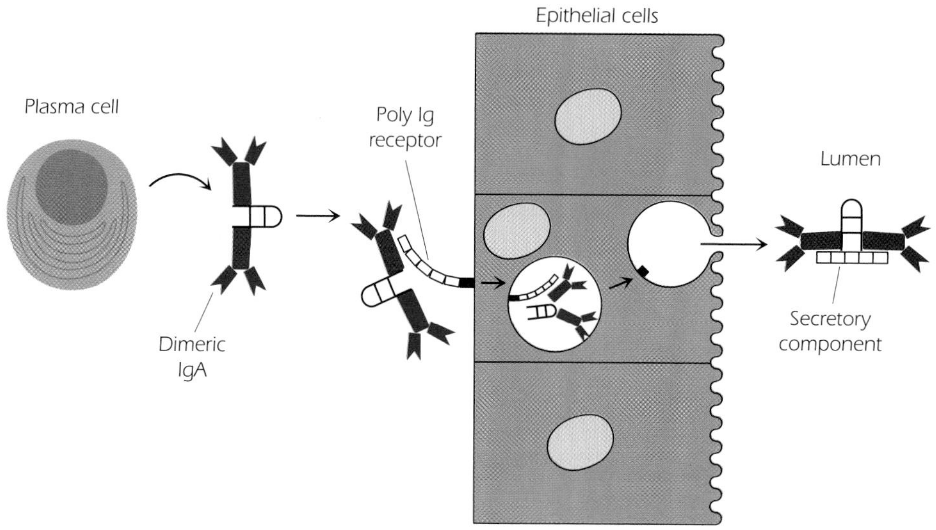

Figure 4.13. Transcytosis of dimeric IgA across epithelia. Plasma cells in close proximity to epithelial basement membranes in the gut, respiratory epithelia, salivary and tear glands, and lactating mammary glands, release dimeric IgA. The IgA binds to the poly-Ig receptor, and the complex undergoes transcytosis within vesicles across the cell. The poly-Ig receptor is cleaved from the complex at the apical surface to release the IgA from the cell. After exiting the cell, a pentameric fragment of the poly-Ig receptor, known as the secretory component, remains attached to the dimeric IgA and is believed to protect the antibody within the lumen of several organs that are in contact with the external environment.

and transports pentameric IgM to mucosal surfaces in small amounts.

Role in Mucosal Infections

Because of its presence in secretions, such as saliva, urine, and gastric fluid, secretory IgA is of importance in the primary immunologic defense against local ***respiratory or gastrointestinal infections.*** Its protective effect is thought to be due to its ability to prevent the invading organism from attaching to and penetrating the epithelial surface. For example, in the case of cholera, the pathogenic *Vibrio* organism attaches to, but never penetrates beyond, the cells that line the gastrointestinal tract, where it secretes an exotoxin responsible for all symptoms. IgA antibody, which can prevent attachment of the organism to the cells, provides protection from the pathogen. Thus, for protection against local infections, routes of immunization that result in local production of IgA are much more effective than routes that primarily produce antibodies in serum.

Bactericidal Activity

The IgA molecule does not contain receptors for complement, and thus ***IgA is not a complement-activating*** or complement-fixing immunoglobulin. Consequently, it does not induce complement-mediated bacterial lysis. However, IgA has been shown to possess bactericidal activity against gram-negative organisms, but only in the presence of lysozyme, which is also present in the same secretions that contain secretory IgA.

Antiviral Activity

Secretory IgA is an efficient antiviral antibody, preventing the viruses from entering host cells. In addition, secretory IgA is an efficient agglutinating antibody.

STRUCTURAL AND BIOLOGIC PROPERTIES OF IgD

The IgD molecule consists of either two κ or two λ light chains and two δ heavy chains (Fig. 4.9). IgD is present as a monomer with a molecular weight of 180,000 Da, it has a sedimentation coefficient of 7S, and it migrates to the fast γ-region of serum globulins. No heavy chain allotypes (see below) or subclasses have been reported for the IgD molecule.

IgD is present in serum in very low and variable amounts, probably because it is not secreted by plasma cells and because, among immunoglobulins, it is uniquely susceptible to proteolytic degradation. In addition, following B cell activation, transcription of the δ heavy chain protein is rapidly downregulated—a phenomenon that also helps explain the low serum IgD levels.

IgD is co-expressed with IgM on the surface of mature B cells and, like IgM, functions as an antigen-specific BCR.

Its presence there serves as a marker of the differentiation of B cells to a more mature form. Thus, during ontogeny of B cells, expression of IgD lags behind that of IgM (see Chapter 7).

While the function of IgD has not been fully elucidated, expression of membrane IgD appears to correlate with the elimination of B cells with the capacity to generate self-reactive antibodies. Thus, during development, the major biologic significance of IgD may be in silencing autoreactive B cells. In mature B cells, IgD serves as an antigen-binding surface immunoglobulin together with co-expressed IgM.

STRUCTURAL AND BIOLOGIC PROPERTIES OF IgE

The IgE molecule consists of two light chains (κ or λ) and two heavy chains (ε). Like the IgM molecule, IgE has an extra C_H domain (Fig. 4.9). IgE has a molecular weight of ~200,000 Da, its sedimentation coefficient is 8S, and it migrates electrophoretically to the fast γ-region of serum globulins. To date, no heavy chain allotypes or subclasses of IgE have been reported.

Importance of IgE in Parasitic Infections and Hypersensitivity Reactions

IgE, also termed ***reaginic antibody,*** has a ***half-life in serum of 2 days,*** the shortest half-life of all classes of immunoglobulins. It is present in serum in the lowest concentration of all immunoglobulins. These low levels are, in part, due to a low rate of synthesis and to the unique ability of the Fc portion of IgE, containing the extra C_H domain, to bind with very high affinity to receptors (Fcε receptors) found on mast cells and basophils. Once bound to these high-affinity receptors, IgE may be retained by these cells for weeks or months. When antigen reappears, it combines with the Fab portion of the IgE attached to these cells, causing it to be cross-linked. The cells become activated and release the contents of their granules: histamine, heparin, leukotrienes, and other pharmacologically active compounds that trigger the immediate hypersensitivity reactions. These reactions may be mild, as in the case of a mosquito bite, or severe, as in the case of bronchial asthma; they may even result in systemic anaphylaxis, which can cause death within minutes (Chapter 14).

IgE is not an agglutinating or complement-activating antibody; nevertheless, it has a role in protection against certain parasites, such as helminths (worms), a protection achieved by activation of the same acute inflammatory response seen in a more pathologic form of immediate hypersensitivity responses. Elevated levels of IgE in serum have been shown to occur during infections with ascaris (a roundworm). In fact, immunization with ascaris antigen induces the formation of IgE.

KINETICS OF THE ANTIBODY RESPONSE AFTER IMMUNIZATION

Primary Response

As mentioned in Chapter 3, the first exposure of an individual to a particular immunogen is referred to as the *priming immunization,* and the measurable response that ensues is called the *primary response.* As shown in Figure 4.12, the primary antibody response may be divided into several phases, as follows:

1. ***Latent, or lag, phase:*** After initial exposure to antigen, a significant amount of time elapses before antibody is detectable in the serum. The length of this period is generally 1 to 2 weeks, depending on the species immunized, the antigen, and other factors (discussed subsequent chapters). The length of the latent period also greatly depends on the sensitivity of the assay used to measure the product of the response. As we shall see in more detail later, the latent period includes the time taken for T and B cells to make contact with the antigen, to proliferate, and to differentiate. B cells must also secrete antibody in sufficient quantity so that it can be detected in the serum. The less sensitive the assay used for detection of antibody, the more antibody will be required for detection and the longer the apparent latent period will be.
2. ***Exponential phase:*** During this phase, the concentration of antibody in the serum increases exponentially.
3. ***Steady state:*** During this period, production and degradation of antibody are balanced.
4. ***Declining phase:*** Finally, the immune response begins to shut down, and the concentration of antibody in serum declines rapidly.

In the primary response, the first class of antibody detected is generally IgM, which in some instances may be the only class of immunoglobulin that is made. If production of IgG antibody ensues, its appearance is generally accompanied by a rapid cessation of production of IgM (Fig. 4.12).

Secondary Response

Although production of antibody after a priming contact with antigen may cease entirely within a few weeks (Fig. 4.12), the immunized individual is left with a ***cellular memory*** (i.e., long-lasting memory cells) of this contact. This memory response (also called ***anamnestic response***) becomes apparent when a response is triggered by a second injection of the same antigen. After the second injection, the lag phase is considerably shorter and antibody may appear in less than half the time required for the primary response. The production of antibody is much greater, and higher concentrations of antibody are detectable in the serum. The production of antibody may also continue for a longer period, with persistent levels remaining in the serum months, or even years, later.

There is a marked change in the type and quality of antibody produced in the secondary response. There is a shift in class response, known as ***class switching,*** with IgG antibodies appearing at higher concentrations and with greater persistence than IgM, which may be greatly reduced or disappear altogether. This may be also accompanied by the appearance of IgA and IgE. In addition, ***affinity maturation*** occurs—a phenomenon in which the average affinity (binding constant) of the antibodies for the antigen increases as the secondary response develops. The driving force for this increase in affinity may be a selection process during which B cells compete with free antibody to capture a decreasing amount of antigen. Thus only those B cell clones with high-affinity immunoglobulin receptors on their surfaces will bind enough antigen to ensure that the B cells are triggered to differentiate into plasma cells. These plasma cells, which arise from preferentially selected B cells, synthesize this antibody with high affinity for antigen.

The capacity to make a secondary response may persist for a long time (years in humans), and it provides an obvious selective advantage for individuals who survive the first contact with an invading pathogen. Establishment of this memory for generating a specific response is, of course, the purpose of public health immunization programs.

THE IMMUNOGLOBULIN SUPERFAMILY

The shared structural features of immunoglobulin heavy and light chains which include the ***immunoglobulin-fold domains*** (Fig. 4.3) are also seen in a large number of proteins. Most of these have been found to be membrane-bound glycoproteins. Because of this structural similarity, these proteins are classified as members of the ***immunoglobulin superfamily.*** The redundant structural characteristic seen in these proteins suggests that the genes that encode them arose from a common primordial gene—one that generated the basic domain structure. Duplication and subsequent divergence of this primordial gene would explain the existence of the large number of membrane proteins that possess one or more regions homologous to the immunoglobulin-fold domain. Genetic and functional analyses of these immunoglobulin superfamily proteins have indicated that these genes have evolved independently, since they do not share genetic linkage or function. Figure 4.14 provides some examples of proteins that are members of the immunoglobulin superfamily. Numerous other examples are discussed in other chapters. As can be seen, each molecule contains the characteristic immunoglobulin-fold structure (loops) formed as a result of intrachain disulfide bonds and consisting of approximately 110 amino acids. These domains are believed to facilitate interactions between membrane proteins (e.g., CD4 molecules on helper T cells and MHC class II molecules on antigen-presenting cells).

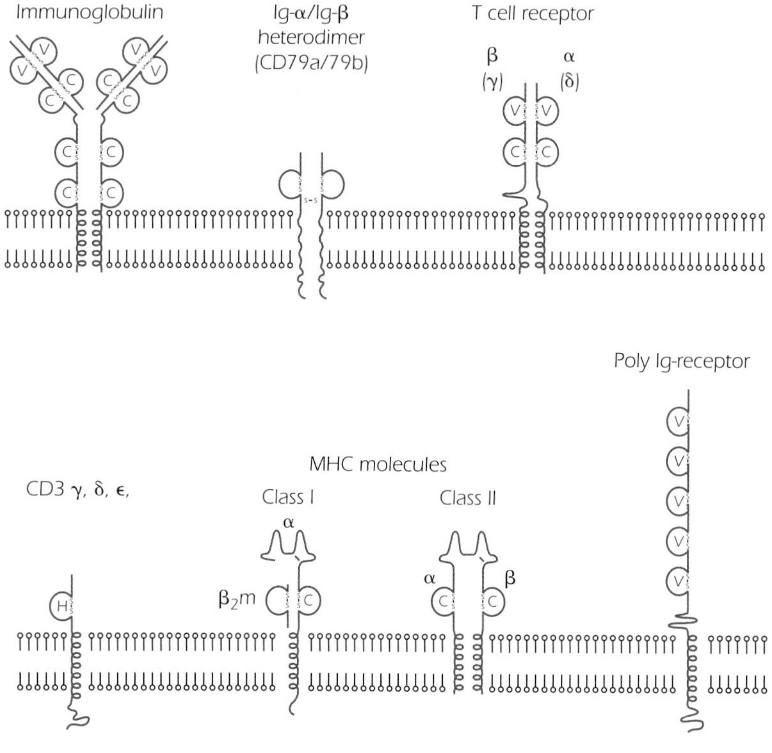

Figure 4.14. Representative members of the immunoglobulin superfamily. The immunoglobulin-fold domains (shown as circular loops in blue) form the common structural features of these molecules. In all cases, the carboxyl-terminal end of the molecules are anchored in the membrane.

SUMMARY

1. Immunoglobulins of all classes have a fundamental four-chain structure, consisting of two identical light (L) and two identical heavy (H) chains. Through disulfide bonds, each light chain is linked to a heavy chain and the two heavy chains are linked to each other.

2. In the native state, the chains are coiled into domains stabilized by an intrachain disulfide bond. A group of other proteins (e.g., TCR, CD4, and MHC class I and class II molecules) also contain these immunoglobulin-fold domains, making them all members of the immunoglobulin superfamily.

3. Immunoglobulins are expressed in two forms: a membrane-bound antibody present on the surface of B cells and a secreted antibody produced by plasma cells. Membrane-bound antibodies associate with a heterodimer called Igα/Igβ to form the B cell receptor.

4. The N-terminal domains of both heavy and light chains are the variable (V) regions and contain the hypervariable regions, also called complementarity-determining regions, which make up the combining site of the antibody and vary according to the specificity of the antibody.

5. The other domains are the constant (C) regions; these domains are similar within each class of immunoglobulin molecule.

6. The Fc regions of the heavy chains are responsible for the different biologic functions carried out by each class of antibody.

7. Immunoglobulin heavy chain isotypes are distinguished by the structure of their constant regions. Immunoglobulins with differences in their alleles for these regions, even a one or two amino acid change, are called allotypes and distinguish individuals within a species. By contrast, idiotypic markers are represented by the unique combinations of amino acids that make up the combining site of an antibody molecule; they are unique for that particular antibody.

8. IgG is a class of antibody capable of carrying out numerous biologic functions that range from neutralization of toxin to activation of complement and opsonization. IgG is the only class of immunoglobulin that passes through the placenta and confers maternal immunity on the fetus. The half-life of IgG (23 days) is the longest of all immunoglobulin classes.

9. IgM is expressed on the surface of mature B cells (as a monomer) and is secreted as a pentameric antibody; of all classes of immunoglobulin, it functions as the best agglutinating and complement-activating antibody.

10. IgA is present in monomeric and dimeric forms. The dimeric IgA, found in secretions and referred to as secretory IgA, is an important antiviral immunoglobulin.

11. IgD is present on the surface of mature B cells and is co-expressed and shares antigen-specificity with IgM. The functional properties of IgD have not been fully elucidated.

12. IgE, also called reaginic antibody, is of paramount importance in allergic reactions. It also appears to be of importance in protection against parasitic infections. The Fc portion of IgE binds with high affinity to receptors on certain cells, including mast cells. On contact with antigen, IgE triggers the degranulation of such cells, resulting in the release of pharmacologically active substances that mediate the hypersensitivity (allergic) reactions.

13. Following the first immunization, the primary response consists mainly of the production of IgM antibodies. The second exposure to the same antigen results in a secondary or anamnestic (memory) response, which is more rapid than the primary response, and the response shifts from IgM production to the synthesis of IgG and other isotypes. The secondary response lasts much longer than the primary response.

REFERENCES

Alzari PM, Lascombe MB, Poljak RJ (1988): Three dimensional structure of antibodies. *Annu Rev Immunol* 6:555.

Capra D, Edmundson AB (1977): The antibody combining site. *Sci Am* 236:50.

Carayannopoulos L, Capra JD (1998): Immunoglobulins: structure and function. In Paul WE (ed): Fundamental Immunology, 4th ed. New York: Raven.

Davies DR, Metzger H (1983): Structural basis of antibody function. *Annu Rev Immunol* 1:87.

Eisen HN (2001): Specificity and degeneracy in antigen

recognition: yin and yang in the immune response. *Ann Rev Immunol* 19:1.

Jefferis R (1993): What is an idiotype? *Immunol Today* 14:19.

Junghans RP, Anderson CL (1996): The protection receptor for IgG catabolism is the β2-microglobulin-containing neonatal intestinal transport receptor. *Proc Natl Acad Sci USA* 93:5512.

Koshland ME (1985): The coming of age of the immunoglobulin J chain. *Annu Rev Immunol* 3:425.

Mestecky J, McGhee JR (1987): Immunoglobulin A (IgA): molecular and cellular interactions involved in IgA biosynthesis and immune response. *Adv Immunol* 40:153.

Stanfield RL, Fisher TM, Lerner R, Wilson IA (1990): Crystal structure of an antibody to a peptide and its complex with peptide antigen at 2.8 D. *Science* 248:712.

Tomasi TB (1992): The discovery of secretory IgA and the mucosal immune system. *Immunol Today* 13:416.

Williams AF, Barclay AN (1988): The immunoglobulin superfamily. *Annu Rev Immuno*l 6:381.

REVIEW QUESTIONS

For each question, choose the ONE BEST answer or completion.

1. Functional properties of immunoglobulins, such as binding to Fc receptors, are associated with
A) light chains.
B) J chains.
C) disulfide bonds.
D) heavy chains.
E) variable regions.

2. The idiotype of an antibody molecule is determined by the amino acid sequence of the
A) constant region of the light chain.
B) variable region of the light chain.
C) constant region of the heavy chain.
D) constant regions of the heavy and light chains.
E) variable regions of the heavy and light chains.

3. Which of the following would generate a polyclonal rabbit antiserum specific for human γ heavy chain, κ chain, λ chain, and Fc regions of immunoglobulin?
A) Bench Jones proteins
B) pooled IgG
C) pepsin-digested IgG
D) purified Fab
E) purified $F(ab')_2$

4. A polyclonal antiserum raised against pooled human IgA will react with
A) human IgM.
B) κ light chains.
C) human IgG.
D) J chain.
E) all of the above.

5. An individual was found to be heterzygous for IgG_1 allotypes 3 and 12. The different possible IgG_1 antibodies produced by this individual will never have
A) two heavy chains of allotype 12.
B) two light chains of either κ or λ.
C) two heavy chains of allotype 3.
D) two heavy chains, one of allotype 3 and one of allotype 12.

6. Papain digestion of an IgG preparation of antibody specific for the antigen hen egg albumin (HEA) will
A) lose its antigen specificity.
B) precipitate with HEA.
C) lose all interchain disulfide bonds.
D) produce two Fab molecules and one Fc molecule.
E) None of the above.

7. In the serum of most normal individuals, the class of immunoglobulin that increases in chronic infections is which?
A) IgA
B) IgE
C) IgG
D) IgM
E) IgD

8. Which of the following immunoglobulins can activate complement as a single molecule when bound to an antigen?
A) IgA
B) B) IgE
C) IgG
D) IgM
E) IgD

9. The relative level of pathogen-specific IgM antibodies can be of diagnostic significance because
A) IgM is easier to detect than the other isotypes.
B) viral infection often results in very high IgM responses.
C) IgM antibodies are more often protective against reinfections than are the other isotypes.
D) relatively high levels of IgM often correlate with a first recent exposure to the inducing agent.

10. Primary and secondary antibody responses differ in
A) the predominant isotype generated.
B) the number of lymphocytes responding to antigen.
C) the speed at which antibodies appear in the serum.
D) the biologic functions manifested by the immunoglobulin isotypes produced.
E) All of the above.

ANSWERS TO REVIEW QUESTIONS

1. D The C-terminal end of the constant region of the heavy contains the domains that are associated with biologic activity of immunoglobulins.

2. E The idiotype is the antigenic determinant of an immunoglobulin molecule, which involves its antigen-combining site, which in turn consists of contributions from the variable regions of both L and H chains.

3. B Only pooled IgG, containing the a mixture of IgG molecules each expressing the γ heavy chain (thus the Fc region) and either the κ or λ light chains would generate an antiserum to each of these immunoglobulin components. None of the other answer choices would stimulate antibodies to all of these components. Bench Jones proteins are dimers of light chains found in the urine of patients with multiple myeloma. Pepsin treatment of IgG results in the digestion of the Fc region. Purified Fab and $F(ab')_2$ regions lack the γ heavy chain (thus the Fc region).

4. E All are correct statements. Antibody to IgA will have antibody specific for κ and λ light chains, which, of course, will react with IgG and IgM, both of which have κ and λ chains. Antibody will also be present against J chain if the IgA used for immunization was dimeric.

5. D In any immunoglobulin produced by a single cell, the two H chains and the two L chains are identical. Therefore, any antibody molecule in this individual would have either allotype 3 H chains or allotype 12 H chains, not a mixture. Similarly, the antibody would have either two κ or two λ chains.

6. D Papain digestion cleaves the IgG molecules above the hinge region, generating two Fab molecules and an Fc part. The Fab regions can still bind to HEA, but, since they are not held together by disulfide binds, they cannot precipitate the antigen. This contrasts with the effects of pepsin treatment of IgG, which cleaves below the hinge region, leaving intact one divalent $F(ab')_2$ molecule capable of precipitating the antigen. Fragments of pepsin-treated HEA-specific antibody will have the same affinity for the antigen as the original Fab regions of the antibody, since the CDR regions of the molecules are preserved.

7. C Chronic infections result in repeated stimulation of B cells engaged in an immune response to the pathogen causing the infection. Thus, in normal individuals, serum levels of IgG will increase during the course of the infection.

8. D Only IgM can activate or fix complement when a single molecule is bound to antigen. This is due to the pentameric form of this immunoglobulin class.

9. D Only the last statement is correct. Relatively high levels of IgM often correlate with first recent exposure to an inducing agent, since IgM is the first isotype synthesized in response to an immunogen. All other statements are not true.

10. E All are correct. The statements are self-explanatory.

5

ANTIGEN–ANTIBODY INTERACTIONS, IMMUNE ASSAYS, AND EXPERIMENTAL SYSTEMS

INTRODUCTION

In previous chapters, we have, by necessity, touched on several techniques and assays that have been used to help us understand some fundamental aspects of innate and adaptive immunity. In this chapter, we discuss, in greater detail, in vitro techniques, assays, and experimental systems that are used in research and diagnostic laboratories. Some of these are strictly antibody-based (e.g., serological methods), whereas others employ molecular biologic methods, genetic engineering, cell culture techniques, and in vivo animal models that have greatly contributed to our understanding of the physiology and pathophysiology of the immune system. Since the sequencing of the human genome in 2000 and with aggressive efforts to sequence microbial genomes, approaches that use bioinformatics and computational biology (so-called ***in silica*** analyses) have emerged as promising methods for the study of our immune system. Based on information derived from genomic and proteomic databases, powerful software tools, and algorithms, these technologies hold great promise for the field of immunology. This is particularly true in regard to important efforts to identify immunogenic epitopes expressed by pathogens that can be studied further as candidate vaccines. Although this topic is beyond the scope of this chapter, it is important to keep in mind that future progress in the field of immunology will come from a combination of in vitro, in vivo, and in silica approaches.

We begin this chapter with a discussion of the physical dynamics of antigen–antibody interactions.

ANTIGEN–ANTIBODY INTERACTIONS

The reaction between antigen and serum antibodies (***serology***) serves as the basis for many immune assays. Because of the exquisite specificity of the immune response, the interaction between antigen and antibody in vitro is widely used for diagnostic purposes, for the detection and identification of either antigen or antibody. An example of the use of serology for the identification and classification of antigens is the ***serotyping*** of various microorganisms by the use of specific antisera.

The interaction of antigen with antibodies may result in a variety of consequences, including ***precipitation*** (if the antigen is soluble), ***agglutination*** (if the antigen is particulate), and ***activation of complement.*** All of these outcomes are caused by the interactions between multivalent antigens and antibodies that have at least two combining sites per molecule. The consequences of antigen–antibody interaction listed above do not represent the primary interaction between antibodies and a given epitope but, rather, depend on secondary phenomena, which result from the interactions between multivalent antigens and antibodies. Such phenomena as the formation of precipitates, agglutination, and complement activation would not occur if the antibody with two or more combining sites reacted with a hapten (i.e., a unideterminant, univalent antigen), nor would they occur as a result of the interaction between a univalent fragment of antibody (e.g., Fab) and an antigen, even if the antigen is multivalent. The reasons for these differences are shown in Figure 5.1. ***Cross-linking*** of various antigen molecules by antibody is

Immunology: A Short Course, Fifth Edition, By Richard Coico, Geoffrey Sunshine, and Eli Benjamini
ISBN 0-471-22689-0

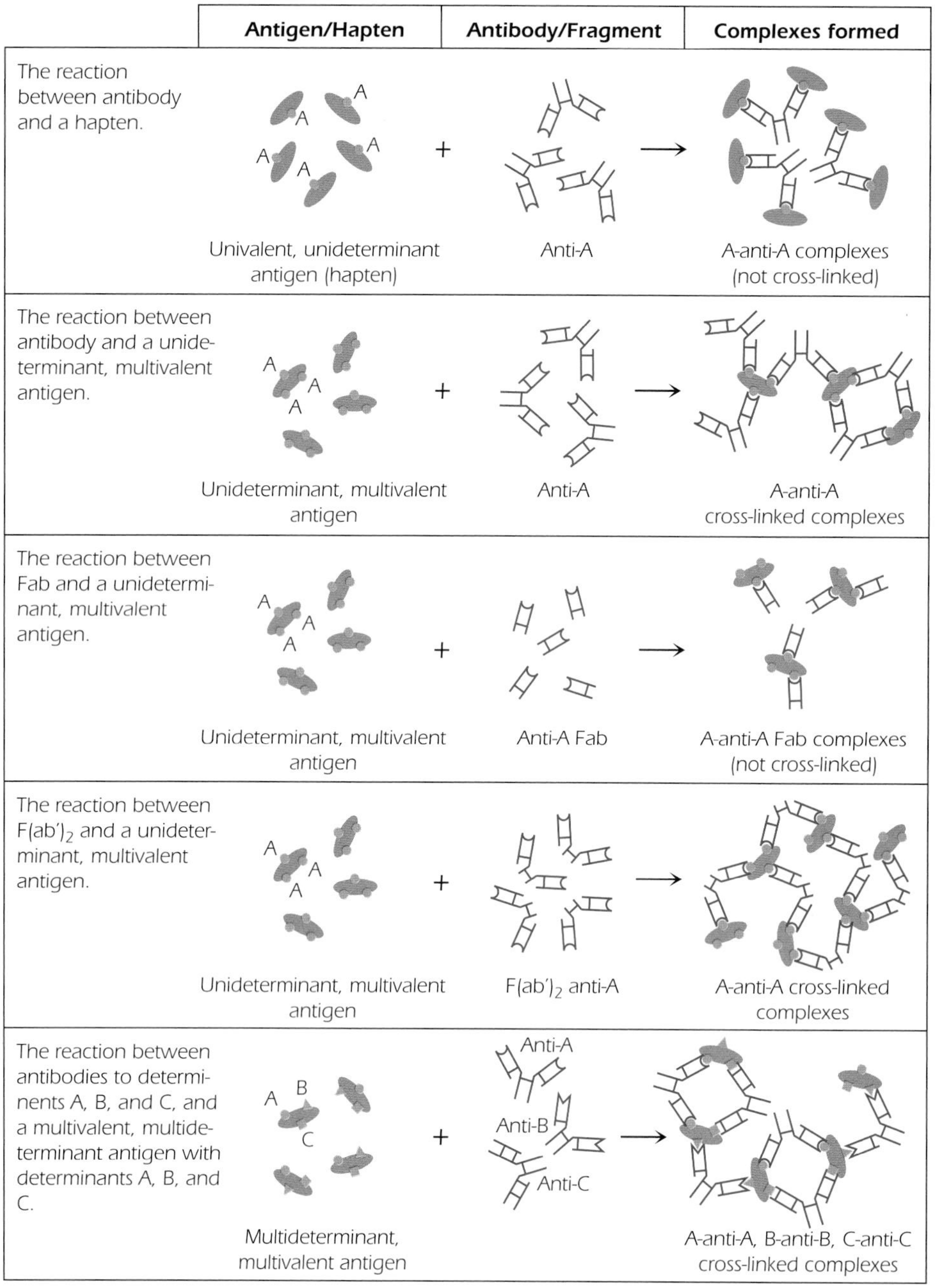

Antigen/Hapten
Antibody/Fragment
Complexes formed
The reaction between antibody and a hapten.
Univalent, unideterminant antigen (hapten)
Anti-A
A-anti-A complexes (not cross-linked)
The reaction between antibody and a unideterminant, multivalent antigen.
Unideterminant, multivalent antigen
Anti-A
A-anti-A cross-linked complexes
The reaction between Fab and a unideterminant, multivalent antigen.
Unideterminant, multivalent antigen
Anti-A Fab
A-anti-A Fab complexes (not cross-linked)
The reaction between F(ab')2 and a unideterminant, multivalent antigen.
Unideterminant, multivalent antigen
F(ab')2 anti-A
A-anti-A cross-linked complexes
The reaction between antibodies to determinents A, B, and C, and a multivalent, multideterminant antigen with determinants A, B, and C.
Multideterminant, multivalent antigen
Anti-A
Anti-B
Anti-C
A-anti-A, B-anti-B, C-anti-C cross-linked complexes

Figure 5.1. Reactions between antibody or antibody fragments and antigens or hapten.

required for precipitation, agglutination, or complement activation, and it is possible only if the antigen is multivalent and the antibody is divalent, either intact, or $F(ab')_2$ (Fig. 5.1). By contrast, no cross-linking is possible if the antigen or the antibody is univalent.

PRIMARY INTERACTIONS BETWEEN ANTIBODY AND ANTIGEN

No covalent bonds are involved in the interaction between antibody and an epitope. Consequently, the binding forces are relatively weak. They consist mainly of ***van der Waals forces, electrostatic forces,*** and ***hydrophobic forces,*** all of which require a very close proximity between the interacting moieties. Thus the interaction requires a close fit between an epitope and the antibody, a fit that is often compared to that of a lock and a key. Because of the low levels of energy involved in the interaction between antigen and antibody, antigen–antibody complexes can be readily dissociated by low or high pH, by high salt concentrations, or by chaotropic ions (e.g., cyanates), which efficiently interfere with the hydrogen bonding of water molecules.

Association Constant

The reaction between an antibody and an epitope of an antigen is exemplified by the reaction between antibody and a univalent hapten. Because an antibody molecule is symmetric, with two identical Fab antigen-combining sites, one antibody molecule binds with two identical monovalent hapten molecules, each Fab binding in an independent fashion with one hapten molecule. The binding of a monovalent antigen (Ag) with each site can be represented by the following equation:

$$\mathrm{Ag} + \mathrm{Ab} \underset{k_{-1}}{\overset{k_1}{\rightleftharpoons}} \mathrm{Ab} - \mathrm{Ag}$$

where k_1 represents the forward (association) rate constant and, k_{-1} represents the reverse (dissociation) rate constant, and Ab is antibody. The ratio of $k_1{:}k_{-1}$ is the association constant K, a measure of affinity. It can be calculated by determining the ratio of bound antibody–antigen complex to the concentration of unbound antigen and antibody:

$$K = \frac{k_1}{k_{-1}} = \frac{[\mathrm{Ab} - \mathrm{Ag}]}{[Ab][Ag]}$$

The association constant (K) is really a measure of the affinity of the antibody for the epitope. When all the antibody molecules that bind a given hapten or epitope are identical (as in the case of monoclonal antibodies), then K represents the intrinsic association constant. However, because serum antibodies—even those binding to a single epitope—are heterogeneous, an average ***association constant*** of all the antibodies to the epitope is referred to as K_0. The interaction between antibodies and each epitope of a multivalent antigen follows the same kinetics and energetics as those involved in the interaction between antibodies and haptens, because each epitope of the antigen reacts with its corresponding antibody in the same manner as that described above.

The association constant (K) can be determined using the method of ***equilibrium dialysis.*** In this procedure, a dialysis chamber is used in which two compartments are separated by a semipermeable membrane that allows the free passage of appropriately sized molecules from one side to the other. Antibody is placed on one side of the semipermeable membrane and cannot pass through because of its size. On the antigen side of the membrane, a known amount of small, permeable, radiolabeled hapten molecules, oligosaccharides, or oligopeptides, making up the epitope of the complex carbohydrate or protein, is added. At time zero, the hapten or antigenic epitope used (referred to as the *ligand* hereafter) will then diffuse across the membrane; at equilibrium, the concentration of free ligand will be the same on both sides. However, the total amount of ligand will be greater on the antibody-containing side because some of the ligand will be bound to the antibody molecules. The difference in the ligand concentration in the two compartments represents the concentration of the ligand bound to antibody (i.e., the [AgAb] complex). The higher the affinity of the antibody, the more ligand that is bound.

Since the concentration of antibody added to the equilibrium dialysis chamber can be predetermined and kept constant, varying concentrations of ligand can also be used in this analysis. This approach facilitates the so-called ***Scatchard analysis*** of the antibody. This is useful in determining whether a given antibody preparation is homogeneous (e.g., monoclonal antibody) or heterogeneous (e.g., polyclonal antiserum) and in measuring the average affinity constant (K_0).

Affinity and Avidity

As noted above, the intrinsic association constant that characterizes the binding of an antibody with an epitope or a hapten is termed ***affinity.*** When the antigen consists of many repeating identical epitopes or when antigens are multivalent, the association between the entire antigen molecule and antibodies depends not only on the affinity between each epitope and its corresponding antibody but also on the sum of the affinities of all the epitopes involved. For example, the affinity of binding of anti-A with multivalent A may be four or five orders of magnitude higher than that between the same antibody (i.e., anti-A) and univalent A (Fig. 5.1). This is because the pairing of anti-A with A (where A is multivalent) is influenced by the increased number of sites on A with which anti-A can react.

While the term *affinity* denotes the intrinsic association constant between antibody and a univalent ligand, such as a hapten, the term ***avidity*** is used to denote the overall binding energy between antibodies and a multivalent antigen. Thus, in general, IgM antibodies are of higher avidity than IgG antibodies, although the binding of each Fab in the IgM antibody with ligand may be of the same affinity as that of the Fab from IgG.

SECONDARY INTERACTIONS BETWEEN ANTIBODY AND ANTIGEN

Agglutination Reactions

Refer again to Figure 5.1; the reactions of antibody with a multivalent antigen that is ***particulate*** (i.e., an insoluble particle) results in the cross-linking of the various antigen particles by the antibodies. This cross-linking eventually results in the clumping or ***agglutination*** of the antigen particles by the antibodies.

Titer. The agglutination of an antigen as a result of cross-linking by antibodies depends on the correct proportion of antigen to antibody. A method sometimes used to measure the level of serum antibody specific for a particulate antigen is the agglutination assay. More sensitive, quantitative assays (e.g., enzyme-linked immunosorbent assay, discussed later in this chapter) have largely replaced this approach for measuring antibody levels in serum. Indeed, the agglutinating titer of a certain serum is only a semiquantitative expression

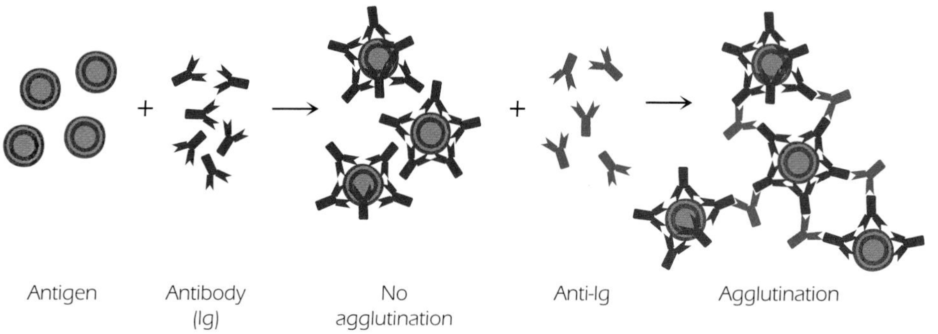

Figure 5.2. The anti-immunoglobulin (Coombs) test.

of the antibodies present in the serum; it is not a quantitative measure of the concentration of antibody (weight to volume). The assay is performed by mixing twofold serial dilutions of serum with a fixed concentration of antigen. High dilutions of serum usually do not cause antigen agglutination because at such dilutions there are not enough antibodies to cause appreciable, visible agglutination. The highest dilution of serum that still causes agglutination, but beyond which no agglutination occurs, is termed the ***titer.*** It is a common observation that agglutination may not occur at high concentrations of antibody, even though it does take place at higher dilutions of serum. The tubes with high concentrations of serum, where agglutination does not occur, represent a ***prozone.*** In the prozone, antibodies are present in excess. Agglutination may not occur at high ratio of antibody to antigen because every epitope on one particle may bind only to a single antibody molecule, preventing cross-linking between different particles.

Because of the prozone phenomenon, in testing for the presence of agglutinating antibodies to a certain antigen, it is imperative that the antiserum be tested at several dilutions. Testing serum at only one concentration may give misleading conclusions if no agglutination occurs, because the absence of agglutination might reflect either a prozone or a lack of antibody.

Zeta Potential. The surfaces of certain particulate antigens may possess an electrical charge, as, for example, the net negative charge on the surface of red blood cells caused by the presence of sialic acid. When such charged particles are suspended in saline solution, an electrical potential, termed the ***zeta potential,*** is created between particles, preventing them from getting very close to each other. This introduces a difficulty in agglutinating charged particles by antibodies, in particular red blood cells by IgG antibodies. The distance between the Fab arms of the IgG molecule, even in its most extended form, is too short to allow effective bridging between two red blood cells across the zeta potential. Thus, although IgG antibodies may be directed against antigens on the charged erythrocyte, agglutination may not occur because of the repulsion by the zeta potential. On the other hand, some of the Fab areas of IgM pentamers are far enough apart and can bridge red blood cells separated by the zeta potential. This property of IgM antibodies, together with their pentavalence, is a major reason for their effectiveness as agglutinating antibodies.

Through the years, attempts were made to improve agglutination reactions by decreasing the zeta potential in various ways, none of which was universally applicable or effective. However, an ingenious method was devised in the 1950s by Coombs to overcome this problem. This method, described next, facilitates the agglutination of erythrocytes by IgG antibodies specific for erythrocyte antigens. It is also useful for the detection of nonagglutinating antibodies that are present on the surface of erythrocytes.

The Coombs Test. The Coombs test employs antibodies to immunoglobulins (hence it is also called the ***anti-immunoglobulin test***). It is based on two important facts: (1) that immunoglobulins of one species (e.g., human) are immunogenic when injected into another species (e.g., rabbit) and lead to the production of antibodies against the immunoglobulins, and (2) that many of the anti-immunoglobulins (e.g., rabbit anti-human Ig) bind with antigenic determinants present on the Fc portion of the antibody and leave the Fab portions free to react with antigen. Thus, for example, if human IgG antibodies are attached to their respective epitopes on erythrocytes, then the addition of rabbit antibodies to human IgG will result in their binding with the Fc portions of the human antibodies bound to the erythrocytes by their Fab portion (Fig. 5.2). These rabbit antibodies not only bind with the human antibodies that are bound to the erythrocyte but also, by so doing, form cross-links (bridges) between human IgG on relatively distant erythrocytes, across the separation caused by the zeta potential, and cause agglutination. The addition of anti-immunoglobulin brings about agglutination, even if the antibodies directed against the erythrocytes are present at sufficiently high concentrations to cause the prozone phenomenon.

There are two versions of the Coombs test: the ***direct Coombs test*** and the ***indirect Coombs test.*** The two versions differ somewhat in the mechanics of the test, but both are based on the same principle: using heterologous anti-immunoglobulins to detect a reaction between immunoglobulins and antigen. In the direct Coombs test, anti-immunoglobulins are added to the particles (e.g., red blood cells) that are suspected of having antibodies bound to antigens on their surfaces. For example, a newborn baby is suspected of having hemolytic disease of the newborn caused by maternal anti-Rh IgG antibodies that are bound to the baby's erythrocytes. If that suspicion proved to be correct, the direct Coombs test would have the following results: The addition of anti-immunoglobulin to a suspension of the baby's erythrocytes causes binding of the anti-immunoglobulin to the maternal IgG on the surface of the erythrocytes, leading to agglutination. The indirect Coombs test is used to detect the presence, in the serum, of antibodies specific to antigens on the particle. The serum antibodies, when added to the particles, may fail to cause agglutination because of the zeta potential. The subsequent addition of anti-immunoglobulin will cause agglutination. A common application of the indirect Coombs test is to detect anti-Rh IgG antibodies in the blood of an Rh^- woman (see Chapter 15). This consists, first, of the reaction of the woman's serum with Rh^+ erythrocytes and, then the addition of the anti-immunoglobulin reagents (as in the direct Coombs test). Thus the direct Coombs test measures bound antibody, whereas the indirect test measures serum antibody.

Originally, the Coombs test was used for the detection of human antibodies on the surface of erythrocytes. Today, the term is applied to the detection, by the use of anti-immunoglobulin, of any immunoglobulin that is bound to antigen.

Passive Agglutination. The agglutination reaction can be used with particulate antigens (e.g., erythrocytes or bacteria) and with soluble antigens, provided that the soluble antigen can be firmly attached to insoluble particles. For example, the soluble antigen thyroglobulin can be attached to latex particles, so that the addition of antibodies to the thyroglobulin antigen will cause agglutination of the latex particles coated with thyroglobulin. Of course, the addition of soluble antigen to the antibodies before the introduction of the thyroglobulin-coated latex particles will inhibit the agglutination, because the antibodies will first combine with the soluble antigen; if the soluble antigen is present in excess, the antibodies will not be able to bind with the particulate antigen. This latter example is referred to as ***agglutination inhibition.*** It should be distinguished from agglutination inhibition in which antibodies to certain viruses inhibit the agglutination of red blood cells by the virus. In these cases, the antibodies are directed to the area or areas on the virus that bind with the appropriate virus receptors on the red blood cells.

When the antigen is a natural constituent of a particle, the agglutination reaction is referred to as ***direct agglutination.*** When the agglutination reaction takes place between antibodies and soluble antigen that has been attached to an insoluble particle, the reaction is referred to as ***passive agglutination.***

The agglutination reaction (direct or passive, employing or not employing the Coombs test) is widely used clinically. In addition to the examples already given, major applications include erythrocyte typing in blood banks, diagnosis of various immunologically mediated hemolytic diseases (such as drug-induced autohemolytic anemia), tests for rheumatoid factor (human IgM, anti-human IgG), confirmatory test for syphilis, and the latex test for pregnancy. The latter involves the detection of human chorionic gonadotropin (hCG) in the urine of pregnant women.

Precipitation Reactions

Reaction in Solutions. In contrast to the agglutination reaction, which takes place between antibodies and particulate antigen, the ***precipitation reaction*** takes place when antibodies and soluble antigen are mixed. As in the case of agglutination, precipitation of antigen–antibody complexes occurs because the divalent antibody molecules cross-link multivalent antigen molecules to form a ***lattice.*** When it reaches a certain size, this antigen–antibody complex loses its solubility and precipitates out of solution.

Figure 5.3 depicts a qualitative precipitin reaction. When increasing concentrations of antigen are added to a series of

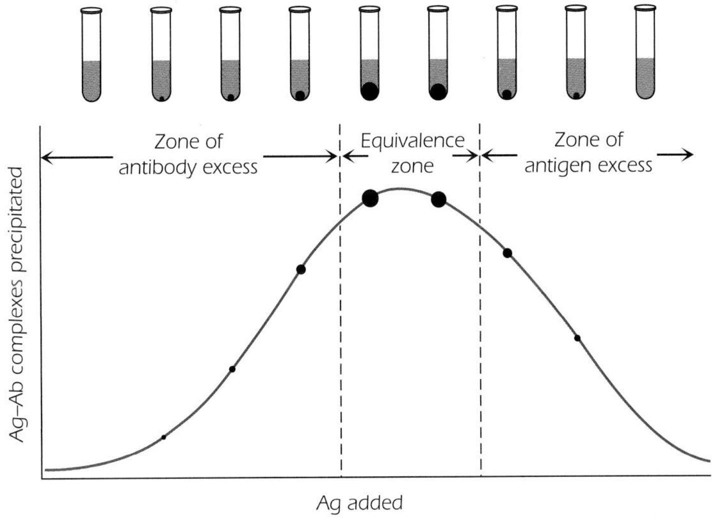

Figure 5.3. The precipitin reaction.

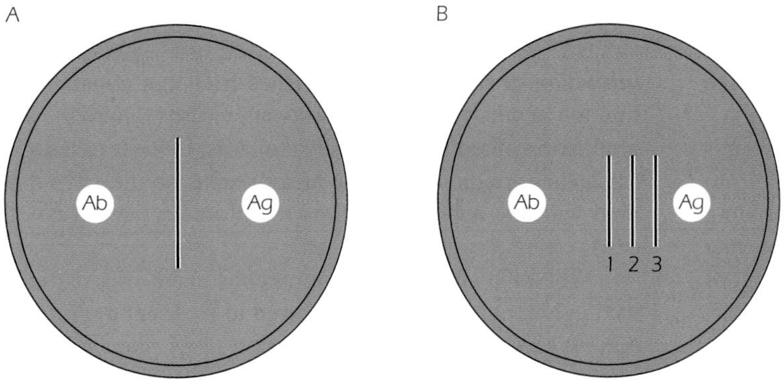

Figure 5.4. **(A)** Gel diffusion by antibodies and a single antigen. **(B)** Gel diffusion by antibodies to antigens 1, 2, 3.

tubes that contain a constant concentration of antibodies, variable amounts of precipitate form. The weight of the precipitate in each tube may be determined by a variety of methods. If the amount of the precipitate is plotted against the amount of antigen added, a precipitin curve, like the one shown in Figure 5.3, is obtained.

There are three important areas under the curve shown in Figure 5.3: (1) the zone of antibody excess, (2) the equivalence zone, and (3) the zone of antigen excess. In the equivalence zone, the proportion of antigen to antibody is optimal for maximal precipitation; in the zones of antibody excess or antigen excess, the proportions of the reactants do not lead to efficient cross-linking and formation of precipitate.

It should be emphasized that the zones of the precipitin curve are based on the amount of antigen–antibody complexes precipitated. However, the zones of antigen or antibody excess may contain soluble antigen–antibody complexes, particularly the zone of antigen excess, in which a minimal amount of precipitate is formed, but large amounts of ***antigen–antibody complexes*** are present in the supernatant. Thus the amount of precipitate formed depends on the proportions of the reactant antigens and antibodies: The correct proportion of the reactions results in maximal formation of precipitate; excess of antigen (or antibody) results in soluble complexes.

Precipitation Reactions in Gels. Precipitation reactions between soluble antigens and antibodies can take place not only in solution but also in semisolid media, such as agar gels. When soluble antigen and antibodies are placed in wells cut in the gel (Fig. 5.4A), the reactants diffuse in the gel and form gradients of concentration, with the highest concentrations closest to the wells. Somewhere between the two wells, the reacting antigen and antibodies will be present at proportions that are optimal for formation of a precipitate.

If the antibody well contains antibodies 1, 2, and 3 specific for antigens 1, 2, and 3, respectively, and diffuse at different rates (with diffusion rates of $1 > 2 > 3$), then three distinct precipitin lines will form. These three lines form because anti-1, anti-2, and anti-3, which diffuse at the same rate, react independently with antigens 1, 2, and 3, respectively, to form three equivalence zones and thus three separate lines of precipitate (Fig. 5.4B). Different rates of diffusion of both antibody and antibody and antigen result from differences in concentration, molecular size, or shape.

This ***double-diffusion method,*** developed by ***Ouchterlony*** (a name sometimes used to describe the assay in lieu of the term *double-diffusion*), by which antigen and antibody diffuse toward each other, is very useful for establishing the antigenic relationship between various substances. Three reaction patterns are seen in gel diffusion, each of which is shown in Figure 5.5: patterns of identity, patterns of nonidentity, and patterns of partial identity. Patterns of identity form when the two antigens are identical. A pattern in which the precipitin lines cross each other denotes nonidentity of the two antigens. Finally, patterns of partial identity form when the test antiserum reacts positively with antigens containing epitopes that match and do not match, causing a precipitin spur to appear in the gel.

Radial Immunodiffusion. The radial immunodiffusion test represents a variation of the double-diffusion test (Fig. 5.6). The wells contain antigen at different concentrations, and the antibodies are distributed uniformly in the agar

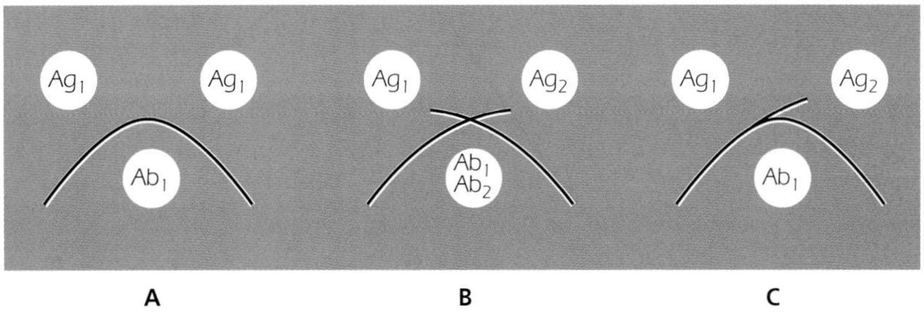

Figure 5.5. Double gel-diffusion patterns showing pattern of identity **(A)** pattern of nonidentity **(B)**, and pattern of partial identity **(C)**.

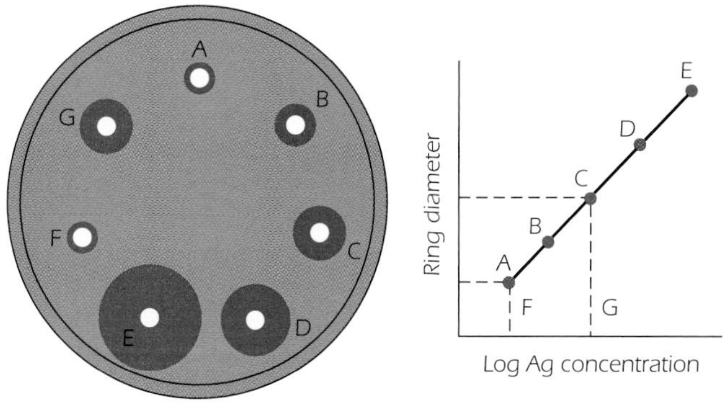

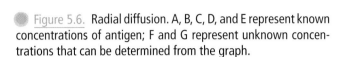

Figure 5.6. Radial diffusion. A, B, C, D, and E represent known concentrations of antigen; F and G represent unknown concentrations that can be determined from the graph.

gel. Thus the precipitin line is replaced by a precipitin ring around the well. The distance the precipitin ring migrates from the center of the antigen well is directly proportional to the concentration of antigen in the well. The relationship between concentration of antigen in a well and the diameter of the precipitin ring can be plotted (Fig. 5.6). If wells, such as F and G, contain unknown amounts of the same antigen, the concentration of that antigen in those wells can be determined by comparing the diameter of the precipitin ring with the diameter of the ring formed by a known concentration of the antigen.

An important application of radial immunodiffusion is its use clinically to measure concentrations of serum proteins. To do so, antiserum to various serum proteins is incorporated in the gel; concentration of a particular protein in a serum sample is determined by comparing the diameter of the resulting precipitin ring with the diameter obtained by known concentrations of the protein in question.

Immunoelectrophoresis. Immunoelectrophoresis involves separating a mixture of proteins in an electrical field (electrophoresis) followed by their detection with antibodies diffusing into the gel. It is very useful for the analysis of a mixture of antigens by antiserum that contains antibodies to the antigens in the mixture. For example, in the clinical characterization of human serum proteins, a small drop of human serum is placed in a well cut in the center of a slide that is coated with agar gel. The serum is then subjected to electrophoresis, which separates the various components according to their mobilities in the electrical field. After electrophoresis, a trough is cut along the side of the slides, and antibodies to human serum proteins are placed in the trough. The antibodies diffuse in the agar, as do the separated serum proteins. At an optimal antigen to antibody ratio for each antigen and its corresponding antibodies, precipitin lines from. The result is a pattern similar to that depicted in Figure 5.7. Comparison of the pattern and intensity of lines of normal human serum with the patterns and intensity of lines obtained with sera of patients may reveal an absence, overabundance, or other abnormality of one or more serum proteins. In fact, it was through the use of the immunoelectrophoresis assay that the first antibody-deficiency syndrome was identified in 1952 (Bruton's agammaglobulinemia) (see Chapter 17).

Western Blots (Immunoblots). In the Western blot (immunoblot) technique, antigen (or a mixture of antigens) is first separated in a gel. The separated material is then transferred onto protein-binding sheets (e.g., nitrocellulose) by using an electroblotting method. Antibody, which is then applied to the nitrocellulose sheet, binds with its specific antigen. The antibody may be labeled (e.g., with radioactivity), or a labeled anti-immunoglobulin may be used to localize the antibody and the antigen to which the first antibody is bound. These so-called Western blots are used widely in research and clinical laboratories for the detection and characterization of antigens. A particularly useful example is the confirmatory diagnosis of HIV infection by the application of a patient's serum to the nitrocellulose sheets on which HIV antigens are bound. The finding of specific antibody is strong evidence of infection by the virus (Fig. 5.8).

IMMUNOASSAYS

Direct Binding Immunoassays

Radioimmunoassay (RIA) employs isotopically labeled molecules and permits measurements of extremely small

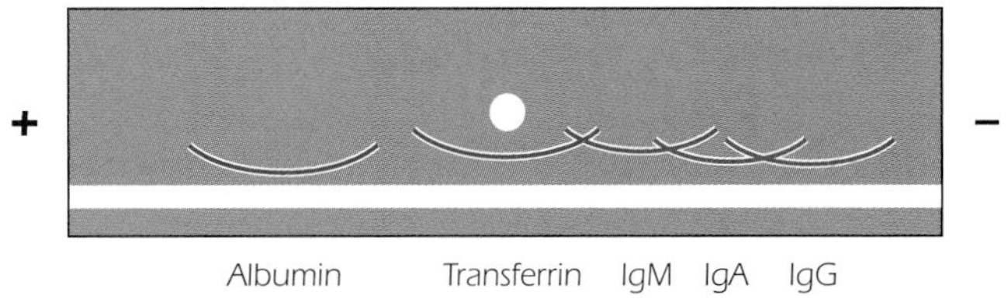

Figure 5.7. Patterns of immunoelectrophoresis of serum proteins.

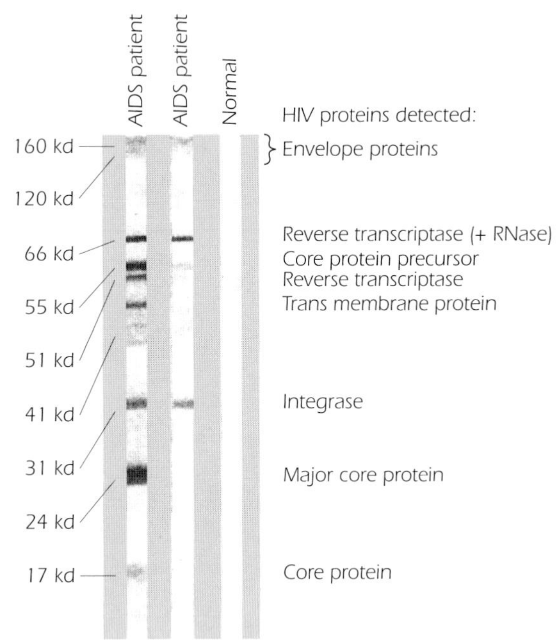

Figure 5.8. Western blots of serum samples from two HIV-infected individuals and one control subject.

amounts of antigen, antibody, or antigen–antibody complexes. The concentration of such labeled molecules is determined by measuring their radioactivity, rather than by chemical analysis. The sensitivity of detection is thus increased by several orders of magnitude. For the development of this highly sensitive analytical method, which has tremendous application in hormone assays as well as assays of other substances found at low levels in biologic fluids, Rosalyn Yalow received the Nobel Prize.

The principle of radioimmunoassay is shown in Figure 5.9. A known amount of radioactively labeled antigen is reacted with a limited amount of antibody. The solution now contains antibody-bound labeled antigen, as well as some unbound labeled antigen. After separating the antigen bound to antibody from free antigen, the amount of radioactivity bound to antibody is determined. The test continues with performance of a similar procedure in which the same amount of labeled antigen is premixed with unlabeled antigen (Fig. 5.10). The mixture is reacted with the same amount of antibody as before, and the antibody-bound antigen is separated from the unbound antigen. The unlabeled antigen competes with the labeled antigen for the antibody; as a result, less label is bound to antibody than in the absence of unlabeled antigen. The more unlabeled antigen present in the reaction mixture, the smaller the ratio of antibody-bound radiolabeled antigen to free radiolabeled antigen. This ratio can be plotted as a function of the concentration of the unlabeled antigen used for competition.

To determine an unknown concentration of antigen in a solution, a sample of the solution is mixed with predetermined amounts of labeled antigen and antibody. The ratio of bound to free radioactivity is compared with that obtained in the absence of unlabeled antigen (the latter value is set at 100%).

An important step in performing a radioimmunoassay, as described above, is the separation of free antigen from that bound to antibody. Depending on the antigen, this separation can be achieved in a variety of ways, principal among which is the anti-immunoglobulin procedure. This procedure is based on the fact that antigen (labeled or unlabeled) bound to immunoglobulin will also be precipitated, following the addition of anti-immunoglobulin antibodies, so that only unbound antigen remains in the supernatant. Radioimmunoassays commonly employ rabbit antibodies to the desired antigens. These rabbit antibody–antigen complexes may be precipitated by the addition of goat antibodies raised against rabbit immunoglobulins.

Since the amounts of antigen and antibody required for radioimmunoassay are extremely small, the antigen–antibody complexes reacted with anti-immunoglobulin would form only tiny precipitates. It is difficult, if not impossible, to recover these precipitates quantitatively by conventional means to determine their radioactivity. To overcome this problem, it is customary to add immunoglobulins that are not specific for the antigen in the reaction mixture, thereby increasing the amount of total immunoglobulins to a level that can easily be precipitated by anti-immunoglobulins and recovered quantitatively. Such precipitates consist mainly of nonspecific immunoglobulins to which radioactive antigen does not bind. However, they also contain the extremely small amount of antigen-specific immunoglobulin and any radioactive antigen bound to it.

An alternative method of separating complexes of antigen bound to antibody from free antigen is based on the fact that immunoglobulins become insoluble and precipitate in

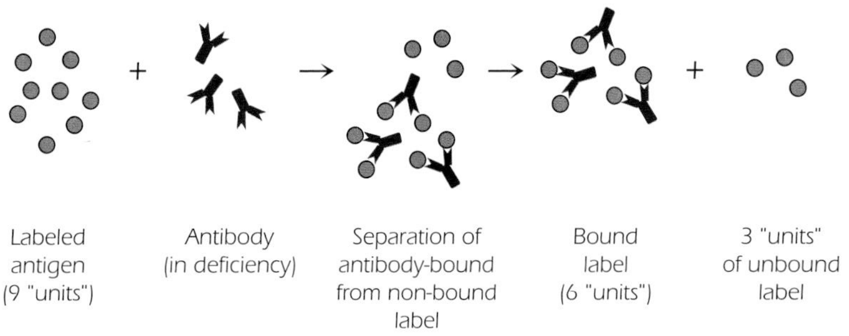

Figure 5.9. Amount of label bound to antibody after incubation of constant amounts of antibody and labeled antigen.

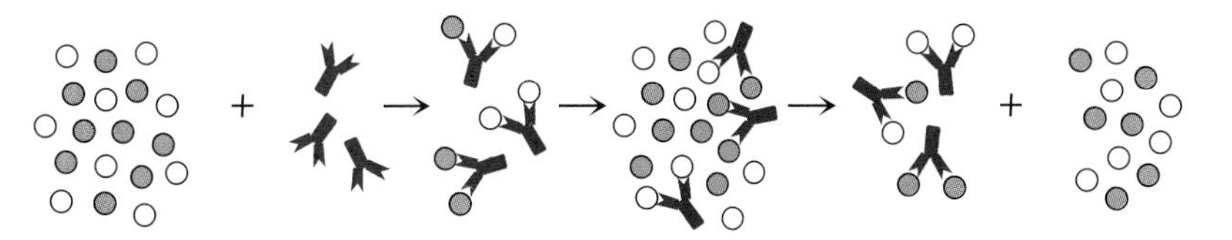

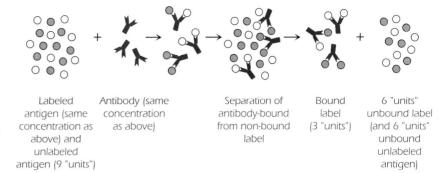

Figure 5.10. Radioimmunoassay, based on the competition of nonlabeled and labeled antigens for antibody.

a solution containing 33% saturated ammonium sulfate. If the antigen does not precipitate under these conditions, additional ammonium sulfate is added to cause the antibody complexed to antigen to precipitate, leaving the free antigen in solution. Here again, the amounts of antibodies reacting with antigen (or free antibodies) are small and unable to form precipitates. As described for the radioimmunoassay in which anti-immunoglobulins are used for the separation of antibody-bound antigen from free antigen, a sufficient amount of nonspecific immunoglobulin is added to the mixture; an appreciable precipitate will form at 33% saturation ammonium sulfate to enable the separation of free antigen from antigen bound to antibody.

Solid-Phase Immunoassays

Solid-phase immunoassay is one of the most widely used immunologic techniques. It is now automated and is widely used in clinical medicine for the detection of antigen or antibody. A good example is the use of solid-phase immunoassay for the detection of antibodies to HIV (see Chapter 17).

Solid-phase immunoassays employ the property of various plastics (e.g., polyvinyl or polystyrene) to adsorb monomolecular layers of proteins onto their surface. Although the adsorbed molecules may lose some of their antigenic determinants, enough remain unaltered and can still react with their corresponding antibodies. The presence of these antibodies, bound to antigen adsorbed onto the plastic, may be detected by the use of anti-immunoglobulins (Fig. 5.11) labeled with a radioactive tracer or with an enzyme. If the test uses anti-immunoglobulins that are labeled with an enzyme that can be detected by the appearance of a color on addition of substrate, the test is called an ***enzyme-linked immunosorbent assay*** (ELISA).

It should be emphasized that after coating the plastic surface with antigen, it is imperative to block any uncoated plastic surface to prevent it from absorbing the other reagents, especially the labeled reagent. Such blocking is achieved by coating the plastic surface with a high concentration of an unrelated protein, such as gelatin, after the application of the antigen.

Solid-phase immunoassay may be used to detect the presence of antibodies to the antigen that coats the plastic. Since the plastic wells are usually coated with relatively large amounts of antigen, the higher the concentration of antibodies bound with the antigen, the higher the amount of

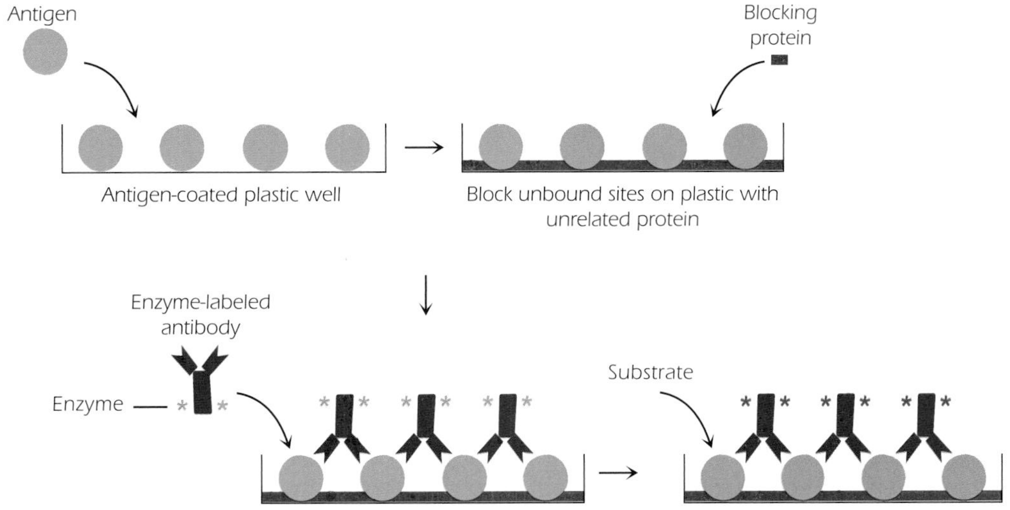

Figure 5.11. A representative ELISA using a well coated directly with antigen.

labeled anti-immunoglobulin that can bind to the antibodies. Thus it is important always to use an excess of labeled anti-immunoglobulin to ensure saturation.

Solid-phase immunoassay may be used for the qualitative or quantitative determinations of antigen. Such determinations are performed by mixing the antiserum with varying known amounts of antigen before adding the antiserum to the antigen-coated plastic wells. This preliminary procedure results in the binding of the antibodies with the soluble antigen, decreasing the availability of free antibodies for binding with the antigen that is coating the plastic. The higher the concentration of the soluble antigen that reacts with antibodies before the addition of the antibody to the wells, the lower the number of antibodies that can bind with the antigen on the plate, and the lower the number of labeled anti-immunoglobulin that can bind to these antibodies. The decrease in the amount of bound label as a function of the concentration of antigen used to cause this decrease can be plotted, and the amount of antigen in an unknown solution can then be determined from the graph by comparing the decrease in bound label caused by the unknown solution to the decrease caused by known concentrations of pure antigen.

IMMUNOFLUORESCENCE

A fluorescent compound has the property of emitting light of a certain wavelength when it is excited by exposure to light of a shorter wavelength. Immunofluorescence is a method for localizing an antigen by the use of fluorescently labeled antibodies. The procedure, originally described by Coombs, employs antibodies to which fluorescent groups have been covalently linked without any appreciable change in antibody activity.

One fluorescent compound that is widely used in immunology is fluorescein isothiocyanate (FITC), which fluoresces with a visible greenish color when excited by ultraviolet light. FITC is easily coupled to free amino groups. Another widely used fluorescent compound is phycoerythrin (PE), which fluoresces red and is also easily coupled to free amino groups. Fluorescence microscopes equipped with an ultraviolet (UV) light source permit visualization of fluorescent antibody on a microscopic specimen, and fluorescent antibodies are widely used to localize antigens on various tissues and microorganisms.

There are two important and related procedures that employ fluorescent antibodies: direct immunofluorescence and indirect immunofluorescence.

Direct Immunofluorescence

Direct immunofluorescence is used to directly detect antigen and involves reacting the target tissue (or microorganism) with fluorescently labeled antigen-specific antibodies. It is widely used clinically for identifying lymphocytic subsets and for demonstrating the presence of specific protein deposition in certain tissues such as kidney and skin in cases of systemic lupus erythematosus (SLE) (see Chapter 12).

Indirect Immunofluorescence

Indirect immunofluorescence involves first reacting the target with unlabeled specific antibodies. This reaction is followed by subsequent reaction with fluorescently labeled anti-immunoglobulin.

The indirect immunofluorescence method is more widely used than the direct method, because a single fluorescent anti-immunoglobulin antibody can be used to localize antibody of many different specificities. Moreover, since the anti-immunoglobulins contain antibodies to many epitopes on the specific immunoglobulin, the use of fluorescent anti-immunoglobulins significantly amplifies the fluorescent signal. An excellent example for the use of indirect immunofluorescence is the screening of patients' sera for anti-DNA antibodies in cases of SLE.

FLUORESCENCE-ACTIVATED CELL-SORTING ANALYSIS

A very powerful tool has been developed around the use of fluorescent antibody specific for cell-surface antigens. This is the technique of ***fluorescence-activated cell sorting*** (FACS). A cell suspension labeled with specific fluorescent antibody is passed through an apparatus that forms a stream of small droplets, each containing one cell. These droplets are passed between a laser beam of UV light and a detector for picking up emitted fluorescence when a labeled cell is present in the droplet. This emitted signal is passed to an electrode, which charges the droplet, leading to its deflection in an electromagnetic field (Fig. 5.12). Thus as the droplets fall past the laser beam, they are counted and can be sorted (e.g., unlabeled versus labeled) according to whether they emit a signal. The intensity of fluorescein staining on each cell, which reflects the density of antigen expressed on the cell, may be determined by sophisticated electronics.

With this type of apparatus, it is now possible to rapidly develop a profile of a pool of lymphocytes based on their differential expression of cell-surface molecules, the relative amount of cell-surface molecule expressed on each cell, and the size distribution and numbers of each cell type. It is also possible to use the apparatus to *sort* a collection of cells stained with five or more different fluorescent labels and obtain a very homogeneous sample of a particular cell type. A variation of this technique uses fluorescent antibodies coupled to magnetic beads to separate cell populations. Cells that bind to the fluorescent antibody can be separated from unstained cells by a magnet. Both FACS and magnetic bead separation methods have resulted in the isolation of very rare cells such as hematopoietic stem cells.

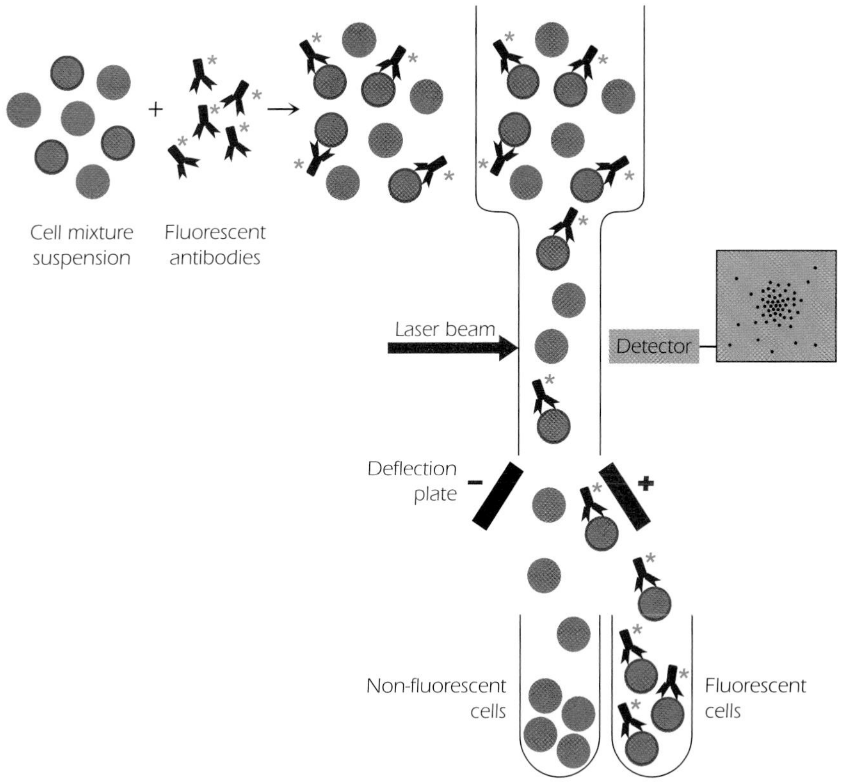

Figure 5.12. FACS analysis.

The most common method for phenotyping and sorting cells involves the use of antibodies that react with cell-surface proteins identified as ***clusters of differentiation*** (CD) ***antigens.*** The CD nomenclature originates from studies using monoclonal antibodies (discussed later in this chapter) to phenotypically characterize cells. It was found that cell-surface markers (CD antigens) are associated with distinct developmental stages. Moreover, these proteins have important biologic functions required for normal cell physiology. The developmental stages of B and T cells and functional subsets of these cells can now be phenotyped based on their expression of CD markers. It is also worth noting, however, that surface expression of a particular molecule may not be specific for just one cell or even for a cell lineage. Nonetheless, cell-surface expression can be exploited for purification, as well as characterization, of cells. For practical purposes, the CD acronym is followed by an arbitrary number that identifies a specific cell-surface protein. CD numbers are assigned by the Nomenclature Committee of the International Union of Immunologic Sciences. A list some of some of the more important CD antigens expressed by B cells, various T cell subsets, and other cells can be found in the appendix.

IMMUNOABSORPTION AND IMMUNOADSORPTION

Because of the specific binding between antigen and antibody, it is possible to trap, or selectively remove, an antigen against which an antibody is directed from a mixture of antigens in solution. Similarly, it is possible to trap or selectively remove the antigen-specific antibodies from a mixture of antibodies, using the specific antigen.

There are two general methods by which this removal can be achieved. The methods are related: In one method, the absorption is done with both reagents in solution ***(immunoabsorption)***; in the second method, it is performed with one reagent attached to an insoluble support ***(immunoadsorption).*** Immunoadsorption is of particular value because the adsorbed material can be recovered from the complex by careful treatments that dissociate antigen–antibody complexes, such as lowering the pH (HCl-glycine or acetic acid, pH 2-3) or adding chaotropic ions. This enables the effective purification of antigens or antibodies of interest.

CELLULAR ASSAYS

Other immune assays used in the evaluation and study of the cellular components of the immune system are also described in this chapter. Among these are the routine methods used to measure lymphocyte function. Assays designed to measure responses of B cells to antigenic or ***mitogenic stimulation*** are sometimes used clinically to assess humoral immunocompenence. In experimental settings, these assays help us understand the regulatory and molecular mechanisms associated with B cell activation. Similarly, assays for measuring T cell function are used both clinically and experimentally to measure T cell proliferative and effector responses and T cell cytokine profiles. T cell assays have contributed significantly to our understanding of T cell functional diversity and to the identification of the many cytokines produced by cells belonging to a particular subset.

Assays to Assess Lymphocyte Function

Assays used to assess lymphocyte function generally attempt to answer one of the following questions: (1) Do the B or T cells respond normally to mitogenic stimuli that activate cells to undergo a proliferative response? (2) Does mitogenic or antigen-driven stimulation result in antibody production (for B cells) or cytokine production (for T cells)? In addition, given the functional heterogeneity of T cells, T cell assays can also be used to evaluate the functional integrity of particular subsets. This is particularly useful in the clinical evaluation of patients with suspected immunodeficiency diseases (see Chapter 17). In the case of T helper cell assays, the target cell receiving the T cell help generally determines the functional parameter to be measured. For example, the target population might be B cells in an assay designed to test the ability of T cells to help induce antibody responses. In this example, the assay would quantitate the level of antibody produced. Similarly, if one were interested in knowing whether T cells provide help needed to optimally activate macrophages, the parameters measured would focus on functional properties associated with these phagocytic cells. It is important to note that many of the assays used to assess helper T cell function also rely on the measurement of specific cytokines, since the cells receiving help may be activated to produce cytokines themselves.

B Cell and T Cell Proliferation Assays

Mitogen-stimulated lymphocyte activation triggers biochemical signaling pathways that lead to gene expression, protein synthesis, cell proliferation, and differentiation. The proliferative responses generated in response to mitogens are polyclonal in nature. Moreover, mitogens have been identified that selectively stimulate either B or T cell populations. Therefore, unlike immunogens that activate only the lymphocyte clones bearing the appropriate antigen receptor, polyclonal activators stimulate many B or T cell clones regardless of their antigenic specificity. Mitogens that selectively activate B cells, such as the ***lipopolysaccharide*** (LPS) component of gram-negative bacterial cell walls, will cause polyclonal stimulation of B cells in mice. The magnitude of cell proliferation in response to mitogenic stimulation can be measured by adding radiolabeled nucleosides (e.g., tritiated thymidine) to the medium during cell culture and then quantitating its incorporation into the DNA of dividing cells using a liquid scintillation counter. Similarly, several sugar-binding proteins, called lectins, including ***concanavalin A*** (Con A) and ***phytohemagglutinin*** (PHA), are very effective T cell mitogens. ***Pokeweed mitogen*** (PWM) is another example of a lectin with potent mitogenic properties. However, unlike Con A and PHA, PWM stimulates polyclonal activation of both B and T cells.

Antibody Production by B Cells

Mitogenic stimulation of B and T cells results in the proliferation and differentiation of many clones of cells. Therefore, in the case of B cells, the polyclonal activators LPS or PWM can be used to assess the ability of a population of B cells to produce antibody. ELISA is the most commonly used quantitative assay for measuring antibody levels. Alternatively, B cells can be stimulated with mitogens or specific antigens in vitro, then temporarily cultured in chambers directly on nitrocellulose membranes in a so-called ***ELISPOT*** assay. The protein-binding property of nitrocellulose facilitates the capture of secreted antibody by individual B cells. This yields discrete foci of antibody bound to the nitrocellulose that can be detected using a secondary, enzyme-labeled antibody specific for the bound antibody, allowing for the enumeration of antibody-secreting cells.

Effector Cell Assays for T Cells and Natural-Killer Cells

As noted above, the choice of effector cell assay used depends on the questions that need to be answered. T cell assays are as varied as the functionally diverse T cell subsets known to exist. Thus various assays that measure T helper cell function have been developed to focus on helper activity for B cells and macrophage activation; even other T cells can be used to measure the helper properties of $CD4^+$ T cells. Similarly, several assays that measure cytotoxic activity of $CD8^+$ T cells are available. One such assay ***(cytotoxicity assay)*** measures the ability of cytotoxic T cells or natural-killer (NK) cells to kill radiolabeled target cells expressing the antigen to which the cytotoxic T cells were sensitized. In a related assay, the NK cells are cultured with radiolabeled target cells bound to target cell-specific antibodies. The rationale for this approach is based on the fact that NK cells express membrane Fc receptors that bind to the Fc region of certain immunoglobulin isotypes. This method measures an important functional property of NK cells, known as ***antibody-dependent, cell-mediated cytotoxicity*** (ADCC).

CELL CULTURE

Several experimental systems have revolutionized our ability to investigate a myriad of questions about the development of the immune system, its functional and regulatory properties, and the pathologic mechanisms associated with immunodeficiency and autoimmune diseases. Many of these experimental systems depend on cell culture methods used to maintain cells in vitro. Cell culture systems have facilitated several major scientific breakthroughs, including the development in the 1970s of B cell ***hybridoma/monoclonal antibody technology*** by Kohler and Milstein. Knowledge of the growth factors required to maintain lymphoid cells has made it possible to clone and grow functionally competent cells in vitro. Moreover, recombinant DNA techniques have permitted the transfer of genes to cloned cell lines, thereby allowing researchers to answer many questions related to the gene under investigation. Similarly, recombinant DNA techniques have made it possible to develop genetically engineered immune molecules and receptors, which can then be transferred into cells that are then used to elucidate the biologic consequences of receptor expression and receptor triggering (e.g., ligand binding). These in vitro systems continue to be used to advance our knowledge of the immune system and, in some cases, to develop new biologic therapies and vaccines for clinical use.

Primary Cell Cultures and Cloned Lymphoid Cell Lines

As with many other fields of biologic science, cell culture systems have served as an essential investigational tool to facilitate our understanding of many developmental/maturational and physiologic properties of cells. The ability to culture primary lymphoid cells consisting of heterogeneous populations of T and/or B cells (albeit for limited periods of time) has allowed immunologists to study the biochemical and molecular mechanisms controlling many important biologic features of B and T cells, including gene rearrangement. Advances in cell culture systems have evolved rapidly during the past few decades leading to the development of cell cloning techniques. Transformation of B and T cells derived from a specific parent cell to generate cloned, immortalized cell lines has been achieved using a variety of methods, including exposure of cells to certain carcinogens or viruses (e.g., Epstein-Barr virus for the transformation of B cells; human T cell leukemia virus *type 1* for the transformation of T cells). It should be noted that many cell lines are derived from tumors arising either spontaneously or experimentally (as a result of administration of carcinogens or virus infection). The major advantage of using cloned cell lines is that large numbers of cells can be generated for investigation. A disadvantage in the use of carcinogen- or virus-transformed cells is that they are, by definition, abnormal. Indeed, many transformed cells have abnormal numbers of chromosomes and often display phenotypic and functional properties not seen in normal cells.

A major advance in the generation of cloned lymphoid cells came in the late 1970s with the discovery that nontransformed antigen-specific T cell lines and antigen-specific T cell clones could be grown for long periods of time when a T cell growth factor (interleukin-2) was included in the culture together with a source of antigen and antigen-presenting cells. This approach offered several advantages over the use of transformed cells, since the cells derived from such cultures were, for all intents and purposes, normal. Thus large numbers of nontransformed antigen-specific T cells could be generated for investigation. Indeed, many of these cloned T cell lines have been used in the identification and biochemical characterization of cytokines, leading to the ultimate cloning of genes that encode these proteins.

The combined use of cell-cloning systems, gene-transfer methods, and animal models has helped us understand how lymphoid cells develop self-tolerance as well as how they can escape tolerance-inducing mechanisms to become disease-causing autoreactive cells. In short, cell culture systems have served as a gateway for research endeavors to shed light on both the physiologic and pathophysiologic properties of lymphoid cells. As will be discussed below, cell culture systems have also been productively exploited with the development of many useful diagnostic and therapeutic reagents, such as monoclonal antibodies.

B Cell Hybridomas and Monoclonal Antibodies

The specificity of the immune response has served as the basis for serologic reactions in which antibody specificity is used for the qualitative and quantitative determination of antigen. The discriminating power of serum antibody is not without limitations, however, because the immunizing antigen, which usually has many epitopes, leads to production of antisera that contain a mixture of antibodies with varying specificity for all the epitopes. Indeed, even antibodies to a single epitope are usually mixtures of immunoglobulins with different fine specificities, and therefore different affinities for the determinant. Furthermore, immunization with an antigen expands various populations of antibody-forming B lymphocytes. These cells can be maintained in culture for only a short time (on the order of days), so it is impractical, if not impossible, to grow normal cells and obtain clones that produce antibodies of a single specificity. A quantum leap in the resolution and discriminating power of antibodies took place in the 1970s with the development of methods for the generation of ***monoclonal antibodies*** by Köhler and Milstein, who shared the Nobel Prize for this development. Monoclonal antibodies are homogeneous populations of antibody molecules, derived from a single antibody-producing cell, in which all antibodies are identical and of the same precise specificity for a given epitope.

In this procedure, transformed plasma cells (immortal in cell culture) that do not produce immunoglobulin are used. The cells are engineered to be deficient in an enzyme—hypoxanthine guanine phosphoribosyl transferase (HGPRT)—and therefore will not survive in culture unless this enzyme is added to the media in which the cells are grown. These cells are fused (hybridized) with a source of freshly harvested B cells from a mouse recently immunized with antigen (e.g., spleen cells) (Fig. 5.13). The fusion is often accomplished by the use of polyethylene glycol (PEG). Following fusion, the cells are cultured in media lacking HGPRT. Since the antibody-producing B cells produce HGPRT, hybridoma cells consisting of immortalized plasma cells fused with B cells will survive in the absence of supplemented HGPRT in the culture medium. Within days, non-fused

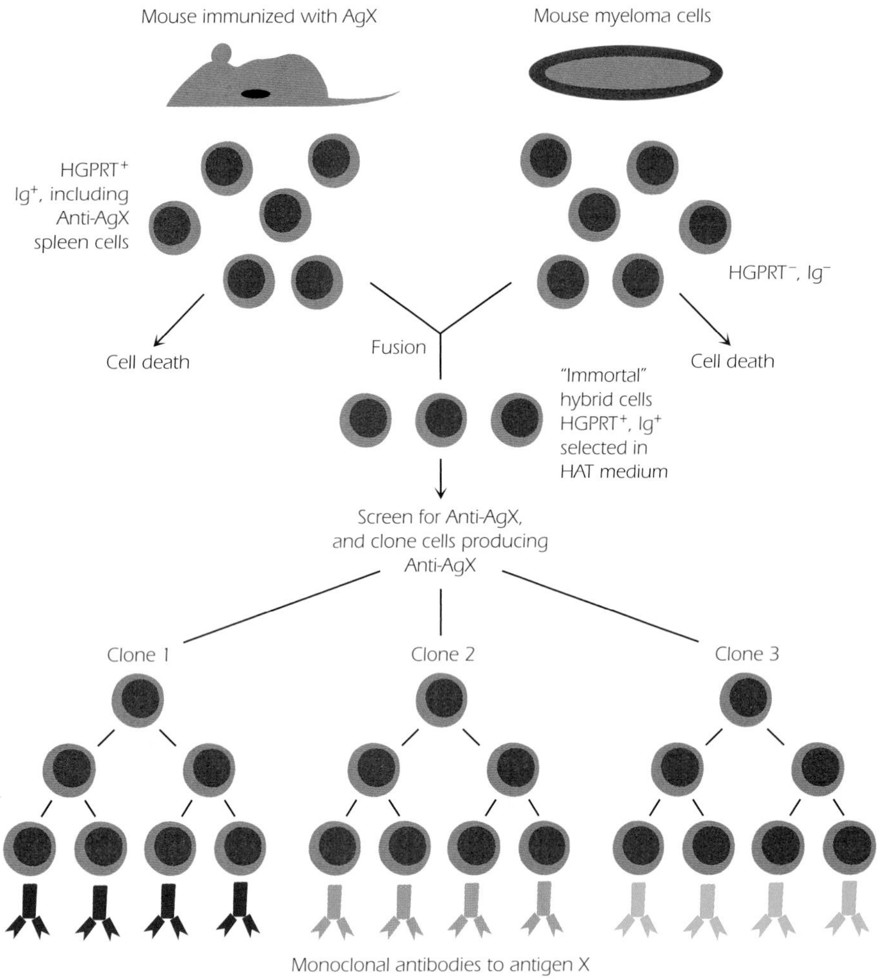

Figure 5.13. The production of monoclonal antibodies.

HGPRT-negative plasma cells soon die, as do all nonfused B cells. Those hybrid cells synthesizing specific antibody are selected by some test for antigen reactivity (e.g., ELISA) and then cloned from single cells and propagated in cell culture, each clone synthesizing antibodies of a single specificity. These highly specific, monoclonal antibodies are used for numerous procedures, ranging from specific diagnostic tests to biologic agents used in immunotherapy of cancer (see Chapter 19). In immunotherapy, various drugs or toxins are conjugated to monoclonal antibodies, which, in turn, deliver these substances to the tumor cells against which the antibodies are specifically directed.

T Cell Hybridomas

It is important to note that hybridoma technology is not limited to the production of monoclonal immunoglobulins. In the late 1970s, methods for producing hybridomas were also developed for T cells, fusing lines of malignant T cells with nonmalignant, antigen-specific T lymphocytes whose populations were expanded by immunization with antigen. T cell hybridomas have been very useful for studying the relationship between T cells of a single specificity with their corresponding epitope.

Genetically Engineered Molecules and Receptors

To date, most of the monoclonal antibodies are made in mouse cells. These are suitable for diagnostic and many other purposes. However, their administration into humans carries the complication that the patient will form antibodies to the mouse immunoglobulins. Attempts to develop in vitro human monoclonal antibodies have, by and large, not been very successful.

Human monoclonal antibodies are currently being produced by genetic engineering using several approaches. One method uses the technology of recombinant DNA to produce a chimeric mouse–human monoclonal antibody. These so-called ***humanized antibodies*** consist of the constant region of human immunoglobulin and a variable region of a mouse immunoglobulin. A similar method is used to construct humanized antibodies consisting of a human constant region and a variable region, which contains a mouse hypervariable region and a human framework region. Another method uses the polymerase chain reaction (PCR) to generate gene libraries of heavy and light chains from DNA obtained from hybridoma cells or plasma cells, joining at random numerous heavy and light chains and screening the resulting Fab clones for antibody activity against a desired antigen. With this technology, it is now possible to produce millions of clones of different specificities, to rapidly screen them for the desired specificity, and to generate the desired monoclonal Fab constructs without immunization and without the difficulties encountered with the production of monoclonal antibodies, especially human monoclonal antibodies.

Genetic engineering of immune proteins is not limited to the production of monoclonal antibodies. Many genes encoding membrane receptors expressed on lymphoid and nonlymphoid cells have been cloned and, in some cases, genetically engineered to allow for gene transfer to cells that do not normally express these receptors. The expression of certain costimulator molecules facilitates cell–cell interactions (e.g., the physical contact between cytotoxic T cells and target cells, which results in the killing of the latter). The expression, through gene transfer, of such costimulator molecules (e.g., B7.1, *a.k.a.* CD80) on tumor cells significantly enhances the ability of T cells to recognize and kill these cells. Experimental vaccination strategies (a form of immunotherapy) have demonstrated that immunization of tumor-bearing animals with their own tumor cells, which have been removed and transfected with the B7.1 gene, can potentiate T cells to recognize and destroy the parent tumor cells. It should be noted that a similar strategy using tumor cells transfected with certain cytokine genes has also been used with some success in animal models. Immunotherapeutic strategies used to treat a variety of diseases are discussed in several chapters of this book (see Chapters 17–19).

EXPERIMENTAL ANIMAL MODELS

Several important in vivo animal models have been developed with experimental value and clinical payoffs similar to those emerging from the use of the in vitro systems noted above. These in vivo systems rely on the use of inbred mouse strains with a variety of genetic profiles, some of which are genetically engineered. Some inbred stains have an innate predisposition for developing a particular disease (e.g., mammary cancer, leukemia, autoimmune disease, severe combined immunodeficiency disease). Genetically altered animals, on the other hand, have been developed to express a particular cloned foreign gene (transgenic mice) or to interfere with the expression of targeted genes (knockout mice). Such strains are useful in the study of the expression of a particular transgene or in determining the consequences of gene silencing in knockout mice. We begin with a discussion of inbred strains of animals.

Inbred Strains

Many of the classic experiments in the field of immunology have been performed using inbred strains of animals such as mice, rats, and guinea pigs. Selective inbreeding of littermates for >20 generations usually leads to the production of an inbred strain. All members of inbred strains of animals are genetically identical. Therefore, like identical twins, they are said to be ***syngeneic.*** Immune responses of inbred strains can be studied in the absence of variables associated with genetic differences between animals. As will be discussed in Chapter 18, organ transplants between members of inbred stains are always accepted since their major histocompatibility complex (MHC) antigens are identical. Indeed, knowledge of the laws of transplantation and the fact that the MHC is the major genetic barrier to transplantation was made possible through the use of inbred strains. Experiments using inbred strains led to the identification of MHC class I and class II genes whose main function is to deliver peptide fragments of antigen to the cell surface, thus allowing them to be recognized by antigen-specific T cells. Subsequent chapters elaborate on the important role of the MHC in the generation of normal immune responses, T cell development, disease susceptibility, and organ transplantation.

Adoptive Transfer and Passive Immunization

Protection against many diseases is conferred through ***cell-mediated immunity*** by antigen-specific T cells as opposed to antibody-mediated (humoral) immunity. The distinction between these two arms of the immune system can be readily demonstrated by ***adoptive transfer*** of T cells or by *passive* administration of antiserum or purified antibodies. Adoptive *transfer* of T cells is usually performed using genetically identical donor and recipients (e.g., inbred strains) and results in long-term adoptive immunization following antigen priming. By contrast, passive transfer of serum which contains antibodies can be performed across MHC barriers and is effective as long as the transferred antibodies remain active in the recipient. This type of transfer is therefore called ***passive immunization.***

SCID Mice

Severe combined immunodeficiency disease (SCID) is a disorder in which B and T cells fail to develop, causing the individual to be compromised with respect to lymphoid defense mechanisms. Chapter 17 discusses various causes of SCID in humans. In the 1980s, an inbred strain of mice spontaneously developed an autosomal recessive mutation, resulting in SCID in homozygous *scid/scid* mice. Because of the absence of functional T and B cells, SCID mice are able to accept cells and tissue grafts from other strains of mice or other species. SCID mice can be engrafted with human hematopoietic stem cells to create ***SCID–human chimeras.*** Such chimeric mice develop mature, functional T and B cells derived from the infused human hematopoietic stem cell precursors. This animal model has become a valuable research tool, since it allows immunologists to manipulate the human immune system in vivo and to investigate the development of various lymphoid cells. Moreover, SCID–human mice can be used to test candidate vaccines, including those that might useful in protecting humans from HIV infection.

Thymectomized and Congenically Athymic (Nude) Mice

The importance of the thymus in the development of mature T cells can be demonstrated by using mice that have been neonatally thymectomized, irradiated, and then reconstituted with syngeneic bone marrow. Such mice fail to develop mature T cells. Similarly, mice homozygous for the recessive *nu/nu* mutation also fail to develop mature T cells because the mutation results in an athymic (and hairlessness, hence the term *nude*) phenotype. In both situations, T cell development can be restored by grafting these mice with thymic epithelial tissue. Like SCID mice, these animal models have been useful in the study of T cell development. They have also been useful for the in vivo propagation of tumor cell lines and fresh tumor explants from other strains and other species owing to the absence of T cells required to reject such foreign cells.

TRANSGENIC MICE AND GENE TARGETING

Transgenic Mice

Another significant animal system used extensively in immunologic research is the ***transgenic mouse.*** Transgenic mice are made by injecting a cloned gene ***(transgene)*** into fertilized mouse eggs. The eggs are then microinjected into pseudopregnant mice (Fig. 5.14). The success rate of this technique is rather low, with 10–30% of the offspring expressing the transgene. Since the transgene is integrated into both somatic and germ-line cells, it is transmitted to the offspring as a Mendelian trait. By constructing a transgene with a particular promoter, it is possible to control the gene's expression. For example, some promoters function only in certain tissues (e.g., the insulin promoter functions only in the pancreas), whereas others function in response to biochemical signals that can be supplied, in some cases, as a dietary supplement (e.g., the metallothionine promoter that functions in response to zinc, which can be added to the drinking water). Transgenic mice have been used to study genes that are not usually expressed in vivo (e.g., oncogenes), as well as the effects of transgenes encoding particular immunoglobulin molecules, T cell receptors, MHC class I or class II molecules, and a variety of cytokines. Trasgenic mice have also been developed in which the entire mouse immunoglobulin locus has been replaced by human immunoglobulin genes. These are useful in generating "human" antibodies in the mouse. It should be noted that a disadvantage of the transgenic method is that the transgene integrates randomly within the genome. This limitation, together with the fact that it is unphysiologic to express high quantities of transgenes in the wrong tissues, forces investigators to use great care in interpreting results obtained in transgenic mice.

Knockout Mice

Sometimes, it is of interest to determine how the removal of a particular gene product affects the immune system. Using

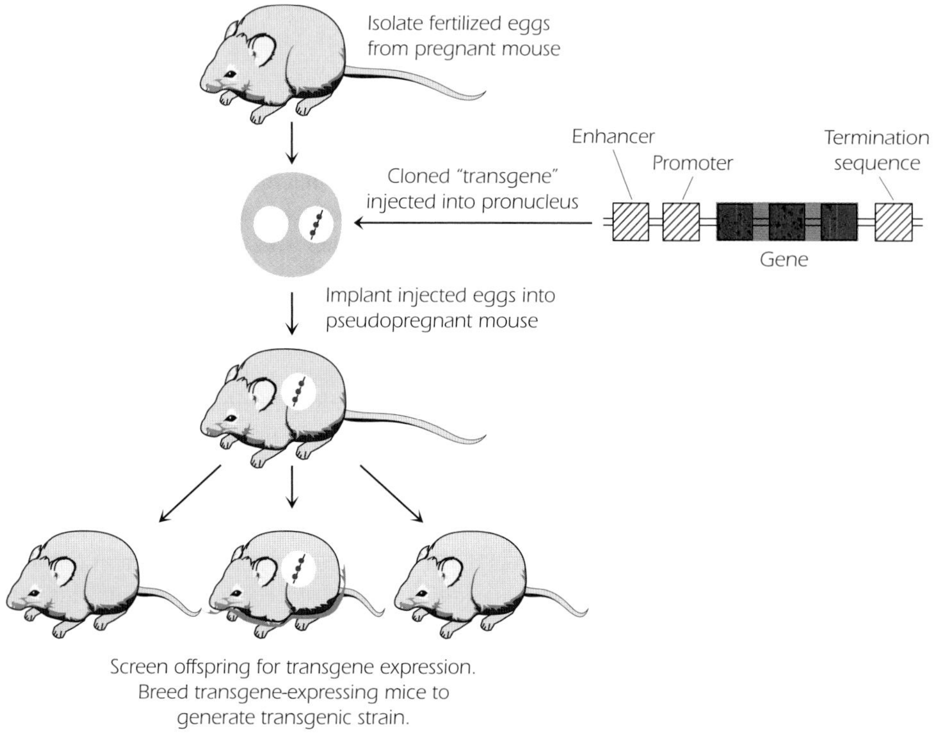

Isolate fertilized eggs from pregnant mouse
Cloned "transgene" injected into pronucleus
Enhancer
Promoter
Termination sequence
Gene
Implant injected eggs into pseudopregnant mouse
Screen offspring for transgene expression. Breed transgene-expressing mice to generate transgenic strain.

Figure 5.14. A general procedure for producing transgenic mice.

a ***gene targeting*** method, it is possible to replace a normal gene with one that has been mutated or disrupted to generate ***knockout mice.*** Thus, unlike the method used to generate transgenic mice, knockout mice express transgenes that integrate at specific endogenous genes through a process known as *homologous recombination.* Virtually any gene for which a mutated or altered transgene exists can be targeted this way. Knockout mice have been generated by using mutated or altered transgenes that target, and therefore silence, the expression of a variety of important genes, including those encoding particular cytokines and MHC molecules. They have also been used to identify the parts of genes essential for normal gene function. This is done by determining whether function can be restored by introducing different mutated copies of the gene back into the genome by transgenesis.

ANALYSIS OF GENE EXPRESSION

Microarrays to Assess Gene Expression

Microarrays, or ***gene chips,*** are powerful tools for examining the level of expression of thousands of genes simultaneously. The microarray is made up of thousands of DNA fragments, each with a unique sequence, attached in an ordered arrangement to a glass slide or other surface. These DNA fragments, in the form of complementary DNA (cDNA; generally 500–5000 base pairs long) or oligonucleotides (20–80 base pairs long), can represent genes from all parts of the genome; alternatively, specialized microarrays can be prepared that use DNA from genes of particular interest. To perform a microarray assay, a sample of total messenger RNA (mRNA)—the product obtained from transcription of all active genes—from a cell or tissue is commonly tested with a reference sample to compare gene expression among various samples. For example, different cell types or tissues can be compared, cells can be compared at different stages of differentiation, or tumor cells can be compared with their normal counterparts, with the goal of assessing differential gene expression within the tested samples. The samples that are added to the microarray are generally not mRNA; rather, the total mRNA is reverse-transcribed into cDNA, which is then labeled with a fluorescent material (a fluorochrome). Different colored fluorochromes are used to distinctly label the different sources of cDNAs. Figure 5.15 demonstrates how microarrays are used to compare gene expression in a lymphoid tumor cell population and a normal cell counterpart. A red fluorochrome is used to label experimental tumor cell cDNAs, and a green fluorochrome is used for cDNAs prepared from their control normal counterparts. The labeled cDNAs are washed over the microarray and allowed to hybridize by base pairing with matching fragments. cDNA samples derived from both control samples and experimental samples are added to the microarray so that they compete for binding to the microarray surface. Unhybridized material is washed away, leaving pockets of fluorescence where matching has occurred. At the end of the hybridization reaction, the microarray is laser-scanned to reveal red, green,

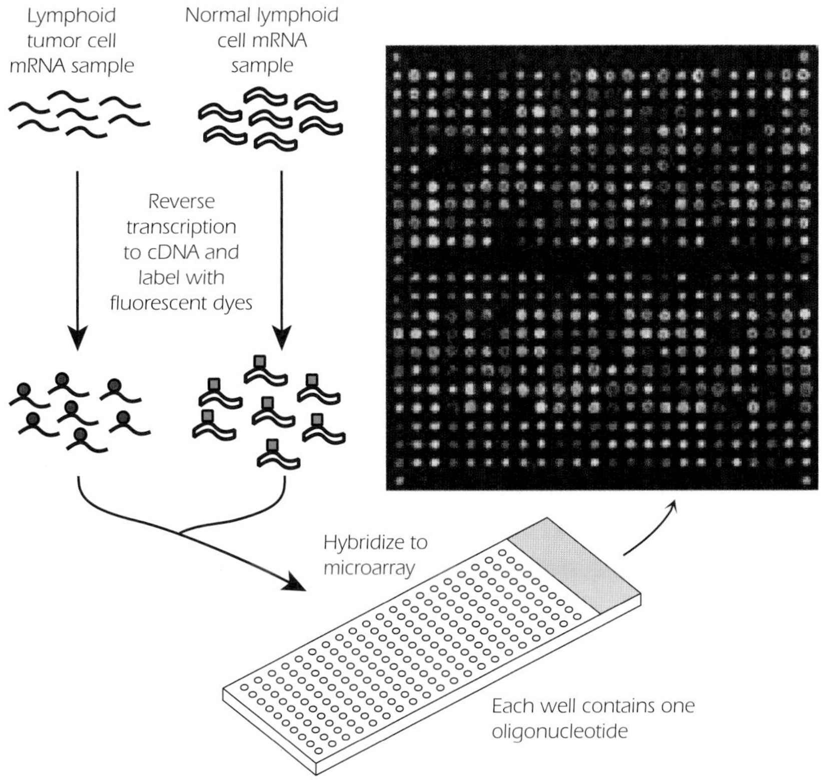

Figure 5.15. Microarray assay comparing samples of mRNA from lymphoid tumor cells and normal lymphoid cells.

or yellow spots, indicating higher levels of the experimental tumor cell cDNA (which was labeled with a red fluorochrome in the example given), higher levels of the control cDNA (labeled green), or equal levels of DNA in the two samples (yellow), respectively. To interpret the results, a fluorescence scanner examines each spot on the slide for the precise level of fluorescence. The data are then analyzed by a computer program, which typically combines the fluorescence information with a genetic database to determine which genes are overexpressed or underexpressed in the tested samples. Characterizing the pattern and amount of binding to the microarray has many potential uses in the field of immunology, including clinical diagnosis of lymphoid tumors, drug development (e.g., testing candidate immunosuppressive drugs for their effects on cytokine gene expression), and new gene discovery.

SUMMARY

1. The reaction between an antibody and an antigen does not involve covalent forces; it involves weak forces of interaction, such as electrostatic, hydrophobic, and van der Waals forces. Consequently, for a significant interaction, the antibody-combining site and the antigen require a close steric fit, like a lock and key.

2. Only the reaction between a multivalent antigen and at least a bivalent antibody can bring about antigen–antibody reactions that result in the cross-linking of antigen molecules by antibodies. These reactions do not take place with haptens or monovalent Fab.

3. The interaction between a soluble antibody and an insoluble particulate antigen results in agglutination. The extent of agglutination depends on the proportions of the interacting antibody and antigen. At high antibody levels, agglutination may not occur. This is referred to as a prozone. The term titer refers to the highest serum dilution at which agglutination still takes place and beyond which, at higher dilution, no agglutination occurs.

4. Precipitation reactions occur on mixing, at the right proportions, of soluble multivalent antigen and (at least) divalent antibodies. The precipitation reaction may take place in aqueous media or in gels.

5. The reaction in gels, between soluble antigen and antibodies, may be used for the qualitative and quantitative analysis of antigen or antibody. Examples of such reactions are seen in gel diffusion, radial diffusion, and immunoelectrophoresis.

6. Radioimmunoassay is a very sensitive test used to quantitate antibody or antigen. It employs the use of radiolabeled antigen or antibody and is based on competitive inhibition of nonlabeled and labeled antigen. Antibody-bound antigen must be separated from nonbound labeled antigen. Separation is usually achieved by precipitation with anti-immunoglobulins.

7. Solid-phase immunoassay is a test that employs the property of many proteins to adhere to plastic and form a monomolecular layer. Antigen is applied to plastic wells, antibodies are added, the well is washed, and any antibodies bound to antigen are measured by the use of radiolabeled or enzyme-linked anti-immunoglobulins.

8. The enzyme-linked immunosorbent assay is essentially a solid-phase immunoassay in which an enzyme is linked to the anti-immunoglobulin. Quantitation is achieved by colorimetric evaluation after the addition of a substrate, which changes color on the action of the enzyme.

9. Immunofluorescence is a method by which an antigen is detected by the use of fluorescence-labeled immunoglobulins. In direct immunofluorescence, the antibody to the antigen in question carries a fluorescent label. In indirect immunofluorescence, the antigen-specific antibody is not labeled; it is detected by the addition of fluorescently labeled anti-immunoglobulin. Fluorescence-activated cell sorters are instruments that can be used to quantitate and sort fluorescently labeled cells.

10. Assays used to assess lymphocyte function typically measure their proliferative responses or effector functions. For example, B cells can be functionally assessed by measuring their ability to proliferate and produce antibodies in response to B cell mitogens, such as lipopolysaccharide or pokeweed mitogen. T cells are often assessed by measuring their ability to provide help for other cells (in the case of $CD4^+$ cells) or to kill antigen-bearing targets (in the case of $CD8^+$ cells). In addition, T cells can be assessed by measuring their ability to proliferate and produce certain cytokines in response to T cell mitogens, such as phytohemagglutinin and concanvalin A.

11. Monoclonal antibodies are highly specific reagents consisting of homogeneous populations of antibodies, all of precisely the same specificity toward an epitope.

REFERENCES

Camper SA (1987): Research applications of transgenic mice. *Biotechniques* 5:638.

Channing-Rodgers RP (1994): Clinical laboratory methods for detection of antigens and antibodies. In Stites DP, Terr AI, Parslow TG (eds): Basic and Clinical Immunology, 8th ed. E Norwalk, CT: Appleton & Lange.

Harlow E, Lane D (1988): Antibodies: A Laboratory Manual. Cold Spring Harbor, NY: Cold Spring Harbor Laboratory.

Hudson L, Hay FC (1989): Practical Immunology, 3rd ed. Oxford, UK: Blackwell.

Johnstone A, Thorpe R (1987): Immunochemistry in Practice. Oxford, UK: Blackwell.

Köhler G, Milstein, C (1975). Continuous cultures of fused cells secreting antibody of predefined specificity. *Nature* 256:495

Koller BH, Smithies O (1992): Altering genes in animals by gene targeting. *Annu Rev Immunol* 10:705.

Mayforth RD (1993): Designing Antibodies. San Diego, CA: Academic Press.

Mishell BB, Shiigi SM (1980): Selected Methods in Cellular Immunology. New York: Freeman.

Thompson KM (1988): Human monoclonal antibodies. *Immunol Today* 9:113.

Weir DM (1986): Handbook of Experimental Immunology, Vol 12, 4th ed. Oxford, UK: Blackwell.

Winter G, Griffith AD, Hawkins RE, Hoogenboom HR (1994): Making antibodies by phage display technology. *Annu Rev Immunol* 12:433.

REVIEW QUESTIONS

For each question, choose the ONE BEST answer or completion.

1. Primary interactions between antigens and antibodies involve all of the following except which?
- A) covalent bonds
- B) van der Waals forces
- C) hydrophobic forces
- D) electrostatic forces
- E) a very close fit between an epitope and the antibody

2. If an IgG antibody preparation specific for hen egg lysosome (HEL) is treated with papain to generate Fab regions, which of the following statements concerning the avidity of such fragments is true?
- A) They will have a lower avidity for HEL than the intact IgG.
- B) They will have a higher avidity for HEL than the intact IgG.
- C) They will have the same avidity for HEL as the intact IgG.
- D) They will have lost their avidity to bind to HEL.
- E) They will have the same avidity but will have a lower affinity for HEL.

3. Western assays used to test serum samples for the presence of antibodies to infectious agents, such as HIV, are particularly useful as diagnostic assays because
- A) they are more sensitive than ELISA.
- B) antibodies specific for multiple antigenic epitopes can be detected.
- C) they provide quantitative data for sample analysis.
- D) they allow multiple samples to be tested simultaneously.
- E) they are less expensive and take less time to perform than ELISA.

4. The major difference between transgenic mice and knockout mice is that
- A) transgenic mice always employ the use of cloned genes derived from other species.
- B) transgenic mice have foreign genes that integrate at targeted loci through homologous recombination.
- C) transgenic mice have a functional foreign gene added to their genome.
- D) knockout mice always have a unique phenotype.

5. SCID mice have a genetic defect that prevents development of functional
- A) hematopoietic cells.
- B) B cells and T cells.
- C) T cells and NK cells.
- D) pluripotential stem cells.
- E) myeloid cells.

6. Which of the following statements regarding B cell hybridomas is false?
- A) They are immortalized cell lines that produce antibodies of a single specificity.
- B) They are derived from B cells that are first cloned and grown in cell culture for short periods.
- C) They contain a large nucleus formed by the fusion of two nuclei.
- D) They can be used to manufacture diagnostic or therapeutic monoclonal antibodies.
- E) They are derived by fusing B cells with transformed plasma cells that are unable to secrete immunoglobulin.

7. An ELISA designed to test for the presence of serum antibody for a new strain of pathogenic bacteria is under development. Initially, a monoclonal antibody specific for a single epitope of the organism was used both to sensitize the wells of the ELISA plate and as the enzyme-labeled detecting antibody in a conventional sandwich ELISA. The

ELISA failed to detect the antigen, despite the use of a wide range of antibody concentrations. What is the most probable cause of this problem?

A) The antigen used in the assay is too large.
B) The antibody has a low affinity for the antigen.
C) The monoclonal antibody used to sensitize the wells is blocking access of the epitope; thus when the same antibody is enzyme labeled, it cannot bind to the antigen.
D) The enzyme-labeled antibody used should have been a different isotype than the sensitizing antibody.
E) The monoclonal antibody used is probably unstable.

ANSWERS TO REVIEW QUESTIONS

1. A No covalent bonds are involved in the interaction between antibody and antigen. The binding forces are relatively weak and include van der Waals forces, hydrophobic forces, and electrostatic forces. A very close fit between an epitope and the antibody is required.

2. A Avidity denotes the overall binding energy between antigens and multivalent antigens. Since the valency of the Fab regions is 1, compared to the HEL-specific IgG molecule, which has a valence of 2 (due to the presence of two Fab regions), the avidity of the fragments will be lower. Choice E is incorrect since the affinity of the Fab fragments will be the same as each of the Fab regions of the intact IgG molecule.

3. B In Western assays, electrophoretic separation techniques are used to resolve the molecular mass of a given antigen or mixtures of antigens. Since antibody responses to infectious agents generate polyclonal responses by virtue of the complex antigenic determinants expressed by such agents, Western assays can confirm the presence of these antibodies, which react with the electrophoretically separated antigens of known molecular weights.

4. C Cloned foreign genes from either the same or other species are introduced into mice to generate a transgenic strain. Integration is random and occurs in both somatic and germ line cells. Choice D is incorrect because sometimes knockout mice do not have a phenotype unique caused by the replacement of a functional gene with one that is nonfunctional, probably due to the activity of redundant or compensatory mechanisms.

5. B SCID mice possess an autosomal recessive mutation that causes a disorder in which B and T cells fail to develop. Like their human counterparts, SCID mice are compromised with respect to lymphoid defense mechanisms. Pluripotential stem cells present in SCID mice can give rise to other hematopoietic lineages, including cells in the myeloid lineage and NK cells.

6. B The method used to generate B cell hybridomas employs the fusion of B cells (e.g., from the spleen and lymph nodes) harvested from immunized mice with a selected population of transformed plasma cells unable to secrete immunoglobulin. Antigen-specific B cells are not cloned first and then fused with such plasma cells.

7. C In a sandwich ELISA, an antibody (often monoclonal) used to coat ELISA wells will bind to the epitope for which it is specific. In the example given, the same epitope-specific monoclonal antibody is used as enzyme-labeled detecting antibody. The sensitizing monoclonal is blocking access to the epitope by the enzyme-labeled monoclonal antibody; therefore it will not bind.

6

THE GENETIC BASIS OF ANTIBODY STRUCTURE

INTRODUCTION

In previous chapters we have described the enormous diversity of the immune response, focusing on the diversity of antibodies—immunoglobulin (Ig) molecules that are the secreted forms of the antigen-specific receptors found on individual B lymphocytes. Estimates of the number of B and T cells with different antigenic specificities that can be generated in a single individual range from 10^{15} to 10^{18}; that is, every person has the ability to generate 10^{15} to 10^{18} different Ig or T-cell receptor (TCR) molecules. Since the ***genomes*** (inherited DNA) of many species have now been sequenced and found to contain only 30,000–40,000 genes, how do so few genes produce so many different antigen receptor molecules?

The work of several investigators over the last 30 years has shown that Ig and TCR genes use a unique strategy involving *combinations* of genes to achieve the degree of diversity required of the immune response. The first key finding was that the variable and constant regions of an Ig molecule are coded for by different genes. In fact, many different variable (V) region genes can be linked up to a single constant (C) region gene. A subsequent crucial finding by Susumu Tonegawa (who was awarded the Nobel Prize) was that antibody genes can move and ***rearrange*** themselves within the genome of a differentiating cell: A V region gene can be located in one position in the DNA of an inherited chromosome (***the germ line***) but then move to another position on the chromosome during lymphocyte differentiation. This process of rearrangement during differentiation brings together a set of genes that codes for the V and C regions. The set of rearranged genes is then transcribed and translated into a complete heavy (H) or light (L) chain.

Subsequent studies (discussed in more detail in Chapter 8), show that TCR genes and the mechanisms used to generate TCR diversity share many common features with Ig genes and the generation of diversity of Ig molecules. To date, the rearrangement strategies used to generate antigen-specific receptors on T and B cells appear unique in the entire body: No other genes have been found to rearrange. In the remainder of this chapter we describe how Ig genes are organized and rearrange, and show how a huge number of Ig polypeptides can be made from a small number of genes.

A BRIEF REVIEW OF NONIMMUNOGLOBULIN GENE STRUCTURE AND GENE EXPRESSION

Before discussing the molecular arrangement and rearrangement of the genes involved in Ig synthesis, we review the organization and expression of nonimmunoglobulin genes. We focus on the components of genes that code for a typical protein expressed at the cell surface, which is illustrated in Figure 6.1.

- The genome (total inherited DNA) of an individual consists of linear arrays of genes in the DNA strands of the various chromosomes. A gene is transcribed into RNA, and RNA is translated into protein.

Immunology: A Short Course, Fifth Edition, By Richard Coico, Geoffrey Sunshine, and Eli Benjamini
ISBN 0-471-22689-0 © 2003 John Wiley & Sons, Inc.

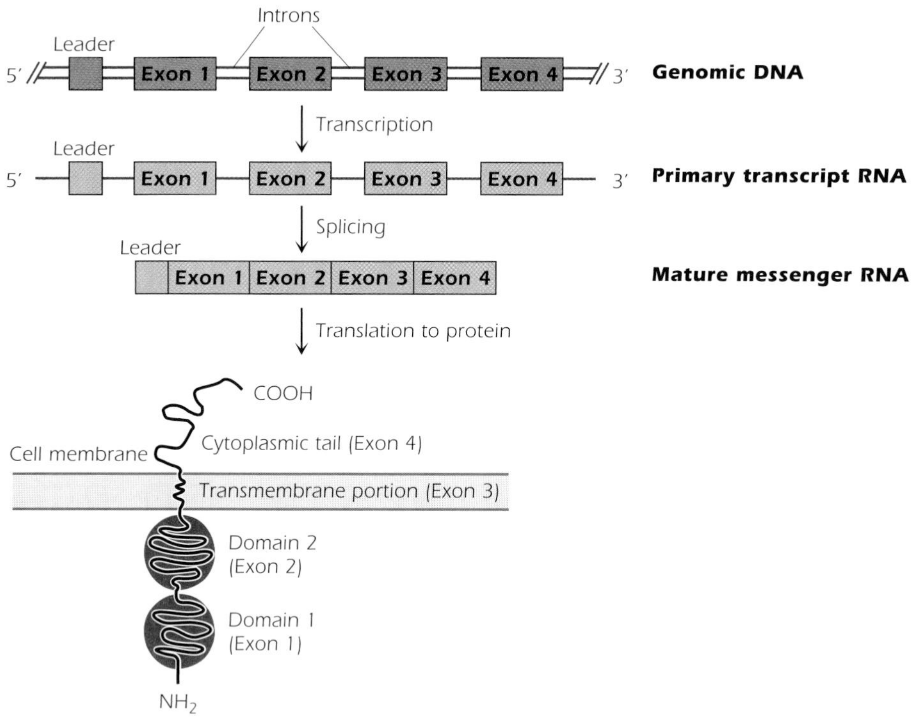

Figure 6.1. A prototypical gene coding for a transmembrane protein.

- Every diploid cell in the human body contains the same set of genes as every other cell. The only exceptions are lymphocytes, which, as we discuss shortly, differ from other cells and each other in the actual content of genes coding for their antigen-specific receptor. Cells within an individual differ from each other because they transcribe and translate different genes. We say that these cells ***express*** different patterns of genes.
- The expression of a specific pattern of genes determines the cell's function. Thus, for example, while every cell contains an insulin gene, only pancreatic β cells express that gene, enabling them to make insulin. Similarly, all cells contain Ig genes; however, only B lymphocytes (and their differentiated form, plasma cells) express Ig genes and therefore synthesize Ig molecules. Like all other cells except B cells, T cells contain Ig genes but do not express them.

  Control of gene expression exists at multiple levels, including the activity of ***transcription factors*** (proteins that initiate or modulate transcription, generally by binding to regulatory DNA sequences close to the 5′ end of genes), the rate of transcription, and the half-life of messenger RNA (mRNA). Understanding the mechanisms that regulate gene expression and, in particular, how genes are turned on and off in different cell types is an area of intense research interest.
- Most genes coding for a protein have a characteristic structure of ***exons*** and ***introns.*** Exons are sequences of base pairs that are later transcribed into mature mRNA. Exons are separated from each other by introns—noncoding regions of base pairs.
- When a gene is transcribed into RNA, the entire stretch of DNA (exons plus introns) is transcribed into a primary RNA transcript. Enzymes modify this primary RNA transcript by ***splicing*** out the noncoding introns and bringing together all the coding exons. This yields a processed mature mRNA segment that is much shorter than the original transcript. This mRNA is translated into protein on ribosomes. Notice in Figure 6.1 that exons generally code for a discrete region of the protein, such as an extracellular ***domain,*** a transmembrane piece, or a cytoplasmic tail. Thus proteins are assembled by putting together multiple functional regions, and each region is coded for by a separate gene segment.
- Genes coding for proteins expressed at the cell surface have a ***leader sequence*** (L exon) at the 5′ end. This codes for a sequence of about 10 mainly hydrophobic amino acids—the ***signal peptide***—at the amino (NH_2-) terminus of the protein. When the mRNA for a cell membrane-associated protein is translated on ribosomes, the signal peptide directs the synthesis of the polypeptide chain to the endoplasmic reticulum. The nascent polypeptide chain is fed from the ribosomes into the interior of endoplasmic reticulum, where the signal peptide is cleaved off. The newly synthesized protein moves from the endoplasmic reticulum into the Golgi apparatus and then to the cell membrane.

The surface molecule depicted in Figure 6.1 is shown with its amino terminus and two domains outside the cell, a single transmembrane region, and a large carboxy-terminal region inside the cell. The structure of a membrane Ig molecule expressed at the surface of a B cell has some similarities to the structure of the molecule depicted in Figure 6.1; in particular, the extracellular N-terminal domains and transmembrane region. Membrane Ig also differs in important ways from the structure of the depicted molecule. First, Ig is a four-chain glycoprotein. To make a complete Ig, the newly synthesized individual H and L chains must be assembled and glycosylated inside the cell before the four-chain molecule reaches the cell surface. Second, each Ig chain has a very short cytoplasmic tail.

Other molecules involved in the immune response are expressed at the cell surface with different configurations, for example, with their C-terminus extracellular and their N-terminus intracellular. Other membrane molecules, such as CD81 expressed on B cells, loop multiple times through the membrane (see Chapters 7 and 10). Yet others, such as leukocyte function–associated antigen 1 (LFA-1; CD58) and decay-accelerating factor (DAF; CD55), are completely extracellular but are linked to the surface of the cell via a covalent bond to an oligosaccharide, which in turn is bound to a phospholipid in the membrane, phosphatidylinositol. Thus these molecules are referred to as glycosylphosphatidylinositol (GPI) linked membrane molecules. (The functions of CD58 and CD55 are discussed in Chapters 10 and 13, respectively.)

GENETIC EVENTS IN THE SYNTHESIS OF Ig CHAINS

Organization and Rearrangement of Light Chain Genes

As we saw in Chapter 4, each κ and λ L-chain polypeptide consists of two major domains, a variable region and a constant region (V_L and C_L). The V_L is the approximately 108-residue amino-terminal portion of the light chain. V_L is coded for by ***two separate gene segments: a variable*** (V) ***segment,*** which codes for the amino-terminal 95 residues, and a small ***joining*** (J) ***segment,*** coding for about 13 residues (96–108) at the carboxy-terminal end of the variable region. One V gene and one J gene are brought together in the genome to create a gene unit that, together with the C region gene, codes for an entire Ig L chain. This unique ***gene rearrangement*** mechanism—referred to as ***V(D)J recombination*** (D gene segments are discussed below with H-chain genes)—is used only by genes coding for Ig L and H chains and genes coding for TCRs.

The complex, tightly regulated sequence of molecular events involved in gene rearrangement is only just beginning to be understood. We do know though that defects in the mechanism or regulation of V(D)J recombination can lead to disease (see Chaper 17). Many of the steps in rearrangement appear to be common to both B cells and T cells. An enzyme complex, known as ***V(D)J recombinase,*** mediates the rearrangement of receptor genes in B and T cells. The products of two genes, ***RAG-1 and RAG-2*** (recombination-activating genes) are, as their name implies, critical in initiating recombination in lymphocyte precursor cells. Both RAG-1 and RAG-2 proteins are required in the first stages of cutting Ig- and TCR-DNA: mice lacking one of these genes ("RAG knockout mice") are deficient in both B and T cells. While the V(D)J recombinase is found in all cells and is involved in the repair of DNA strands, RAG-1 and RAG-2 gene products are expressed exclusively in lymphocytes.

κ Chain Synthesis. We will first examine the synthesis of κ light chains. Figure 6.2 shows the set of human genes coding for κ chains—referred to as the κ ***locus***—that is found on chromosome 2. Genetic analysis has shown that the arrangement of κ genes in the germ line—that is, in *any* cell in the body—is as follows: There are approximately 40 different V_κ genes, each of which can code for the N-terminal 95 amino acids of a κ variable region. As shown in Figure 6.2, the V_κ genes are arranged linearly in the genome, separated by introns. Each V_κ gene has its own L (leader) sequence, which, for simplicity, has been omitted from the figure. A series of 5 J_κ gene segments is found downstream (i.e., 3′) of this region. Each J_κ gene segment can encode the remaining 13 amino acid residues (96–108) of the κ variable region. A long intron separates the C_κ gene segment—the gene coding for the single constant region of the κ chain—from the J_κ gene segments.

To make a κ chain, an early cell in the B lymphocyte lineage selects one of the V_κ genes from its DNA and physically joins it to one of the J_κ segments (in Fig. 6.2, V_2 rearranges to J_4). How this selection of V and J genes is made is not known but is probably a random process. Joining involves the linking of ***recognition sequences,*** which are found at the ends of all genes (both Ig and TCR) that use rearranging gene segments to generate polypeptides. Figure 6.3 shows this V_2 to J_4 rearrangement in more detail; note that the DNA in this cell still contains the unrearranged gene segments V_1 and J_5. When joining occurs during rearrangement, in most cases the intervening DNA is looped, cut out, and ultimately broken down.

Figure 6.2 also indicates that after a cell in the B cell lineage rearranges its DNA, it makes a primary RNA transcript. This transcript is then spliced to remove all intervening noncoding sequences, bringing the V_κ, J_κ, and C_κ exons together in a mature mRNA. At the cell's rough endoplasmic reticulum, the leader sequence is cleaved off, and the mRNA is translated into the κ polypeptide chain. The κ chain moves into the lumen of the endoplasmic reticulum, where it can join with a newly synthesized H chain to form an Ig molecule.

λ Chain Synthesis. The λ genes are found on chromosome 22 in the human—that is, on a chromosome distinct from the κ and from the H chain genes. The synthesis of λ

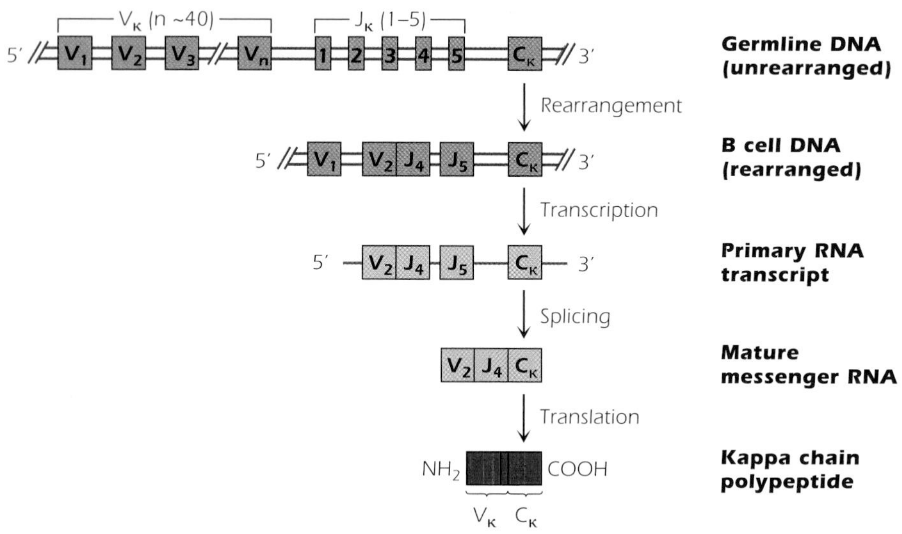

Figure 6.2. The genetic events leading to the synthesis of a kappa light chain.

chains is similar in principle to the synthesis of κ chains in that it involves rearrangement of DNA, which joins a V_λ gene (coding for the N-terminal region of a λ variable region) with a J_λ segment (coding for the remaining 13 amino acids of the λ variable region). The human λ locus comprises about 40 V_λ and 4 J_λ genes, which are known to be functional. (The J_λ region also contains sequences known as ***pseudogenes,*** long stretches of DNA that have some defect that prevents them from being transcribed or translated.) The organization of the λ gene locus is slightly different from the organization of the κ gene locus, which contains only one C_κ gene: By contrast, each J_λ is associated with a different C_λ gene. Thus there are four different types of C_λ polypeptides in the human.

Organization and Rearrangement of Heavy Chain Genes

H chain genes are found on a chromosome distinct from either L chain (chromosome 14 in humans). Figure 6.4 shows the organization of genes coding for the H chain and illustrates the similarities and differences of this locus with the L chain loci. In contrast to the variable region of a light chain that is constructed from two gene segments, the variable region of a heavy chain is constructed from three gene segments (V_H, D_H, and J_H). Thus, in addition to V and J segments, genes coding for the variable region of a H chain also use a ***diversity*** (D) ***segment.*** The D and J segments code for amino acid sequences in the third hypervariable, or ***complementarity determining region*** (CDR) 3 of the heavy chain (see Chapter 4). Figure 6.4 indicates that the human H chain locus includes approximately 50 V_H genes, about 20 D_H gene segments, and 6 J_H gene segments.

The second key feature of the H chain genes is the presence in the germ line of multiple genes coding for the C region of the Ig. As described in Chapter 4, the C region determines the class and hence biologic function of the particular antibody. The C genes, each flanked by introns, are separated from the V_H genes by a large intron. The order of C genes in the human is shown in Figure 6.4. The C genes closest to the V region genes are μ and δ, which are transcribed first during B cell development.

Heavy chain synthesis uses the same mechanisms of rearrangement described for light chains—namely, the use of the V(D)J recombinase to mediate the joining of different gene segments. In the early stages of the life of a particular B cell, two rearrangements of germ line DNA must occur. The first brings one D segment alongside one J segment. The

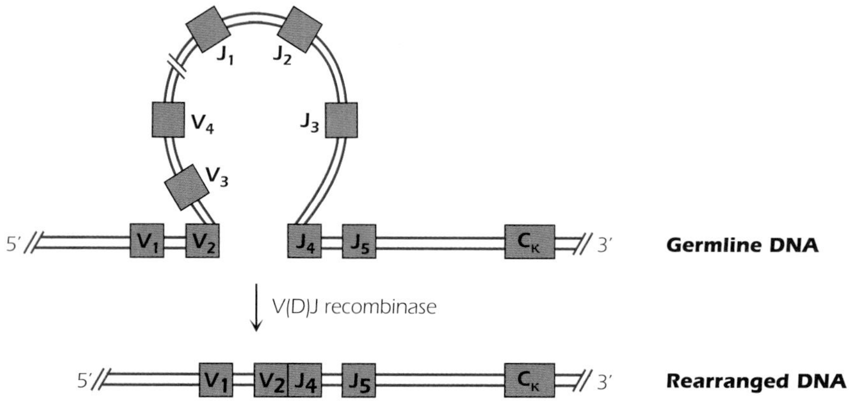

Figure 6.3. Rearrangement of DNA coding for a kappa light chain.

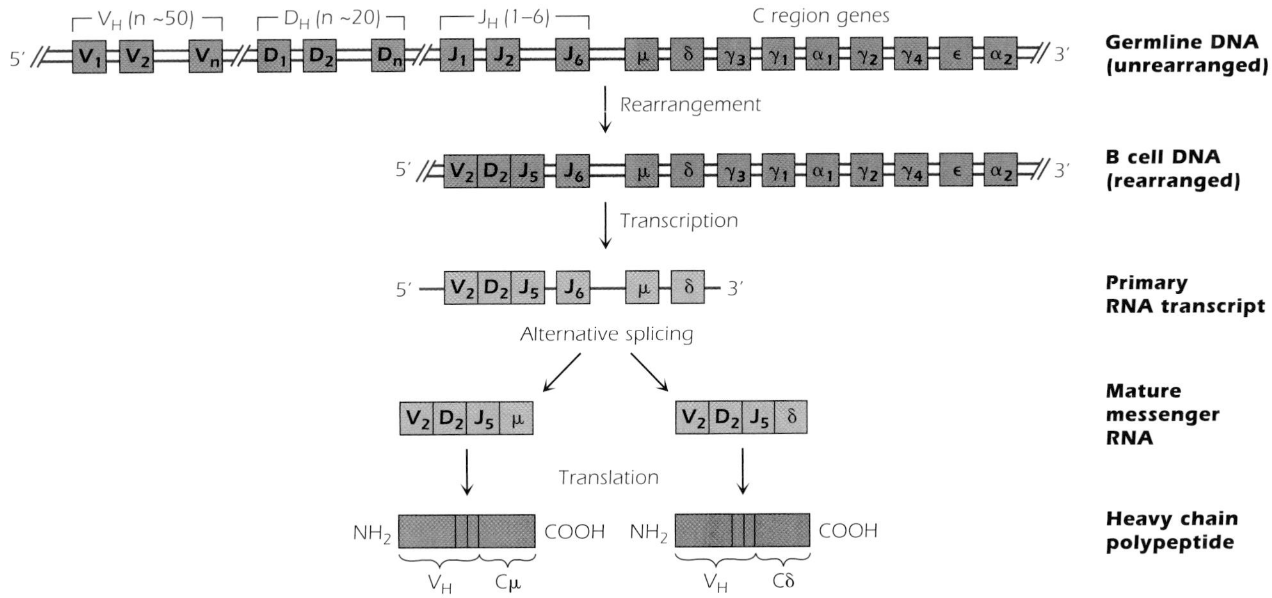

Figure 6.4. The genetic events leading to the synthesis of a human heavy chain.

second brings one V segment next to the DJ unit (V_2 D_2 J_5 in Fig. 6.4), fixing the antigen specificity of the H chain. The rearranged DNA is then transcribed along with the closest C region genes μ and δ. This primary transcript can be spliced in two different ways (***alternative splicing***) to yield either a VDJ-μ or a VDJ-δ mRNA. These two messages may then be translated in rough endoplasmic reticulum to yield either a μ or δ polypeptide. In this way, an individual resting B cell may express both μ and δ with identical antigenic specificity.

Alternative splicing of the heavy chain primary transcript also generates membrane and secreted forms of a heavy chain polypeptide. Two additional exons (not shown in Figure 6.4) are found at the 3′ end of each C_H gene, for example at the 3′ end of C_μ. These exons code for a) the transmembrane plus cytoplasmic tail of the membrane form of the molecule, and b) the C-terminal end of the secreted form of the molecule. Both exons are transcribed into the primary transcript, but one or other of the transcribed exons is spliced out in the mature mRNA. In this way, either the membrane or the secreted form of the heavy chain polypeptide is synthesized.

Regulation of Ig Gene Expression

Theoretically, any one B cell has many genes from which to choose to synthesize an Ig molecule: multiple V, D, and J genes to form the variable regions, and different genes for the light chains, κ and λ. In reality, each B cell uses only one set of VDJ genes and one type of light chain. As a result, ***a single B cell produces an Ig of only one antigenic specificity***.

Furthermore, a given B cell has two sets of chromosomes, one set from each parent, so theoretically, Ig genes located on both chromosomes could synthesize Ig molecules. This does not occur. In contrast to almost all other gene products, which are derived from genes from both parental chromosomes, Ig chains are coded for by only one set of genes, either from the maternal or the paternal chromosome. For example, the H chain may be coded for by genes on the paternal chromosome and the L chain (either κ or λ) by genes on the maternal chromosome. This phenomenon of using genes from only one parental chromosome is known as ***allelic exclusion.***

The steps in rearrangement, allelic exclusion, and hence the synthesis of a complete Ig molecule, are very tightly controlled, although all the control mechanisms are not yet completely clear. If a successful or ***productive*** rearrangement of V, D, and J gene DNA occurs on one of the parental chromosomes, and an H chain polypeptide is produced, the other parental H-chain locus stops rearranging as a result of some kind of suppressive mechanism. If the attempt to rearrange the V, D, and J genes on the first parental chromosome is unsuccessful (i.e., if it fails to produce a polypeptide chain), then the second parental chromosome continues H-chain locus rearrangement. The same process then occurs with the L chain loci, first with the κ and then with the λ chain genes. Productive rearrangement resulting from the joining of a V segment to a J segment of any one of these genes causes the others to remain in germ line form. In this way, the cell progresses through some or all of its chromosomal copies until it has successfully completed the productive rearrangement of genes for one H and one L chain. These chains then become the basis of the antibody specificity of that particular cell.

In summary, only one H chain and one L chain are functionally expressed in a B cell, even though every B cell contains two chromosomes (paternally and maternally derived) that could code for the heavy chain and two chromosomes that could code for the light chain. This mechanism of gene exclusion ensures that every B cell and the antibody it synthesizes are ***monospecific***—that is, are specific for only one epitope. In this way, an individual B cell is prevented from forming and expressing Ig molecules with different antigenic specificities on its cell surface.

CLASS OR ISOTYPE SWITCHING

As we have described above, one B cell makes antibody of just a single specificity that is fixed by the nature of VJ (L chain) and VDJ (H chain) rearrangements. These rearrangements occur in the absence of antigen in the early stages of B cell differentiation. We have also described how a single B cell can synthesize IgM and IgD with the same antigenic specificity. In the paragraphs that follow, we show how an individual B cell can switch to make a different class of antibody, such as IgG, IgE, or IgA. This phenomenon is known as ***class*** or ***isotype switching.*** Class switching changes the effector function of the B cell but does not change the cell's antigenic specificity.

Class switching occurs in antigen-stimulated mature B cells synthesizing IgM and IgD (discussed in Chapter 7) and involves further DNA rearrangement, juxtaposing the rearranged VDJ genes with a different heavy-chain C region gene (see Figure 6.5). In addition to antigen, class switching is dependent on the presence of factors known as ***cytokines*** released by T cells (see below and further discussion in Chapters 10 and 11). There is little or no class switching by B cells in the absence of such T cell–derived cytokines.

The cytokines that affect class switching induce further rearrangement of B cell DNA and produce switching to other Ig classes in a downstream progression (e.g., to IgG_4 or IgE). Thus a single B cell with a unique specificity is capable of making an antibody of all possible classes, depending on the switches occurring in the DNA coding for its H chain.

The mechanism by which mature B cells undergo class switching is shown in Figure 6.5. At the 5′ end of every H chain C region (C_H) gene, apart from C_δ, is a stretch of repeating base sequences called a ***switch*** (S) ***region.*** This S region permits any of the C_H genes (other than C_δ) to associate with the VDJ unit; in the figure, only the C_H genes γ_3, γ_1, and α_2 are shown, but other C_H genes may also be used. Under the stimulating influence of antigen and T cell–derived cytokines, a B cell with a VDJ unit linked to C_μ and C_δ further rearranges its DNA to link the VDJ to an S region in front of another C_H region gene (γ_1 in Fig. 6.5). After a primary RNA transcript is made from the rearranged DNA, the introns are spliced out to give an mRNA coding for the IgG_1 H chain. In so doing, the intervening C region DNA is removed. Thus, at this stage, the cell loses its ability to revert to making a class of antibody whose C region gene has been deleted (IgM, IgD, or IgG_3 in this example).

Class switching is a mechanism unique to Ig H chains of B cells. It allows an antibody with a single antigenic specificity to associate with a variety of different constant region chains and thus have different effector functions. For example, an antibody with a VDJ unit specific for a bacterial antigen may be linked to $C\gamma$ to produce an IgG molecule; this IgG antibody interacts with cells such as macrophages that express receptors for $Fc\gamma$. Alternatively, the same VDJ unit may be linked to $C\varepsilon$ to produce an IgE molecule; IgE antibody interacts with cells such as mast cells that express receptors for $Fc\varepsilon$.

Cytokines present when antigen activates B cells play a key role in C_H gene selection during isotype switching. For example, in the presence of the cytokine interferon-γ, the B cell can rearrange its VDJ to the $C\gamma_2$ heavy chain, and the cell switches to IgG_2 synthesis. By contrast, in the presence of the cytokine interleukin-4 (IL-4), a B cell can rearrange its VDJ

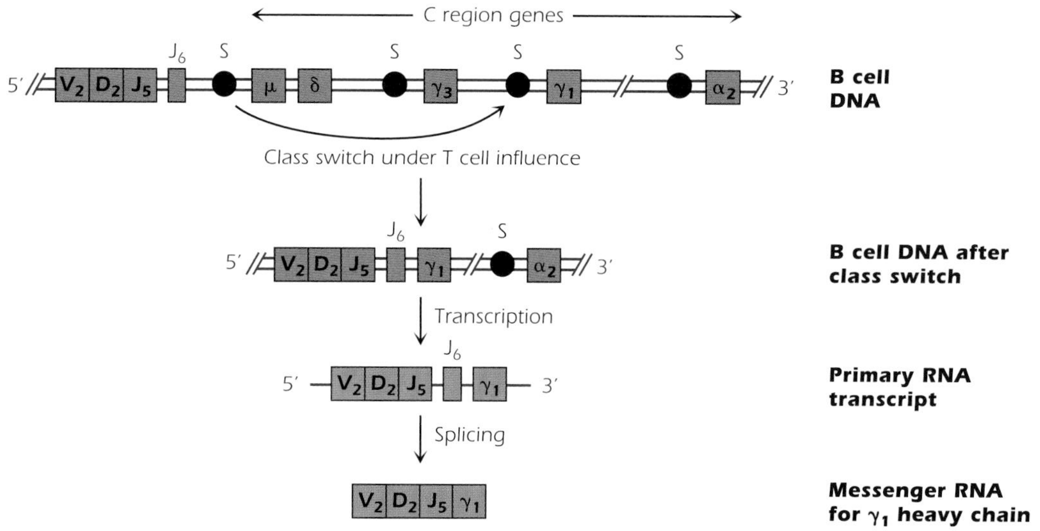

Figure 6.5. Mechanism of class switching in Ig synthesis. S = switch region, upstream of each heavy-chain constant region.

to $C\gamma_4$ or $C\varepsilon$, and the cell switches to IgG_4 or IgE synthesis, respectively. Each cytokine is thought to loosen the structure of the DNA double helix at only certain points along the Ig locus, allowing an enzyme known as a "switch recombinase" to recognize DNA coding for specific C regions.

GENERATION OF ANTIBODY DIVERSITY

Thus far we have described the unique genetic mechanisms involved in generating an enormously varied set of antibodies to cope with the universe of antigens without using a great deal of DNA. Still more mechanisms for generating diversity exist, some of which are discussed briefly below.

Presence of Multiple V Genes in the Germ Line

The number of different genes for the V region in the germ line constitutes the baseline from which antibody is derived and represents the minimum number of different antibodies that can be produced.

VJ and VDJ Combinatorial Association

As we have already seen, the association of any V gene segment with any J gene segment can occur to form an L chain variable region, and similarly, any V can associate with any D or J gene segments in H chain gene rearrangement. All these distinct segments contribute to the structure of the variable region. As there are about 40 V_κ and 5 J_κ genes coding for the κ chain variable region, assuming random association, then 40×5 or 200 κ chains can be formed; with 40 V_κ and 4 J_λ genes, 160 λ chains can be formed. Similarly, if there are about 50 V genes, 20 D genes, and 6 J genes that can code for an H chain variable region, and these may also associate in any combination, $50 \times 20 \times 6$ or 6000 different heavy chains can be formed.

Random Assortment of H and L Chains

In addition to VJ and VDJ combinatorial association, any H chain may associate with any L chain. Thus if any H chain can associate with any κ or λ chain, a total of 1.2×10^6 different κ-containing Ig molecules (200×6000), and 0.96×10^6(160×6000) λ-containing molecules can be generated from just 165 different genes (adding up all the H, κ, and λ segments)! This illustrates very effectively how a limited set of genes can generate a large number of different antibodies.

Junctional and Insertional Diversity

The precise positions at which the genes for the V and J (or V, D, and J) segments are fused together are not constant, and imprecise DNA recombination can lead to changes in the amino acids at these junction sites. The absence of precision in joining during DNA rearrangement leads to deletions or changes of amino acids (***junctional diversity***) that affect the antigen-binding site, since they occur in parts of the hypervariable region where complementarity to antigen is determined. In addition, small sets of nucleotides may be inserted (***insertional diversity***) at the V–D and D–J junctions. The major mechanism for inserting nucleotides into the DNA sequence is mediated by the enzyme ***terminal deoxynucleotidyltransferase*** (TdT). The additional diversity generated is termed ***N region diversity.***

Somatic Hypermutation

Mutations that occur in V genes of heavy and/or light chains during the lifetime of a B cell also increase the variety of antibodies produced by the B cell population. Generally, an antibody of low affinity is produced in the primary response to antigen. DNA and polypeptide sequencing of antibodies formed in the primary response indicate that the sequences closely match the sequences encoded by germ line DNA. As the response matures, however, and especially after secondary stimulation by the antigen, the affinity for antigen of the antibodies synthesized increases, and the amino acid sequences of these antibodies diverge from those coded for in the germ line DNA.

This divergence results predominantly from point mutations in the VDJ recombined unit of antibody V genes, which result in changes in individual amino acids. This phenomenon is referred to as ***somatic hypermutation*** because it occurs at a rate at least 10,000-fold higher than the normal rate of mutation. Somatic hypermutation results in the observed increased affinity of antibodies for antigen in the secondary response. As a consequence of this fine-tuning of the immune response, somatic hypermutation increases the variety of antibodies produced by the B cell population. The evidence suggests that there is a narrow window for somatic hypermutation to occur—that is, after antigenic stimulation in the germinal centers of spleen and lymph node (see Chapter 7).

Somatic Gene Conversion

The paradigm that Ig diversity is generated by VDJ recombination and somatic hypermutation evolved from studies of mouse and human B cells. Subsequent studies in other species, most notably in birds and rabbits, however, revealed that these animals use a mechanism known as ***somatic gene conversion*** to generate a repertoire of diverse B cell specificities. Somatic gene conversion involves the nonreciprocal exchange of sequences among genes: Part of the donor gene or genes is "copied" into an acceptor gene, but only the acceptor gene is altered. The precise mechanism by which this occurs is currently not clear. Figure 6.6 shows the chicken H chain locus, which includes a single functional V_H gene that rearranges in all B cells and approximately 20 defective V_H genes (pseudogenes) that cannot rearrange. The bottom line

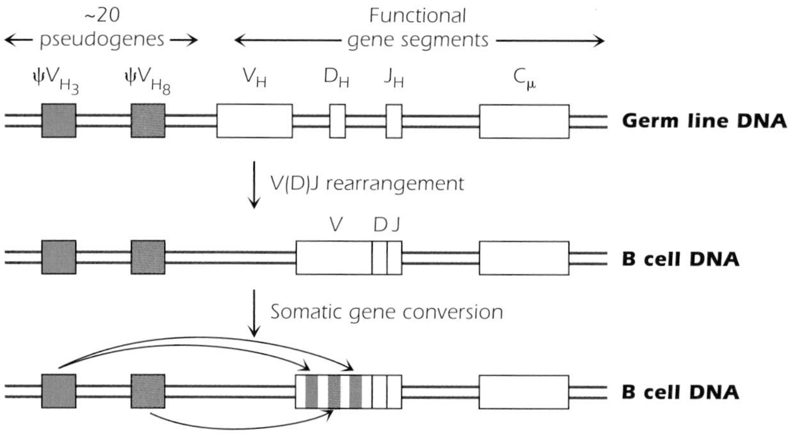

Figure 6.6. Somatic gene conversion generates diversity in Ig genes of several species. The figure illustrates the phenomenon in the chicken Ig heavy-chain locus: short sequences of DNA from one or more pseudogenes (3 and 8 in the figure) are copied into the rearranged B-cell VDJ unit.

of the figure shows that in this particular B cell a diversified variable gene unit is generated by incorporating two short sequences from pseudogene 3 and one from pseudogene 8 into the rearranged VDJ gene. Somatic gene conversion can also generate L chain diversity.

Many species other than humans and mice rely on somatic gene conversion and somatic hypermutation to generate diversity within the *primary* Ig repertoire—that is, before antigen stimulation. For example, chickens use somatic gene conversion as a major mechanism to generate the primary repertoire, whereas sheep use somatic hypermutation. Other species, such as rabbit, cattle, and swine, use very limited VDJ recombination plus somatic gene conversion and somatic hypermutation to generate their primary Ig diversity.

Receptor Editing

Under some circumstances, a cell in the B cell lineage can undergo a second rearrangement of its L chain variable gene segments, after it has formed a recombined VJ unit. This process is known as ***receptor editing,*** (described in Chapter 7). The mechanism of receptor editing can be understood by looking at Figure 6.3. The rearranged DNA of this particular B cell contains the unrearranged elements V_1 and J_5, which can be used in a second rearrangement. Receptor editing can occur when a B cell with a receptor specific for a self-antigen interacts with that self-antigen. One outcome of this interaction is that the V and J genes of the B cell undergo a second rearrangement, which may generate a VJ recognition unit specific for a foreign, rather than a self, antigen. Thus receptor editing may increase the diversity of the overall response to foreign antigens.

All these mechanisms contribute to the formation of a huge ***library*** or ***repertoire*** of B lymphocytes that contain all the specificities required to deal with the universe of diverse epitopes. Estimates of the number of total Ig specificities that can be generated in an individual are on the order of 10^{15}, which is increased even more by somatic hypermutation.

SUMMARY

1. Every individual synthesizes an enormous number of different Ig molecules, each of which can act as a receptor on the B cell surface, specific for a particular epitope.

2. The variable region of the H chain in an Ig molecule is coded for by three separate genes, referred to as V_H (variable), D_H (diversity), and J_H (joining) gene segments. A distinct gene segment codes for the constant region of the heavy chain, C_H. The variable region of the L chain is coded for by two gene segments, V_L and J_L, distinct from the gene segments used for heavy chain synthesis. DNA from every cell in the body (the germ line) contains multiple V, D, and J gene segments for Ig H and L chain synthesis.

3. In the course of differentiation, a B cell rearranges its H chain DNA so as to join one V_H gene segment to one D_H gene segment and one J_H gene segment. The joined VDJ unit codes for the entire variable region of the heavy chain. These gene rearrangements put the VDJ unit close to the H chain constant region genes, C_μ and C_δ.

4. The same type of rearrangement produces a gene unit coding for the entire V region of an Ig L chain; one V_L gene segment is joined to one J_L segment, putting the VJ unit close to a L chain constant region gene. In a B cell committed to making a κ chain, the $V_\kappa J_\kappa$ unit is juxtaposed to the C_κ gene, and in a B cell committed to making a λ chain, the $V_\lambda J_\lambda$ unit is juxtaposed to a C_λ gene.

5. Primary RNA transcripts are made from the rearranged DNA. Noncoding RNA is spliced out of the primary transcripts, resulting in mRNA for light and heavy chains, which are then translated into the L and H chains of IgM and IgD.

6. In a B cell, the H chain is coded for by the H chain gene segments found on either the maternally or the paternally derived chromosome; the L chain is also coded for by the L chain gene segments found on one or other chromosome. This phenomenon, allelic exclusion, ensures that a single B cell produces an Ig of only one antigenic specificity.

7. After antigenic stimulation, a B cell can further rearrange its H chain DNA. The VDJ unit, which has joined to the C_μ and C_δ genes, can rearrange to join another C region gene, such as $C\gamma$, $C\alpha$ or $C\varepsilon$. This phenomenon is known as class switching. As a result, the B cell that was synthesizing IgM and IgD can now synthesize antibody of a different isotype (IgG, IgA, or IgE) but with the same antigenic specificity.

8. Diversity in antibody specificity is achieved by the following:
   - Multiple inherited genes for the V regions of both L and H chains.
   - Rearrangement of V, D, and J segments in different combinations, and random assortment of H and L chains.
   - Junctional and insertional diversity when V, D, and J genes are joined.
   - Somatic hypermutation, which primarily occurs after stimulation by antigen, leading to selection for mutations that endow the antibody with higher affinity for the antigen.
   - Somatic gene conversion in species other than the human or mouse: Short DNA sequences from nonrearranging genes are copied into a rearranged VDJ gene unit.

   These mechanisms allow a small number of genes to generate a vast number of antibody molecules with different antigenic specificities.

REFERENCES

Bassing CH, Swat W, Alt FW (2002): The mechanism and regulation of chromosomal V(D)J recombination. *Cell 109*(Suppl):S45.

Flajnik MF (2002): Comparative analyses of immunoglobulin genes: surprises and portents. *Nat Rev Immunol* 2:688.

Guttmacher AE, Collins FS (2002): Genomic medicine—a primer *N Engl J Med* 347:1512.

Honjo T, Kinoshita K, Muramatsu M (2002): Molecular mechanism of class switch recombination: linkage with somatic hypermutation. *Annu Rev Immunol* 20:165.

Schlissel M (2002): Allelic exclusion of immunoglobulin gene rearrangement and expression: why and how? *Semin Immunol* 14:207.

Seagal J, Melamed D (2002): Role of receptor revision in forming a B cell repertoire. *Clin Immunol* 105:1.

REVIEW QUESTIONS

For each question, choose the ONE BEST answer or completion.

1. The DNA for an H chain in a B cell making IgG_2 antibody for diphtheria toxoid has the following structure: 5′–$V_{17}D_5J_2$ $C\gamma_2$—$C\gamma_4$—$C\varepsilon$—$C\alpha_2$–3′ How many individual rearrangements were required to go from the embryonic DNA to this B-cell DNA?
   A) 1
   B) 2
   C) 3
   D) 4
   E) none

2. If you had 50 V, 20 D, and 6 J regions able to code for a heavy chain, and 40 V and 5 J region genes able to code for a light chain, you could have a maximum repertoire of
   A) $76 + 45 = 121$ antibody specificities
   B) $76 \times 45 = 3420$ specificities
   C) $(40 \times 5) + (50 \times 20 \times 6) = 6200$ specificities
   D) $(40 \times 5) \times (50 \times 20 \times 6) = 1{,}200{,}000$ specificities
   E) more than 1,200,000 specificities

3. The antigen specificity of a particular B cell
   A) is induced by interaction with antigen.
   B) is determined only by the L-chain sequence.
   C) is determined by H + L-chain variable region sequences.
   D) changes after isotype switching.
   E) is determined by the heavy-chain constant region.

4. If you could analyze, at the molecular level, a plasma cell making IgA antibody, you would find all of the following *except*

A) a DNA sequence for V, D, and J genes translocated near the $C\alpha$ DNA exon.
B) mRNA specific for either κ or λ light chains.
C) mRNA specific for J chains.
D) mRNA specific for μ chains.
E) a DNA sequence coding for the T-cell receptor for antigen.

5. The ability of a single B cell to express both IgM and IgD molecules on its surface at the same time is made possible by

A) allelic exclusion.
B) isotype switching.
C) simultaneous recognition of two distinct antigens.
D) selective RNA splicing.
E) use of genes from both parental chromosomes.

6. Which of the following statements concerning the organization of Ig genes is correct?

A) V and J regions of embryonic DNA have already undergone a rearrangement.
B) Light-chain genes undergo further rearrangement after surface IgM is expressed.
C) V_H gene segments can rearrange with $J\kappa$ or $J\lambda$ gene segments.
D) The VDJ segments coding for an Ig V_H region may associate with different heavy-chain constant region genes.
E) After VDJ joining has occurred, a further rearrangement is required to bring the VDJ unit next to the $C\mu$ gene.

7. Which of the following does not contribute to the generation of diversity of B-cell antigen receptors?

A) multiple V genes in the germ line
B) random assortment of L and H chains
C) imprecise recombination of V and J or V, D, and J segments
D) inheritance of multiple C-region genes
E) somatic hypermutation

8. Which of the following concerning Ig expression on a B cell is *incorrect:*

A) The light chains of the IgM and IgD have identical amino acid sequences.
B) The constant parts of the heavy chains of the IgM and IgD have different amino acid sequences.
C) The IgM and IgD have different antigenic specificities.
D) If the B cell is triggered by antigen and T-cell signals to proliferate and differentiate into antibody secreting plasma cells, the cell can potentially secrete IgG, IgE, or IgA antibody.
E) The IgM on the surface will have either κ light chains or λ light chains, but not both.

9. Which of the following plays a role in changing the antigen binding site of a B cell *after* antigenic stimulation?:

A) junctional diversity
B) combinatorial diversity
C) germ-line diversity
D) somatic hypermutation
E) differential splicing of primary RNA transcripts

CASE STUDY

As a member of a research team studying a tribe found in a remote region of New Guinea, you make the astonishing discovery that members of the tribe have only two V genes for the L chain and three V genes for the H chain of Igs. Nevertheless, people seem healthy and able to resist the large number of pathogenic organisms endemic to the area. Suggest how this might be accomplished.

ANSWERS TO REVIEW QUESTIONS

1. *C* Three DNA rearrangements are required. First, $D_5 \rightarrow J_2$ rearrangement occurs, followed by $V_{17} \rightarrow D_5J_2$. This permits synthesis of IgM and IgD molecules using $V_{17}D_5J_2$. The third rearrangement is the class switch of $V_{17}D_5J_2C\mu C\delta$ to $V_{17}D_5J_2C\gamma 2$, leading to the synthesis of IgG_2 molecules.

2. *E* While 1,200,000 would be the product of all possible combinations of genes, the generation of many more antibody specificities is likely as a result of imprecise recombinations of VJ or VDJ segments, insertional diversity, and somatic hypermutation.

3. *C* The antigenic specificity is determined by the sequences and hence the structure formed by the combination of heavy- and light-chain variable regions.

4. *D* As a consequence of the rearrangement of the VDJ to $C\alpha$ in the IgA producing cell, the $C\mu$ gene will have been deleted. The other DNA sequences and mRNA species will be found in the cell.

5. *D* The simultaneous synthesis of IgM and IgD is made possible by the alternate splicing of the primary RNA transcript $5'$–VDJ—$C\mu$—$C\delta$–$3'$; to give either VDJ$C\mu$ or VDJ$C\delta$ messages.

6. *D* This is the basis of isotype or class switching.

7. *D* The presence of multiple C_H region genes, although the basis for functional diversity, does not contribute to the diversity of antigen-specific receptors.

8. *C* The IgM and IgD expressed on a single B cell use the same heavy- and light-chain V(D)J gene units and therefore have the same antigenic specificity.

9. *D* Of the mechanisms described for generating diversity of Ig molecules, only somatic hypermutation affects the antigen binding site *after* antigen stimulation.

ANSWER TO CASE STUDY

Despite their paucity of V-region genes, members of the tribe presumably retain other mechanisms for generating diversity of their antibody genes. These mechanisms include: the presence of multiple J and D gene segments in the germ line, junctional diversity due to deletion or insertion of bases at joining sites, random assortment of H and L chains, and somatic hypermutation. Thus, even with their limited V-gene repertoire, these individuals generate sufficient diversity of antibody specificity to survive.

7

BIOLOGY OF THE B LYMPHOCYTE

INTRODUCTION

In Chapter 6 we described how B lymphocytes can develop a vast repertoire of different antigenic specificities. This explains one of the key features of the adaptive immune response that we initially described in the "Clonal Selection Theory" section of Chapter 2—namely, ***diversity,*** the ability to respond to many different antigenic determinants—epitopes—even if the individual has not previously encountered them. The other important characteristics of the adaptive immune response are as follows:

- **Specificity.** The ability to discriminate among different epitopes.
- **Memory.** The ability to recall previous contact with a particular antigen, so that a subsequent exposure leads to a more rapid and more effective immune response than the first encounter.
- **Discrimination between self and nonself.** The ability to respond to those antigens that are "foreign," or nonself, and to prevent responses to those antigens that are part of self.

This chapter describes the biology of B lymphocytes, the cells that synthesize antibody in response to antigen. It focuses on the critical steps in B cell development and how B cells acquire the features associated with the adaptive immune response—diversity, specificity, memory, and discrimination between self and nonself.

Sites of Early B Cell Differentiation

Our understanding of B cell differentiation has been facilitated by studying different animals in which the early embryonic stages can be manipulated. For this reason, B cell differentiation in chickens and in mammals is particularly well characterized. Many of the differentiation steps are common to humans, chickens, and mice.

B lymphocytes acquired their name from early experiments in birds: the synthesis of antibody was shown to require the presence of an organ called the bursa of Fabricius (an outpouching of the cloacal epithelium). Surgically removing the bursa prevented antibody synthesis. Thus the cells that developed into mature, antibody-forming cells were called ***bursa-derived,*** or ***B cells.*** In contrast to birds, mammals do not appear to have a bursa; rather, B cell differentiation occurs in a restricted number of critical sites. Precursors of the B cell lineage are found early in fetal development, at sites including the fetal liver. Later in fetal development and throughout the rest of life, the bone marrow is the predominant site of B cell differentiation. The bone marrow is therefore considered the ***primary lymphoid organ*** for B cell differentiation in the human and other mammals (see Chapter 2).

Immunology: A Short Course, Fifth Edition, By Richard Coico, Geoffrey Sunshine, and Eli Benjamini
ISBN 0-471-22689-0

ONTOGENY OF THE B LYMPHOCYTE

Early Phases of B Cell Differentiation: Pro-B and Pre-B Cells

Figure 7.1 illustrates the key stages in the B cell differentiation pathway. Many of these stages are defined by specific Ig gene rearrangements that we described in Chapter 6.

B lymphocytes arise from ***hematopoietic stem cells.*** Adhesive interactions with the bone marrow ***stroma,*** the nonlymphoid cells that make up the framework or matrix of the marrow, and the actions of the cytokine interleukin-7 (IL-7), provide signals that promote the survival and enhance proliferation of cells early in the B cell lineage. The earliest distinguishable cell in the B lineage is known as a ***pro-B cell,*** in which a heavy-chain D_H gene segment rearranges to a J_H gene segment. In the next stage, the ***pre-B cell,*** a heavy-chain V_H gene segment rearranges to join the rearranged D_HJ_H segments, forming a VDJ unit. This rearranged VDJ is thus put close to C_μ (see Fig. 6.4), and the pre-B cell synthesizes a μ chain.

The Ig gene rearrangements that occur during these early phases of B cell differentiation follow an ordered sequence, as was described in Chapter 6. The initial D-J rearrangement in the pro-B cell takes place on both H chain chromosomes at the same time. The chromosome that makes a productive DJ rearrangement then rearranges a V region gene to the DJ unit. If this V-DJ rearrangement is productive, the chromosome makes a μ chain, and H chain rearrangement is shut down on the other chromosome. If the V-DJ rearrangement is not productive on the first chromosome, however, rearrangement takes place on the other chromosome. If rearrangement on the second chromosome is productive, then *this* chromosome makes a μ chain. If none of these rearrangements is productive, the cell dies by ***apoptosis,*** also known as ***programmed cell death.***

A key characteristic of the pre-B cell is that it expresses the μ chain as a transmembrane molecule at the cell surface in conjunction with the products of two nonrearranging genes, called λ5 and VpreB; λ5 and VpreB together function as ***surrogate light chains.*** Figure 7.2A shows that the μ chain and surrogate light chains of the pre-B cell are expressed at the cell surface with two closely associated transmembrane molecules known as ***Igα*** (CD79a) and ***Igβ*** (CD79b), which are disulfide-linked to each other. The complex of μ and surrogate light chains in conjunction with Igα and Igβ is referred to as the ***pre-B cell receptor,*** (pre-BCR).

Igα and Igβ are associated with membrane Ig molecules on all cells in the B cell lineage, from the pre-B cell to the memory B cell (Fig. 7.1). The complex of Igα and Igβ associated with membrane Ig molecules of more mature cells in the B lymphocyte lineage is known as the ***B-cell receptor*** (BCR) and is depicted in Figure 7.2B. Igα and Igβ do not bind antigen. Their function is to transmit signals to the cell nucleus, leading to a change in the pattern of genes expressed; for this reason, Igα and Igβ are referred to as ***signal transduction molecules*** associated with the pre-BCR and the BCR. As we discuss in Chapters 8 and 10, signal transduction molecules are also associated with the antigen-specific receptor expressed at different stages of T lymphocyte development.

On mature B cells, the role of Igα and Igβ in the BCR is to transmit signals after antigen binds to the variable domains of surface Ig (discussed in more detail in Chapter 10). By contrast, there is no evidence that the pre-BCR

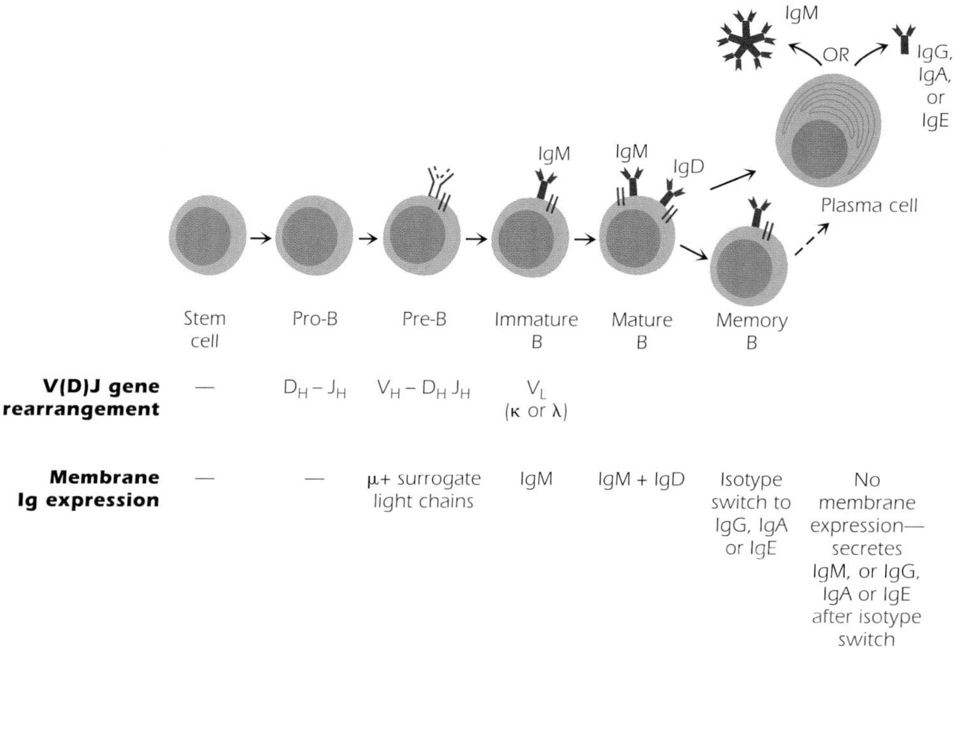

Figure 7.1. Differentiation pathway of B lymphocytes. Dashed lines on the pre-B cell indicate surrogate light chains. The two lines associated with the cell surface heavy chain represent the signaling molecules Igα and Igβ (CD79a and b).

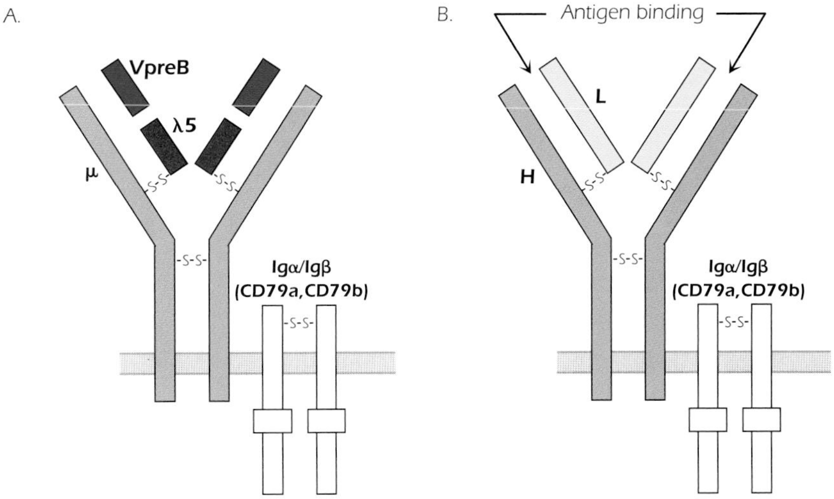

Figure 7.2. A: The pre-B-cell receptor (pre-BCR). B: The B-cell receptor (BCR). The heavy chain of the pre-BCR is a μ chain; the heavy chain of the BCR may be a μ, δ, γ, α, or ε chain. The immunoreceptor tyrosine-based activation motif (ITAM, discussed later in this chapter) is depicted as a rectangle in the Igα and Igβ polypeptides.

binds antigen. Rather, the data suggest that Igα and Igβ associated with the pre-BCR instruct the cell that it has successfully rearranged its Ig H chain genes and has made a functional μ chain. As a result of this signaling, the cell expressing the pre-BCR further differentiates: It proliferates, shuts down surrogate light-chain synthesis, starts L chain gene rearrangement, and stops further H chain gene rearrangement.

Light chain rearrangement in the later phases of pre-B cell development is also sequential: κ chain genes rearrange first, but if neither of the chromosomes coding for κ chains successfully rearranges, λ gene rearrangement takes place. (If no productive L chain rearrangement occurs, the cell dies.) As we pointed out in Chapter 6, the biological consequence of this use of genes from only one chromosome to make an H chain and genes from one chromosome to make an L chain—***allelic exclusion***—ensures that an individual B cell expresses an Ig molecule with only a single antigenic specificity on its cell surface.

Immature B Cells

At the next stage of B cell differentiation, L chains now pair with μ chains to form monomeric IgM, which is inserted in the membrane. The cell bearing only monomeric membrane IgM as its antigen-specific receptor is referred to as an ***immature B cell.*** Early experiments showed that immature B cells can recognize and respond to foreign antigen, but this interaction resulted in long-lasting ***inactivation,*** rather than expansion and differentiation. More recent studies indicate that immature B cells can interact with self-molecules in the bone marrow, which can also result in inactivation of the immature B cell. This interaction of self-molecules and immature B cells is important in the development of ***self-tolerance in the B cell lineage:*** Cells with potential reactivity to self are prevented from responding.

Figure 7.3 depicts the two ways that self-tolerance can develop. If the immature B cell is exposed to a self-molecule expressed on the surface of bone marrow cells, it dies by apoptosis (***deletion***). Alternatively, if the immature B cell is exposed to a non-cell-surface molecule (***soluble antigen***) in the bone marrow, the cell is inactivated but not deleted; it is said to be ***anergized.*** (Deletion and anergy are described further in Chapter 12.) The inactivation of immature B cells with potential reactivity to self through interaction with self-molecules is known as ***negative selection.*** As described in Chapter 8, developing T lymphocytes also undergo negative selection during differentiation in the thymus.

Figure 7.3 also depicts a third possible outcome for the interaction of an immature B cell and a self-molecule—namely, reactivation of the cell's V(D)J recombinase, in the phenomenon known as ***receptor editing*** (see Chapter 6). As

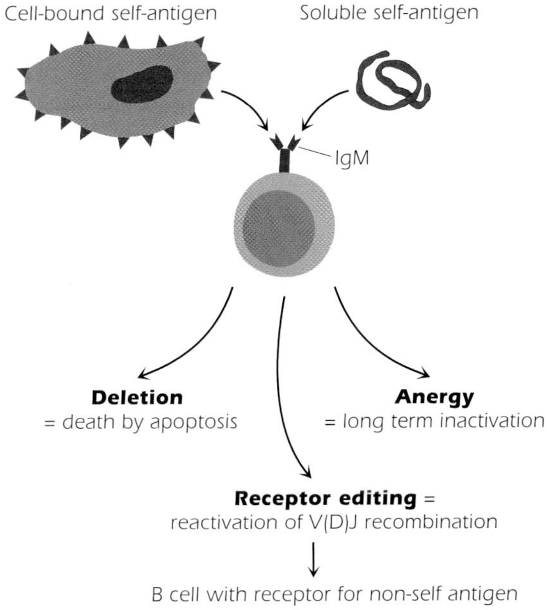

Figure 7.3. Interaction of the immature B cell with self-antigens.

a consequence, the cell's Ig L chain genes undergo secondary rearrangement, using unrearranged V or J elements. For example, in the cell shown in Figure 6.3, which is rearranging its κ locus, V_1 and J_5 are unrearranged genes that may be used in a second rearrangement. Receptor editing may generate a specificity for a non-self (foreign) antigen, and the immature B cell is thus "rescued" from inactivation.

Mature B Cells

The next step in the B cell differentiation pathway is the development of the ***IgM^+IgD^+ mature B cell.*** This is thought to occur predominantly in the bone marrow but may also take place in secondary lymphoid organs. The signals that drive the differentiation of the IgM^+ B cell to the IgM^+IgD^+ stage are not known. The IgM and IgD expressed on a single mature B cell have identical antigenic specificities; this results from the alternative splicing of a single RNA species transcribed from VDJ plus μ and δ genes (discussed in Chapter 6). The function of IgD is not completely understood; as we described in Chapter 4, cells B cells expressing IgD do not make antibodies that react with self-components. Thus the expression of IgD may be a signal to "silence" such autoreactive clones.

Antibody Synthesis and Class Switching. The interaction of antigen with the mature IgM^+IgD^+ B cell generally results in activation, in contrast to the inactivation we described earlier when antigen interacts with an immature IgM^+ B cell. Interaction of antigen with the mature B cell occurs primarily in the secondary lymphoid organs, the lymph nodes, and the spleen. Most antigens, especially proteins, are known as ***thymus dependent*** because they require ***helper T cells*** (described in Chapter 10) for B cells to synthesize antibody. The initial interaction of antigen, helper T cells, and mature B cells occurs at the interface of the B and T cell regions of the secondary lymphoid organ. The B cells enlarge (to become B-cell ***blasts***) and proliferate. Some of the activated B cells may differentiate further into ***plasma cells,*** which are a specialized end stage of B cell development that synthesize and secrete antibody (depicted on the far right of Fig. 7.1). The antibody secreted by an individual plasma cell has the same antigenic specificity as the Ig on the surface of the B cell that was initially triggered by antigen. Plasma cells do not express a membrane form of Ig.

Antibody of the IgM class is synthesized in the early stages of an immune response. Later in the response, progeny of the IgM^+IgD^+ B cell that initially responded to antigen may produce antibody of a different isotype. This ***class (isotype) switch,*** the mechanism of which we described in Chapter 6, occurs as a result of the synthesis of helper T cell derived cytokines and T–B-cell-surface interactions (discussed more fully in Chapter 10). Consequently, an IgM^+IgD^+ B cell switches to synthesizing IgG, IgA, or IgE molecules. Whatever the isotype of the Ig produced, all the daughter cells have the same antigenic specificity.

Affinity Maturation and Memory Cell Formation. Even later in the response to thymus-dependent antigens, some of the activated B cells form a specialized region in the secondary lymphoid organ, known as the ***germinal center*** (see Figs. 2.9 and Fig. 7.4). Figure 7.4 indicates that the germinal center consists predominantly of activated B cells; a few helper T cells; and a small number of specialized cells, known as follicular dendritic cells, which retain antigen on their surface and present it to B cells.

Figure 7.4 also indicates that the germinal center is the site of intense B cell proliferation. During this huge expansion of the initial B cell population, B cells with mutations in their Ig variable region genes are generated at a much higher rate than normal. This ***somatic hypermutation*** (referred to in Chapter 6) produces B cells whose Ig variable region genes can synthesize antibody with *higher affinity* to the activating antigen than can variable region genes of the original antigen-activated B cell. Recent evidence suggests that hypermutation occurs as the result of the action of an enzyme induced in the activated B cells. The enzyme converts cytosine in the antibody V region DNA into uracil; attempts to repair this incorrect base by the cell's repair machinery are highly prone to errors and introduce mutations.

B cells with these higher affinity V region genes are clonally selected and expanded in the germinal center, whereas B cells that do not have mutations in their V regions are not selected and die. Thus somatic hypermutation results in an increase in the production of high-affinity antibodies to a particular antigen, a phenomenon known as ***affinity maturation.*** These cells may also undergo class switch. B cells that are selected in the germinal center exit the lymphoid organ and make antibody of the appropriate class.

B cells activated in the germinal center may also differentiate to become ***memory B cells*** (see also Fig. 7.1), which leave the lymphoid organ and move into tissues. How precisely memory B cells develop in the germinal center is currently not clear, but it is thought that plasma cells do not become memory cells. Memory B cells are nonproliferating, generally long-lived B cells that can be activated for a subsequent (secondary) and more rapid response to antigen. They express isotypes other than IgM and IgD on their surface—namely, IgG, IgA, or IgE. Memory B cells do not appear to express unique molecules on their surface that distinguish them from naive or activated mature B cells. Memory B cells do express higher levels of CD44 than do other B cells; CD44 is involved in adhesion of lymphocytes to cells outside the lymph node.

The overall result of the differentiation steps described above is that the individual builds up a continuously replenished library of diverse B cell antigen specificities (***a repertoire***) directed against a wide array of antigens. The development of a response to antigen therefore depends on

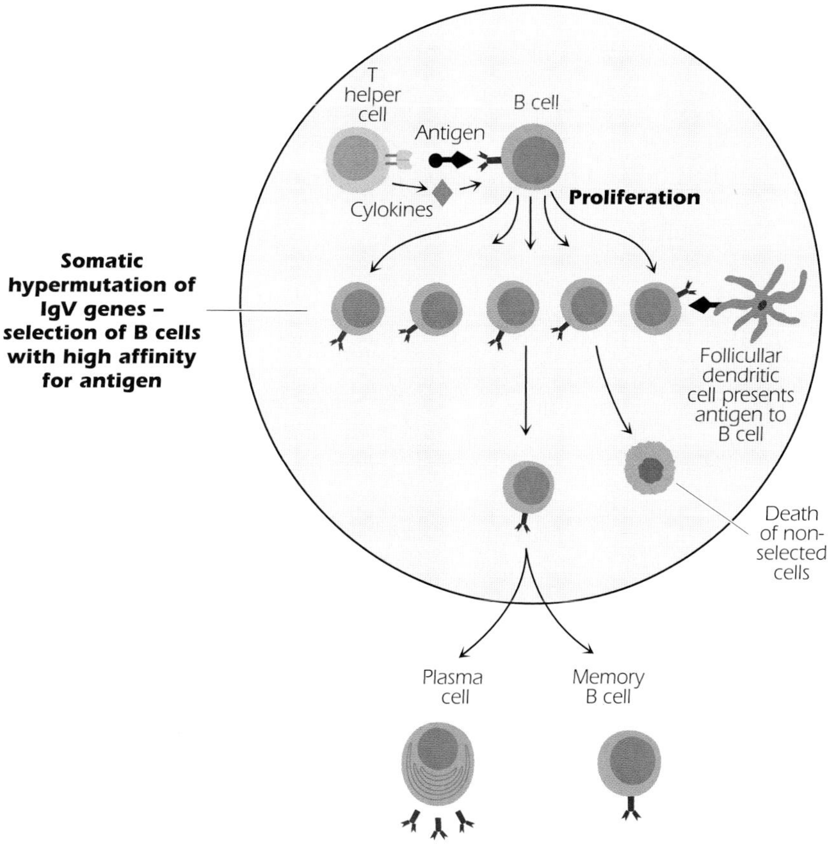

Figure 7.4. Development of B cells in the germinal center: somatic hypermutation, affinity maturation, and memory B cell formation.

the interaction of antigen with an existing B cell clone contained in this library. Most B cells in the vast B cell repertoire, however, do not interact with antigen during their lifetime—estimated to be 4–5 months for a mature B cell found in spleen—but remain as resting unstimulated IgM^+IgD^+ cells.

Anatomical Distribution of B Cell Populations

As described above, the early phases of B cell differentiation take place in bone marrow. Mature B cells circulate through blood to secondary lymphoid organs, primarily lymph nodes, spleen, and Peyer's patches of the intestine. If the B cell does not interact with antigen, either it leaves the lymphoid organ via the lymphatic vessels and continues to circulate or it dies in the organ. If the B cell does interact with antigen and helper T cells in the lymphoid organ, a germinal center is formed as described above. Those B cells that develop into plasma cells secreting IgG migrate through the lymphatic system to the bone marrow and continue to synthesize Ig. Plasma cells secreting IgA are found in mucosal tissue. The migration of naive B cells into secondary lymphoid organs, and of antigen-activated and memory B cells into other tissues, is governed by the same types of "homing" interactions that are described in Chapters 8 and 10 for T cells.

B-1 Cells

The differentiation steps described above form the population of B cells that predominates in blood, lymph, and secondary lymphoid organs. These B cells are referred to as B-2 cells. A second population of B cells known as **B-1 cells** has been described in humans, mice, and other animals. In the adult, B-1 cells are minor populations in spleen and lymph node but predominate in the peritoneal and pleural cavities. How exactly B-1 and B-2 cells are related is not fully worked out. B-1 cells appear to use a limited set of V gene segments to form their repertoire. Most but not all B-1 cells are characterized by the surface expression of the molecule CD5 which is not expressed on B-2 cells. $CD5^+$ B-1 cells are the predominant cell type in chronic lymphocytic leukemia (see Chapter 17).

B-1 cells synthesize predominantly low-affinity IgM polyspecific antibodies (i.e. reactive with many different antigens) early in the primary response to many bacteria. B-1 cells make what is referred to as a *thymus-independent* response to bacterial polysaccharides (see Chapter 10); that is, they do not require helper T cells to synthesize antibody and synthesize IgM but little or no other Ig isotypes. For these reasons, B-1 cells are thought to have an important role as a first line of defense against many pathogens, particularly in the mucosal immune system. In addition, B-1 cells are considered responsible for synthesizing most **"natural" antibody;** that is, generally IgM antibodies that are detected in an individual in the absence of antigen priming.

B CELL MEMBRANE PROTEINS

The key characteristic of B cells is their ability to synthesize antibody after antigenic stimulation. As we describe in more detail in subsequent chapters, production of antibody by B cells is a multistep process that generally requires the mutual activation of B and T cells. In the following paragraphs and in Figure 7.5 we briefly describe some of the B cell membrane proteins that play a role in antibody synthesis and some that have other important functions.

Antigen-Binding Molecules: Membrane Immunoglobulin

The quintessential property of the B lymphocyte lineage is the expression of Ig chains at the cell surface. (Note though that the pro-B cell, the most immature cell in the lineage, and the plasma cell, the end-stage cell of B-cell differentiation that secretes Ig, do not express Ig on their surface.) Thus, because membrane-associated Ig binds antigen, the expression of surface Ig can be used both to identify B cells and to separate them from other lymphocytes and mononuclear cells.

Signal Transduction Molecules Associated with Membrane Immunoglobulin

The function of key signal transduction molecules associated with the BCR is described in more detail in Chapter 10, in the section on intracellular events in B cell activation. Here, we identify some of these molecules and briefly outline their function.

Ig H and L chains have very short intracellular domains and do not directly transmit a signal into the B cell after antigen binding. Rather, the previously described Igα (CD79a) and Igβ (CD79b) molecules, which are noncovalently associated in the membrane of B cells with Ig H and L chains (Fig. 7.2), transmit the activation signal into the interior of the B cell. One of the earliest events in B cell activation after antigen binding to the BCR is the phosphorylation of tyrosine residues—the addition of a phosphate group—in the cytoplasmic regions of Igα/Igβ by enzymes known as protein tyrosine kinases. These Igα/Igβ tyrosine residues are contained in a sequence of amino acids referred to as an ***immunoreceptor tyrosine-based activation motif*** (ITAM). The amino acid sequence is referred to as a *motif* because it is found in a number of other signal transduction molecules on cells of the immune system (e.g., those associated with the T cell receptor; discussed in Chapter 8).

Other molecules on the B cell membrane affect the signal that is transmitted through the BCR, and thus play important signal transducing roles in the B cell. ***CD19, CD81*** (also known as TAPA-1), and ***CD21*** are associated in a complex that is known as the ***B cell coreceptor.*** Antigen binding to the coreceptor enhances the activation signal transmitted through the BCR. As a result, much lower levels of an antigen are needed to activate a B cell if the antigen binds to the coreceptor as well as the BCR. A coreceptor with similar

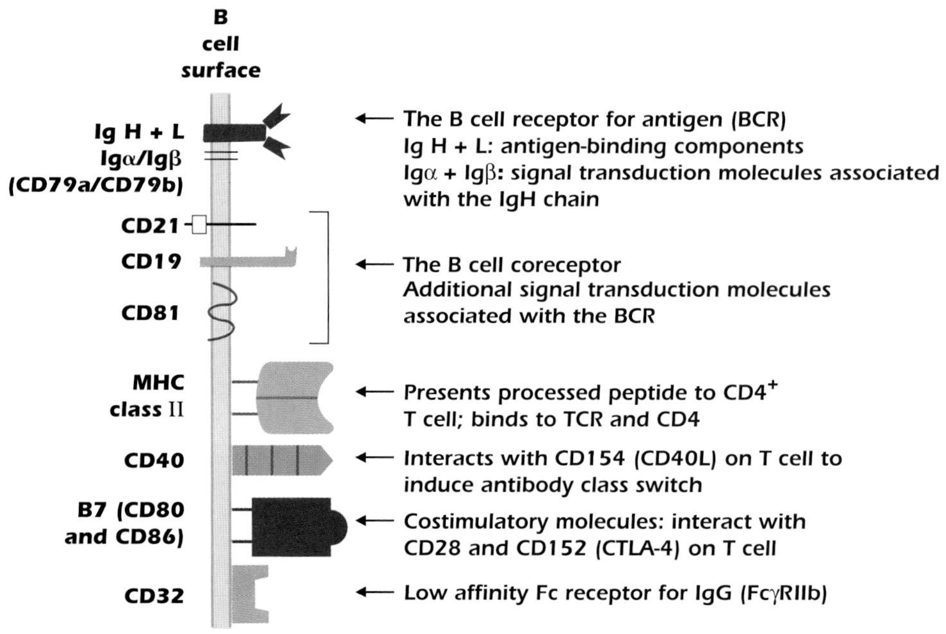

Figure 7.5. Important molecules expressed at the surface of the mature B cell.

function is also associated with the T cell receptor (described in Chapter 8).

CD21 in the B cell coreceptor complex is a receptor for a complement component, C3d, which binds to microbial pathogens (see Chapter 13). In this way, CD21 is thought to play a major role in augmenting B cell responses to pathogens that activate the complement pathway. CD21 also acts as a receptor for ***Epstein-Barr virus*** (EBV), allowing B cells to be infected and proliferate in response to the virus. EBV is responsible for mononucleosis and, in Africa, Burkitt's lymphoma.

Some molecules expressed on the B cell surface have a *negative* effect on signaling to the B cell. These include ***CD22,*** which negatively regulates the CD19, CD81, CD21 coreceptor, and ***CD32.*** CD32 is the low-affinity receptor for the Fc region of IgG (FcγRIIb), expressed on virtually all mature B cells. CD32 binds IgG when it aggregates in the absence of antigen (see Chapter 4) and when the IgG is in the form of an antigen–antibody complex. CD32 plays an important role in ***antibody feedback,*** the inactivation of B cells by antibody, by delivering a negative signal to the B cell (see Chapter 10).

Molecules Involved in T Cell–B Cell Interactions

As described more fully in Chapters 8–10, antigen must be presented by cells referred to as ***antigen-presenting cells*** (APCs) to activate T cells. B cells, and activated B cells in particular, can act as APCs for T cells. B cells share several important characteristics with other APCs: First, B cells express on their surface proteins known as ***major histocompatibility complex*** (MHC) ***class II molecules*** (see Chapter 9). These proteins are essential for presenting antigen to a major set of T cells known as CD4$^+$ T cells. Unlike the expression pattern of many other cell types, B cell expression of MHC class II molecules is ***constitutive***—that is, the molecules are always expressed. B cell expression of MHC class II molecules can be further increased by exposure to certain cytokines, such as IL-4. MHC class II molecules are expressed on all cells in the B cell lineage, except pro-B cells.

Second, activated B cells also express high levels of a family of molecules known as ***B7*** (***CD80/CD86***), which are referred to as ***costimulatory molecules,*** because they are required in addition to antigen to activate naive (unprimed) T cells. Resting mature B cells express low levels of B7 and are poor APCs, whereas activated B cells are very efficient APCs.

Third, B cells express ***CD40,*** which interacts with CD154 (CD40 ligand; CD40L) expressed on activated T cells. This interaction activates B cells and plays a critical role in isotype switching. The importance of the CD40–CD154 interaction is underscored by a condition known as human X-linked hyper-IgM syndrome. Boys who have a mutation in their CD154 gene and whose T cells either do not express or have a nonfunctional CD154 make only IgM antibodies; their B cells cannot switch to synthesize other isotypes.

SUMMARY

1. In mammals, the early stages of B cell differentiation take place in the bone marrow and throughout the life of an individual. The earliest recognizable cell in the B cell lineage is the pro-B cell, in which the first stage of Ig H chain gene rearrangement takes place: A D_H gene segment rearranges to a J_H gene segment.
2. The next stage is the pre-B cell, in which a V_H gene segment rearranges to the joined DJ segments to form a VDJ unit, putting the rearranged VDJ close to the C_μ gene. The pre-B cell transcribes and translates the $VDJC_\mu$ gene unit and thereby synthesizes a μ chain. This μ chain is expressed on the surface of the pre-B cell in association with surrogate light chains.
3. On the surface of the pre-B cell, the μ chain and surrogate light chains are expressed with two closely associated transmembrane molecules: Igα (CD79a) and Igβ (CD79b). The complex of μ and surrogate light chains in conjunction with Igα and Igβ is referred to as the pre-B cell receptor.
4. In the next stage of differentiation, L chain genes start to rearrange; surrogate light-chain synthesis is shut down; and a κ or λ chain is formed, which associates with the cell's μ chain. This results in the formation of an IgM molecule, which is expressed on the surface of the cell. This cell is referred to as an immature B cell.
5. If the immature B cell interacts with antigen, it is generally inactivated. The interaction of immature cells with self-molecules—resulting in inactivation or deletion of cells with potential reactivity to self—is one of the important ways of maintaining self-tolerance (negative selection).
6. In the next phase of B cell differentiation, the mature B cell expresses IgM and IgD—with identical antigenic specificity—on the cell surface.
7. Further development of the mature B cell occurs predominantly outside the bone marrow and as a result of exposure to antigen. Activation of the B cell leads to proliferation and differentiation into a plasma cell,

the cells that synthesize and secrete antibody. In the primary response to antigen, predominantly IgM is synthesized.

8. B cells that interact with T cells and their products—cytokines—undergo isotype (class) switching, i.e., produce antibody of different isotypes—IgG, IgA, or IgE. Isotype switching involves a rearrangement mechanism unique to B cells: The VDJ heavy-chain unit that was joined to the $C\mu$ and $C\delta$ genes rearranges to join another C-region gene, such as $C\gamma$, $C\alpha$, or $C\varepsilon$. The B cell that was synthesizing IgM and IgD can now synthesize antibody of a different isotype (IgG, IgA, or IgE) but with the same antigenic specificity.

9. Somatic hypermutation of genes coding for antibody V regions takes place in the germinal centers of secondary lymphoid organs. This results in the selection of B cells with mutations in their Ig V genes that code for antibodies with higher affinity for the antigen than antibody synthesized by the original antigen-activated B cell ("affinity maturation"). These selected B cells can develop into memory B cells or plasma cells.

10. In a single B cell, the H chain is coded for by the H chain gene segments found on either the maternally derived or the paternally derived chromosome; the L chain is also coded for by the L chain gene segments found on one or other chromosome. This phenomenon, the use of genes on only one chromosome to synthesize an Ig chain, is known as allelic exclusion and ensures that an individual B cell produces an Ig of only one antigenic specificity.

11. Expression of membrane Ig is unique to B cells. The molecules $Ig\alpha$ and $Ig\beta$, and other molecules associated with membrane immunoglobulin, transduce signals into the B cell after antigen binding to Ig. The B cell also expresses an array of molecules on its cell surface that play a vital role in interactions with other cells, particularly T cells. These include MHC class II molecules, B7, and CD40.

REFERENCES

Akashi K, Reya T, Dalma-Weiszhausz D, Weissman IL (2002): Lymphoid precursors. *Curr Opin Immunol* 12:144.

Calame KL (2001) Plasma cells: Finding new light at the end of B cell development. *Nature Immunol* 2:1103–1108.

Gellert M (2002): V(D)J recombination: RAG proteins, repair factors, and regulation. *Annu Rev Biochem* 71:101.

Longo NS, Lipsky PE (2001): Somatic hypermutation in human B cell subsets. *Semin Immunopathol* 23:367.

Martin A, Scharff MD (2002): AID and mismatch repair in antibody diversification. *Nat Rev Immunol* 2:605.

Storb U, Stavnezer J (2002): Immunoglobulin genes: generating diversity with AID and UNG. *Curr Biol* 12:R725.

REVIEW QUESTIONS

For each question, choose the ONE BEST answer or completion.

1. The earliest stages of B-cell differentiation
   A) occur in the embryonic thymus.
   B) require the presence of antigen.
   C) involve rearrangement of κ-chain gene segments.
   D) involve rearrangement of surrogate light-chain gene segments.
   E) involve rearrangement of heavy-chain gene segments.

2. Which of the following is expressed on the surface of the mature B lymphocyte?
   A) CD40
   B) MHC class II molecules
   C) CD32
   D) IgM and IgD
   E) All of the above.

3. Which of the following statements is *incorrect?*
   A) Antibodies in a secondary immune response generally have a higher affinity for antigen than antibodies formed in a primary response.
   B) Somatic hypermutation of V region genes may contribute to changes in antibody affinity observed during secondary responses.
   C) Synthesis of antibody in a secondary response occurs predominantly in the blood.
   D) Isotype switching occurs in the presence of antigen.
   E) Predominantly IgM antibody is produced in the primary response.

4. Immature B lymphocytes
   A) have rearranged only D and J gene segments.
   B) are progenitors of T as well as B lymphocytes.
   C) express both IgM and IgD on their surface.

D) are at a stage of development where contact with antigen may lead to unresponsiveness.
E) must go through the thymus to mature.

5. Antigen binding to the B-cell receptor
A) transduces a signal through the antigen-binding chains.
B) invariably leads to B-cell activation.
C) transduces a signal through the Igα and Igβ molecules.
D) results in macrophage activation.
E) leads to cytokine synthesis, which activates T cells.

6. Which of the following would *not* be found on a memory B cell:
A) Igα and Igβ
B) γ heavy chains
C) ε heavy chains
D) surrogate light chains
E) κ light chains

7. Germinal centers found in lymph nodes and spleen:
A) support the development of immature B and T cells
B) function in the removal of damaged erythrocytes from the circulation
C) act as the major source of stem cells and thus help to maintain hematopoiesis
D) are sites of antigenic stimulation of mature B cells
E) are the sites of T cell differentiation

ANSWERS TO REVIEW QUESTIONS

1. *E* The earliest events in B-cell differentiation take place in fetal liver and bone marrow in the adult and involve rearrangement of heavy-chain V, D, and J gene segments.

2. *E* All the molecules are expressed on the surface of the mature B cell.

3. *C* Antibody synthesis in secondary responses occurs predominantly in lymph nodes, not blood.

4. *D* In immature B cells, which express only IgM, contact with antigen leads to unresponsiveness rather than activation.

5. *C* The molecules Igα and Igβ, which are associated with the surface Ig molecule, transduce a signal following antigen binding to surface Ig.

6. *D* Surrogate light chains are expressed only at the pre-B cell stage of B-cell differentiation.

7. *D* Germinal centers are the areas of lymph node and spleen in which antigen-activated B cells proliferate and undergo somatic hypermutation, ultimately differentiating into memory or plasma cells.

8

BIOLOGY OF THE T LYMPHOCYTE

INTRODUCTION

In the previous chapters, we focused on the characteristics of B lymphocytes and their receptor for antigen, immunoglobulin (Ig). Ig molecules secreted from B cells, antibodies, play a critical role in interacting with antigens when they are found *outside* cells; for example, when viruses are encountered in blood or at mucosal surfaces. Once an antigen gets into a cell, however, antibodies do not generally have access to it, and so antibodies are ineffective in dealing with antigens *inside* cells.

It is generally believed that T cells evolved to deal with the crucial phase of the response to pathogens—such as viruses, bacteria, and parasites—that takes place inside cells of the host. Almost exclusively, T cells respond to protein antigens (some exceptions will be described in Chapters 9 and 10). Because proteins are either major components of pathogens or are synthesized by pathogens, T cells play a critical role in the intracellular phase of the response to nearly all the potentially harmful agents to which an individual is exposed.

T cells, like B cells, express an antigen-specific receptor that is ***clonally distributed***—that is, every clone of T cells expresses a ***T-cell receptor*** (TCR) for antigen with a unique sequence. The huge repertoire of TCR molecules, calculated to be on the order of 10^{15}–10^{18} different possible structures, is generated by the same V(D)J gene rearrangement strategies that we described for Ig molecules in Chapter 6. The unique aspects of TCR gene rearrangement are discussed in more detail later in this chapter. The structures of the TCR and the B cell receptor for antigen Ig and the organization of the genes that code for the TCR and Ig are strikingly similar. These similarities or ***homologies*** suggest that the TCR and Ig (and, indeed, many other molecules expressed at the cell surface) have evolved from a common ancestral gene. These genes are said to belong to the ***immunoglobulin gene superfamily,*** and the molecules are referred to as members of the ***immunoglobulin superfamily.***

In this chapter we describe the characteristics of the TCR, compare them with those of Ig, and describe other important molecules on the T cell surface. We also explain the key steps in T cell development in the thymus, the organ in which the developing T cell acquires its antigen-specific receptor.

NATURE OF THE ANTIGEN-SPECIFIC T CELL RECEPTOR

Molecules That Interact with Antigen

Each T cell expresses at its surface a two-chain molecule, the TCR, that interacts with antigen. The left side of Figure 8.1 shows the form of the TCR, the polypeptide α **and** β chains that are expressed on the majority of mature T cells in humans and many other species. The α and β chains are disulfide-linked, transmembrane glycoproteins with short cytoplasmic tails. The chains contain variable amounts of carbohydrate

Immunology: A Short Course, Fifth Edition, By Richard Coico, Geoffrey Sunshine, and Eli Benjamini
ISBN 0-471-22689-0

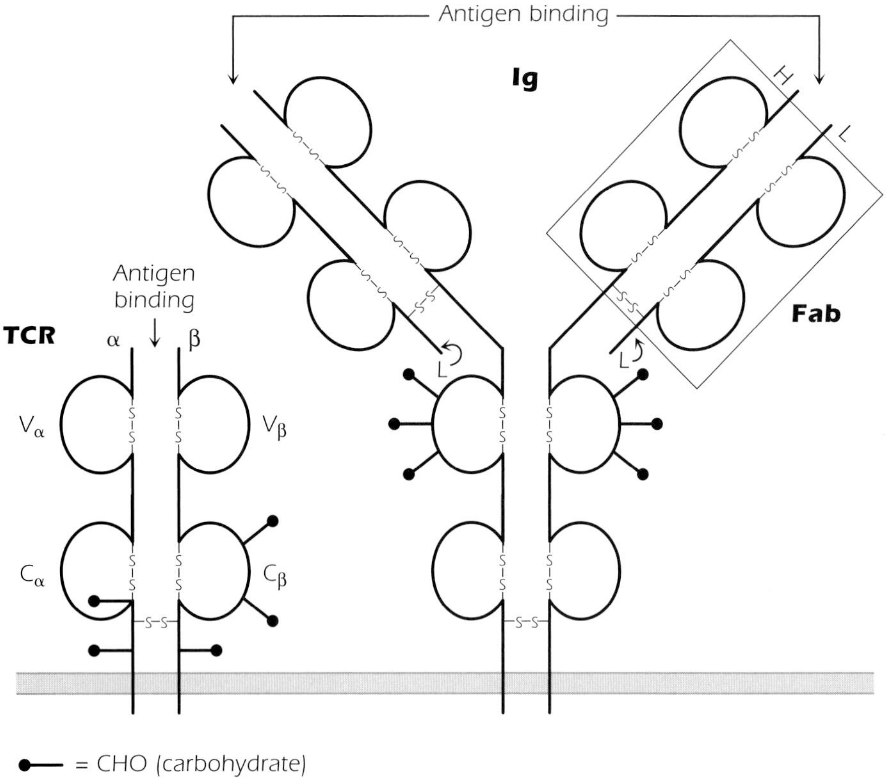

Figure 8.1. The predominant form of the antigen-binding chains of the T-cell receptor (TCR), α and β, and the membrane-bound Ig showing the Fab region.

so the molecular weights of the α and β chains vary between 40 and 60 kDa.

Figure 8.1 compares the structure of the TCR with the structure of membrane Ig. Each chain of the TCR is made up of variable (V) and constant (C) regions, analogous to the V and C regions of Ig molecules. Each TCR V and C region folds into an Ig-like domain. Moreover, like Ig, the TCR V regions contain hypervariable or ***complementarity-determining regions*** (CDRs 1, 2, and 3), which form the antigen-binding site.

The structures of the TCR and Ig differ in several important ways, though.

- **Valence and conformation.** The TCR is a two-chain structure that forms a single binding site for antigen—that is, the TCR is monovalent and resembles the monovalent Fab fragment of an antibody. The extensive interactions between the domains of each TCR chain give the TCR a rigid conformation. By contrast, Ig is a four-chain molecule with a hinge and two antigen-binding sites. These properties give the Ig molecule a flexibility that allows it to bind bivalently to antigens of different shapes and sizes.
- **Antigen recognition.** In Chapters 3 and 4 we described how Ig binds to many different types of antigen (carbohydrates, DNA, lipids, and proteins) that it encounters in fluids, such as serum. We also described that Ig can respond to linear *and* conformational epitopes in an antigen; thus the three-dimensional shape and the sequence of an antigen are important in eliciting antibody responses.

Because T cells interact with protein antigens that come from inside cells, however, they use an antigen-recognition system that differs from that used by B cells. The TCR interacts with small fragments of proteins (peptides) that are expressed on the surface of a host cell. These peptides, generated by enzymatic degradation of the protein inside cells, associate with ***major histocompatibility complex*** (MHC) molecules. Thus, as shown in Figure 8.2, the TCR interacts with a peptide bound to an MHC molecule on the surface of a host cell. (The role of MHC molecules in creating epitopes for T cell responses was briefly referred to in Chapter 3 and Fig. 3.4 and will be discussed in more detail in Chapter 9.) Consequently, in contrast to the variety of structures and shapes recognized by Ig molecules, the antigen recognized by the TCR is a combination of MHC molecule and a small linear sequence of peptide.

Recent crystallographic evidence suggests that different regions of the TCR contact different parts of the peptide–MHC molecule. The common feature of all the different peptide–MHC–TCR structures that have been examined is that the TCR V_α and V_β CDR3 interact with two or three amino acids in the center of the peptide sequence; thus this interaction appears critical in providing the specificity of peptide binding to the TCR. In some crystal structures, the

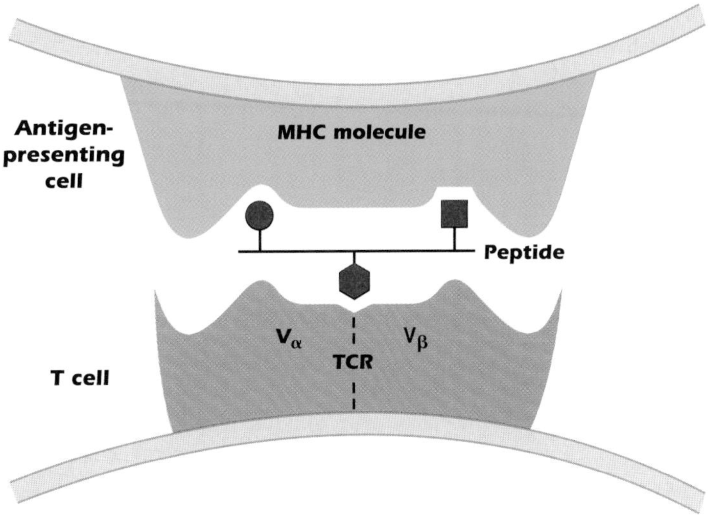

Figure 8.2. The interaction of the TCR with an MHC molecule and bound peptide.

TCR CDR1 and CDR2 of V_α and V_β interact with the MHC component of the peptide–MHC molecule, whereas in others, all three CDRs interact with the MHC.

- **Secretion of the receptor.** Unlike Ig, the TCR does not exist in a specifically secreted form and is not secreted as a consequence of T cell activation. As described in Chapter 10, T cell activation results in cytokine secretion and/or the killing of infected host cells. By contrast, as we described in Chapter 7, after antigen binds to membrane Ig and activates the B cell, the B cell differentiates into a plasma cell that secretes Ig with the same antigenic specificity expressed by the B cell that initially bound antigen.

- **No change in the TCR during the response to antigen** As discussed in Chapters 6 and 7, over the course of a response to antigen, Ig molecules undergo ***somatic hypermutation*** (with associated affinity maturation) and ***class switching,*** the linking of one set of genes coding for a particular V region to different C region genes. These mechanisms are unique to B cells: The TCR does not change during the response to antigen.

Coreceptor Molecules

The TCR is expressed on the T cell surface in association with another transmembrane molecule, referred to as a ***coreceptor.*** Figure 8.3 shows that this coreceptor can be one of two molecules on the mature T cell: either ***CD4*** or the two-chain molecule ***CD8*** (both members of the Ig superfamily.) Thus expression of the coreceptor splits the T-cell population into two major subsets, **CD4$^+$** or **CD8$^+$**. (A cell expressing the gene of interest is referred to as "+," and a cell not expressing this gene is "−.") As described later in this chapter, only immature T cells differentiating in the thymus express *both* CD4 and CD8.

CD4 and CD8 have several important functions:

- The extracellular portions of CD4 and CD8 bind to MHC molecules on the surface of a cell that presents antigen to T cells, an ***antigen presenting cell,*** (APC; described more fully in Chapter 9). CD4 binds selectively to the subset of MHC molecules known as ***MHC class II*** and CD8 binds selectively to the subset of MHC molecules known as ***MHC class I.*** Thus Figure 8.3 shows that CD4$^+$ T cells interact with host cells expressing peptide associated with MHC class II, and CD8$^+$ T cells with cells expressing peptide associated with MHC class I. This forms the basis of MHC restriction of the T cell response (described in Chapter 9).
- The binding of CD4 or CD8 to MHC molecules expressed on the APC helps tighten the binding of T cells to APCs. Thus CD4 and CD8 act as ***adhesion molecules*** in T cell interactions with APC.

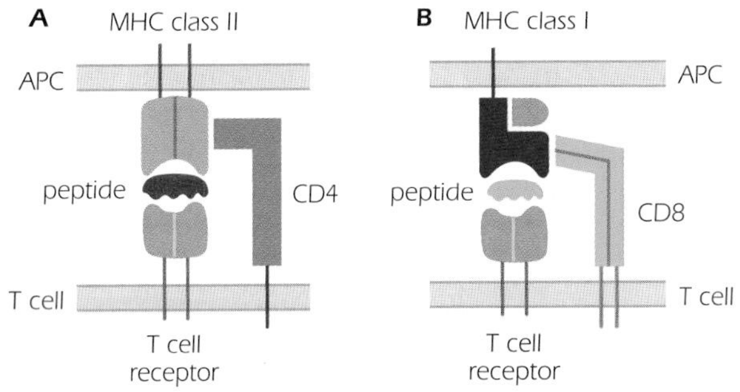

Figure 8.3. The interactions of TCR coreceptors with MHC molecules. (A) CD4 with MHC class II, and (B) CD8 with MHC class I.

- CD4 and CD8 are involved in ***signal transduction*** after antigen binding to the TCR. Specifically, the intracellular portions of CD4 and CD8 are linked to enzymes, known as protein tyrosine kinases, which are important early components of the T cell activation pathways. This is discussed more fully in Chapter 10.
- A unique characteristic of the CD4 molecule is that it binds to HIV. This allows the virus to infect cells expressing CD4, eventually leading to the disease AIDS (see Chapter 17).

The T Cell Receptor Complex

Figure 8.4 shows that the antigen-recognizing α and β chains of the TCR are also expressed on the surface of T cells in tight, noncovalent association with the molecule **CD3** and with two identical **ζ (zeta)** chains (**CD247;** molecular weight 16 kDa). The combination of the α and β chains of the TCR and CD3 and ζ is referred to as the **T cell receptor complex,** analogous to the B cell receptor complex described in Chapter 7.

CD3 is made up of the three distinct polypeptides γ, δ, and ε (molecular weights 25, 20, and 20 kDa, respectively, and all members of the Ig superfamily). It is currently believed that ε associates with both γ and δ chains in the complex (Fig. 8.4). Because CD3 plays a "chaperone" role in transporting the newly synthesized TCR molecule through the cell to the cell surface, it is always found associated with the TCR. CD3 is invariant—that is, it is the same on all T cells—and because it is expressed exclusively on T cells it can be used as a marker to distinguish T cells from all other cells.

CD3 and ζ polypeptides do not bind antigen. They are signal transduction molecules activated after antigen binding to the TCR, analogous to the Igα and Igβ molecules associated with the BCR, described in Chapter 7. Each chain of the CD3 complex contains one tyrosine-containing sequence referred to as an ***immunoreceptor tyrosine-based activation motif*** (ITAM), also found in Igα and Igβ, and the ζ chain contains three. As we discuss in more detail in Chapter 10, after antigen binds to the α and β chains of the TCR, the ITAMs of the CD3 and ζ chains play important roles in the early phases of T cell activation.

Other Important Molecules Expressed on the T Cell Surface

In the following paragraphs and in Figure 8.5 we describe molecules in addition to those associated with the TCR complex and the T cell coreceptors that play important roles in T cell function.

Costimulatory Ligands. In Chapter 7 we referred to the expression of the B7 family of molecules (of which most is known about the molecules B7-1 and B7-2, CD80 and CD86) on B cells and other APCs. The interaction of B7 with ***CD28*** expressed on the mature T cell provides a ***co-stimulatory*** or ***second signal*** for T cell activation. The costimulator interaction is required in addition to the interaction of peptide–MHC with the TCR to activate naive T cells (i.e., T cells that have not previously encountered antigen). Activated T cells also express a molecule closely related to CD28, known as ***CD152 (CTLA-4),*** that interacts with B7 molecules to impart a

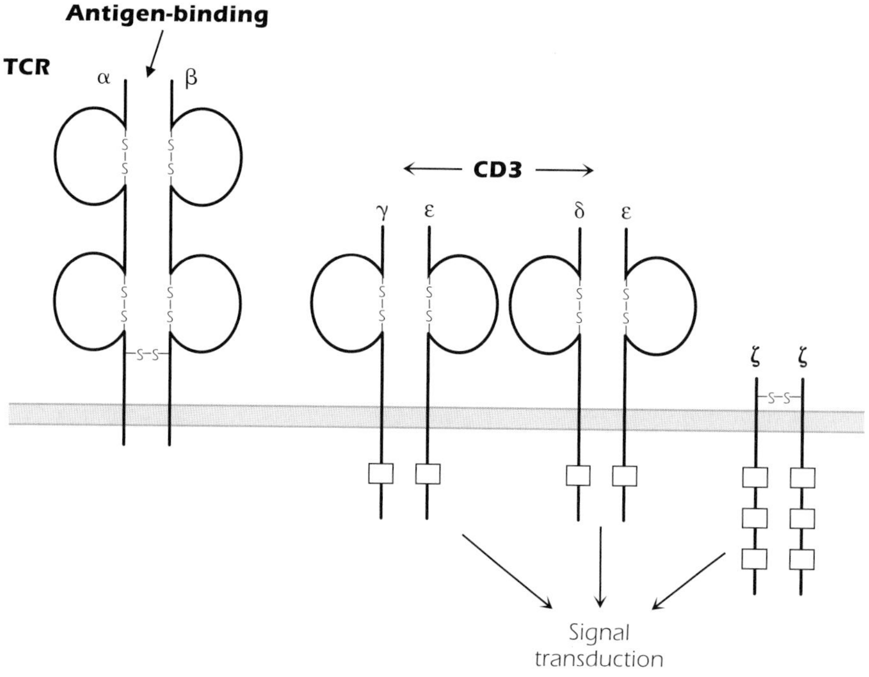

Figure 8.4. The TCR complex. The TCR and associated signal transduction complex, CD3 (γ, δ, and ε chains) plus ζ. Open boxes, ITAMs.

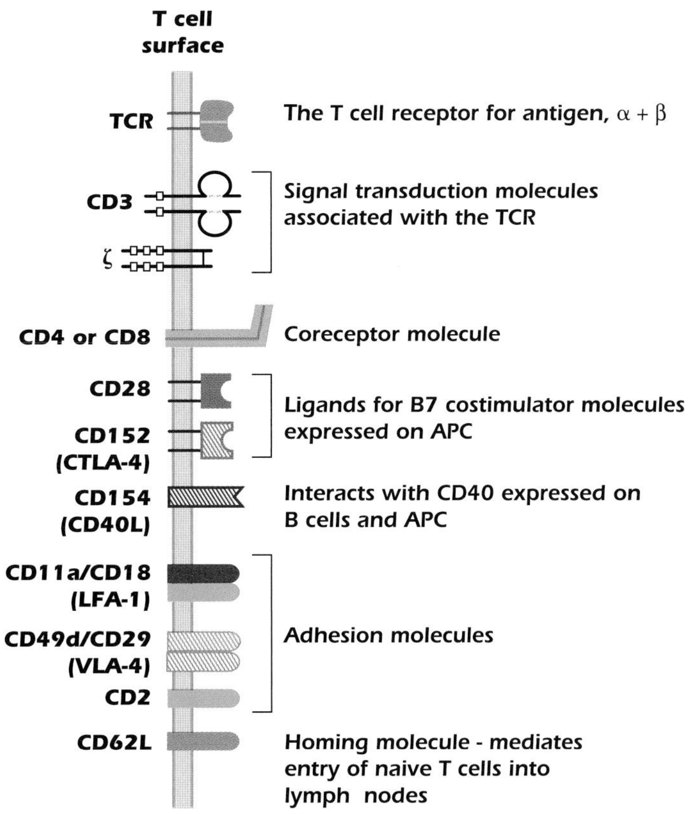

Figure 8.5. Important molecules expressed at the T cell surface.

negative signal to the activated T cell. In Chapter 10 we describe more fully the interaction of B7 molecules with CD28 and CD152.

Adhesion Molecules. We described above how CD4 and CD8 expressed on the T cell act as both adhesion molecules (molecules that tighten the adherence of T cells to APCs) and signal transduction molecules. Nearly all mature T cells express ***CD2,*** which also has adhesive and signal transduction properties. In humans, CD2 interacts with ***CD58*** (LFA-3) expressed on many different cells.

CD2, CD4, and CD8 are expressed almost exclusively on T cells. Other molecules known as ***integrins***—a family of two-chain molecules—are expressed by T cells and other cell types. Integrins play an important role in T cell adhesion to APCs and endothelial cells in blood vessels, and integrin-mediated adhesion is enhanced by chemokines—small cytokines produced during inflammatory responses (see Chapter 11). The major integrin expressed by mature T cells is ***LFA-1 (CD11aCD18),*** which interacts with several ligands, including ICAM-1(CD54), expressed on APCs such as macrophages and dendritic cells and on endothelial cells. Activated T cells express other integrins, including ***VLA-4 (CD49dCD29),*** which interacts with VCAM-1, expressed on activated endothelial cells. It is not clear whether integrins have signal transduction function.

Homing. T cells also express molecules on their surface that are associated with ***homing,*** the preferential entry of different types of lymphocytes into different tissues. Naive T lymphocytes home to peripheral and mucosal lymph nodes. Homing is mediated by the binding of ***CD62L*** (L-selectin or MEL-14) expressed on the naive T cell surface to glycoprotein molecules known as ***addressins,*** expressed on cells in a specialized region of the vascular endothelium at the boundary of the nodes. This interaction triggers further paired interactions that result in the naive lymphocyte leaving the circulation and entering the node by squeezing through adjacent endothelial cells. As we describe in more detail in Chapter 10, antigen-activated and memory T cells move out of the nodes and home to sites in the skin and other tissues. This is mediated by downregulating the expression of CD62L, and upregulating the expression of other cell-surface molecules, such as CD44 and the integrin CD49dCD29 (VLA-4), described above.

Recent evidence indicates that naive and memory T cells differ not only in their expression of homing molecules but also in their expression of chemokine receptors. Thus differences in expression of both homing molecules and of chemokine receptors result in different subsets of T cells selectively migrating to distinct sites in the body.

$\gamma\delta$ T CELLS. Some T cells express a TCR distinct from $\alpha\beta$. This alternative TCR is known as $\boldsymbol{\gamma\delta}$, and the cells expressing this receptor are referred to as **$\gamma\delta$ T cells.** $\gamma\delta$ is expressed in association with CD3 and ζ. (Note that the $\gamma\delta$ chains of the TCR are different from the γ and δ chains of CD3.) Generally, $\gamma\delta$ cells lack the CD4 coreceptor molecule found on $\alpha\beta$-expressing T cells, but some $\gamma\delta$ cells do express CD8.

In normal adult humans, $\gamma\delta$ T cells are found at much lower numbers than $\alpha\beta$ cells, but their numbers are increased by infectious agents. $\gamma\delta$ T cells are present in all mammals at some level; the peripheral blood of ruminant species, such as the cow and deer, can have higher circulating levels of $\gamma\delta$ T cells than $\alpha\beta$ T cells.

The $\alpha\beta$ and $\gamma\delta$ lineages diverge early in intrathymic development, but less is known about the steps in $\gamma\delta$ T cell differentiation than $\alpha\beta$ differentiation. During development of the individual, $\gamma\delta$ cells appear in the thymus before $\alpha\beta$-bearing cells. There are at least two subpopulations of $\gamma\delta$ cells, defined by different V_γ gene usage. The subpopulations migrate to different sites: skin or epithelial areas, such as lung and intestine.

The functions of $\gamma\delta$ T cells are not well understood; in general, $\gamma\delta$ T cells do not respond to a wide range of protein antigens. Some have been found to be activated by mycobacterial antigens and some to heat-shock proteins (proteins that form in cells when they are heated or stressed in different ways). $\gamma\delta$ T cells can produce many of the cytokines synthesized by $\alpha\beta$ TCR cells in response to antigen and may exhibit other functions associated with $\alpha\beta$ T cells, such as cytotoxicity. From this sparse information, it has been suggested that $\gamma\delta$ TCR cells may provide a first line of defense against invading pathogens.

Unlike $\alpha\beta$ T cells, some $\gamma\delta$ T cells do not respond to complexes of peptide and MHC molecules. Some $\gamma\delta$ can recognize native antigen (such as viral proteins) and some interact with other cell surface molecules that can present antigen, such as nonpolymorphic MHC class I molecules and CD1 (discussed in Chapter 9). Crystallographic evidence indicates that the framework structure of a V_δ domain more closely resembles the V region of an Ig H chain than the corresponding regions of an $\alpha\beta$ TCR. This suggests that antigen binding to the $\gamma\delta$ TCR may have more in common with antigen binding to antibody than to $\alpha\beta$ TCRs.

GENES CODING FOR T CELL RECEPTORS

The organization of the human gene loci coding for the α, β, and δ T cell receptor chains is shown in Figure 8.6. (Because of its complexity, the organization of γ genes is not shown.) Several features are noteworthy. First, α and γ chains are constructed from V and J gene segments, like Ig L chains, whereas β and δ chains are constructed from V, D, and J gene segments, like Ig H chains. Second, the β and γ loci are each found on different chromosomes, while gene segments of α and δ loci are interspersed on the same chromosome. Genes coding for the δ chain are flanked on both the 5′ and 3′ sides by genes coding for the α chain. Third, there are many more V_α and V_β genes than V_γ and V_δ genes (5–10) in the germ line. Note too that there are two C_β genes, $C_\beta 1$ and $C_\beta 2$, but these genes and their products are virtually identical and have no known functional differences. Thus they should not be confused with antibody isotypes, in which the Ig H chain constant genes and products differ considerably.

Individual TCR V regions have been given numbers, for example, $V_\alpha 2$ and $V_\beta 7$. The use of certain TCR V regions has been associated in some cases with the response to specific antigens and in particular to ***superantigens***—a set of antigens that activates all T cells expressing a particular V_β as a component of its TCR (see Chapter 9). In humans, superantigens include a number of bacterial toxins, and the massive T cell responses to these bacterial products can have clinical consequences (discussed further in Chapter 11.)

In Chapter 6 we also described how Ig genes show ***allelic exclusion,*** which ensures that a single B cell makes a receptor with only a single antigenic specificity. The situation with TCR genes is somewhat analogous, in that TCR β, γ, and δ genes do show allelic exclusion, but α genes do not. Thus some T cells that use $\alpha\beta$ as their TCR have two different α chains expressed with a single β chain and thus may have two different antigenic specificities. Up to 30% of human and

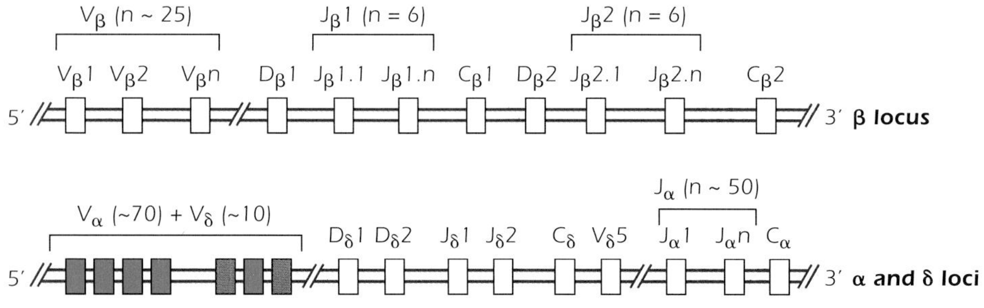

Figure 8.6. Organization of the α, β, and δ genes coding for the human T-cell receptor. The organization of the γ-gene locus is not shown because of its complexity.

mouse $\alpha\beta$ T cells express two α chains, but the functional significance of this finding is currently not clear.

GENERATION OF T CELL RECEPTOR DIVERSITY

The mechanisms for generating diversity in T cell receptors are very similar to the mechanisms of generating diversity in B cell receptors. The same fundamental principles of gene rearrangement, as described in Chapter 6 for Ig, apply in synthesizing the V and C regions of each chain of the T cell receptor α, β, γ, and δ. ***Recombinases*** and ***joining sequences*** are used to link up a VJ or a VDJ unit, generating the variable region specificity of a particular TCR polypeptide chain. The same enzymes are involved in the recombination events in both B and T cells. As described in Chapter 6, two genes known as ***recombination activation genes*** (*RAG*-1 and *RAG*-2) have been shown to play a crucial role in activating the recombinase genes in both early B and T cells. Thus, as in the generation of Ig diversity, TCR diversity is generated by (1) multiple V genes in the germ line, (2) random combination of chains, and (3) junctional and insertional variability. However, we pointed out one important difference between diversity generation in TCRs and Ig molecules earlier in the chapter: Ig but not the TCR undergoes somatic hypermutation following antigenic stimulation.

The repertoire of different TCRs is believed to be as large or larger than the repertoire of Ig molecules (estimated in the range of 10^{15} different potential specificities for $\alpha\beta$ and 10^{18} for $\gamma\delta$ TCRs). Junctional and insertional variability are important contributors to TCR diversity, and these result in an enormous number of different sequences for the part of the hypervariable region of the TCR known as CDR3. (By contrast, the sequences of the TCR CDR1 and CDR2 are not generated by rearrangement but are coded for by the V gene, which is found in the germ line.) Crystallographic evidence indicates that CDR3 is the region of the $\alpha\beta$ TCR binding site that makes contact with amino acids in the center of a peptide bound to an MHC molecule (see Figs. 9.3 and 9.4). Thus the large number of different TCR CDR3 sequences ensures that TCR binding to the peptide portion of the peptide–MHC complex is highly specific.

T CELL DIFFERENTIATION IN THE THYMUS

As described in Chapter 2, the thymus is the ***primary lymphoid organ*** for the development of T cells, analogous to the bone marrow as the primary organ for mammalian B cell differentiation. This signifies that the thymus is absolutely required for the differentiation of immature precursor cells into cells with the characteristics of T cells. The drastic effects of lacking a thymus and consequently not having mature T cells can be seen in children born without a thymus (DiGeorge syndrome, discussed in Chapter 17) or in mice genetically lacking a thymus (known as nude mice because they also lack hair).

T cell differentiation in the thymus occurs throughout the life of the individual but diminishes significantly after puberty. The size of the thymus itself decreases with the onset of puberty in mammals (thymic involution), presumably because of the synthesis of steroid hormones at this time. In some species, particularly the mouse, the mature T cell population is drastically depleted if the thymus is removed shortly after birth. Indeed, these were the pioneering observations that established the crucial role of the thymus in T cell responses. Removing the thymus later in the development of the animal has much less impact on the mature T cell population.

T cell differentiation in the thymus is a complex multistep process. In the paragraphs that follow and in Figure 8.7, we focus on a number of key steps in the differentiation sequence.

Thymocytes Interact with Thymic Nonlymphoid Cells

Figure 8.7 indicates that at every stage of thymic maturation, from precursor to mature T cell, the developing T lymphocytes ***(thymocytes)*** are in contact with, and interact with, a mesh formed by the nonlymphoid (***stromal***) cells of the thymus. The thymocytes trickle through this network of nonlymphoid cells, starting at the outer region of the thymus—***the thymic cortex***—and continuing into the inner region—***the thymic medulla.*** The most important thymic nonlymphoid cells are (1) ***cortical epithelial cells,*** and (2) ***dendritic cells,*** found predominantly at the junction of the cortex and medulla. Thymic dendritic cells are bone marrow derived, and in the same family of cells that present antigens to T cells in other tissues and organs (see Chapter 10).

As we describe in more detail below, the nonlymphoid cells provide critical cell surface interactions required for the development of maturing T cells. They also produce the cytokine interleukin 7, which induces proliferation of cells in the early stages of T (and B) lymphocyte development. Indeed, the thymus is a site of intense proliferation of developing T cells; the vast majority of these cells, however—calculated to be around 95% of the cells produced daily—do not emerge, but die in the thymus.

T CELL RECEPTOR GENE REARRANGEMENTS

Lymphoid precursor cells enter the outermost region of the thymus (the subcapsular region) with their TCR genes in an unrearranged (germ line) configuration. It is generally

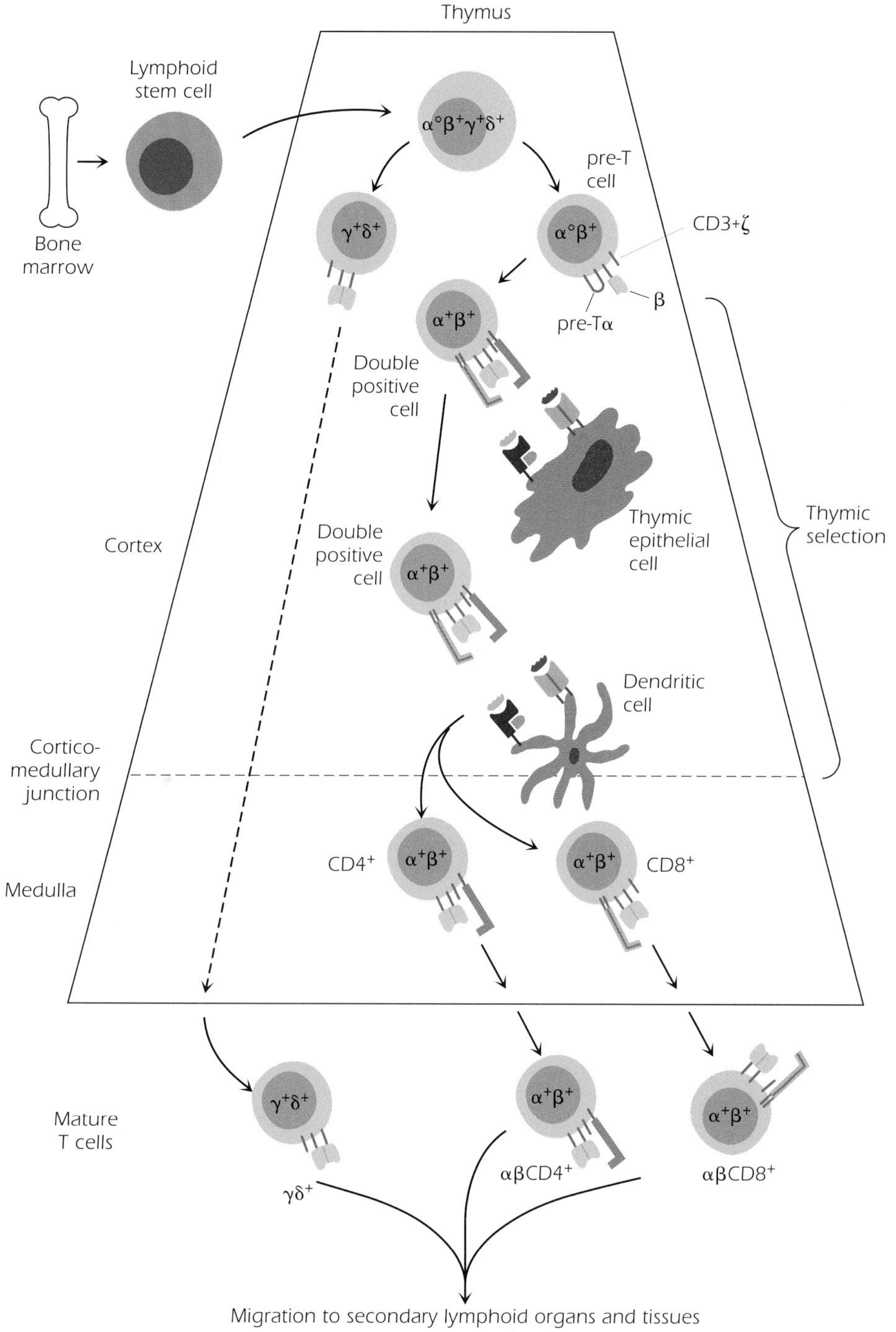

Figure 8.7. The developmental pathways of T cells in the thymus. Genes coding for the α, β, γ, or δ chains of the T-cell receptor are designated as α^0 etc. if unrearranged and α^+ etc. if rearranged.

thought that genes coding for TCR γ, δ, and β chains then start to rearrange more or less simultaneously. Cells that productively rearrange both a γ and a δ gene express TCR γ and δ chains on the cell surface. The sequence of events in the earliest stages of TCR gene rearrangement is still not completely understood, however, and so it is not clear if the cells expressing γ and δ at the surface do or do not productively rearrange a β chain gene. Nonetheless, the evidence suggests that cells expressing γ and δ as their TCR split off from cells that will express α and β as their receptor early in intrathymic development, although the precise stage at which this occurs is still not clear. Cells expressing $\gamma\delta$ as their TCR exit the thymus and form the pool of peripheral $\gamma\delta$ T cells.

Cells that productively rearrange a β gene express the TCR β chain on the surface of the cell in association with an invariant molecule known as ***pre-Tα.*** These cells are referred to as ***pre-T cells,*** and the combination of β chain and pre-Tα (together with CD3 and ζ) constitute the **pre-T cell receptor**

(pre-TCR), analogous to pre-B cells and the pre-B cell receptor discussed in Chapter 7.

Cells expressing the pre-TCR differentiate further. Similar to the steps we described in the differentiation of the pre-B cell in Chapter 7, signaling through the pre-TCR stops further rearrangement of TCR β genes. This ensures that the cell expresses only one type of β chain ***(allelic exclusion).*** In addition, the cell proliferates, and in this expanded population expression of pre-Tα is downregulated, α genes start to rearrange, and expression of both CD4 and CD8 genes starts. As we noted above, gene segments of the α and δ TCR loci are interspersed on the same chromosome, so rearrangement of the α locus on a particular chromosome also deletes the δ locus. (This ensures that a β chain does not pair with a δ chain.) Thus the next important cell in the $\alpha\beta$ lineage expresses both CD4 and CD8 coreceptor molecules on its surface. This ***$\alpha\beta^+CD3^+CD4^+CD8^+$*** thymocyte, referred to as a $CD4^+CD8^+$ or ***double positive*** cell, is found in the thymic cortex and forms the majority of thymocytes in the young mammalian thymus.

THYMIC SELECTION

Positive Selection

The double positive thymocyte undergoes a multistep process known as ***thymic selection*** (shown in Fig. 8.8). (Whether $\gamma\delta$ T cells undergo a similar selection process before they leave the thymus is currently not clear.) In the first stage, ***positive selection,*** the TCR of the double positive thymocyte interacts with MHC molecules expressed on epithelial cells in the thymic cortex. This interaction results in the survival and differentiation of the double positive cell; double positive cells that do not make this critical interaction, and are thus not selected, die by apoptosis. Positive selection also results in the downregulation of *RAG-1* and *RAG-2* gene expression, so no further gene rearrangement occurs. Thus, because as we described above the α gene does not show allelic exclusion, positive selection stops the further attempts of the α chain to rearrange.

Another critical feature of positive selection is that the developing $\alpha\beta$ T cell becomes ***"educated"*** to the MHC molecules expressed by the thymic cortical epithelial cells. This means that for the rest of the life of the T cell, even as a mature cell when it leaves the thymus, it will respond to antigen only when the antigen is bound to the MHC molecules that the developing T cell encountered in the thymus. For this reason, the MHC molecules expressed in a person's thymus and that educate his or her developing T cells are referred to as **self-MHC;** for that person, all other types of MHC molecules are ***non-self.*** This is the origin of the phenomenon known as ***MHC restriction,*** or more specifically, ***self-MHC restriction,*** which is central to T cell responses and is described more fully in Chapter 9.

Negative Selection

Because the recombination events involved in TCR generation are more or less random, T cells expressing TCRs specific for both foreign *and* self antigens can develop in the thymus and survive positive selection. Allowing T cells with strong reactivity to self components to leave the thymus and interact with these antigens in tissues could result in undesirable autoimmune responses. To prevent this from occurring, the double positive cell undergoes a second selection step, known as ***negative selection*** (shown Fig. 8.8).

Figure 8.8 shows negative selection taking place when double positive cells interact with dendritic cells at the corticomedullary junction. The critical interactions are between the TCR, CD4, and CD8 expressed on the double positive cell and the MHC molecules expressed on the dendritic cell. Because dendritic cells have peptides associated with MHC molecules, the double positive cell likely interacts with MHC and peptide expressed on the dendritic cell surface. A T cell expressing a TCR that reacts with too high an affinity to the combination of MHC and peptide is deleted by apoptosis. Thus negative selection removes T cells expressing TCRs with **high** (or strong) **reactivity** to self components.

Double positive cells that survive negative selection downregulate expression of either CD4 or CD8 by a mechanism that is currently not well understood. This results in the development of either $CD4^+CD8^-$ or $CD4^-CD8^+$ (**single positive**) T cells. These two sets of cells are the end point of the complex pathway of $\alpha\beta$ TCR cell differentiation in the thymus. They leave the thymus and make up the ***peripheral*** (i.e., outside the thymus) mature $CD4^+$ and $CD8^+$ T cell lineages.

Role of Peptides in Thymic Selection

A number of questions remain about the mechanisms involved in selection. One is the role and nature of peptides expressed by the thymic nonlymphoid cells at different stages of the selection processes. Current evidence indicates that peptides expressed by cortical epithelial cells play a critical role in the positive selection step. These peptides are derived from self antigens either expressed in the thymus or brought into the thymus. It is not currently clear, however, how these peptides derived from self antigens select T cells with TCR specificities for non-self as well as self antigens. In addition, it is not clear whether the peptides expressed by the cortical epithelial cells in positive selection differ from those expressed by the dendritic cell in negative selection. A further unresolved issue is how the interaction of the TCR expressed on a double positive cell with peptides and MHC molecules of the cortical epithelial cell results in survival and differentiation of the double positive cell, whereas interaction of the double positive cell with a thymic dendritic cell induces a negative signal

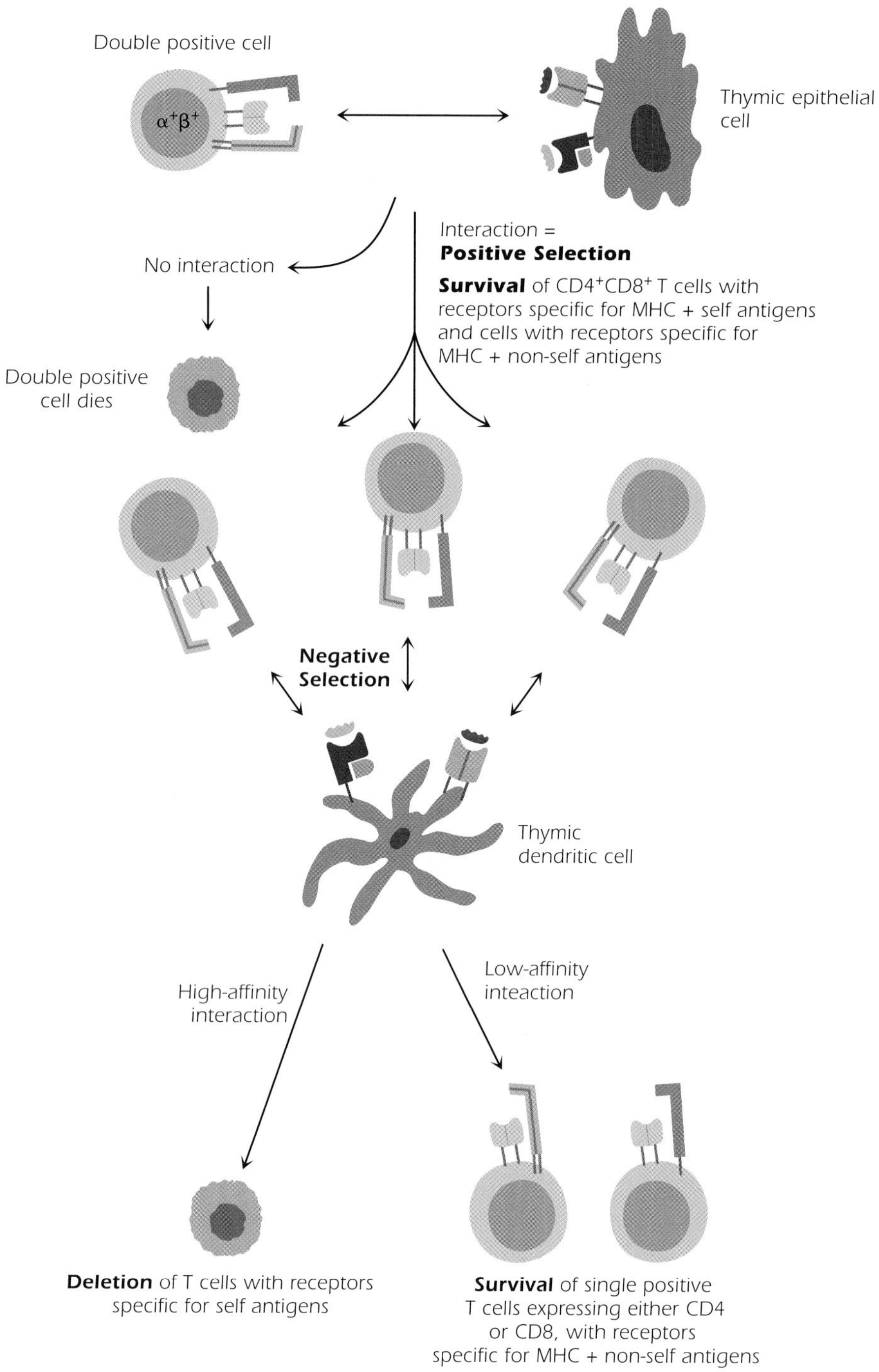

Figure 8.8. Positive and negative selection of $\alpha\beta$TCR$^+$CD4$^+$CD8$^+$ (double positive) T cells in the thymus.

(cell death). These topics are the subject of intense research activity.

Characteristics of T Cells Emerging from the Thymus

Thymic differentiation of T cells expressing $\alpha\beta$ as their TCR generates a repertoire of peripheral CD4$^+$ T cells and CD8$^+$ T cells that is able to respond to the universe of non-self antigens. These CD4$^+$and CD8$^+$ T cells have two other important characteristics:

- **They are self-MHC restricted.** they interact with peptides derived from non-self antigens only when the peptides are associated with the same set of MHC molecules that the developing T cell interacted with during positive selection in the thymus;
- **They are self-tolerant.** CD4$^+$and CD8$^+$ T cells do not respond to self components.

SUMMARY

1. The individual has an enormous number of different T cells. Each T cell bears a unique, clonally distributed receptor for antigen, known as the T-cell receptor. The same rearrangement strategies and recombinase machinery are used to generate a repertoire of T cells with different TCRs as are used by B cells to generate Ig diversity.
2. On the majority of human and mouse T cells, the TCR is a two-chain transmembrane molecule, $\alpha\beta$. The TCR is made up of V and C regions, analogous to those of Ig molecules. The extracellular portion of the TCR resembles the Fab region of an antibody.
3. An $\alpha\beta$ TCR interacts with a peptide bound to an MHC molecule on the surface of a host cell.
4. Coreceptor molecules are associated with the $\alpha\beta$ TCR. On mature T cells, the co-receptor is either CD4 or CD8, dividing T cells into two subsets, either $\alpha\beta^+$CD4$^+$ or $\alpha\beta^+$CD8$^+$. The function of these coreceptor molecules is to (1) bind MHC molecules on an antigen-presenting cell, (2) tighten the adherence between the T cell and antigen presenting cell, and (3) play a role in signal transduction after activation of the TCR.
5. The antigen-binding $\alpha\beta$ chains of the TCR are expressed on the surface of the T cell in a multimolecular complex (the TCR complex) in association with CD3 and ζ polypeptides, which act as a signal transduction unit after antigen binding to $\alpha\beta$.
6. The T cell also expresses molecules on its surface with important costimulatory, adhesion, and/or signal transduction properties. These include CD28 and CD152 (CTLA-4); the integrins CD11aCD18 (LFA-1), CD49dCD29 (VLA-4), and CD2; and molecules involved in homing to different tissues.
7. A different two-chain structure, $\gamma\delta$, is the TCR on a minor population of human and mouse T cells. $\gamma\delta$ is also expressed on the surface of the cell in association with CD3 and ζ. Most $\gamma\delta^+$ T cells do not express CD4 but some express CD8. The functions of $\gamma\delta^+$ T cells are not as well understood as those of $\alpha\beta^+$ T cells.
8. The genes coding for the β, γ and δ chains of the TCR show allelic exclusion—that is, genes from only one chromosome are used to synthesize the polypeptide chain. TCR α genes do not show allelic exclusion.
9. The TCR is initially expressed on the surface of developing T cells during differentiation in the thymus. The divergent development of T cells using $\alpha\beta$ as their receptor from T cells using $\gamma\delta$ as their receptor occurs early in the differentiation pathway in the thymus.
10. $\alpha\beta$TCR$^+$ CD4$^+$CD8$^+$ thymocytes (double positive) cells undergo thymic selection, mediated by interactions of the TCR and coreceptor molecules on the developing T cell with MHC molecules and peptides expressed by the thymic nonlymphoid cells. *Positive selection* on cortical epithelial cells educates the developing T cell: As a mature cell, it responds to antigen only when presented by a cell that expresses the same MHC molecules that the T cell interacted with during differentiation in the thymus (MHC restriction of the T-cell response). *Negative selection* on dendritic cells at the junction of the thymic cortex and medulla removes T cells with potential reactivity to self molecules, ensuring self-tolerance. Thus $\alpha\beta$TCR$^+$ T cells that emerge from the thymus are self-MHC restricted and self-tolerant.
11. $\alpha\beta$TCR$^+$ CD4$^+$ and $\alpha\beta$TCR$^+$CD8$^+$ T cells that survive negative selection, together with $\gamma\delta^+$ T cells, leave the thymus. These cells constitute the repertoire of peripheral T cells in blood, secondary lymphoid organs, and tissues that respond to non-self (foreign) antigen.

REFERENCES

Allison TJ, Garboczi DN (2002): Structure of $\gamma\delta$ T cell receptors and their recognition of non-peptide antigens. *Mol Immunol* 38: 1051.

Anderson G, Jenkinson EJ (2001): Lymphostromal interactions in thymic development and function. *Nat Rev Immunol* 1:31.

Berg LJ, Kang J (2001): Molecular determinants of TCR expression and selection. *Curr Opin Immunol* 13:232.

Borowski C, Martin C, Gounari F, Haughn L, Aifantis I, Grassi F, von Boehmer H (2002): On the brink of becoming a T cell. *Curr Opin Immunol* 14:200.

Carding SR, Egan PJ (2002): $\gamma\delta$ T cells: functional plasticity and heterogeneity. *Nat Rev Immunol* 2:336.

MacDonald HR, Radtke F, Wilson A (2001): T cell fate specification and $\alpha\beta/\gamma\delta$ lineage commitment. *Curr Opin Immunol* 13:219.

Spits H (2002): Development of $\alpha\beta$ T cells in the human thymus. *Nat Rev Immunol* 2:760.

REVIEW QUESTIONS

For each question, choose the ONE BEST answer or completion.

1. Which of the following statements concerning T-cell development is correct?
- A) Progenitor T cells that enter the thymus from the bone marrow have already rearranged their T cell receptor genes.
- B) Interaction with thymic non-lymphoid cells is critical.
- C) Maturation in the thymus requires the presence of foreign antigen.
- D) MHC class II molecules are not involved in positive selection
- E) Mature, fully differentiated T cells are found in the cortex of the thymus.

2. The development of self-tolerance in the T-cell compartment is important for the prevention of autoimmunity. Which of the following results in T-cell self-tolerance?
- A) allelic exclusion
- B) somatic hypermutation
- C) thymocyte proliferation
- D) positive selection
- E) negative selection

3. Which of the following statements is correct?
- A) The TCR $\alpha\beta$ chains transduce a signal into a T cell.
- B) A cell depleted of its CD4 molecule would be unable to recognize antigen.
- C) T cells with fully rearranged $\alpha\beta$ chains are not found in the thymus.
- D) T cells expressing the $\gamma\delta$ receptor are found only in the thymus.
- E) Immature $CD4^+CD8^+$ T cells form the majority of T cells in the thymus.

4. Which of the following is *incorrect* regarding mature T cells that use $\alpha\beta$ as their antigen-specific receptor?
- A) They coexpress CD3 on the cell surface.
- B) They may be either $CD4^+$ or $CD8^+$.
- C) They interact with peptides derived from nonself antigens.
- D) They can further rearrange their TCR genes to express $\gamma\delta$ as their receptor.
- E) They circulate through blood and lymph and migrate to secondary lymphoid organs.

5. CD4
- A) binds directly to peptide antigen.
- B) binds to MHC class I molecules.
- C) binds to MHC class II molecules.
- D) binds to CD8 on the T cell surface.
- E) binds to the peptide-binding site of MHC class II.

6. Which of the following statements is *incorrect* concerning TCR and Ig genes?
- A) In both B- and T-cell precursors, multiple V-, D-, J-, and C-region genes exist in an unrearranged configuration.
- B) Rearrangement of both TCR and Ig genes involves recombinase enzymes that bind to specific regions of the genome.
- C) Both Ig and TCR are able to switch C-region usage.
- D) Both Ig and the TCR use combinatorial association of V, D, and J genes and junctional imprecision to generate diversity.

7. Which of the following statements is *incorrect* concerning antigen-specific receptors on both B and T cells?
- A) They are clonally distributed transmembrane molecules.
- B) They have extensive cytoplasmic domains that interact with intracellular molecules.
- C) They consist of polypeptides with variable and constant regions.
- D) They are associated with signal transduction molecules at the cell surface.
- E) They can interact with peptides derived from nonself antigens.

ANSWERS TO REVIEW QUESTIONS

1. ***B*** Interaction of thymocytes with thymic stromal cells—cortical epithelial cells and interdigitating dendritic cells at the corticomedullary junction—is critical in T cell development.

2. ***E*** Negative selection removes developing T cells with potential reactivity to self-molecules.

3. ***E*** $CD4^+CD8^+$ T cells form the majority of cells in the thymus.

4. ***D*** The genes of T cells that use $\alpha\beta$ as their receptor cannot further rearrange to use $\gamma\delta$ as their receptor; TCR δ gene segments are interspersed with the α locus and are deleted when the α locus rearranges.

5. ***C*** CD4 expressed on T cells binds to MHC class II molecules.

6. ***C*** The ability to change the heavy-chain constant region while retaining the same antigen specificity is a property unique to Ig. The other features are common to both the TCR and Ig.

7. ***B*** Both the TCR and Ig have short cytoplasmic tails. The signal transduction molecules associated with the antigen-binding chains interact with intracellular molecules.

9

THE ROLE OF THE MAJOR HISTOCOMPATIBILITY COMPLEX IN THE IMMUNE RESPONSE

INTRODUCTION

In the previous chapter, we referred to the critical role that major histocompatibility complex (MHC) molecules play in T cell responses to antigen; specifically, that MHC molecules are critical both for the development of immature T cells in the thymus and for the responses of mature T cells to antigen. The centrality of MHC molecules to T cell interactions is referred to as the ***MHC restriction of T-cell responses.*** In this chapter, we shall describe more fully the structure and function of MHC molecules. Before doing so, we shall also discuss the characteristics of MHC genes and how they vary from individual to individual.

The term *major histocompatibility complex* derives from early research into the acceptance or rejection of tissues—literally, ***histocompatibility***—transplanted between different members of the same species (generally mice; see Chapter 19 for more discussion). Originally, researchers interpreted their findings to indicate that rapid rejection of such transplants was determined by one gene, thus that gene was called the *major histocompatibility gene.* Later studies indicated that this "gene" was a ***complex***—a set of closely linked genes inherited as a unit—and so it became known as the *major histocompatibility complex.* Other early studies indicated that T cells played an important role in transplantation rejection. Taken together, these findings from transplantation studies indicated a link between the molecules coded for by MHC genes and T cell responses. Because individuals do not normally undergo transplants, the function of the MHC in "everyday" T cell responses became the focus of intense investigation. Since the 1970s, a clearer picture of the role of MHC molecules in T cell responses within an individual has emerged.

MHC GENES AND PRODUCTS

Nomenclature

Every vertebrate species has MHC genes and products, but the most detailed information is known about the human and mouse systems. Figure 9.1A shows a simplified view of the region of human chromosome 6 containing the human MHC, called ***human leukocyte antigen or HLA***. Generally, the names of the MHCs of other species are similar; for example, BoLA for the bovine system and SLA for swine. By contrast, the name of the mouse MHC—***H-2,*** located on chromosome 17 and shown schematically in Figure 9.1B—is derived from the early studies of histocompatibility genes involved in transplantation responses that we described in the previous section.

Two major sets of MHC genes, known as ***MHC class I*** and ***MHC class II,*** and their cell-surface expressed products (***MHC molecules,*** sometimes referred to as ***MHC antigens,*** because of their role in transplantation), are involved in T cell responses. Figure 9.1A depicts the three independent genes that code for the human MHC class I molecules; the genes and molecules are known as ***HLA-A, HLA-B,*** and ***HLA-C.*** The figure also shows that the human MHC class II region is made up of three sets of genes, known as ***HLA-DP, HLA-DQ,*** and ***HLA-DR.*** Each MHC class II subregion contains an A

Immunology: A Short Course, Fifth Edition, By Richard Coico, Geoffrey Sunshine, and Eli Benjamini
ISBN 0-471-22689-0 © 2003 John Wiley & Sons, Inc.

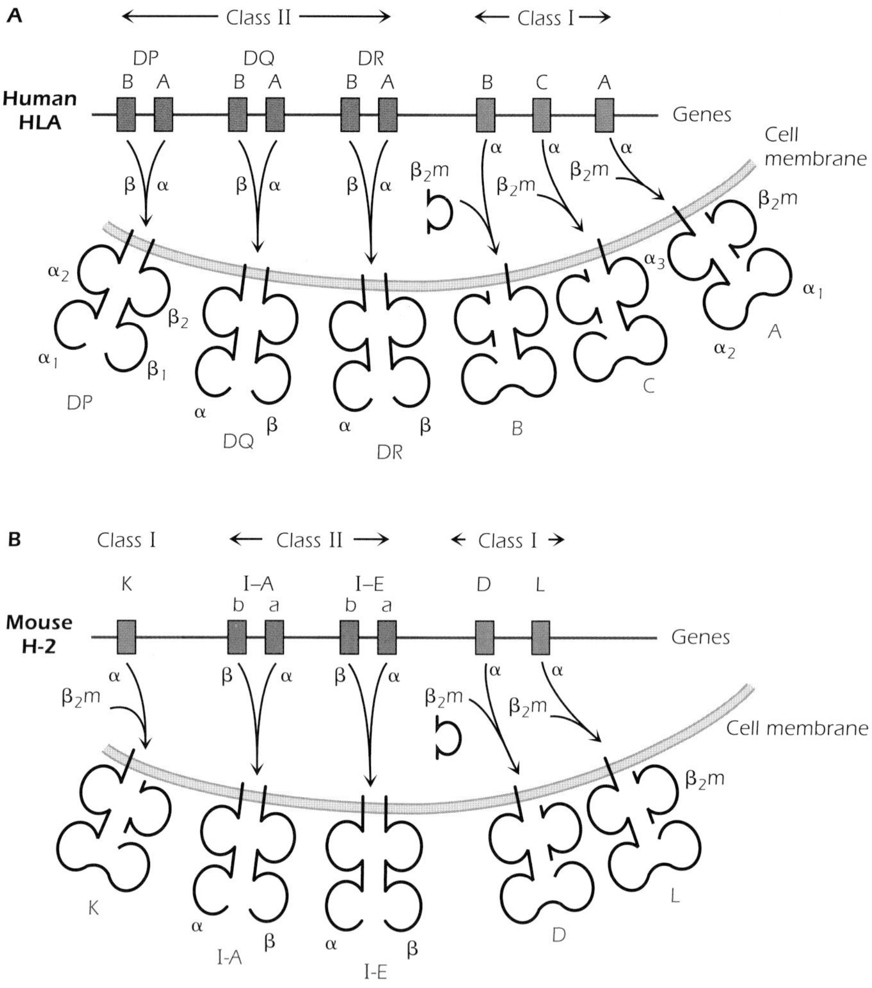

Figure 9.1. Simplified depiction of the human (A) and mouse (B) MHC, showing regions and genes coding for polymorphic MHC class I and II molecules. β_2m $= \beta_2$-microglobulin, encoded outside the MHC.

and a B gene that codes for one chain, α or β, respectively, of a two-chain MHC class II molecule. Thus, for example, the *HLA-DPA* gene codes for DPα of the HLA-DP molecule, and the *HLA-DPB* gene codes for the other chain, DPβ, of the HLA-DP molecule. The two-chain molecules DQ$\alpha\beta$ and DR$\alpha\beta$ are made by similar pairings of gene products of the DQ and DR subregions.

Figure 9.1B shows the mouse MHC, H-2. The figure depicts the three independent genes that code for the murine MHC class I molecules; the genes and molecules are known as ***K, D,*** and ***L.*** H-2 contains two MHC class II regions—rather than three in the human—known as ***I-A*** and ***I-E,*** that code for I-A $\alpha\beta$ and I-E $\alpha\beta$ molecules, respectively. The genes and protein products from the mouse and human MHCs show a high degree of homology, indicating a common ancestral origin.

Pattern of MHC Molecule Expression in Different Cells

MHC class I molecules are expressed at varying levels on almost every nucleated cell in the body. MHC class II molecules have a more limited distribution than class I molecules: They are expressed ***constitutively*** (i.e., under all conditions) only on B lymphocytes, dendritic cells, thymic epithelial cells—and in the human, macrophages and monocytes. These are cells that present antigen to T cells (***antigen-presenting cells;*** APCs). Many other cells, such as fibroblasts and endothelial cells and mouse macrophages, may be ***induced*** to express MHC class II molecules by factors such as the cytokine interferon-γ (IFNγ) that are released during the response to infectious agents.

Expression of MHC class I molecules is ***coordinate,*** in that all three MHC class I molecules are expressed on the cell surface at the same time. Similarly, MHC class II molecules are also coordinately expressed, but under distinct regulation. Thus MHC class I molecules can be expressed in the absence of any MHC class II molecule. The level of MHC class I and II expression at the cell surface can be coordinately upregulated or downregulated by a number of stimuli; for example, IFNγ enhances expression of all MHC class I and class II molecules.

In summary, in the absence of inducing factors, most cells express MHC class I molecules without expressing MHC class II molecules. Certain cells, such as B cells, constitutively express both MHC class I and class II molecules.

By contrast, very few, if any, cells express MHC class II in the absence of MHC class I.

VARIABILITY OF MHC GENES AND PRODUCTS

Genetic Polymorphism

Different individuals within a species have slightly different forms, referred to as ***alleles,*** of each MHC class I or II gene—that is, at a single MHC locus, different individuals have different types of a prototypical gene. In humans, different alleles are given numbers, such as *HLA-B15* or *B27.* (In mice, alleles are given superscripted small letters such as $H\text{-}2K^b$ or K^d.) The phenomenon of having multiple stable forms of one gene in the population is known as ***genetic polymorphism.***

Genetic polymorphism generates diversity of MHC molecules within the population—that is, MHC-distinct individuals express MHC molecules with somewhat different sequences. The MHC is the most highly polymorphic gene system in the body and hence in the population. This extensive polymorphism of MHC genes makes it very unlikely that two random individuals will express identical sets of MHC molecules. As we shall describe in Chapter 19, this polymorphism is the basis for rapid graft rejection between genetically different individuals.

> The advent of polymerase chain reaction (PCR) technology has shown the extent of HLA polymorphism; individuals formerly designated identical at a particular HLA locus by the use of serologic techniques (reaction with antibodies specific for particular HLA alleles) have been shown to differ in their HLA gene sequences. To better define HLA gene variability in the population, a new nomenclature employs a more extensive definition of an HLA allele. For example, in place of the older serological definition of allele ***DR7,*** the newer definition includes the ***locus*** (e.g., DRB1—"B1," because molecular mapping has shown more than one DRB gene) followed by an asterisk, then two digits to define the ***allele group,*** usually the same as the serologically defined specificity (e.g., DRB1*07), and two digits that identify the ***subtype*** (e.g., **DRB1*0701** or **DRB1*0704).** This more extensive and precise characterization of HLA alleles has been invaluable in trying to match transplant donors and recipients, and for identifying individuals who may be at risk for different autoimmune diseases (see Chapters 19 and 12).

Codominant Expression

Both MHC class I and II molecules are ***codominantly expressed***—that is, every cell that expresses MHC molecules expresses proteins transcribed from *both* the maternal and the paternal chromosome (indicated in the top part of Figure 9.2 by arrows from both chromosomes to the cell surface). Note that the same set of MHC gene products is expressed in every cell in a single individual—that is, in one person, the MHC class I molecules expressed on every lymphocyte are the same, and the same as those expressed by every liver cell. This contrasts with the strategy for diversifying antigen-specific T and B cell receptors, discussed in Chapters 6 and 8: Gene rearrangement ensures that each lymphocyte within an individual has a unique set of genes coding for an antigen-specific receptor. As a result, every clone of lymphocytes expresses a different antigen-specific receptor.

Thus, because MHC molecules are expressed codominantly, every cell within one person expresses up to six different HLA class I molecules: three coded for by the HLA class I genes on each chromosome. For example, all the cells in one person may express the molecules HLA-A2 and -A5, HLA-B7 and -B13, and HLA-C6 and -C8 on their surface. Another person may express six completely different HLA class I molecules. Some individuals may express fewer than six different HLA class I molecules because they are ***homozygous*** for a particular allele (i.e., both paternal and maternal chromosomes express the same allele). As we describe in subsequent sections, MHC molecules bind peptides, so individuals who are heterozygous at their MHC alleles bind a more diverse array of peptides than those who are homozygous. This may have clinical significance, which is discussed later in this chapter.

HLA DP, DQ, and DR molecules are also codominantly expressed in the cells that express HLA class II molecules. This results in the expression of at least six HLA class II molecules in individuals heterozygous at all HLA class II alleles. Frequently, more than six different HLA class II molecules are expressed on a human cell. This occurs because in addition to the HLA-DP, DQ, and DR $\alpha\beta$ molecules, gene products from different genetic regions—such as DPα with DQβ—can pair and be expressed at the cell surface. Furthermore, the HLA class II subregions DP and DQ have more than one A and B gene, and the DR subregion has more than one B gene (not shown in Figure 9.1A). Consequently, a subregion can synthesize more than one $\alpha\beta$ polypeptide.

The set of MHC class I plus class II genes expressed on an individual chromosome—referred to as a ***haplotype***—is passed on as a unit into the offspring (Fig. 9.2). The offspring will also inherit a set of MHC class I plus class II genes from their other parent. Because of the diversity of HLA molecules in the population, it can be almost guaranteed that the HLA haplotype contributed by the second parent will differ from the haplotype of the first parent (represented by the different colors of the chromosomes in the figure). Thus Figure 9.2 shows that the HLA haplotypes of any offspring will differ from the haplotypes of the parents and generally will differ from the haplotypes of other offspring (although there is a 1 in 4 chance that any two siblings will have identical HLA haplotypes.) Usually, however, individuals within a family do not express identical MHC molecules; and as we have said previously, the likelihood of finding individuals in the

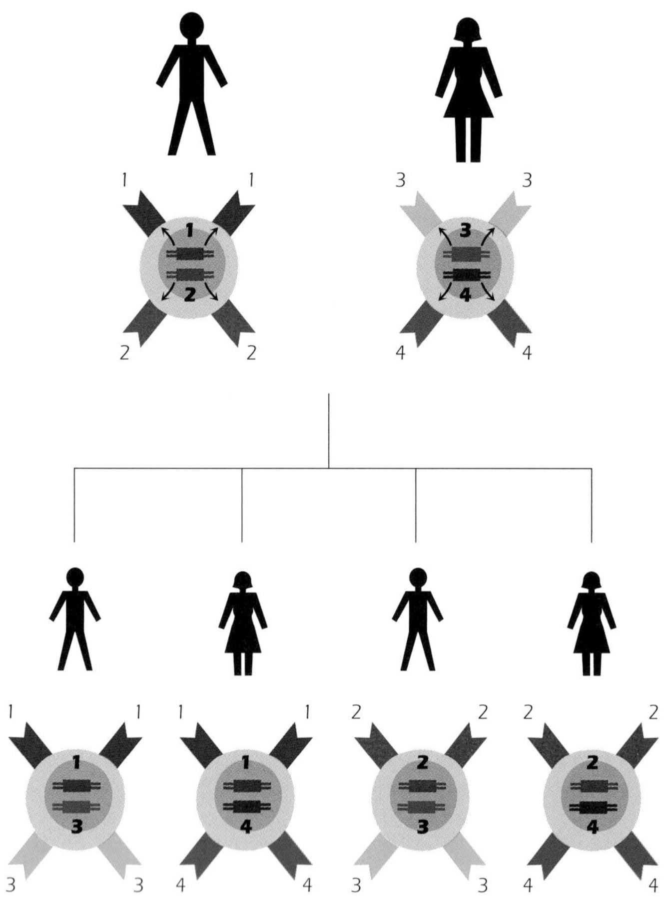

Figure 9.2. A set of HLA genes—the HLA haplotype—is passed on as a unit from parent to child; because HLA genes are so diverse in the population, the HLA haplotypes of children differ from those of their parents.

general population who are matched at all HLA alleles is tiny. By contrast to humans, other species can be selectively bred to create ***inbred strains*** in which all members of the strain are genetically identical. Studies taking advantage of the genetic identity of inbred strains of mice in particular have helped answer many fundamental immunological questions that cannot be addressed easily in humans.

STRUCTURE OF MHC MOLECULES

Structure of MHC Class I Molecules

Figure 9.3A shows the general features of an MHC class I molecule in humans and mice. Each MHC class I gene codes for a transmembrane glycoprotein of approximate molecular weight 43 kDa, which is referred to as the α, or heavy chain. It comprises three extracellular domains: α_1, α_2, and α_3. Every MHC class I molecule is expressed at the surface of a cell in noncovalent association with a small invariant polypeptide called ***β_2-microglobulin (β_2m;*** molecular weight 12 kDa), which is coded for on another chromosome. β_2m has a structure homologous to a single Ig domain, and indeed, β_2m is also a member of the Ig superfamily. Thus, at the cell surface, MHC class I plus β_2m has the appearance of a four-domain molecule, with the α_3 domain of the class I molecule and β_2m juxtaposed closest to the membrane.

The sequences of different allelic forms of MHC class I molecules are very similar. Sequence differences among MHC molecules are confined to a limited region in their extracellular α_1 and α_2 domains. Thus an individual class I molecule can be divided into a ***nonpolymorphic*** or ***invariant region*** (similar in all class I allelic forms) and a ***polymorphic*** or ***variable region*** (sequence unique to that allele). The T cell molecule CD8 binds to the invariant region of all MHC class I molecules (see Fig. 8.3A).

All MHC class I molecules that have been examined by X-ray crystallography have the same general structure, depicted in Figures 9.3B and C. The most striking feature is that the part of the molecule farthest from the membrane, made up of parts of the α_1 and α_2 domains, contains a deep groove or cleft. ***This groove in the MHC class I molecule is the binding site for peptides.*** The cleft resembles a basket with an irregular floor (made up of amino acids in a β-pleated sheet structure), and the surrounding walls form α-helices. The cleft is closed at both ends and thus can fit peptides eight to nine amino acids long in a linear array (see also Fig. 3.4.)

Comparing the sequence and structure of clefts in different MHC class I molecules, we find that the floor of each is different, consisting of a number of ***allele-specific pockets*** (Fig. 9.3D). The shape and charge of these pockets at the bottom of the cleft help determine which peptides bind to a particular allelic form of an MHC molecule. The

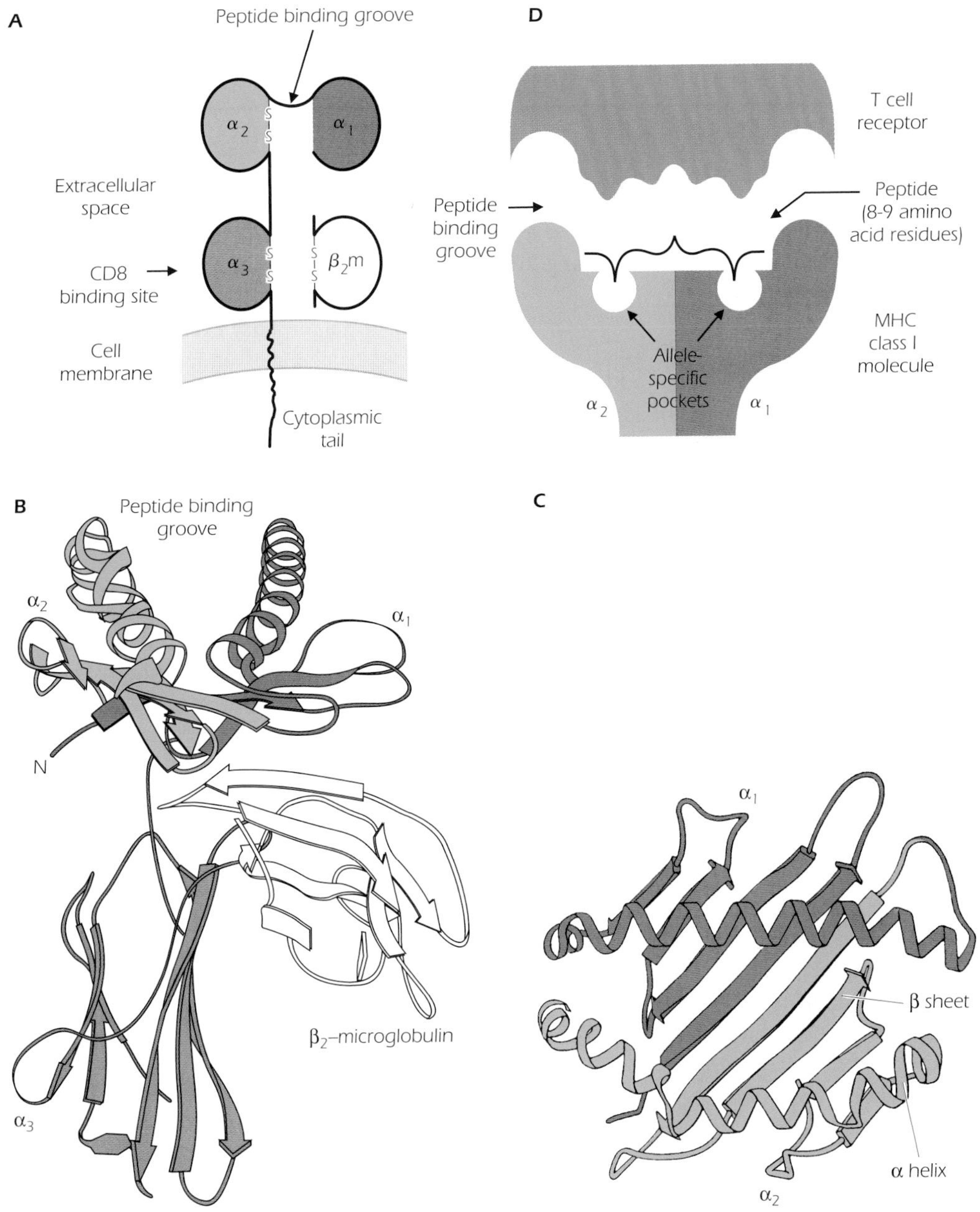

Figure 9.3. Different depictions of an MHC class I molecule. (A) Diagram of the structures of an MHC class I molecule associated at the cell surface with β_2m. (B) Side view of the MHC class I molecule with β_2m, showing the peptide-binding groove. (C) Top view of the peptide-binding groove. (D) Diagram of the interaction of a T-cell receptor with an MHC class I molecule and peptide bound in the peptide-binding groove. (Figures B and C from Bjorkman et al., 1987, with permission; Figure D adapted from Rammensee et al., 1993.)

pockets also help secure peptides in a position in which they can be recognized by specific T cell receptors (TCRs). Figures 9.3D and 8.2 illustrate that peptide bound in this cleft and parts of the MHC class I molecule interact with the T cell receptor. As we described in Chapter 8, the center of the bound peptide—the only part of the peptide not buried in the MHC molecule—interacts with the CDR3 regions of the TCR α and β, the regions of most variability in the TCR. This suggests that limited contacts with amino acids in the center of the peptide are critical for recognition by the TCR.

A single MHC class I molecule can bind to a variety of peptides but binds preferentially to peptides with certain ***motifs***—that is, peptides with either invariant or closely related amino acids at certain positions (***anchor residues***) in the eight- or nine-amino acid sequence but variability at the other positions. Thus, for example, the human class I molecule HLA-A2 binds peptides with leucine at position 2 and valine at position 9 in the peptide sequence; by contrast, another HLA-A molecule may bind peptides with the amino acid anchor residues phenylalanine or tyrosine at position 5 and leucine at position 8. The other positions on the bound peptides can be occupied by a variety of different amino acids. In this way, any one MHC molecule can bind to a large number of peptides with different sequences. This helps explain why T cell responses are made, with very few exceptions, to at least one epitope from almost all proteins and why failing to respond to a protein antigen is so rare.

Structure of MHC Class II Molecules

MHC class II α and β genes code for chains of approximate molecular weight 35,000 and 28,000 Da, respectively. Figure 9.4A shows that MHC class II molecules, like MHC class I molecules, are transmembrane glycoprotein molecules with cytoplasmic tails and extracellular Ig-like domains; the domains are referred to as α_1, α_2, β_1, and β_2. MHC class II molecules are also members of the Ig superfamily. As we described for MHC class I molecules, MHC class II molecules are also made up of variable or polymorphic regions (differing among alleles) and invariant or nonpolymorphic regions (common to all alleles). The T cell molecule CD4 binds to the invariant portion of all MHC class II molecules.

The MHC class II molecule also contains a peptide-binding groove or cleft at the top of the molecule (Figures 9.4B and C), which is structurally analogous to the MHC class I groove. In the MHC class II molecule, however, the cleft is formed by interactions between domains of different chains, the α_1 and β_1 domains. Figure 9.4C indicates that the floor of the MHC class II groove is made up of eight β-pleated sheets, with the α_1 and β_1 domains each contributing four; helical sections of the α_1 and β_1 domains each make up one wall of the cleft. In contrast to the class I groove, however, the class II groove is open at both ends, allowing larger peptides to bind. Thus the MHC class II groove binds peptides varying in length from 12 to approximately 17 amino acids in a linear array, with the ends of the peptide outside the groove. Figure 9.4D shows that the TCR contacts the peptide, bound in the groove of the MHC class II molecule, and parts of the MHC class II molecule. Peptides that bind to different MHC class II molecules also exhibit motifs; because the lengths of the peptides are more variable than those that bind to MHC class I molecules, the motif is generally seen in the central region of the peptide, the region that fits inside the MHC class II binding groove.

THE FUNCTION OF MHC MOLECULES: ANTIGEN PROCESSING AND PRESENTATION

As we mentioned in the previous chapter, pathogens such as bacteria and viruses can penetrate and infect the cells of the body and T cells mount an immune response against the cells harboring the invading organism. How do T cells recognize an infected cell or indeed the presence of any foreign protein antigen that is inside a host cell? In brief, we now know that proteins are broken down inside cells into smaller fragments, peptides. Some of these peptides associate inside the cell with MHC class I or class II molecules, and the peptide-MHC complex moves to the surface of the cell where it can be recognized by a T cell with an appropriate receptor. In the presence of costimulatory signals (described later in this chapter and more fully in Chapter 10), the T cell is activated and mounts a response against the antigen.

The events involved in the generation of peptides from proteins inside cells, the binding of peptides to MHC molecules, and the display of peptide-MHC complexes at the cell surface for T-cell recognition are known collectively as ***antigen processing and presentation.*** MHC molecules play a central role in these phenomena, and for this reason, as we described earlier in this chapter, T-cell responses are said to be ***MHC restricted.*** MHC class I and class II molecules have different functions in T cell responses, however. In every vertebrate species studied, the function of MHC class I molecules is to present peptides derived from protein antigens to $CD8^+$ T cells. Fr this reason, $CD8^+$ T cell responses are said to be MHC class I-restricted. By contrast, the function of MHC class II molecules is to present peptides to $CD4^+$ T cells and thus $CD4^+$ T cells are said to be MHC class II-restricted.

How do peptides derived from protein antigens associate with MHC molecules? In the paragraphs that follow, we describe how the processing of two different sets of protein antigens—known as ***exogenous*** and ***endogenous*** antigens—results in peptides associating with either MHC class II or MHC class I molecules, and thus leads to the activation of different sets of T cells.

Responses to Exogenous Antigens: Generation of MHC Class II–Peptide Complexes

As the term implies, exogenous antigens are those antigens *taken into* cells, normally by endocytosis or phagocytosis (see Fig. 2.2). Exogenous antigens can be derived from pathogens (e.g., bacteria and viruses) and from foreign proteins (e.g., ovalbumin and sheep red blood cells) that do not injure the host but activate an immune response. Responses to exogenous antigens taken up by APCs—dendritic cells, B lymphocytes, or macrophages—are particularly important.

Figure 9.5 shows the processing and presentation of a typical exogenous antigen, a protein injected as a component of an inactivated or "dead" virus vaccine. Once internalized, the protein is contained in an intracellular vesicle that then fuses with existing endosomal or lysosomal vesicles. The endosomal and lysosomal vesicles are highly acidic (pH ~4.0) and contain an array of degradative enzymes, including proteases and peptidases. Proteases, known as cathepsins, that function at low pH are thought to be involved in selective cutting of proteins in these vesicles.

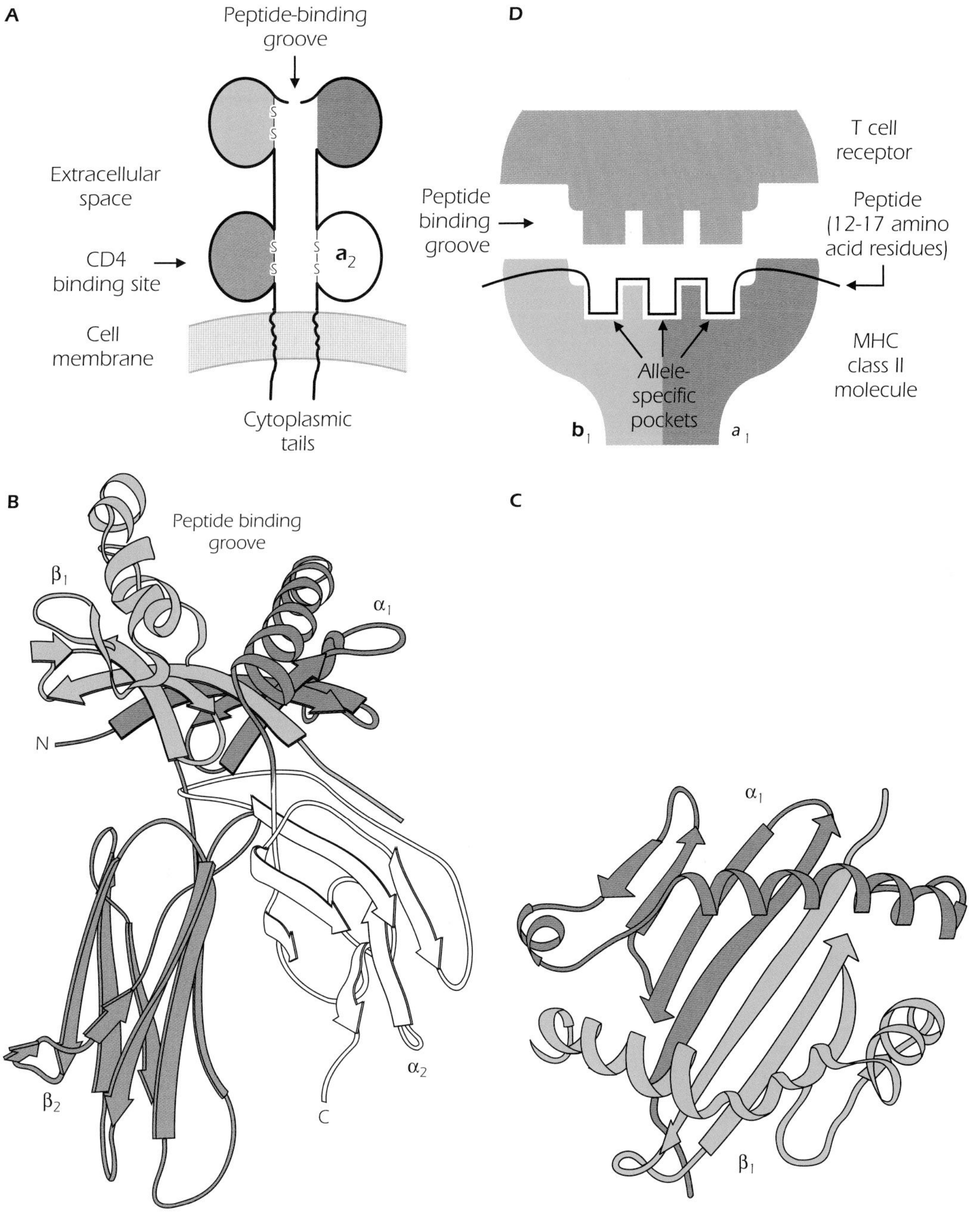

Figure 9.4. Different depictions of an MHC class II molecule. (A) Diagram of the structure of an MHC class II molecule at the cell surface. (B) Side view of the MHC class II molecule showing the peptide-binding groove. (Adapted from Stern and Wiley, 1994, with permission.) (C) Top view of the peptide-binding groove. (Adapted from Stern et al., 1994, with permission.) (D) Diagram of the interaction of a T-cell receptor with an MHC class II molecule and peptide bound in the peptide-binding groove. (From Rammensee et al., 1993.)

Figure 9.5 also illustrates that the acid vesicles containing peptides intersect inside the cell with vesicles containing newly synthesized MHC class II molecules. MHC class II α and β chains are synthesized on ribosomes of the rough endoplasmic reticulum (ER). The chains associate in the ER with a molecule known as ***CD74, invariant chain*** (Ii); a region of CD74 interacts with the groove of the newly formed MHC class II molecule, preventing the binding of peptides that may be present in the ER. (These can arise from the processing of endogenous antigens, described in the next section.) CD74 also acts as a "***chaperone***" for the newly synthesized MHC class II chains: Interaction with CD74 allows the MHC class II α plus β chains to leave the ER and enter the Golgi and from there into the acid

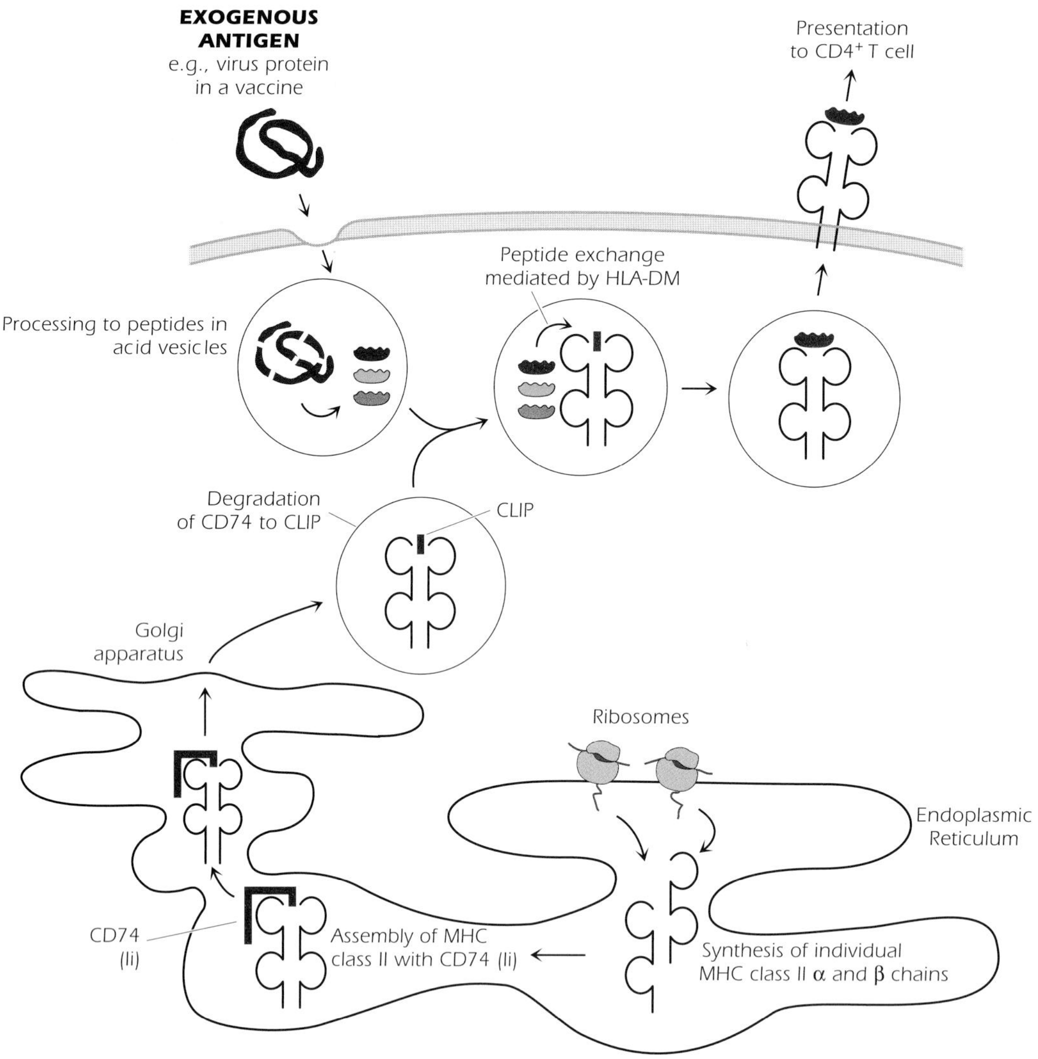

Figure 9.5. Processing of an exogenous antigen in the MHC class II pathway. CD74 (Ii = invariant chain), CLIP = fragment of CD74 bound to MHC class II groove.

vesicle endocytic pathway. Removal of CD74 from the complex occurs in stages in acid vesicles. Initially, CD74 is degraded proteolytically, leaving a fragment known as CLIP bound to the MHC class II groove. Vesicles containing MHC class II bound to CLIP then fuse with acid vesicles (endosomes/lysosomes) containing peptides derived from the catabolism of exogenous antigens. In this compartment, a molecule known as **HLA-DM** facilitates peptide exchange between the MHC class II-CLIP complex and peptides derived from the exogenous antigen. In this way, a peptide-MHC class II complex is generated, which moves to the cell surface where it can interact with a $CD4^+$ T cell expressing the appropriate antigen receptor.

Catabolism of a typical protein antigen yields several peptides (only three are shown in Fig. 9.5). Figure 9.6 indicates that the association of MHC class II molecules and processed peptides is ***selective:*** A single peptide binds with high affinity to some but not all MHC molecules. This selectivity is based on the strength of the interactions between amino acids in the peptide-binding groove of the MHC molecule and in the processed peptide. In Figure 9.6, peptide 35–48 (the numbers refer to the position of an amino acid in the protein sequence) preferentially binds to HLA-DR4, and peptide 110–122 preferentially binds to HLA-DP2 in a person who expresses these MHC class II molecules. Thus we call the peptides 35–48 and 110–122 the ***immunodominant*** T cell epitopes of the protein in this person, because they bind to MHC molecules and are presented to and activate $CD4^+$ T cells.

Peptides that do not bind to MHC molecules do not activate T cell responses. In Figure 9.6, peptide 1–13 does not bind to the HLA molecules of the individual shown and, therefore, does not trigger a T cell response. Peptide 1–13, however, is quite probably the immunodominant epitope of this protein in an individual expressing a completely different set of HLA molecules. Thus we can say almost without fail that *every* person will make a T cell response to this viral protein.

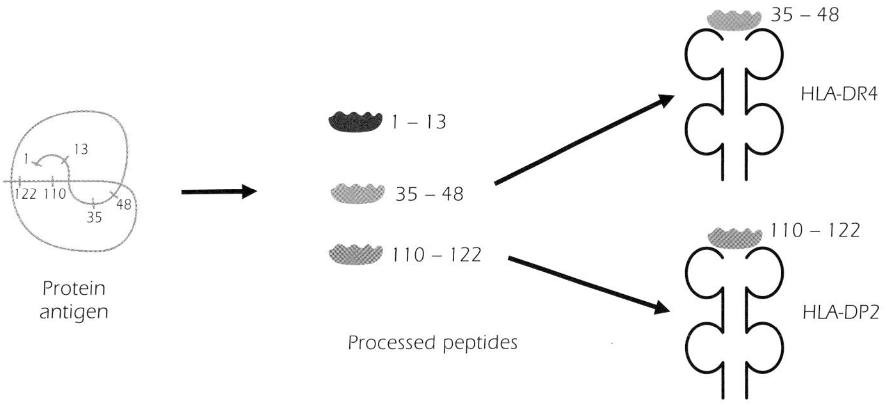

Figure 9.6. Selective binding of processed peptides by different MHC class II alleles. The numbers refer to positions of amino acids in the sequence of the protein antigen.

Because of the selectivity of peptide–MHC binding, however, individuals who express different allelic forms of MHC molecules respond to different parts of the same protein.

Endogenous Antigens: Generation of MHC Class I–peptide Complexes

Endogenous antigens are synthesized inside a cell; typically, they are derived from pathogens (e.g., viruses, bacteria, and parasites) that have *infected* the cell. Figure 9.7 illustrates the processing and presentation of a viral protein that has been synthesized after the cell has been infected by a virus. Processing of endogenous antigens occurs in the cytoplasm rather than in the acid vesicles in which exogenous antigens are processed. The major mechanism for generating peptide fragments in the cytoplasm is via a giant protein complex known as the ***proteasome.*** This cleaves proteins into peptides about 15 amino acids in length. Cytosolic enzymes (aminopeptidases) remove even more amino acids from the peptides. Some peptides are destroyed, but some, 8–15 amino acids in length, are selectively transported into the ER by a peptide transporter, the product of two genes, *TAP-1* and *TAP-2.*

In the ER, peptides transported from the cytosol into the ER bind to newly synthesized MHC class I molecules: Figure 9.7 also shows that MHC class I and β2-microglobulin chains are synthesized separately in the ER and associate in this compartment. As we described for newly synthesized MHC class II molecules, additional proteins help to stabilize the structure of the assembled MHC class I plus β2-microglobulin chains in the ER and direct the complex of peptide, MHC class I, and β2-microglobulin through the cell. Among the best characterized of the additional proteins that are unique to the MHC class I pathway in the ER are *tapasin* and the chaperone *calreticulin.*

MHC class I molecules preferentially bind peptides eight to nine amino acids long—shorter than the peptides that bind to MHC class II—because the groove in the MHC class I binding site is closed at both ends. Recent evidence indicates that the normal fate of peptides that reach the ER is to be degraded by an aminopeptidase that trims amino acids one at a time until the peptides are completely degraded; only peptides eight to nine amino acids long are "rescued" by binding to an available newly synthesized MHC class I molecule.

As we described for peptide–MHC class II interactions, binding of peptides to MHC class I molecules is also ***selective*** and based on the sequence and structure of the peptide and the MHC class I binding groove. A peptide that binds to an MHC class I molecule in the ER moves via the Golgi apparatus to the cell surface, where it is presented to a $CD8^+$ T cell expressing the appropriate antigen receptor.

Other Pathways of Antigen-Processing and Presentation

The foregoing sections have described how peptides from endogenous and exogenous antigens interact with newly synthesized MHC class I and class II molecules on their way to the cell surface. Evidence also suggests that peptides can bind to some MHC molecules at the cell surface, either to MHC molecules not containing peptide or by displacing previously bound peptide. Peptides can also intersect with MHC molecules that have been expressed on the surface of the cell and then recycle from the surface back into the cell.

APCs such as dendritic cells and macrophages also have a unique pathway, known as ***cross-priming,*** for generating peptides that are presented to $CD8^+$ T cells. These APCs can take up exogenous protein antigens and process them in the *MHC class I pathway* (in addition to the MHC class II pathway). This pathway is thought to play an important role in activating $CD8^+$ T cells to respond to virus-infected cells and to some tumors (see Chapters 10 and 20, respectively.)

Table 9.1 compares the properties of MHC class I and class II molecules and the roles of these molecules in processing and presenting antigens.

Which Antigens Trigger Which T Cell Responses?

We have described how exogenous protein antigens are taken up by antigen presenting cells, are processed in acid compartments that intersect with the MHC class II pathway, and activate $CD4^+$ T cells. Thus we can say that almost without

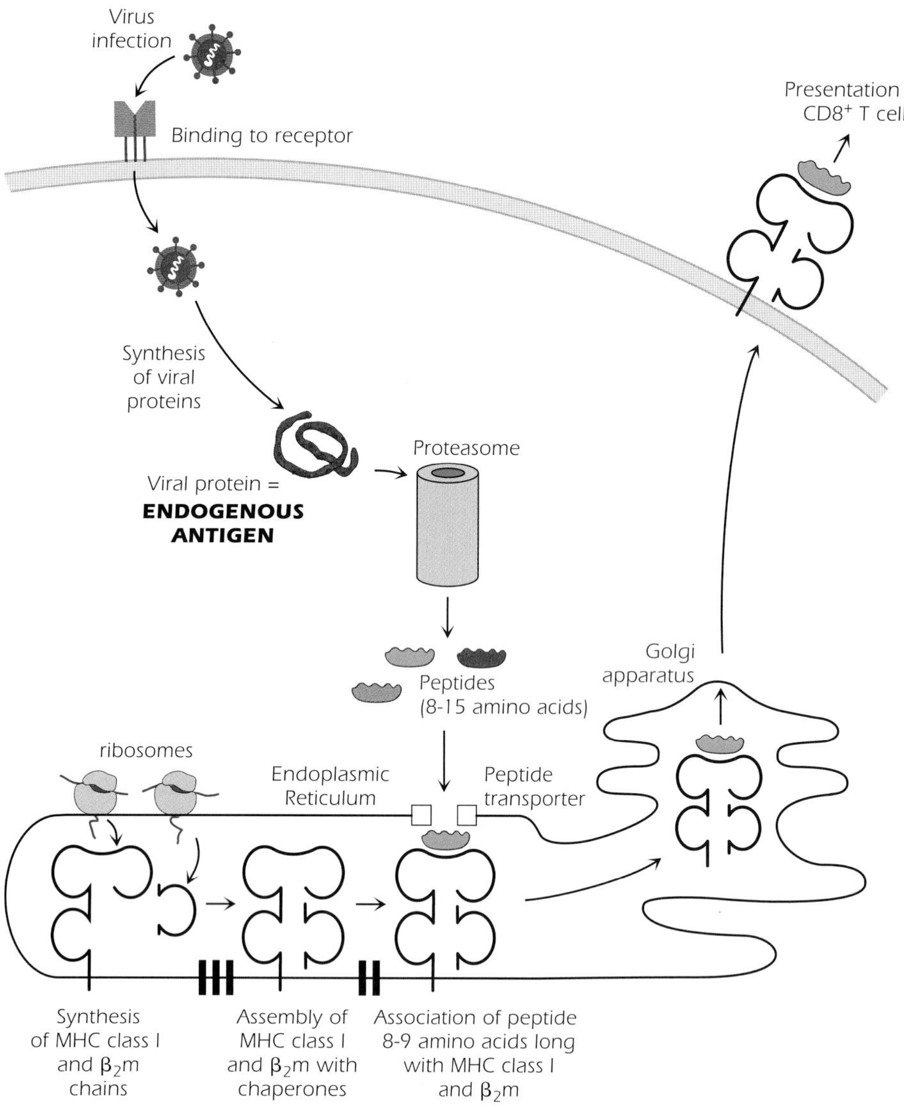

Figure 9.7. Processing of an endogenous antigen in the MHC class I pathway. β_2m = β_2-microglobulin.

TABLE 9.1. Comparison of the Properties and Function of MHC Class I and Class II Molecules

Characteristic	MHC Class I	MHC Class II
Structure	α chain + β_2m	α and β chains
Domains	α_1, α_2 and α_3 + β_2m	$\alpha_1 + \alpha_2$ and $\beta_1 + \beta_2$
Constitutive cellular expression	Nearly all nucleated cells	APCs (B cells, dendritic cells, macrophages)
Peptide-binding groove	Closed, binds 8–9 amino acid peptides; formed by α_1 and α_2 domains	Open, binds 12–17 amino acid peptides; formed by α_1 and β_1 domains
Peptides derived from	Endogenous antigens, catabolized in the cytoplasm. Antigens derived from cross-priming	Exogenous antigens, catabolized in acid compartments
Peptide presented to	CD8$^+$ T cells	CD4$^+$ T cells

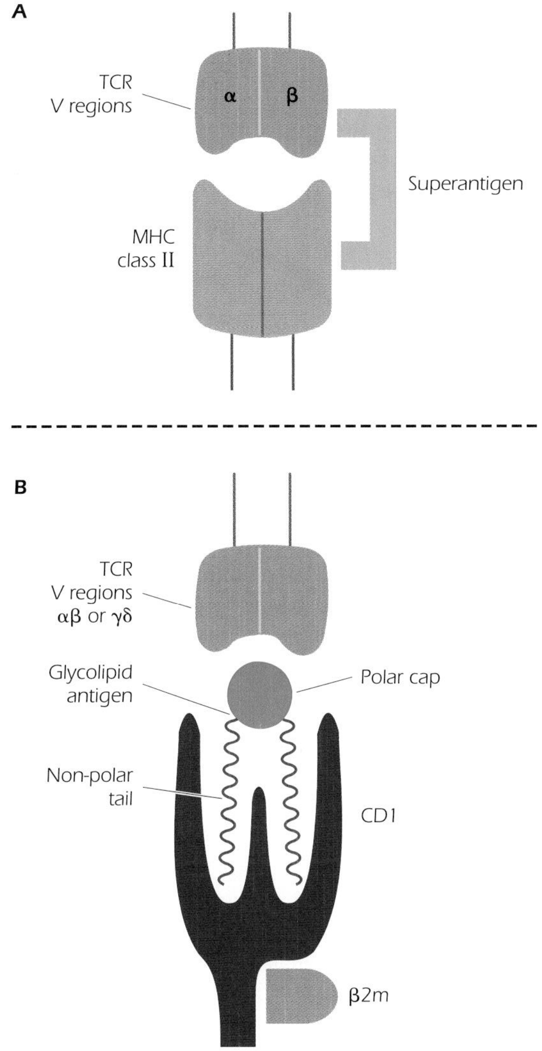

Figure 9.8. The interaction of TCRs with different types of antigen. (A) Superantigens bind outside the MHC class II peptide-binding groove and to the TCR V_β; (B) CD1 presents glycolipid antigens.

exception that proteins from bacteria, viruses, allergens (the proteins that induce allergic responses), or completely harmless antigens, trigger $CD4^+$ T cell responses. We have also described how proteins derived from pathogens that infect cells—such as bacteria and viruses—create epitopes via the endogenous or the cross-priming pathways that are presented to $CD8^+$ T cells. Thus proteins derived from these infectious agents activate $CD4^+$ *and* $CD8^+$ T cells.

Note that the processing pathway, rather than inherent properties of the antigen, determines whether a protein is presented to $CD4^+$ or $CD8^+$ T cells. This is illustrated by the cross-priming pathway that we described above, in which an exogenous antigen is processed in the MHC class I pathway and is presented to $CD8^+$ T cells. In addition, antigens that are injected or introduced into the cytoplasm can create peptides for presentation to $CD8^+$ T cells; this approach may be useful for generating responses to tumor antigens (see Chapter 20).

Superantigens are another category of protein antigens. In humans, these are predominantly bacterial toxins, such as staphylococcal enterotoxin, but in mice they can also be the products of some viruses. Superantigens bind to MHC class II molecules without being processed, but as shown in Figure 9.8A, bacterial superantigens bind to a region of the MHC class II molecule outside the peptide-binding groove. Figure 9.8A also shows that superantigens bind to the V_β region of a TCR, irrespective of the V_α expressed by the TCR. Specifically, superantigens bind to the part of the TCR V_β region that is coded for in the germ line and not to a part of the V_β that is formed by rearrangement of TCR_β V, D, or J segments. Thus, because there are only about 25 V_β germ line genes (see Chapter 8) and each superantigen binds to one or a few of these V_β germ line sequences, a superantigen can activate a huge number of an individual's T cells—up to 10% of a person's total T cells—many more than are triggered by conventional antigens. In Chapters 10 and 11, we shall describe more fully the clinical consequences of activating so many T cells.

RECOGNITION OF LIPIDS

In the last 10 years we have learned that T cells can recognize lipids and glycolipids as well as protein-derived antigens. The T cell response to the lipid and glycolipid cell wall products derived from mycobacteria has been well documented. Figure 9.8B shows that the genes and products of a family known as ***CD1*** play a role in the presentation of these lipids and glycolipids. CD1 molecules are distantly related to MHC class I and II molecules, and it is believed that they constitute a third family of antigen-presenting molecules that have evolved to present lipid and glycolipid antigens derived from microbial pathogens to T cells.

CD1 molecules are cell-surface glycoproteins that are non-MHC and nonpolymorphic. They are expressed in association with β_2m on APCs such as dendritic cells and B cells. Binding of lipid antigens to CD1 is believed to take place in acidic cellular compartments, similar to the loading of exogenous peptides to MHC class II molecules. Figure 9.8B shows that the structure of a recently crystallized CD1 molecule is similar to the structure of an MHC class I molecule, but CD1 contains a larger binding groove with a deep cavity. The cavity probably binds the hydrophobic backbone of a lipid antigen, and the polar region of the lipid or glycolipid is exposed in the groove for binding to the T cell receptor. Different members of the CD1 family have been shown to present antigens to $\gamma\delta^+$ T cells, to $\alpha\beta^+$ $CD8^+$ T cells, and to a subset of $\alpha\beta^+$ T cells known as NK1.1 T cells—cells with very limited TCR V region usage that express natural killer (NK) as well as T cell surface molecules (see pages 15–16).

MHC Molecules Bind Peptides Derived from Self-Molecules

We now understand that the phenomena of antigen processing and presentation are aspects of normal cell physiologic pathways; in other words, the proteins normally found inside cells—self-proteins—"turn over" and are metabolized in the same pathways we have described in this chapter. For example, ribosomal and mitochondrial proteins are also broken down inside cells, and peptides derived from these molecules can associate with MHC molecules. Indeed, MHC molecules extracted from cells nearly always contain peptides derived from such self-proteins.

Self-peptides bound to MHC molecules, however, do not normally activate T cells; one reason is that T cells reactive to many self-molecules are removed or inactivated during differentiation in the thymus (see Chapter 8). However, we know that mature T cells with the potential to react with self-molecules are detectable outside the thymus (see Chapter 12). Why are these T cells not activated? Equally important, since an individual's cells are bathed in a sea of self-proteins which they are continually processing and binding to their MHC molecules, how can a person respond to a tiny amount of foreign protein? These are critical issues, because a T cell must be able to distinguish between a normal host cell, to which no response is required, and a cell that has been infected by a pathogen, to which a T cell must respond to eliminate the pathogen.

The answer appears to be that pathogens induce effects that activate the immune response, over and above their ability to generate peptides for binding to MHC molecules. The major effect that pathogens induce is ***costimulator function***—also referred to as ***second signals***—in specialized cells that present antigen to T cells (discussed further in Chapter 10). Costimulator signals are required to activate naive T cells (T cells that have not previously encountered antigen). By contrast to peptides derived from pathogens, peptides derived from self-molecules generally encounter T cells on the surface of normal tissue cells (e.g., of the liver or pancreas), which do not express costimulator function; in this case, T cells are not activated. Even if peptides derived from a self-molecule are presented by an APC in the tissue, T cells are not activated. This is because APCs in tissue do not normally express costimulator signals in the absence of foreign antigen or of an inflammatory response (see Chapter 10). This requirement for signals in addition to MHC plus peptide ensures that T cells do not respond to peptides derived from self-components but do respond to peptides derived from nonself, potentially harmful, antigens.

Some scientists have proposed that exposure to a foreign antigen induces tissue damage (the ***danger hypothesis***) and that the "danger signals" so generated activate T cells. This hypothesis has been invoked to explain why T cells respond to foreign antigens but not to self-molecules—self-molecules do not generate danger signals. Further studies are needed to evaluate the hypothesis.

Inability to Respond to an Antigen

As we have described in the preceding sections, a limited number of different MHC class I molecules (6) and MHC class II molecules (usually between 10 and 20 in the human; 6 in the mouse) is expressed on the cells of any one individual. For an antigen to generate a T cell response, at least one peptide derived during processing must bind to one of these MHC molecules. A peptide that does not bind to an MHC molecule does not activate a T cell response. Thus it is possible that some individuals may respond to a small peptide, but other MHC-distinct individuals may not. This situation can occur if many people are injected with a peptide vaccine—some will make a response but others will not.

If an entire antigen fails to generate a single peptide able to bind to an MHC molecule, the individual will not mount a T cell response to that particular antigen. This kind of unresponsiveness to an entire antigen can occur, for example, in the response to synthetic polymers of amino acids that contain a very limited number of epitopes. Pathogens generally contain multiple epitopes, so an inability to respond to naturally occurring pathogens is very rare.

DIVERSITY OF MHC MOLECULES: MHC ASSOCIATION WITH RESISTANCE AND SUSCEPTIBILITY TO DISEASE

In this chapter we have described the extensive polymorphism of MHC genes and molecules. We have indicated that such polymorphism is a great impediment to the acceptance of tissue transplanted between individuals, because it is highly unlikely that two random individuals are genetically identical (discussed more fully in Chapter 19). Because nearly every vertebrate species has developed a similarly diverse array of MHC genes and molecules, the maintenance of MHC diversity must have some major benefit to the species.

The maintenance of diversity of MHC molecules is thought to be an important mechanism that the species uses to protect itself from the surrounding array of pathogenic organisms. To illustrate this point, imagine the situation if there were only one MHC molecule in the population and a new pathogen emerged that did not produce an epitope able to bind to the single MHC molecule. In this extreme case, no T cell response would be mounted, and the entire species could be wiped out. Thus maintaining a large number of MHC genes and molecules in the species would greatly reduce the risk of one pathogen having such a negative effect.

A recent example of how diversity among HLA alleles may affect the progress of a disease was reported in a study of HIV-1-infected patients. Individuals who were HLA heterozygotes (expressing different paternal and maternal chromosome products) at one or more HLA class I loci progressed more slowly to AIDS than individuals who were homozygotes (expressing the same gene product). One possible explanation of these findings is that HLA heterozygotes are able to present a wider range of pathogen-derived peptides to their T cells than homozygotes and thus may be more likely to induce some type of protective response.

Over the last few years it has also become apparent that the expression of a specific MHC allele is one of the important factors associated with ***susceptibility*** and with ***resistance*** to different infectious agents. In humans, expression of specific HLA alleles has been associated with either susceptibility or resistance to a number of different infectious diseases, such as human T lymphotropic virus 1 (HTLV-1), hepatitis B, leprosy, malaria, tuberculosis, and rapid progression to AIDS. Similar MHC associations with susceptibility or resistance have also been shown in infectious diseases of other species. These include Marek's disease (a viral disease in chickens) and bovine leukemia virus infection in cows. For almost all known examples of diseases or conditions associated with a particular MHC allele, definitive mechanisms connecting possession of the gene with the onset or progress of the disease have not been established. Individuals with certain HLA alleles have a higher risk of developing certain autoimmune or inflammatory diseases. This is discussed in more detail in Chapter 12.

OTHER GENES WITHIN THE MHC REGION

The MHC regions of the human and of the mouse have been mapped and shown to contain many more genes (and pseudogenes) than the polymorphic MHC class I and class II molecules that we have described in the chapter. The MHC region between the class I and class II genes contains ***MHC class III genes*** that code for serum complement components C2, C4, and factor B (described in Chapter 13). In the human, this region also contains several different genes: two cytokines (tumor necrosis factor-α and β), two heat-shock proteins (hsp 70-1 and 70-2), and 21-hydroxylase (an enzyme involved in steroid metabolism). Additional human (HLA-E, F, and G) and murine (Qa and TLa) MHC class I genes have been identified that are much less polymorphic than the class I genes we have described in the chapter. The function of the products of most of these less-polymorphic class I genes is not well understood, but they may be involved in the presentation of antigens to T cells. The expression of HLA-G by placental trophoblast cells has been suggested as a potential mechanism by which rejection of the fetus by the maternal host is prevented.

The MHC class II region includes genes other than those coding for the cell-surface molecules described earlier in the chapter. These include genes known as HLA-DM and HLA-DO in the human class II region (M and O in the mouse region). As described earlier in the chapter, HLA-DM catalyzes peptide exchange between foreign peptides and the invariant chain-derived CLIP protein. HLA-DO is expressed only in B cells and thymic epithelial cells and acts as a negative regulator of HLA-DM-mediated peptide exchange. Genes coding for molecules involved in the MHC class I pathway of antigen presentation—the peptide transporter molecules TAP-1 and TAP-2 and the major subunits (LMP-2 and LMP-7) of the proteasome—are also found in the MHC class II region. Why all these genes are linked in a complex that is passed down as a unit with genes coding for crucial cell interaction molecules is currently not known.

SUMMARY

1. MHC molecules play a crucial role in the response of T cells to antigens that penetrate or live inside cells of the body. MHC molecules bind peptides derived from proteins and present them to T cells with the appropriate receptor. Thus T cell responses are said to be MHC restricted.

2. The MHC codes for two major categories of cell-surface transmembrane molecules, MHC class I and class II molecules. MHC class I molecules are expressed on all nucleated cells; MHC class II molecules are expressed constitutively only on APCs such as B cells and dendritic cells. The expression of MHC molecules is inducible on many cell types, particularly in response to cytokines released during the response to infectious agents.

3. Each individual expresses a distinct array of MHC class I and class II molecules. This diversity comes about because different individuals within a species have a range of slightly different forms (alleles) of MHC class I and class II genes (genetic polymorphism). Because of the extensive polymorphism of MHC genes, every individual has an almost unique array of inherited MHC genes.

4. Within one individual, the MHC class I and II molecules expressed are the same on all cells of the body, and they are codominantly expressed at the cell surface (i.e., products of both maternal and paternal chromosomes).

5. The outer region of every MHC class I and class II molecule contains a deep groove that binds peptides

derived from the catabolism (processing) of protein antigens. The binding of peptides to MHC molecules is selective. Each MHC molecule binds a distinct subset of peptides with a particular motif.

6. Exogenous protein antigens are taken into APCs and processed to peptides in acid compartments where they interact with MHC class II molecules. The peptide–MHC class II complex is transported to the cell surface where it interacts with the TCR expressed by a $CD4^+$ T cell. The response of $CD4^+$ T cells is referred to as restricted by MHC class II molecules (self-MHC class II molecules).

7. Endogenous protein antigens, generally derived from infectious pathogens, come from within cells and are processed to peptides in the cytosol. Peptides derived from these proteins interact with MHC class I molecules in the endoplasmic reticulum. The peptide–MHC class I complex is transported to the cell surface where it interacts with the T cell receptor expressed by a $CD8^+$ T cell. The response of $CD8^+$ T cells is referred to as restricted by MHC class I molecules (self-MHC class I molecules).

8. Since proteins are generally structurally complex, they usually generate at least one peptide able to bind to an MHC molecule, ensuring that a T cell response is made to at least some part of a foreign antigen.

9. MHC molecules bind peptides derived from self-components as well as from foreign antigens, but complexes of MHC molecules with self-peptides do not normally activate a T cell response. This is because self-molecules do not normally generate the costimulatory (second) signals needed to activate naive T cells. The T-cell response is focused on the response to foreign (non-self) molecules, particularly components of microorganisms, which induce costimulatory function.

10. Susceptibility and resistance to many diseases in humans and other species are associated with the expression of a particular MHC allele.

REFERENCES

Beck S, Trowsdale J (2000): The human major histocompatibility complex: lessons from the DNA sequence. *Annu Rev Genomics Hum Genet* 1:117.

Bjorkman PJ, Saper MA, Samraoui B, Bennett WS, Strominger JL, Wiley DC (1987): Structure of the human class I histocompatibility antigen, HLA-A2. Nature 329:506–12.

Bryant PW, Lennon-Dumenil AM, Fiebiger E, Lagaudriere-Gesbert C, Ploegh HL (2002): Proteolysis and antigen presentation by MHC class II molecules. *Adv Immunol* 80:71.

Heath WR, Carbone FR (2001): Cross-presentation in viral immunity and self-tolerance. *Nat Rev Immunol* 1:126.

Hoots K, O'Brien SJ (1999): HLA and HIV-1: heterozygote advantage and B*35-Cw*04 disadvantage. *Science* 283:1748.

Klein J, Sato A (2000): The HLA system *N Engl J Med* 343:702, 782.

Matzinger P (2002): The danger model: a renewed sense of self. *Science* 296:301.

Pieters J (2000): MHC class II-restricted antigen processing and presentation. *Adv Immunol* 75:159.

Rammensee HG, Falk K, Rötzschke O (1993): Current Opinion in Immunology 5:35–44. MHC molecules as peptide receptors.

Robinson JH, Delvig AA (2002): Diversity in MHC class II antigen presentation. *Immunology* 105:252.

Rudolph MG, Wilson IA (2002): The specificity of TCR/pMHC interaction. *Curr Opin Immunol* 14:52.

Stern LJ, Wiley DC (1994): Antigenic peptide binding by class I and class II histocompatibility proteins. Structure 2:245–251

Stern LJ, Brown JH, Jardetzky TS, Gorga JC, Urban RG, Strominger JL, Wiley DC (1994): Crystal structure of the human class II MHC protein HLA-DR1 complexed with an influenza virus peptide. Nature 368:215–21.

Wang JH, Reinherz EL (2002): Structural basis of T cell recognition of peptides bound to MHC molecules. *Mol Immunol* 38: 1039.

Yewdell JW, Bennink JR (2001): Cut and trim: generating MHC class I peptide ligands. *Curr Opin Immunol* 13:13.

REVIEW QUESTIONS

For each question, choose the ONE BEST answer or completion.

1. All the following are characteristics of both MHC class I and class II molecules *except:*
   A) They are expressed codominantly.
   B) They are expressed constitutively on all nucleated cells.
   C) They are glycosylated polypeptides with domain structure.
   D) They are involved in presentation of antigen fragments to T cells.
   E) They are expressed on the surface membrane of B cells.

2. MHC class I molecules are important for which of the following?
A) binding to CD8 molecules on T cells
B) presenting exogenous antigen (e.g., bacterial protein) to B cells
C) presenting intact viral proteins to T cells
D) binding to CD4 molecules on T cells
E) binding to Ig on B cells

3. Which of the following is *incorrect* concerning MHC class II molecules?
A) B cells may express different allelic forms of MHC class molecules on their surface.
B) MHC class II molecules are synthesized in the endoplasmic reticulum of many cell types.
C) Genetically different individuals express different MHC class II alleles.
D) MHC class II molecules are associated with β2-microglobulin on the cell surface.
E) A peptide that does not bind to an MHC class II molecule will not trigger a CD4$^+$ T cell response.

4. Products of TAP-1 and -2 genes
A) bind β2-microglobulin.
B) prevent peptide binding to MHC molecules.
C) are part of the proteasome.
D) transport peptides into the endoplasmic reticulum for binding to MHC class I.
E) transport peptides into the endoplasmic reticulum for binding to MHC class II.

5. Which of the following is *incorrect* concerning the processing of an antigen, such as a bacterial protein, in the acid compartments of the cell?
A) It results in production of potentially immunogenic peptides that associate with MHC class II molecules.
B) Predominantly exogenous antigens are processed by this pathway.
C) It may lead to activation of CD4$^+$ T cells.
D) It may lead to the activation of CD8$^+$ T cells.
E) Bacterially derived peptides displace a fragment of the invariant chain from the MHC class II binding groove.

6. Which of the following statements about the MHC is *incorrect?*
A) It codes for complement components.
B) It codes for both chains of the MHC class I molecule.
C) It codes for both chains of the MHC class II molecule.
D) It is associated with susceptibility and resistance to different diseases.
E) The total set of MHC alleles on the chromosome is known as the MHC haplotype.

7. The synthesis of which of the following molecules does *not* require V(D)J recombination?
A) TCR α
B) TCR β
C) Ig heavy chain
D) Ig light chain
E) MHC class II α chain

8. A virus is taken up by a dendritic cell and processed via the endogenous pathway. Which one of the following statements about this pathway is *incorrect?*
A) some peptides derived from viral proteins associate with MHC class I molecules
B) the T cell that recognizes the combination of MHC molecule and viral peptide processed in this pathway underwent positive selection in the thymus
C) the processing of viral proteins into peptide fragments takes place in the proteasome
D) following processing, the peptides presented to the T cell will be approximately 12–20 amino acids long
E) the end result of this pathway is presentation to a CD8$^+$ T cell

ANSWERS TO REVIEW QUESTIONS

1. ***B*** MHC class I molecules are expressed on nearly all nucleated cells, but the constitutive expression of MHC class II molecules is limited to APC such as B cells and dendritic cells. MHC class II expression can be induced on other cell types such as endothelial cells and fibroblasts by cytokines.

2. ***A*** The interaction of CD8 expressed on the T cell and an invariant region of an MHC class I molecule expressed on an antigen-presenting cell or target cell tightens the interaction between the two cells and plays a critical role in the triggering of CD8$^+$ T cells (see also Chapter 10).

3. ***D*** The MHC class I molecule, not the MHC class II molecule, associates with β2-microglobulin.

4. ***D*** The products of the TAP-1 and -2 genes selectively transport peptides generated in the cytoplasm into the ER where they may bind to MHC class I molecules.

5. ***D*** CD8$^+$ T cells are generally not activated by processing in acid compartments; exogenous antigen processing in acid compartments results in the generation of peptides, some of which can displace the CLIP fragment of the invariant chain from the MHC class II binding groove. The peptide–MHC class II complexes move to the cell surface and can interact with a CD4$^+$ T cell with the appropriate receptor.

6. ***B*** The β2-microglobulin gene is located outside the MHC, on a different chromosome.

7. ***E*** Ig and TCR chains are generated by V(D)J recombination, but MHC chains are synthesized by individual genes in the genome.

8. ***D*** The peptides generated in the endogenous pathway (involving both degradation via the proteasome in the cytoplasm and transport into the endoplasmic reticulum) and that associate with MHC class I molecules are 8–9 amino acids long.

10

ACTIVATION AND FUNCTION OF T AND B CELLS

INTRODUCTION

Activating T and B cells expressing appropriate antigen-specific receptors results in ***proliferation***—the expansion of the lymphocyte clone size—and further differentiation into ***effector cells;*** a small fraction of the expanded cells also becomes ***memory cells.*** The effector functions of T and B cells, are completely different however. For T cells, activation and differentiation lead to the synthesis and secretion of an array of cytokines that affect many different cell types or, alternatively, to the development of effector cells that are directly cytotoxic to cells of the host. By contrast, the activation and differentiation of B cells results in antibody production. In this chapter we describe in more detail how T and B cells are activated and how they exert their effector functions.

ACTIVATING CD4$^+$ T CELLS

In this section we describe how CD4$^+$ T cells, the cells that play a central role in the response to nearly all protein antigens, are activated by exogenous antigens. First, we describe how these exogenous antigens are taken up by ***antigen presenting cells*** (APCs) in vivo and how the APCs subsequently interact with CD4$^+$ T cells.

Specialized Cells Present Antigen to T Cells

Antigen can enter the body via several different routes, and specialized, or ***professional,*** APCs are found at these entry sites—especially in the airways, gastrointestinal tract, and skin—as well as in lymphoid organs and other tissues throughout the body. The most important of these APCs are bone marrow–derived cells of the myeloid lineage, ***dendritic cells*** and ***macrophages.*** As we described in Chapter 9, the functions of APCs are to take up antigen, process and present it to T cells, and provide costimulator signals that activate naive T cells. We will describe this latter function in more detail in this chapter.

Dendritic cells, a heterogeneous family of cells found in many tissues including the thymus (as described in Chapter 8), are the principal APCs for initiating ***primary*** or ***naive T cell responses***—that is, the first activation of T cells by foreign antigen. Many attributes contribute to the effectiveness of dendritic cells as APC: As we discussed in Chapter 9, they constitutively express high levels of MHC class II (as well as class I). In addition, they are highly motile, moving rapidly from sites where they are exposed to antigen to lymph nodes, where they can interact with T cells. Furthermore, dendritic cells' uptake and processing of antigens—and microbial pathogens in particular—induce costimulatory signals that are required to activate naive T cells. These properties are described in more detail below.

Immunology: A Short Course, Fifth Edition, By Richard Coico, Geoffrey Sunshine, and Eli Benjamini
ISBN 0-471-22689-0

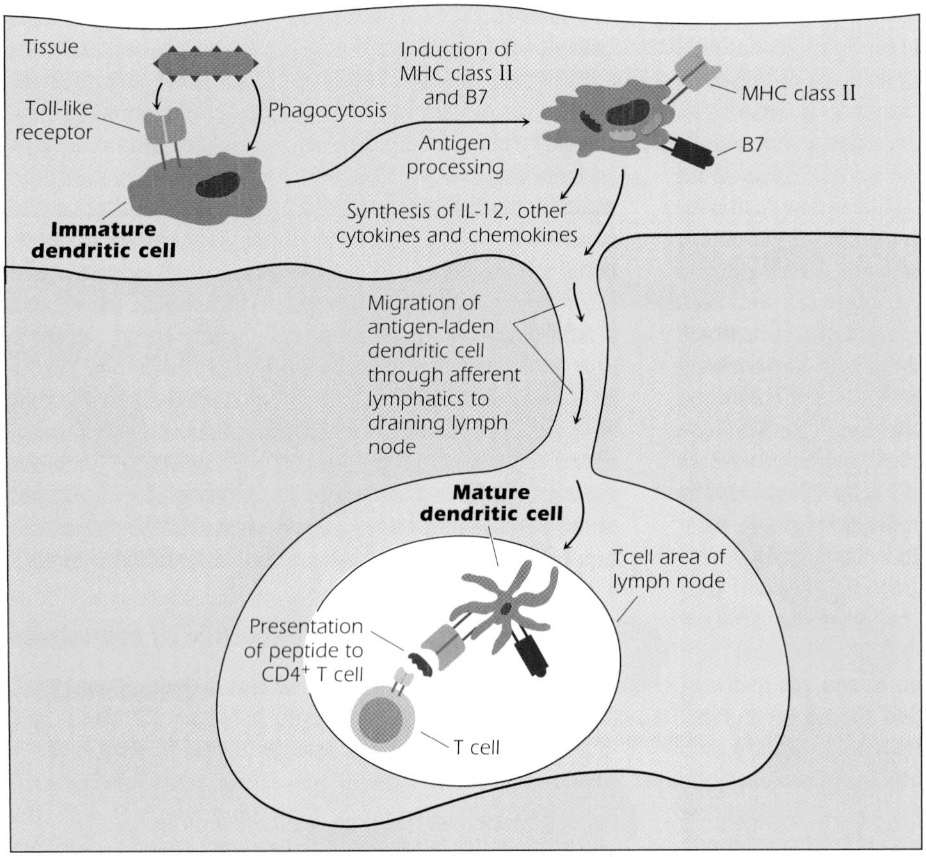

Figure 10.1. Dendritic cell maturation after interacting with a bacterium in a tissue.

Figure 10.1 shows that the interaction of antigen with dendritic cells in a tissue results in the ***maturation*** of the dendritic cell, ultimately leading to the antigen-bearing cell moving out of the tissue and to the lymph node draining this tissue site. The antigen shown in the figure is a gram-negative bacterium taken up by the ***immature dendritic cell*** in the tissue. The bacterium interacts with ***Toll-like receptors (TLRs,*** see Chapter 2) expressed by the dendritic cell. TLRs are a family of ***pattern-recognition molecules*** expressed on cells of the innate immune system. TLRs interact with infectious microorganisms or components of microorganisms—particularly bacterial products such as DNA, lipoprotein, and lipopolysaccharide. Some TLRs interact with different bacterial components while others are believed to interact with viral products. The cell walls of gram-negative bacteria contain lipopolysaccharide and interact with TLR-4 expressed on the dendritic cell. This interaction, coupled with the uptake of the bacterium into the cell, activates the phenomena we describe below.

The protein components of the bacterium are processed into peptides in the acid vesicle, MHC class II pathway of the cell that we described in Chapter 9. High levels of the ***B7 family (CD80/CD86)*** of costimulatory molecules are induced on the cell surface, and levels of MHC class II molecules are also increased. The dendritic cell also synthesizes high levels of chemokines and what are referred to as ***pro-inflammatory cytokines,*** that is, soluble factors that enhance or induce an inflammatory response in the tissue. These cytokines include tumor necrosis factor (TNF)-α, and IL-12, and their functions are described later in this chapter and in Chapter 12. Finally, the dendritic cell containing processed peptides leaves the tissue where it encountered the antigen and migrates via the lymph to the lymph node draining the tissue. (Migration out of the tissue is associated with the dendritic cell's upregulating the expression of the chemokine receptor known as CCR7; see Chapter 12.) In the T cell area of the node, the now ***mature dendritic cell***— expressing high levels of MHC class II and costimulator molecules—presents the peptides to a naive $CD4^+$ T cell expressing a TCR specific for a particular combination of MHC and peptide.

Note that in the absence of the signal induced by antigen, immature dendritic cells express low levels of costimulatory molecules. Thus antigens that do not induce high levels of costimulator function do not activate naive T cells. This is why we believe that, as described in Chapter 9, the encounter of a dendritic cell with ***self-molecules*** in normal tissue does not lead to activation of the dendritic cell or of T cells—costimulator function is not induced. Similarly, we pointed out in Chapter 3 that T cell and antibody responses to many "harmless" antigens (e.g., the protein ovalbumin when injected into mice) require the presence of an ***adjuvant***—such as complete Freund's adjuvant—that includes bacteria or bacterial components. The bacterial components of the adjuvant activate the APC, in particular to express costimulatory molecules. In the absence of this additional signal, even a foreign antigen may evoke little or no response.

The migration of an antigen-bearing APC to the draining node combined with the ability of naive T cells to recirculate through lymph to the lymph nodes (Chapter 2) increase the likelihood that the rare T cell expressing the "correct" TCR—estimated to be about 1 in 10^5–10^6 of the total population—interacts with an antigen-bearing APC. Indeed, studies suggest that this interaction occurs in vivo within hours of exposure to antigen.

Although we have stressed in this section the interaction of antigen-bearing APCs and naive T cells in a lymph node, the interaction of antigen-bearing APCs and T cells—especially activated and memory T cells—can take place in any tissue that has been exposed to or damaged by antigen. The cascade of events that occurs after an APC with bound peptide interacts with a $CD4^+$ T cell is described below.

Paired Interactions at the Surface of the APC and the $CD4^+$ T Cell

In this section, and shown in Figure 10.2, we describe the multiple interactions that take place between the surfaces of the APC and the $CD4^+$ T cell.

Peptide/MHC and the TCR. The interaction between peptide + MHC class II molecule expressed on the APCs and the variable regions, $V_\alpha + V_\beta$, of the TCR of a T cell is known as the ***first signal*** for T cell activation. This interaction is necessary but generally not sufficient for T cell activation—in particular for the activation of naive $CD4^+$ T cells—because of the low affinity of the interaction between the TCR and the peptide–MHC complex.

MHC Class II and CD4. The interaction of the nonpolymorphic region of an MHC class II molecule (i.e., outside the peptide-binding groove) with the coreceptor CD4 greatly enhances the ability of the T cell to respond to antigen. It has been estimated that the CD4–MHC class II interaction makes a cell 100-fold more responsive to antigen than in the absence of the interaction. In addition, as we describe in more detail in the following section, CD4 plays an important role in T cell signal transduction: After the peptide–MHC complex binds to the TCR, CD4 is believed to move closer to the TCR. The cytoplasmic tail of CD4 is associated with an enzyme involved in T cell activation; "clustering" of CD4 with the TCR brings this enzyme into a signal transduction complex.

Costimulator Pairs: B7 with CD28 and CD152, CD40 with CD154. We described earlier in the chapter how interaction with foreign antigen induces ***costimulator*** molecules on the surface of APCs. Costimulator, or ***second signals,*** enhance and sustain signals delivered by the MHC–peptide–TCR interaction (we describe below how they are believed to do this). Costimulators are required for activation of naive (unprimed) T cells but are probably less important for the activation of previously activated (primed) T cells.

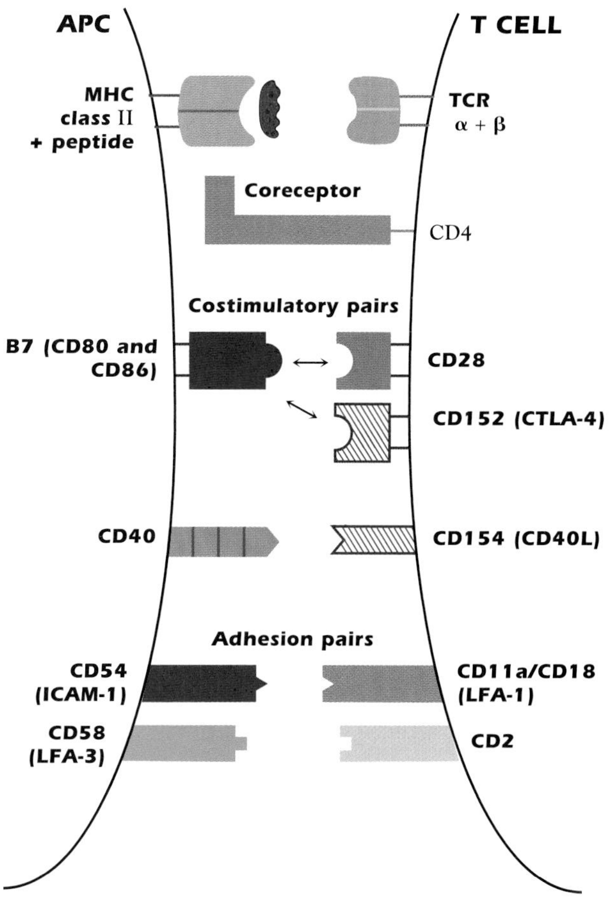

Figure 10.2. Key cell surface interactions leading to T-cell activation and cytokine secretion. Hatching indicates expression upregulated by activation.

The best characterized costimulator interactions are between a family of molecules known as ***B7,*** expressed on professional APCs such as dendritic cells and macrophages and activated B cells, and ***CD28,*** expressed constitutively on T cells. Within the B7 family, most is known about ***CD80*** and ***CD86*** (***B7.1*** and ***B7.2,*** respectively), both of which bind to CD28. It is currently not clear if CD80 and CD86 have distinct functions. CD80 and CD86 also interact with another molecule on the T cell surface, ***CD152*** (known as ***CTLA-4***), which is induced by T cell activation. CD152 is in the same family of molecules as CD28 but plays a role in T cell activation distinct from CD28 (discussed later in the chapter). The costimulator function of other molecules in the B7 and CD28 families is currently being evaluated.

The interaction of peptide–MHC with the TCR also upregulates the expression of ***CD154*** (CD40 ligand [CD40L]) on the T cell. CD154 interacts with ***CD40*** expressed constitutively by APC, such as dendritic cells and macrophages, and also by B cells. The CD40–CD154 interaction induces increased expression of B7 on the APC and thus enhances the B7–CD28 interaction between the APC and the T cell. The interaction of CD154 on activated T cells with CD40 expressed on B cells has an additional critical role in T cell–B cell interactions (described later in the chapter).

Adhesion Molecules: CD54 with CD11a/CD18, CD58 with CD2. Two pairs of adhesive interactions strengthen and stabilize the interaction of the APC and T cell over the several hours that the cells need to be in contact to ensure T cell activation. These are (1) ***CD54*** (***intercellular adhesion molecule 1;*** ICAM-1) expressed on the APC and the integrin ***CD11a/CD18*** (***leukocyte function-associated antigen 1;*** LFA-1) expressed on the T cell and (2) ***CD58*** (***LFA-3***) expressed on the APC and ***CD2*** expressed on the T cell. In addition, these adhesive interactions are thought to slow down the movement apart of the APC and T cell when the cells first interact; this allows time for the TCR to "scan" the APC for the appropriate MHC class II plus peptide.

The Immunological Synapse

In our current view, the interaction of APC and peptide with the $CD4^+$ T cell forms an area of contact between the cells that is known as the ***immunological synapse.*** In addition to the MHC–peptide and TCR, the synapse incorporates the adhesion pairs described above and B7–CD28 on the surface of the T cell and APC. (The inclusion of CD40–CD154 in the synapse has not been fully explored.) In addition, on the T cell side, the synapse includes signaling molecules that are recruited from inside the T cell (described below) and proteins of the cytoskeleton. The synapse appears to be required for sustained intracellular signaling, lasting until the APC and T cell split apart after approximately 8 hours in contact. The formation and development of the synapse is dynamic, its composition and structure changing with time after initial contact. For example, the paired adhesion molecules CD54 (ICAM-1) and CD11a/CD18 (LFA-1) are found in different regions of the synapse at different times after initial contact between the cells. In addition, other molecules are included or excluded from the synapse at different times after initial contact.

Several experiments suggest that the T cell reorganizes its structure, both of its internal cytoskeleton and of the cell membrane, as a consequence of activation. In the T cell membrane, the structure of the lipids is not homogeneous; rather, they form what are referred to as "microdomains" or ***lipid rafts,*** enriched in cholesterol and glycosphingolipids. When the T cell is activated, these lipid rafts—which had been dispersed throughout the membrane—are mobilized to the synapse and draw with them the intracellular signaling components that we describe below. This redistribution also pushes molecules not involved in the APC–T cell interaction out of the contact area.

Intracellular Events in $CD4^+$ T Cell Activation

Much recent research has focused on identifying the sequence of activation events inside the $CD4^+$ T cell after initial contact with an APC expressing an MHC class II–associated peptide. As yet, we do not completely understand all the steps in these complicated and interconnected pathways. We do know though that activation cascades spread in an ordered manner from the surface of the cell, through the cytoplasm, and into the nucleus. We also know that some events occur within seconds, others within minutes, and yet others within hours of the initial interaction. The critical events in T cell activation are described in the following paragraphs and in Figure 10.3.

Initial Signal. The binding of peptide–MHC to the extracellular variable regions ($V_\alpha + V_\beta$) of the TCR transmits a signal via the tightly associated CD3 and ζ molecules into the interior of the T cell. The nature of the signal across the membrane is not currently clear: It may involve the aggregation of multiple TCR molecules in the cell membrane (similar to the initial steps in activation through the B cell receptor, described later in the chapter) or a conformational change in the transmembrane region of the TCR chains.

Phosphorylation of Kinases and the Assembly and Activation of Signaling Complexes at the Cell Membrane. One of the earliest detectable events inside the T cell after binding to the TCR is the activation within seconds of ***tyrosine kinases***—enzymes that activate proteins by adding phosphate groups to tyrosine residues—which are associated with the cytoplasmic regions of the TCR complex and CD4 molecules. (The membrane protein CD45, a tyrosine phosphatase, is thought to activate these kinases by removing inhibitory phosphate groups.) The tyrosine kinase associated with CD3 and ζ is ***Fyn*** and the tyrosine kinase associated with CD4 is ***Lck.*** Fyn and Lck belong to a family of tyrosine kinases known as ***Src*** (pronounced "sark"). When Fyn and Lck are activated, they cluster with the regions of the CD3 and ζ chains that contain the previously described ***immunoreceptor tyrosine-based activation motifs*** (ITAMs), and phosphorylate them. This clustering also pulls CD4 into closer association with the TCR complex, as we described earlier in the chapter. The phosphorylated ITAMs in CD3 and ζ then act as docking sites for another tyrosine kinase, ***ZAP-70*** (belonging to a second tyrosine kinase family known as ***Syk***). This step appears critical for T cell activation, because T cells from the rare individuals who lack ZAP-70 do not respond to antigen. Because CD3 and ζ contain multiple ITAMs, more than one molecule of ZAP-70 is recruited into this complex of signaling proteins.

Lck activates ZAP-70 when it has joined the multiprotein signaling protein complex. Activated ZAP-70 phosphorylates multiple proteins inside the cell: Among the most important substrates of activated ZAP-70 are ***adapter molecules***—proteins that do not have enzymatic activity but contain multiple binding domains for other proteins. Two of the

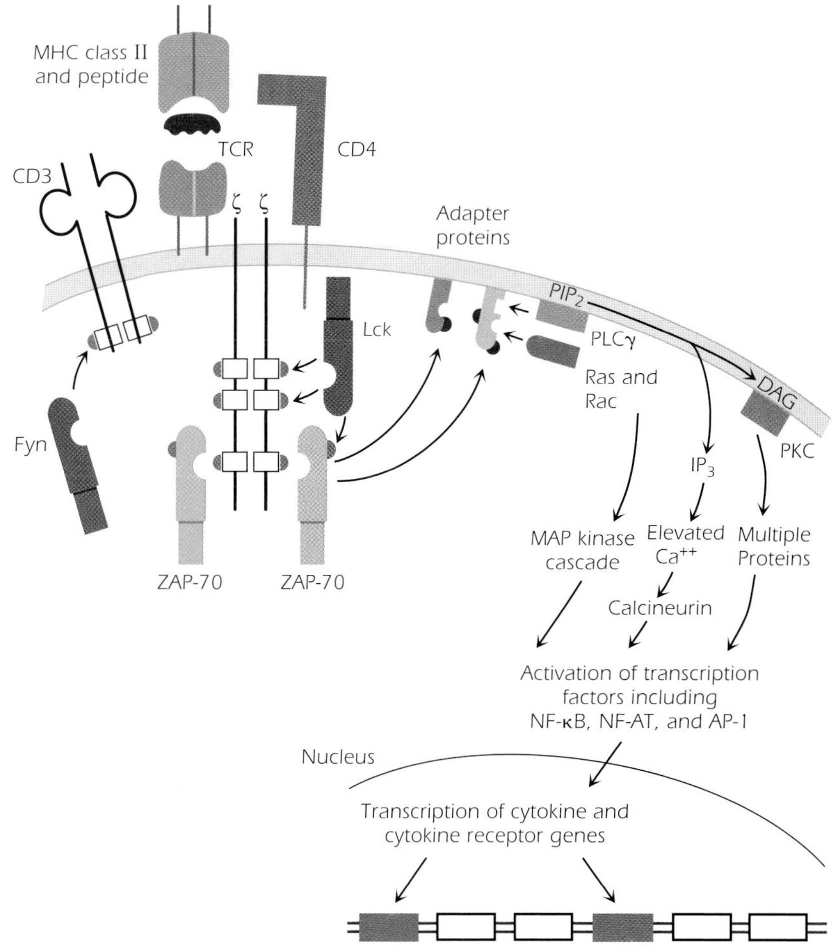

Figure 10.3. Intracellular events in T-cell activation. For simplicity, only one chain of CD3 and ζ (zeta) and one phosphorylated ITAM are shown. Orange semicircles indicate phosphate groups added to activated molecules.

important adapter molecules phosphorylated after T cell activation—LAT and SLP-76—are shown in Figure 10.3. The phosphorylated adapters are recruited to the cell membrane, forming an even larger complex of signal transduction molecules at the immunological synapse. In summary, a multiprotein complex of signal transduction molecules is assembled in sequence and activated on the cytoplasmic side of the T cell membrane.

Activation of Intracellular Signaling Pathways. Activated adapter molecules that are recruited to the immunological synapse bind enzymes and other adapters, activating several major intracellular signaling pathways. The adapter molecules bind ***phospholipase C-γ (PLCγ)***, which, after being phosphorylated by ZAP-70, catalyzes the breakdown of the membrane phospholipid phosphatidylinositol bisphosphate (PIP_2). PIP_2 is split into two components: one is diacylglycerol (DAG), which activates the membrane-associated enzyme ***protein kinase C (PKC),*** which in turn activates a cascade of kinases, ultimately leading to the activation in the cytoplasm of a transcription factor, ***NF-κB***. Inositol triphosphate (IP_3) is the second component formed when PIP_2 is split. IP_3 increases intracellular free calcium levels, which in turn activates the cytoplasmic molecule calcineurin, ultimately activating the transcription factor ***NF-AT.*** This pathway is clinically significant because the immunosuppressive agent cyclosporin A—used to prevent graft rejection when tissues are transplanted between genetically different individuals—binds to calcineurin and thereby inhibits the subsequent steps in T cell activation (see Chapter 18).

In addition, activated adapter molecules bind to and activate guanosine-nucleotide binding proteins known as ***Ras*** and ***Rac,*** which in turn activate a cytoplasmic cascade of mitogen-activated protein (MAP) kinases, leading to the activation of the transcription factor ***AP-1.***

Cytokine Secretion and Proliferation. As shown in Figure 10.3, NF-κB, NF-AT, AP-1, and other activated transcription factors enter the nucleus of the T cell and bind selectively to regulatory sequences of several different genes. As a result, genes coding for the cytokine IL-2 and one chain of the IL-2 receptor (IL-2Rα; CD25) are transcribed and translated (Fig. 10.4). IL-2Rα joins with the other chains of the IL-2 receptor to form a high-affinity receptor for IL-2 on the activated T cell (Chapter 11). Within 24 hours, the cell enlarges (becoming a ***T cell blast***), and IL-2 protein is secreted from the cell. IL-2 is a growth factor for T cells and binds to the high-affinity IL-2 receptor on the same or on a different T cell. After about 48 hours, DNA is synthesized, and approximately 24 hours later, the activated CD4+ T cells

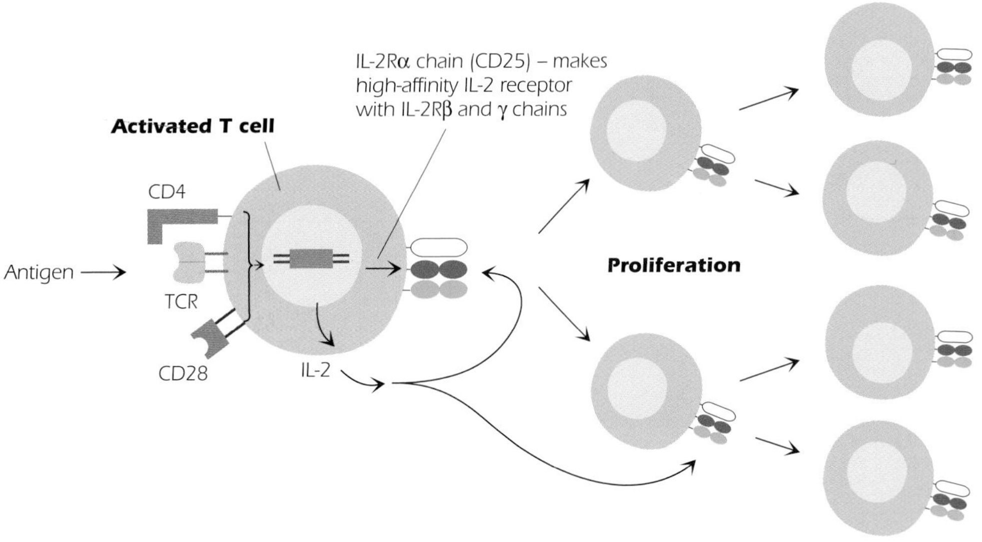

Figure 10.4. Secretion of IL-2 and interaction with the high-affinity IL-2 receptor results in expansion of the $CD4^+$ T cell clone.

start to proliferate, expanding the number of cells in this particular clone of T cells. Some of these activated cells develop into $CD4^+$ memory cells.

Distinct Roles of B7-CD28 and B7-CD152 in T Cell Activation

We have previously stressed the importance of the interaction of B7 family members with CD28 in enhancing and sustaining the signal from the peptide/MHC with the TCR on the naive $CD4^+$ T cell. As we have mentioned previously, we believe that in the absence of the B7-CD28 costimulatory signal the naive $CD4^+$ T cell does not make IL-2 and may be *inactivated* (*anergized,* discussed further in Chapter 12).

How the B7-CD28 interaction leads to "full" activation of the T cell is not completely understood, but seems to involve several different mechanisms. One important pathway is that activating the T cell through CD28 increases the lifetime of certain mRNAs, in particular IL-2 mRNA. This results in enhanced IL-2 protein synthesis in T cells activated by both the first and second signals compared to cells activated only through the TCR. Studies also suggest that the CD28 signal enhances the survival of activated T cells by inducing the expression of a protein, Bcl-x, that inhibits apoptosis. Recent studies also indicate that the B7-CD28 interaction mobilizes lipid rafts inside the T cell; in this way, CD28 brings molecules such as the tyrosine kinases that are involved in T-cell activation inside the T cell to the area where the TCR is in contact with the APC. The B7-CD28 interaction has also been shown to activate a kinase known as phosphatidylinositol-3 kinase; activation of subsequent steps in this kinase pathway is thought to enhance the intracellular pathways activated by signals through the TCR.

We have also previously referred to the interaction of the B7 ligands on the APC (CD80 and CD86) with a T-cell surface molecule that is closely related to CD28, ***CD152*** (known as ***CTLA-4***). In contrast to CD28 which is expressed on resting T cells, CD152 expression is induced as a consequence of T cell activation. The interaction of B7 with CD152 transmits a *negative* signal to the activated T cell. This turns off the production of IL-2 and thus T cell proliferation, limiting the extent of the immune response. The mechanism of B7-CD152's negative effect is not fully elucidated; like the B7-CD28 interaction, multiple biochemical pathways are probably involved. Recent studies suggest that CD152 acts in the immunological synapse by displacing critical components of the signaling complex and/or by limiting their function.

Migration Out of the Lymph Node. Days after the initial activation steps, activated—and memory—T cells leave the node and move to different sites in the body and in particular to sites in the body that have been exposed to or have been infected by pathogens. Migration from the node is mediated by a change in expression of cell surface molecules that we referred to in Chapter 8. Most activated T cells downregulate expression of ***CD62L*** (L-Selectin or MEL-14), the homing receptor for naive T cells that allows the cell to enter the node. Activated T cells upregulate expression of other cell-surface molecules, such as the integrin CD49dCD29 (VLA-4) and CD44; ligands for these molecules are expressed outside the node, in tissues such as the skin or sites of inflammation. Recent evidence also indicates that naive and activated T cells differ in their expression of chemokine receptors. Thus, as a consequence of this change in pattern of expression of homing molecules and chemokine receptors, activated and memory T cells exit from the node and home to tissues.

OTHER WAYS TO ACTIVATE T CELLS

In the preceding sections, we focused on how a peptide–MHC complex expressed on an APC activates a specific clone of

T cells. Since naive T cells expressing any one particular peptide specificity are rare, approximately 1 in 10^5–10^6 T cells, only a small fraction of the total T cell pool is activated by any one peptide–MHC complex. Detecting and studying the response to antigen of those rare antigen-specific cells in the total T cell population has thus proved challenging. To address questions about T cell activation and function, immunologists have developed many tools for studying the response of isolated antigen-specific T cells. These include growing clones of individual antigen-activated T cells in vitro and using transgenic mice that have T cells expressing only one TCR. These approaches have provided important information (see Chapter 5 for further discussion).

Naive T cells can be activated in a number of different ways, however, in addition to being activated by peptide–MHC complexes. This allows us to evaluate the function of more than just a rare subpopulation of unprimed antigen-specific T cells. Some alternative ways of activating the population of unprimed T cells are described below. Generally, the consequences of activating T cells in these alternative ways—most notably cytokine production and cell proliferation—are very similar to those we have described above when T cells are activated by peptide–MHC complexes.

Superantigens

Figure 9.8 showed the unique MHC-TCR binding properties of ***superantigens.*** In the human, superantigens are predominantly bacterial toxins from disease-causing organisms, such as *Staphylococcus aureus.* Superantigens activate $CD4^+$ T cells expressing a particular V_β molecule as one chain of its TCR. Since individual V_β segments (e.g., $V_\beta 3$ or $V_\beta 11$) may be expressed in up to 10% of the T cell population, a high percentage of T cells of various antigenic specificities may become activated when a superantigen interacts with an individual's T cells. The massive release of cytokines following superantigen action can result in injury to the host (see Chapter 12).

Plant Proteins and Antibodies to T Cell Surface Molecules

Several naturally occurring materials have the ability to trigger the proliferation and differentiation of many if not all clones of T lymphocytes. These substances are referred to as ***polyclonal activators*** or ***mitogens*** because of their ability to induce mitosis of the cell population. The plant glycoproteins ***concanavalin A*** (Con A) and ***phytohemagglutinin*** (PHA) are particularly potent mitogens for T cells. These molecules are lectins, molecules that bind to carbohydrate moieties on proteins. Both Con A and PHA are thought to act through the TCR. Because the T cell response to Con A and PHA of blood from healthy people falls in a well-defined range, a low response to Con A or PHA frequently indicates that a person is immunosuppressed. Another plant lectin, ***pokeweed mitogen,*** activates both T and B cells.

Some antibodies specific for CD3 have the ability to activate T cells. Since CD3 is expressed on all T cells in association with the T cell receptor, these anti-CD3 antibodies thereby induce all T cells to proliferate.

Lipids

In Chapter 9, we described how some T cells recognize and respond to lipid and glycolipid antigens presented by $CD1^+$ APC, such as dendritic cells. NK1.1 T cells are one of the T cell subsets activated. These are $\alpha\beta^+$ T cells that express natural killer (NK) as well as T cell surface molecules and use only a very limited number of V regions to form their T cell receptor (see pages 15–16). Once activated, they synthesize high levels of cytokines, particularly IL-4 and IFN_γ, and are thought to play a role in responses to infectious organisms and in regulating many other immune responses.

T CELL FUNCTION

One of the key effector functions of activated $CD4^+$ T cells is the synthesis of antigen-nonspecific soluble factors known as ***cytokines.*** The cytokines produced by $CD4^+$ T cells affect the function of multiple cell types, including $CD8^+$ T cells, B cells, myeloid cells (such as macrophages and eosinophils), and the differentiation of bone marrow precursors. For this reason, the loss of $CD4^+$ T cells in AIDS is devastating. The properties of cytokines produced by T cells and other cells and the nature of cytokine receptors are discussed in detail in Chapter 12. Many important functions of T cells will be discussed in subsequent chapters on cell-mediated immunity and transplantation. In the following sections, we shall focus first on the heterogeneity of cytokines produced by $CD4^+$ T cells, then describe the important features of the interaction between $CD4^+$ T cells and B cells, and finally discuss the function of $CD8^+$ T cells.

Subsets of $CD4^+$ T Cells Defined by Cytokine Production

Earlier in the chapter, we described how the naive $CD4^+$ T cell initially synthesizes IL-2 after stimulation by peptide associated with MHC molecules. The activated $CD4^+$ T cell can differentiate further to synthesize a large number of cytokines. Not all activated $CD4^+$ T cells synthesize the same cytokines following antigenic stimulation, however. Studies of the function of mouse and human T cells indicate that antigen-primed $CD4^+$ T cells can be divided into at least three subsets based on the different cytokines they produce; these subsets are known as ***T_H0, T_H1*** and ***T_H2.*** As shown in Figure 10.5, T_H1 and T_H2 are generated from the antigen-driven differentiation of T_H0 cells, which synthesize IL-2, interferon-γ (IFNγ), and IL-4.

T_H1 cells which synthesize IL-2, IFNγ, and TNFβ and T_H2 cells which synthesize IL-4, IL-5, IL-10, and IL-13

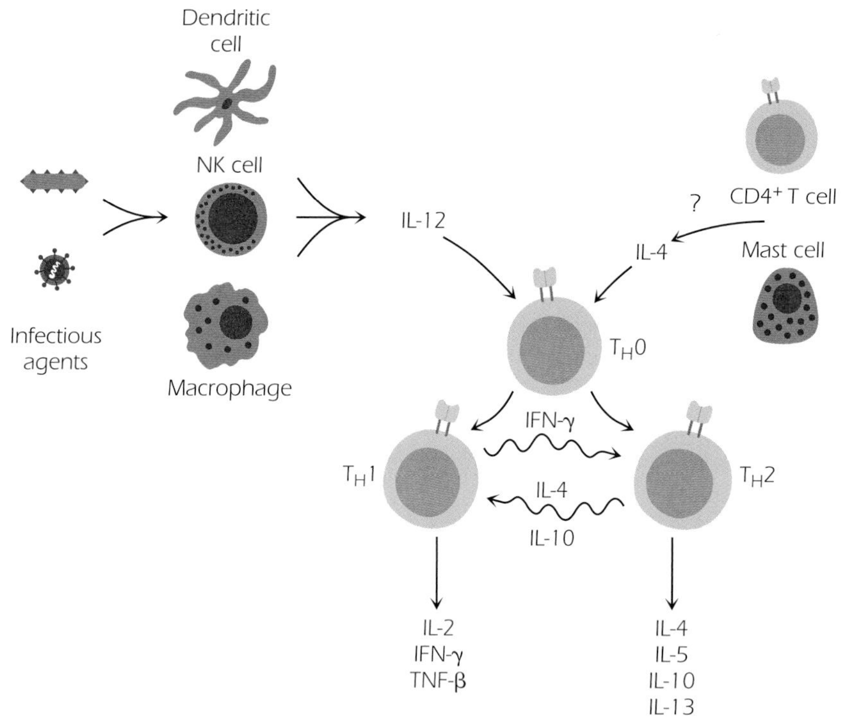

Figure 10.5. Cytokine control of T_H1 and T_H2 $CD4^+$ T cell subset generation. Wavy lines indicate inhibition.

play important but distinct roles in the immune response. Since different cytokines interact with different target cells, a major consequence of the production of unique sets of cytokines by T_H1 and T_H2 cells is that ***each subset induces different effector functions.*** Thus the cytokines synthesized by T_H1 cells activate cells involved in cell-mediated immunity: $CD8^+$ T cells, NK cells, and macrophages. In addition, the cytokines produced by T_H1 cells induce B cells to synthesize Ig isotypes, such as IgG3, that enhance the phagocytosis of pathogens by phagocytic cells (see Chapter 4 and the discussion of T–B cooperation later in this chapter). By contrast, the cytokines synthesized by T_H2 cells trigger B cells to class switch to IgE production and to activate eosinophils, a pattern found in the response to allergens and to parasitic worms. Many of these T cell functions will be discussed in subsequent chapters.

To date, the results of studies attempting to characterize cell surface molecules whose expression would distinguish T_H1 from T_H2 subsets have been controversial and are an area of intense research interest. Some recent studies suggest that T_H1 and T_H2 cells may express different molecules expressed in homing interactions, including different chemokine receptors, but further research is needed either to confirm or to modify these conclusions.

Many antigens give rise to T_H0, T_H1, and T_H2 subsets of $CD4^+$ T cells, but some antigens produce more of one subset than the others. In particular, ***viruses and bacteria favor the production of T_H1 cells, whereas allergens and parasites favor T_H2 cell induction.*** Figure 10.5 indicates that one of the major factors driving the differentiation to either T_H1 or T_H2 cells by different antigens is the presence of cytokines at the time of T cell stimulation.

T_H1 cells develop when IL-12 is present during antigen stimulation of T cells. As we showed at the beginning of this chapter, IL-12 and other proinflammatory cytokines are made by dendritic cells and other APC early in the response to pathogens, such as bacteria and viruses. These cytokines are also synthesized by other cells of the innate immune system, including NK cells. By contrast, the presence of IL-4 early in the response results in differentiation to T_H2 cells. The source of this IL-4 is currently not clear; it may be produced by either activated $CD4^+$ T cells or mast cells. Other factors, such as the concentration and route of exposure to antigen, the affinity of interaction between peptide–MHC and the TCR, and the nature of the APC in the response, have also been suggested to play a role in determining which subset of $CD4^+$ T cell develops.

Figure 10.5 also shows that cytokines produced by T_H1 can inhibit the function of T_H2 and vice versa. For example, IFNγ produced by T_H1 cells inhibits the generation of T_H2 cells, and IL-4 and IL-10 produced by T_H2 cells inhibit the generation of T_H1 cells. Table 10.1 demontrates two other important points about the T_H1 and T_H2 subsets of $CD4^+$ T cells. First, the subsets synthesize a number of cytokines in common, including IL-3 and granulocyte-macrophage colony-stimulating factor (GM-CSF). Second, mouse T_H1 and T_H2 $CD4^+$ T subsets show more clearcut differences in cytokine production than human subsets.

The functional differences between the $CD4^+$ T cell subsets may have some clinical significance in humans. In particular, a preponderance of T_H1 cells and T_H1-produced cytokines has been found in the response to many viruses and bacteria, delayed-type hypersensitivity (described in Chapter 16), and in diseases such as the tuberculoid form

TABLE 10.1. The Synthesis of Cytokines by the T_H1 and T_H2 Subsets of $CD4^+$

Cytokine	T_H1^a	T_H2^a
IL-2	+	−
IFNγ	+	−
TNFβ (lymphotoxin)	+	−
IL-4	−	+
IL-5	−	+
IL-6	−(+)	+(++)
IL-10	−(+)	+(++)
IL-13	−(+)	+(++)
IL-3	+	+
GM-CSF	+	+

[a]The pluses in parentheses indicate that in humans IL-6, IL-10, and IL-13 are also made by T_H1 cells but at lower levels than by T_H2 cells.

of leprosy. By contrast, the presence of T_H2 cells and increases in levels of cytokines synthesized by T_H2 cells have been linked to allergic and parasitic responses (see Chapter 14). These observations suggest that regulating the balance of T_H1 and T_H2 subsets may be a way to treat different diseases.

T–B Cooperation

Nearly all proteins are ***thymus-dependent*** (TD) ***antigens,*** so called because they require $CD4^+$ T cells to "help" or cooperate with B cells to synthesize antibodies. For this reason, the set of $CD4^+$ T cells that participates in antibody responses to TD antigens is referred to as ***helper T cells*** (T_H). The helper T cell and B cell that cooperate in the response to a particular TD antigen must be specific for that antigen. The T_H cell and the B cell generally respond to different epitopes in the antigen, but for the helper T and B cells to cooperate effectively the epitopes must be part of the same protein sequence. For this reason, T–B cooperation in the response to a TD antigen is also known as ***linked recognition.***

The key steps in T–B cell cooperation leading to antibody synthesis are shown in Figures 10.6 and 10.7. Figure 10.6 indicates how the B cell acts as an antigen-presenting cell for the $CD4^+$ T cell. Initially, a B cell expressing an Ig specific for a particular protein antigen "captures" the antigen by binding it to the cell's membrane Ig. After antigen binds, the complex of antigen and Ig is taken into the cell, and the antigen is processed in acid compartments (described in Chapter 9). Some of the peptides formed by the degradation of antigen selectively bind to MHC class II molecules also found in these acid compartments. The peptide–MHC class II complexes traffic through the cell to the B cell surface, where they interact with a $CD4^+$ T cell with the appropriate TCR (top of Fig. 10.7).

In addition to the peptide–MHC presented by the B cell to the TCR of the appropriate T cell, paired molecules interact at the surface of the B and T cells (Fig. 10.7). These interactions are critical for the mutual activation of T and B cells; as a result, the T cell synthesizes cytokines, and the B cell synthesizes antibodies. The paired adhesion molecules ***CD11a/CD18-CD54 (LFA-1-ICAM-1)*** and ***CD2-CD58*** we described earlier in the chapter in APC-T cell interactions maintain contact between the T cell and the B cell. The costimulator pairs ***B7-CD28*** and ***CD40-CD154*** also play key roles in the B cell-T cell interaction.

B cell presentation of peptide-MHC class II to the TCR upregulates expression of CD154 (CD40Ligand, or CD40L) on the T helper cell. The CD40-CD154 interaction in turn upregulates the expression of the costimulatory molecule B7 on the B cell, and B7 interacts with CD28 expressed on the T cell. As we described earlier in the chapter for APC-$CD4^+$ T cell interactions, the CD40-CD154 and B7-CD28 interactions result in the activated T cell synthesizing cytokines that induce proliferation. Cytokine production by the T helper cell leads to both T helper cell proliferation and, via upregulation of cytokine receptors on the activated B cell, B cell proliferation and Ig synthesis.

The CD40-CD154 interaction is also required for the B cell to switch from synthesizing IgM to other isotypes, such as IgG (***isotype switch***). In the absence of this interaction,

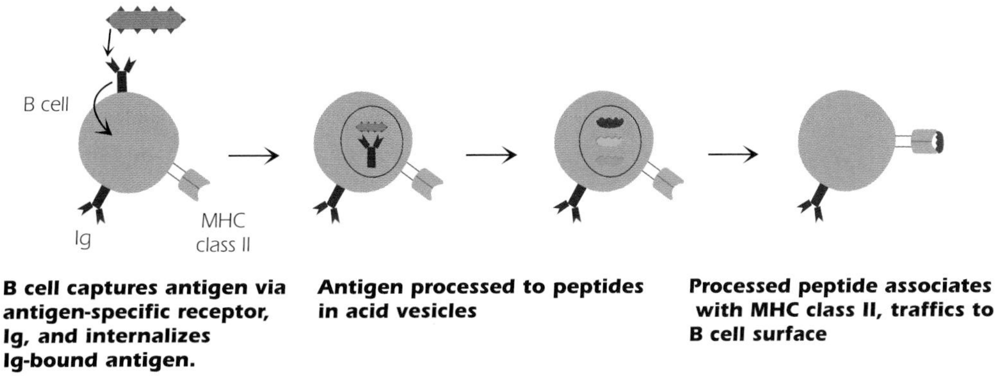

B cell
MHC
class II
Ig
B cell captures antigen via antigen-specific receptor, Ig, and internalizes Ig-bound antigen.
Antigen processed to peptides in acid vesicles
Processed peptide associates with MHC class II, traffics to B cell surface

Figure 10.6. A B cell takes up antigen that binds to surface Ig, processes the antigen in acid vesicles, and presents peptides associated with MHC class II molecules to $CD4^+$ T cells.

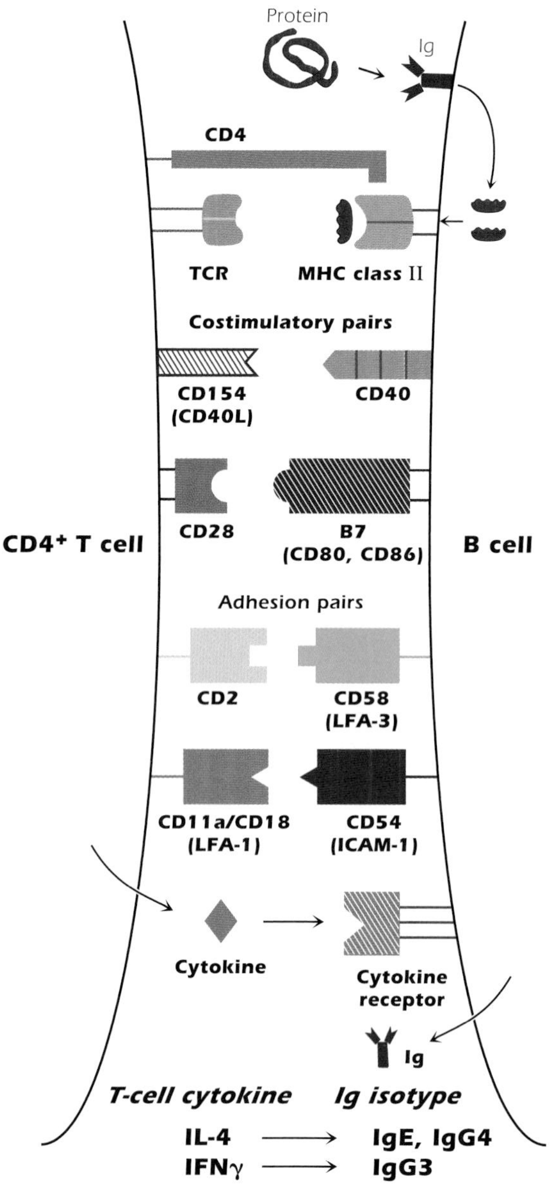

Figure 10.7. Key interactions involved in T-B cooperation. Hatching indicates expression upregulated by activation. T-cell derived cytokines associated with specific B cell isotypes are also shown.

only IgM is made. This is demonstrated in humans with nonfunctional CD154, a clinical condition known as hyper-IgM syndrome (see Chapter 17), and in so-called CD154 knockout mice: IgM antibody, but no other isotype, is made in these two situations.

Isotype switching by the B cell also requires cytokines synthesized by the activated T cell. Figure 10.7 shows that the cytokine produced by the T cell determines the antibody isotype that the B cell synthesizes. Thus if the T cell makes IL-4, B cells switch to producing predominantly IgE and IgG4; if the T cell produces IFNγ, B cells switch to producing IgG subtypes such as IgG3 that activate complement (see Chapters 4 and 13).

B cells are particularly effective APCs for CD4$^+$ T cells in responses in which both cells have already been primed by antigen. In Chapter 7 we described how this interaction generally takes place in specialized areas of the lymph node—the follicles—with further B cell activation, somatic hypermutation, and memory B cell induction occurring in the germinal center. As we described earlier in this chapter, however, *naive* CD4$^+$ T cells are most effectively activated by antigen processed and presented by dendritic cells. T cells activated by dendritic cells in the primary response are then likely to interact with and activate B cells that have captured antigen using the mechanisms that we described above.

The importance of T cell involvement in B cell antibody synthesis can be gauged from findings with antigens that do not use T cell help, so-called ***T-independent*** (TI) ***antigens,*** discussed later in the chapter. These TI antigens do not induce memory B cells, and B cells do not undergo Ig class switching from IgM to other isotypes.

FUNCTION OF CD8$^+$ T CELLS

In the sections above we described the function of one of the major sets of T cells, CD4$^+$ T cells, which produce a plethora of cytokines and thus interact with a vast array of cells. We now turn our attention to the other major population of T cells, CD8$^+$ T cells. The principal function of CD8$^+$ T cells is to kill cells that have been infected by bacteria and viruses. CD8$^+$ T cells are also involved in killing transplanted foreign cells during graft rejection and tumor cells (see Chapters 18 and 19). For this reason, CD8$^+$ T cells are frequently referred to as ***T killer*** or ***cytotoxic T lymphocytes*** (CTLs). The cell killed by a CTL is known as a **target,** which can be a specialized antigen-presenting cell such as a dendritic cell, or any other cell in the body. In contrast to the TCR of CD4$^+$ T cells, the TCR of a CD8$^+$ T cell recognizes a combination of peptide in association with an MHC class I molecule on the surface of a cell. This interaction, in the presence of appropriate second signals (discussed below), results in the death of the cell presenting the peptide.

CD8$^+$ T cells also synthesize cytokines; many produce cytokines associated with the T_H1 CD4$^+$ phenotype. These include IFNγ, which regulates certain viral and bacterial infections, as well as TNFβ, which plays a role in target cell killing. Other CD8$^+$ T cells, however, synthesize cytokines such as IL-4, which are associated with the T_H2 CD4$^+$ T cell pattern.

Activating CD8$^+$ T Cells

CD8$^+$ T cells that emerge from the thymus do not kill targets; they must first be activated to proliferate and differentiate. Activation requires both the first signal—peptide–MHC interacting with the TCR—and second or costimulatory signals, which we will describe below. The development of cytolytic function also requires the synthesis of cytokines, including IL-2, IFNγ, and IL-12.

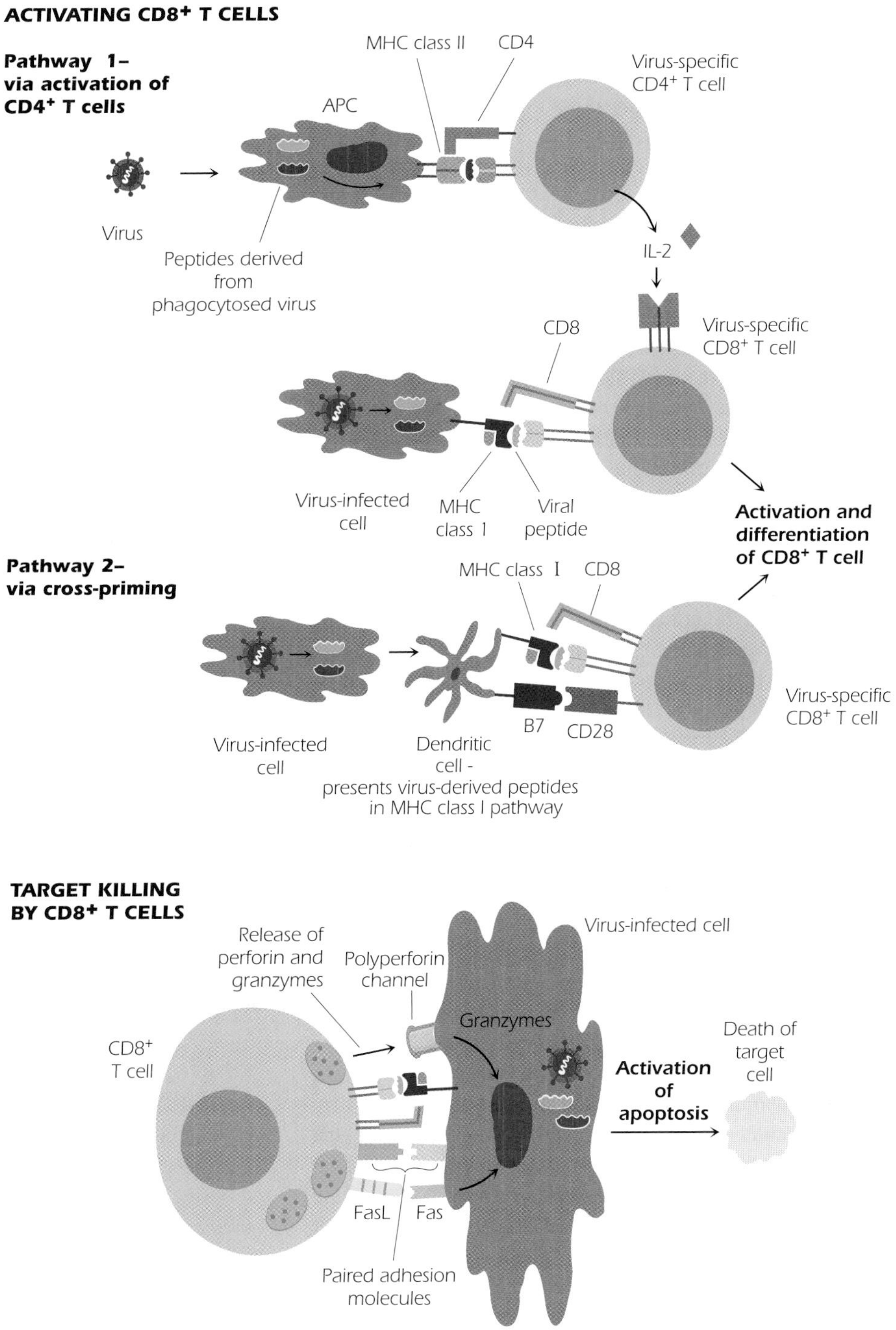

Figure 10.8. $CD8^+$ T cells: Pathways of activation (top two panels) and target cell killing (bottom panel).

Figure 10.8 shows two of the major pathways for activating CTL in the response to a virus infection. The top part of the figure shows the first pathway, which involves the participation of virus-specific $CD4^+$ T cells and the production of IL-2. The combination of virus-infected target and IL-2 produced from $CD4^+$ T cells induces $CD8^+$ T cell proliferation and differentiation. The virus-specific $CD4^+$ T cells in this response are activated by virus antigens presented by the MHC class II molecules of an APC, such as a dendritic cell or macrophage. In this pathway, the virus epitope that activates $CD4^+$ T cells is quite probably different from the epitope that activates $CD8^+$ T cells.

The middle part of Figure 10.8 indicates how $CD8^+$ T cells can be activated without activating $CD4^+$ T cells, as has been described in the response to some viruses. This pathway involves ***cross-priming,*** mentioned in Chapter 9. In this pathway, virus-derived antigens are transferred from virus-infected cells that are dead or dying to professional APCs, such as dendritic cells. Dendritic cells then process the viral antigens in the *MHC class I* pathway and present peptides to virus-specific CD8$^+$ T cells. Because dendritic cells also express costimulatory molecules such as B7, they can activate the virus-specific CD8$^+$ T cell. In this pathway, the activated CD8$^+$ T cell itself probably provides the cytokines necessary for proliferation and differentiation. Cross-priming is thought to be important in activating CD8$^+$ T cell responses to infected tissue cells which lack co-stimulatory molecules and in the response to some tumors (see Chapter 19).

Whatever the cellular interactions involved in activating the CD8$^+$ T cell, it is likely that the early intracellular events in CD8$^+$ T cell activation are similar to those we described above for CD4$^+$ T cell activation. Like CD4, CD8 is associated with the tyrosine kinase Lck. In addition, the same pairs of costimulatory and adhesion molecules we described in the activation of CD4$^+$ T cells—CD28-B7, CD11a/CD18-CD54 (LFA-1–ICAM-1), and CD2–CD58—are involved in the activation of CD8$^+$ T cells.

CD8$^+$ T Cell Killing of Target Cells

Once activated, the now mature CD8$^+$ T cell initiates killing by attaching to the target cell. The bottom panel of Figure 10.8 indicates that paired adhesion molecules expressed on the T-cell and target cell surfaces help to maintain contact between the cells for several hours. The figure also shows that the activated CD8$^+$ T cell contains ***granules that contain cytotoxic proteins*** and expresses the cell surface molecule ***CD178 (Fas Ligand).*** As we describe below, these molecules are critical in target cell killing.

Killing by CD8$^+$ T cells is thought to occur by two pathways. The first, and considered to be the predominant pathway for CD8$^+$ T cell killing of most targets, involves the action of the cytotoxic substances contained in granules inside the T cell. After attaching to the target cell, the CD8$^+$ T cell mobilizes its granules directionally toward the target and, by a process known as ***exocytosis,*** releases the contents of these granules onto the target cell. These cytotoxic substances produce lesions in the membranes of target cells. The major constituents of the granules involved in target-cell killing are ***perforin*** and ***granzymes.*** Perforin is a molecule that polymerizes to form ringlike transmembrane channels or pores in the target-cell membrane. The resulting increase in permeability of the cell membrane contributes to the eventual death of the cell. The action of perforin on cell membranes is similar to that of the complement membrane attack complex, described in Chapter 13. CTL killing via this pathway also involves granzymes, a set of serine proteases. Granzymes pass into the target cell through the pores created by polyperforin molecules and interact with intracellular components of the target cell to induce apoptosis. Since death by apoptosis does not result in the release of the cell's contents, killing infected cells by apoptotic mechanisms may prevent the spread of infectious virus into other cells.

A second pathway of target cell killing occurs via the interaction of the molecule ***CD178*** (***Fas ligand***) on the CD8$^+$ T cell with ***CD95 (Fas),*** a surface molecule expressed on many host cells. This interaction activates the apoptosis of the target cell via a sequential activation of proteolytic enzymes known as ***caspases*** inside the target cell. As a result, the cell dies within hours. Once the CD8$^+$ T cell has initiated one or both of the killing mechanisms we have described, it detaches from the target cell to attack and kill additional target cells.

As the foregoing paragraphs illustrate, activation of CD8$^+$ T cells and killing of the target cell are separable events. This can be demonstrated by preparing CD8$^+$ T cells from an individual who has been infected with a virus. These virus-specific cytotoxic cells are able to kill virus-infected targets outside the body. (The assay for CD8$^+$ T cell killing of targets is described in Chapter 5.) In vitro killing of the infected target does not require the addition of any further factors.

We stress again the concept of *MHC restriction of T-cell responses* that we have referred to in previous chapters: A virus-specific CD8$^+$ CTL recognizes, and subsequently kills, a target cell expressing a specific combination of viral peptide and a particular MHC class I molecule. This means that a CD8$^+$ CTL specific for a flu virus peptide and HLA-A2, for example, kills a target that expresses HLA-A2 that has bound the flu-derived peptide. This CTL does not kill uninfected or normal cells from an individual expressing HLA-A2 in the absence of the flu peptide. In addition, this virus-specific CD8$^+$ T cell does not kill targets expressing different combinations of peptides plus MHC molecules, such as a measles virus–derived peptide bound to HLA-A2 or even the same flu peptide bound to HLA-B3. These findings, by Rolf Zinkernagel and Peter Doherty (both awarded the Nobel Prize), established the concept of MHC restriction of T cell responses, indicating that T cells recognize the combination of antigen plus MHC molecule rather than antigen alone.

Note too that the recognition of peptide–MHC class I by a CD8$^+$ T cell occurs irrespective of the expression of any MHC class II molecule by the target cell. This has important biological consequences, because, as we described in Chapter 9, MHC class I molecules are expressed on almost every cell in the body. Since an infectious pathogen (such as a virus, parasite, or bacterium) may infect *any* nucleated cell in the body, a pathogen generates peptides that associate with MHC class I molecules that are expressed on the surface of any nucleated host cell. Expression of the pathogen-derived peptide–MHC class I complexes at the cell surface leads to recognition by CD8$^+$ T cells, followed by the killing of the infected cell. Thus killing by CD8$^+$ T cells provides a mechanism to eliminate any cell in the body that becomes infected with a pathogen. Clearly, elimination of the pathogen does result in the destruction of host cells, but this is the bearable price the individual pays to remove the source of infection.

To repeat and extend the concept we referred to in Chapter 9: Generally, only pathogens such as viruses, parasites, and bacteria that *infect* cells generate peptides that associate with MHC class I molecules and evoke CD8$^+$ T cell

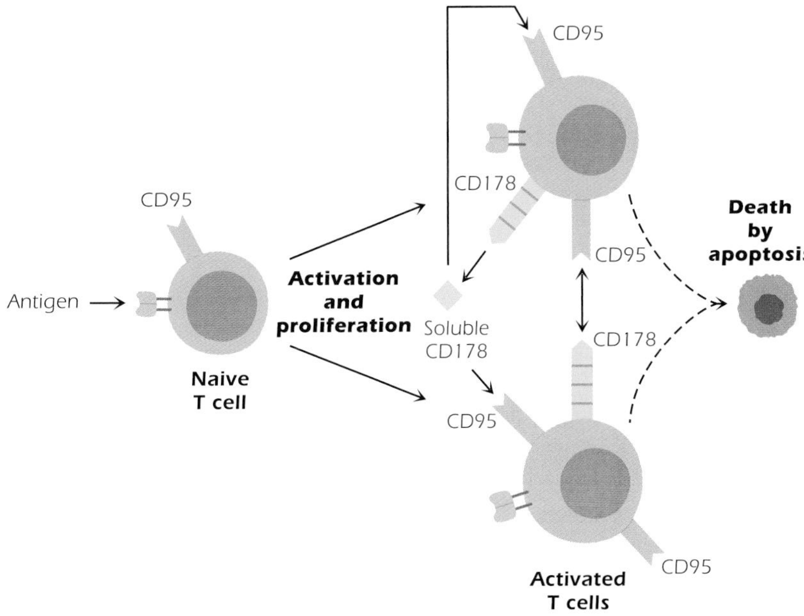

Figure 10.9. Activation-induced cell death. Activated T cells express CD95 (Fas), upregulate surface expression of CD178 (FasL), and can secrete a soluble form of CD178. Death of the activated cell results when either soluble or surface CD178 interacts with CD95.

responses. These pathogens also activate pathogen-specific $CD4^+$ T cells and induce antibody synthesis because they are taken up by APCs, such as dendritic cells and macrophages. In this way, $CD4^+$ T cells, $CD8^+$ T cells (and $\gamma\delta$ T cells, too), and antibody are all likely to be involved in the host's protective immune response against a particular pathogen (discussed further in Chapter 21). In contrast, harmless or noninfectious antigens (such as a killed virus protein in a vaccine) do not generally trigger $CD8^+$ T cell responses. These exogenous antigens are taken up into an APC's acidic compartments, interact with MHC class II molecules, and activate $CD4^+$ T cell and antibody responses.

$CD8^+$ T cells almost invariably function as cytotoxic T cells in both the human and mouse. A considerable proportion of human $CD4^+$ T cells and some mouse $CD4^+$ T cells, however, also display cytotoxic function. As might be expected from our foregoing discussion of MHC restriction, these cytotoxic $CD4^+$ T cells are activated to kill by the recognition of peptide–MHC class II complexes on the APC or target cell. Because activated $CD4^+$ T cells express CD178 but are not thought to contain granules with cytotoxic function, $CD4^+$ T cells probably use the CD95-CD178 pathway as the predominant method of killing target cells.

Termination of the Response: Induction of Memory Cells

Antigen stimulation increases the number of lymphocytes specific for the stimulating antigen, as well as the numbers of lymphocytes and other effector cells that are "recruited" by cytokine synthesis during the course of the response. Once the antigen has been eliminated, however, it is critical to decrease the size of this pool of activated cells, otherwise the body would fill quickly with expanded populations of cells. Figure 10.9 shows the predominant mechanism that eliminates activated T cells, ***activation-induced cell death*** (AICD). Studies indicate that T cells are susceptible to apoptosis after they have been activated and particularly after repeated antigenic stimulation. Apoptosis results as a consequence of the CD95-CD178 interaction, described earlier in this chapter. Activated T cells express both CD95 *and* CD178, which is induced by activation. Once antigen has been removed, for example, after activated CTLs have killed their infected targets, the CTLs interact with each other via CD95-CD178 and induce apoptosis. Figure 10.9 also shows that activated cells secrete CD178, and the secreted molecule can also interact with surface-expressed CD95 to induce apoptosis. The CD95-CD178 interaction is believed to play a critical role in the elimination of the majority of activated $CD4^+$ and $CD8^+$ T cells following antigen stimulation.

Not all the antigen-activated cells die, however; a minor population of long-lived antigen-specific cells survives. This constitutes the ***memory*** T cell population for that antigen, either $CD4^+$ or $CD8^+$ memory T cells. Memory and (secondary) T cell responses are more effective than primary responses. One reason is that the clonal size of the memory population specific for a particular antigen is still larger than the size of the unprimed population, even after AICD removes many of the expanded cells. It is also thought that the memory cell does not need B7–CD28 co-stimulatory interactions to induce full T cell activation.

No surface molecules have been defined that uniquely characterize memory T cells. Rather, some differences in level from high to low expression or vice versa have been found between unprimed and memory T cells; for example, the increase in CD44 and decrease in CD62L that was described earlier in the chapter. Changes in the membrane phosphatase CD45 have also been described; activation is thought to change CD45 from a form known as CD45RA to CD45RO caused by alternative splicing of the CD45 gene transcript. It is not clear whether the persistence of memory cells requires the presence of antigen, even at some very low level; some studies indicate that in the absence of the priming antigen, memory cells die.

B-CELL FUNCTION IN THE ABSENCE OF T CELL HELP

We have focused until now on the major set of antigens—T-dependent antigens—that require helper T cells to evoke an antibody response by B cells. Some antigens, however, activate B cells to produce antibody in the absence of T cells or cytokines produced by T cells. These antigens, referred to as ***thymus-independent*** (***TI***) ***antigens***, are generally large polymeric molecules with multiple, repeating, antigenic determinants; for example, the components of bacterial cell walls such as lipopolysaccharides and the capsule polysaccharide component of *Haemophilus influenzae.* The mechanism by which these antigens activate B cells is described below.

A subset of TI antigens referred to as TI-1 are ***mitogenic*** at high concentrations—that is, they are able to activate multiple B cell clones to proliferate and to produce antibody. Because of this antigen-nonspecific activation property, such antigens are called ***polyclonal B cell activators.*** In mice, lipopolysaccharide derived from a number of gram-negative bacteria such as *E. coli* are TI-1 antigens; in humans, however, these lipopolysaccharides do not activate B cells to proliferate. A second subset of TI antigens, known as TI-2, which includes bacterial and fungal polysaccharides (e.g., pneumococcal polysaccharide, dextrans, and ficoll) is not mitogenic at high concentrations.

There are two biologically relevant features of TI responses. First, unlike responses involving T-dependent antigens, ***responses to TI antigens generate primarily IgM and do not give rise to memory.*** In other words, a second injection of a TI antigen leads to the same level of production of IgM as the first, with no increase in level, speed of onset, or class switch. This finding reinforces the importance of T cell–derived cytokines in the development of memory cells and B cell isotype switch. Second, a immune response can still be made against TI antigens even if an individual lacks T cells. Thus patients with T cell immune deficiencies can still make protective IgM responses against extracellular bacteria, even if they cannot make significant responses to viruses that are T cell dependent.

Intracellular Pathways in B Cell Activation

Multivalent antigens with repeating epitopes, such as are found in many TI antigens, directly activate the B cell (Fig. 10.10). Activation is initiated by ***receptor cross-linking***—that is, by bringing together more than one

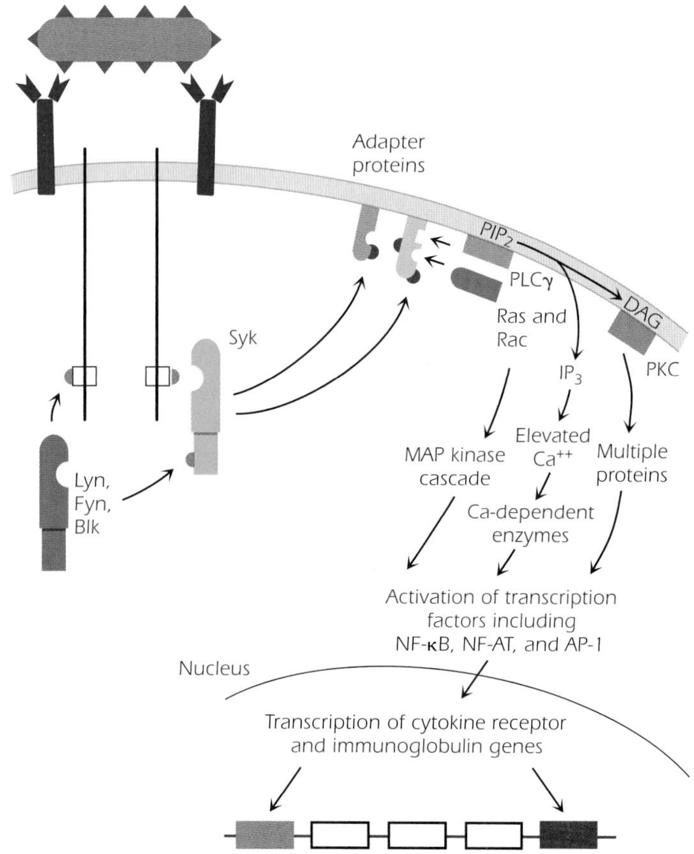

Figure 10.10. Intracellular events in B-cell activation. For simplicity, only one chain of Igα and Igβ associated with each Ig molecule is shown. Orange semicircles indicate phosphate groups added to activated molecules.

B cell receptor (BCR) complex in the cell membrane. Like the antigen-binding chains of the TCR, Ig H and L chains have very short intracellular domains and do not play a direct role in signal transduction after they bind antigen.

Figure 10.10 indicates that cross-linking activates pathways at the inner surface and inside the B cell very similar to the pathways we described earlier in the chapter for $CD4^+$ T cell activation. These are: phosphorylation of kinases, the assembly and activation of signaling complexes at the cell membrane; and activation of intracellular signaling pathways. The end result of B cell activation, however, is the transcription and translation of Ig and cytokine receptor genes, rather than the transcription and translation of cytokine genes that were key features of T cell activation. We shall briefly describe some of the key similarities and differences between the pathways of B cell and T cell activation.

Figure 10.10 shows, as we described above for the activation of T cells, that one of the earliest events in B cell activation is the activation of Src family tyrosine kinases—Lyn, Blk, Lck, and Fyn—associated with the BCR. (These kinases are also believed to be activated by CD45, as we described for T cell activation.) The activated kinases phosphorylate tyrosine residues in ITAMs of the Igα and Igβ molecules (CD79a and b) associated with Ig chains in the membrane. Phosphorylation of these ITAMs recruits another kinase, Syk, to the cluster of molecules, and Syk is phosphorylated and activated. Syk is in the same family of kinases as ZAP-70, which plays a central role in T cell activation.

Activated Syk recruits and activates adapter molecules, which in turn activate intracellular signaling pathways similar to those we described in activated T cells. These are: the activation of ***PLCγ***, leading to the activation of protein kinase C, increases in ***intracellular calcium ion levels*** and the subsequent activation of multiple cytoplasmic enzymes; and the activation of ***Ras and Rac,*** which in turn activate a cytoplasmic cascade of MAP kinases. As a result of this sequence of intracellular signaling pathways, transcription factors (including NF-AT, AP-1, and NF-κB) enter the nucleus of the B cell and promote the transcription of several genes, the most important of which are Ig and cytokine receptor genes. Approximately 12 hours after antigenic stimulation, the B cell increases in size (becoming a ***B cell blast***), which proliferates and differentiates into a cell that synthesizes and secretes Ig (a plasma cell). In the absence of T cell cytokines, the B cell makes IgM. As described in the section on T–B cooperation, the presence of T cell derived cytokines induces isotype switch to particular isotypes and, as described in Chapter 7, induces affinity maturation and memory B cell formation in the germinal center.

Modulation of the BCR Signal

Another feature of the BCR that it shares with the TCR is a ***coreceptor*** that enhances the signal through the antigen-binding receptor. For the T cell, the co-receptor is CD4 or CD8, and these molecules enhance the binding of an APC or target to a T cell, thereby decreasing the amount of antigen needed to trigger the T cell. The molecules CD19, CD81, and CD21 (discussed in Chapter 7)—which are noncovalently associated in the B cell membrane function—play a similar role as a coreceptor for the BCR (Fig. 10.11). The BCR coreceptor role has been characterized best in the response to microbial antigens; estimates indicate that 100- to 1000-fold less antigen is needed to stimulate an antibody response by activating the B cell via the coreceptor plus BCR compared to activating via the BCR alone.

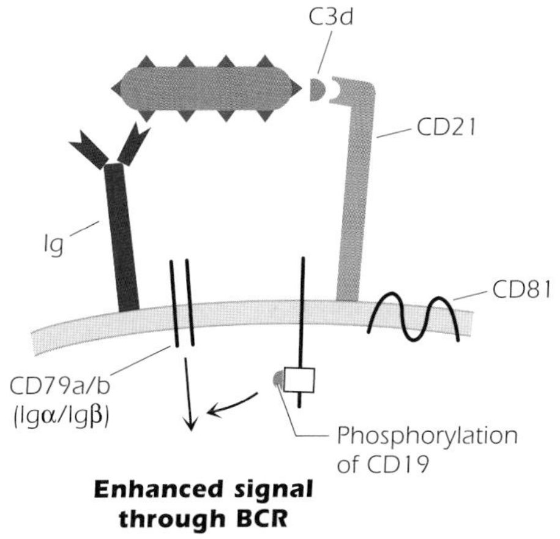

Figure 10.11. Signaling through the B cell coreceptor CD19/CD21/CD81 lowers the threshold for antigen needed to activate B cells through the BCR: activation signals are enhanced when a bacterium binds simultaneously to Ig and to complement component C3d, whose receptor is CD21, part of the B cell coreceptor.

Figure 10.11 indicates how the coreceptor lowers the threshold for stimulating B cell responses to microbial pathogens. Microbial pathogens activate the complement pathways found in plasma (see Chapter 13), and become coated or "tagged" with complement component C3d. The receptor for C3d is the B cell coreceptor molecule CD21. Thus, the pathogen bound to C3d becomes attached via CD21 to the B cell. The pathogen can also bind to IgM on the same B cell. This cross-linking of antigen via IgM and C3d on the B cell surface delivers simultaneous activating signals to the B cell; CD19 in the coreceptor complex is phosphorylated and activates the ITAMs in Igα/Igβ (CD 79a/b). Thus activating the B cell via the coreceptor as well as the BCR augments the signal induced when antigen interacts only via the BCR.

The signal through the BCR can also be modulated *negatively.* This occurs as a result of ***antibody feedback*** when antibody has been synthesized in response to an antigen; the antibody produced inhibits further B cell response to that antigen. Antibody feedback can also be induced by injecting an antibody into an individual shortly before or during an immune response to the antigen for which the antibody is specific; the injected antibody shuts off the response to the antigen. Antibody feedback has been used clinically to treat a condition in newborns in which antibody responses are made to the erythrocyte antigen Rh (see Chapter 15 for a fuller description.)

One important way in which the presence of antibody inhibits B cell function is by forming antigen–antibody complexes that interact with the low-affinity F_c receptor for IgG ***(FcRγIIb, CD32)*** expressed on the B cell. How this leads to negative signaling to the B cell is shown in Figure 10.12: The Fc end of the antigen–antibody complex binds to CD32, while the antigen end of the complex simultaneously binds to the Ig on the same cell. This simultaneous binding to Ig and to the FcR results in a *negative* signal to the B cell. Ig binding to the extracellular portion of CD32 recruits a phosphatase to an intracellular portion of CD32, which contains a tyrosine-containing sequence of amino acids. By analogy to the previously described ITAMs, the sequence in CD32 and other molecules is known as ***immunoreceptor tyrosine-based inhibitory motif*** (ITIM). The phosphatase that binds to the CD32 ITIM removes phosphate groups from tyrosine residues in the signal transduction polypeptides associated with the BCR. As a result, the activating signal through the BCR is inhibited.

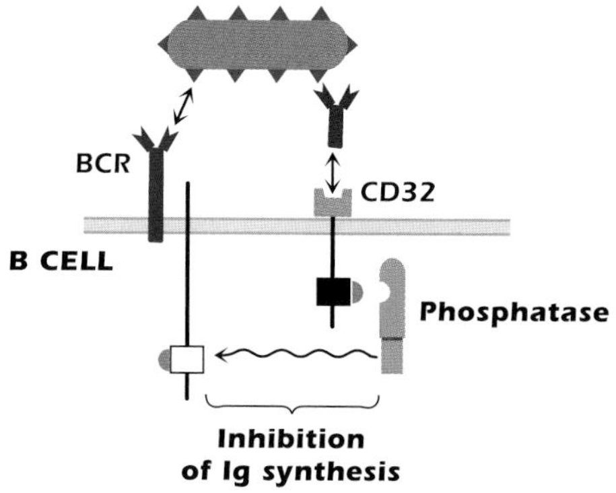

Figure 10.12. Antibody feedback inhibits B-cell activation. Simultaneous binding of the antigen and antibody components of an antigen–antibody complex to receptors on a B cell (antigen to the Ig, and the Fc portion of the antibody component to the FcR, CD32) results in a negative signal to the cell. The rectangle in the cytoplasmic region of CD32 represents the immunoreceptor tyrosine-based inhibitory motif (ITIM).

SUMMARY

1. Activating naive CD4$^+$ T cells requires a first signal (peptide–MHC class II with the TCR) and the interaction of costimulatory (second) signals and adhesion pairs on the surface of an APC and the T cell. Dendritic cells are the principal APCs for activating naive CD4$^+$ T cell responses.

2. T cell activation involves a cascade of events spreading from the area of contact between the APC and the T cell (the immunological synapse) through the cytoplasm and into the nucleus. The critical pathways include the phosphorylation of kinases, the assembly and activation of signaling complexes at the cell membrane, and activation of intracellular signaling pathways. Among the most important genes transcribed and translated are those coding for cytokines, such as IL-2, and cytokine receptors. Ultimately, the activation of these genes results in the proliferation and differentiation of the T cell clone.

3. As a consequence of activation by antigen, CD4$^+$ T cells secrete cytokines that affect CD8$^+$ T cells, B cells, and many other cell types. Subsets of CD4$^+$ T cells have been defined by the range of cytokines they produce. T_H1 cells secrete IL-2, IFNγ, and TNFβ but not IL-4, IL-5, IL-10, and IL-13. Cytokines produced by T_H1 cells activate other T cells, NK cells, and macrophages and induce B cells to switch to producing Ig isotypes that enhance the phagocytosis of microorganisms. By contrast, a second subset of CD4$^+$ T cells, T_H2, secretes IL-4, IL-5, IL-10, and IL-13 but not IL-2, IFNγ, or TNFβ. The cytokines synthesized by T_H2 cells result in B cell class switch to IgE synthesis and in eosinophil activation.

4. CD8$^+$ T cells (CTL) interact with and kill target cells infected by microorganisms such as bacteria or viruses. The TCR of the CD8$^+$ T cell interacts with peptide derived from the pathogen bound to an MHC class I molecule on the surface of the target cell. CTLs must be activated before they kill their targets. The two main pathways of CTL killing of targets involve (1) secretion of perforin and granzymes and (2) interaction of CD95 and CD178 (Fas and Fas ligand). Some CD4$^+$ T cells are also cytotoxic; they recognize peptide and MHC class II.

5. T cells respond to material other than MHC-peptide complexes. Superantigens activate all T cells that use a specific Vβ segment to form its TCR. Lectins such as concanavalin A and phytohemagglutinin activate proliferation of multiple T cell clones by binding to cell-surface glycoproteins. T cells also recognize lipids and glycolipids presented by CD1.

6. The generation of antibody in the response to TD antigens (the vast majority of responses to proteins) requires antigen, CD4$^+$ T cells, and B cells. This T–B cell cooperation involves (1) interaction between pairs of molecules on the surface of the CD4$^+$ T cell and the

B cell, resulting in mutual activation, and (2) cytokine secretion by T cells.

7. Class or isotype switching to IgG, IgA, or IgE requires the interaction of CD40 on the B cell with its ligand CD40L on the T cell. The cytokine produced by the T cell determines the isotype of antibody synthesized by the switched B cell.

8. Some antigens, such as polysaccharides that have many repeating, identical epitopes on each molecule, are capable of triggering B cells without significant help from T cells. These so-called T-independent responses involve predominantly the production of IgM and do not include the development of immunological memory.

REFERENCES

Akira S, Takeda K, Kaisho T (2001): Toll-like receptors: critical proteins linking innate and acquired immunity. *Nat Immunol* 2:675.

Bromley SK, Burack WR, Johnson KG, Somersalo K, Sims TN, Sumen C, Davis MM, Shaw AS, Allen PM, Dustin ML (2001): The immunological synapse. *Annu Rev Immunol* 19:375.

Dong C, Davis RJ, Flavell RA (2002): MAP kinases in the immune response. *Annu Rev Immunol* 20:55.

Fearon DT, Carroll MC (2000): Regulation of B lymphocyte responses to foreign and self-antigens by the CD19/CD21 complex. *Annu Rev Immunol* 18:393.

Fonteneau JF, Larsson M, Bhardwaj N (2002): Interactions between dead cells and dendritic cells in the induction of antiviral CTL responses. *Curr Opin Immunol* 14:471.

Guermonprez P, Valladeau J, Zitvogel L, Thery C, Amigorena S (2002): Antigen presentation and T cell stimulation by dendritic cells. *Annu Rev Immunol* 20:621.

Janeway CA Jr, Medzhitov R (2002): Innate immune recognition. *Annu Rev Immunol* 20:197.

Kurosaki T (2002): Regulation of B-cell signal transduction by adaptor proteins. *Nat Rev Immunol* 2:354.

Luster AD (2002): The role of chemokines in linking innate and adaptive immunity. *Curr Opin Immunol* 14:129.

Russell JH, Ley TJ (2002): Lymphocyte-mediated cytotoxicity. *Annu Rev Immunol* 20:323.

Samelson LE (2002): Signal transduction mediated by the T cell antigen receptor: the role of adapter proteins. *Annu Rev Immunol* 20:371.

Sharpe AH, Freeman GJ (2002): The B7-CD28 superfamily. *Nat Rev Immunol* 2:116.

Shortman K, Liu YJ (2002): Mouse and human dendritic cell subtypes. *Nat Rev Immunol* 2:151.

REVIEW QUESTIONS

For each question, choose the ONE BEST answer or completion.

1. The role of the antigen-presenting cell in the immune response is all of the following *except*
   A) the limited catabolism of polypeptide antigens.
   B) to allow selective association of MHC gene products and peptides.
   C) to supply second signals required to fully activate T cells.
   D) to present non-self peptides associated with MHC class II molecules to B cells.
   E) to present peptide-MHC complexes to T cells with the appropriate receptor.

2. Which of the following statements about interleukin-2 (IL-2) is *incorrect?*
   A) It is produced primarily by activated macrophages.
   B) It is produced by $CD4^+$ T cells.
   C) It can induce the proliferation of $CD4^+$ T cells.
   D) It binds to a specific receptor on $CD4^+$ T cells.
   E) It can activate $CD8^+$ T cells in the presence of antigen.

3. An interaction between which of the following pairs on the surface of B and T cells is required for isotype switching by the B cell:
   A) LFA-3 (CD58) on the B cell and CD2 on the T cell
   B) ICAM-1 (CD54) on the B cell and LFA-1 (CD11a/CD18) on the T cell
   C) B7 on the B cell and CD28 on the T cell
   D) CD40 on the B cell and CD40 Ligand (CD154) on the T cell
   E) membrane Ig on the B cell and CD4 on the T cell

4. Which of the following statements about the activation of $CD4^+$ T cells is *incorrect?*
   A) Activation results in rapid phosphorylation of tyrosine residues in proteins associated with the TCR.
   B) Intracellular calcium levels rise rapidly following activation.
   C) Peptide bound in the groove of MHC class I molecules activates the $CD4^+$ T cell.
   D) Interaction of B7 and CD28 stabilizes IL-2 mRNA so effective IL-2 translation occurs.
   E) The activated cell synthesizes IL-2 and a receptor for IL-2.

5. Which of the following statements about cytokines synthesized by $CD4^+$ T_H1 and T_H2 subsets is *incorrect?*

A) Cytokines produced by T_H1 cells include IFNγ and TNFβ.
B) Cytokines produced by T_H2 cells are important in allergic responses.
C) T_H1 cells secrete cytokines that induce macrophage and NK cell activation.
D) The presence of IL-12 during the activation and differentiation of $CD4^+$ T cells favors the development of T_H2 cells.
E) T_H2 cell cytokines may inhibit the action of T_H1 cells.

6. Which of the following statements about $CD8^+$ CTL is *incorrect?*

A) They lyse targets by synthesizing perforin and granzymes.
B) They cause target cell apoptosis.
C) They cannot kill $CD4^+$ T cells.
D) They interact with their target through paired cell surface molecules.
E) They must be activated before exerting their cytotoxic function.

7. Infection with vaccinia virus results in the priming of virus-specific $CD8^+$ T cells. If these vaccinia virus-specific $CD8^+$ T cells are subsequently removed from the individual, which of the following cells will they kill in virto?

A) vaccinia-infected cells expressing MHC class II molecules from any individual
B) influenza-infected cells expressing the same MHC class I molecules as the individual
C) uninfected cells expressing the same MHC class I molecules as the individual
D) vaccinia-infected cells expressing the same MHC class I molecules as the individual
E) vaccinia-infected cells expressing the same MHC class II molecules as the individual

8. Bacterial lipopolysaccharide (LPS), a T-independent antigen, stimulates antibody production in mice. Which of the following is *incorrect?*

A) The antibody produced will be predominantly IgM.
B) Memory B cells will not be induced.
C) IL-4 and IL-5 are required for the production of antibody during response.
D) The polymeric nature of the antigen crosslinks B-cell surface receptors.
E) B cell activation involves phosphorylation of intracellular molecules.

CASE STUDY

Great effort is still being directed at developing safe and effective vaccines for a variety of diseases. In one study, many individuals given a candidate protein vaccine for a bacterial infection developed antibodies specific for one particular epitope on a protein of the pathogen's surface membrane. The structure of this epitope was determined to be a peptide 10 amino acids in length. This peptide was synthesized and used to immunize individuals who were at risk of subsequent exposure to the bacterium. Disappointingly, no protection was seen. Can you suggest why this may have occurred?

ANSWERS TO REVIEW QUESTIONS

1. ***D*** The antigen-presenting cell does not present peptide + MHC class II to B cells. The other statements are all features of the antigen-presenting cell.

2. ***A*** IL-2 is produced almost exclusively by activated T cells.

3. ***D*** The pairs of molecules in answers A-D are all important in adhesion and/or costimulation, but only the interaction between CD40 and CD40 Ligand is critical for isotype switching; it is not thought that Ig interacts with CD4.

4. ***C*** Peptides bound in the groove of MHC class II, or superantigens—which bind outside the MHC class II groove—activate $CD4^+$ T cells.

5. ***D*** The presence of IL-4 during the activation and differentiation of $CD4^+$ T cells favors the development of T_H2 cells; IL-12 favors the development of T_H1 cells.

6. ***C*** A $CD8^+$ CTL can kill any cell expressing an MHC class 1 molecule in association with a non-self peptide, including, for example, a $CD4^+$ T cell infected with HIV.

7. ***D*** The principle of MHC restriction indicates that the TCR of $CD8^+$ T cells interacts with target cells that express specific peptide bound to self-MHC class I molecules. Thus, vaccinia-primed $CD8^+$ T cells recognize and hence kill only vaccinia-infected targets that express self MHC class I.

8. ***C*** T-independent antigens, because they do not generate T cell-derived cytokines, do not produce IL-4 or IL-5. Thus, no isotype switching or memory cell induction occurs in the response to T-independent antigens.

ANSWER TO CASE STUDY

The small size and potential lack of complexity of the peptide—features that are required for immunogenicity (see Chapter 3)—may not have evoked an immune response. Moreover, the response to the membrane protein of the bacterium was almost certainly thymus-dependent, and so individuals would need to be immunized with an epitope recognized by T helper cells linked to an epitope recognized by B cells. A vaccine comprising sequences recognized both by T and B cells would induce helper and memory responses that would provide a better chance of protecting the individual after exposure to the pathogen.

Although the vaccine protein that was injected induced an antibody response, we do not know if this response was protective. For example, in the response to some infectious agents, such as the Human Immunodeficiency virus (HIV), the antibody response that develops does not appear to be protective (see Chapter 17). In such cases, it will probably be important to include epitopes in potential vaccines that are recognized by cytotoxic $CD8^+$ lymphocytes, as well as epitopes recognized by helper T and B cells.

11

CYTOKINES

INTRODUCTION

As discussed in preceding chapters, the immune system is regulated by soluble mediators, collectively called ***cytokines.*** These low molecular weight proteins are produced by virtually all cells of the innate and adaptive immune systems and, in particular, by $CD4^+$ T cells, which orchestrate many effector mechanisms. Their major functional activities are concerned with the regulation of the development and behavior of immune effector cells. Some cytokines possess direct effector functions of their own. A simple way to understand how cytokines work is to compare them to hormones—the chemical messengers of the endocrine system. Cytokines serve as chemical messengers within the immune system, although they also communicate with certain cells in other systems, including those of the nervous system. Thus they can function in an integrated fashion to facilitate homeostasis. By contrast, they also play a significant role in driving hypersensitivity and inflammatory responses, and in some cases they can promote acute or chronic distress in tissues and organ systems.

As we will discuss later in this chapter, cells regulated by a particular cytokine must express a receptor for that factor. Cells are positively and/or negatively regulated by the quantity and type of cytokines to which they are exposed and by the expression or downregulation of cytokine receptors. Normal regulation of innate and adaptive immune responses is largely controlled by a combination of these methods.

THE HISTORY OF CYTOKINES

In the late 1960s, when the activities of cytokines were first discovered, it was believed that they served as amplification factors that acted in an antigen-dependent fashion to elevate proliferative responses of T cells. Gery and colleagues were the first to demonstrate that macrophages released a thymocyte mitogenic factor, termed ***lymphocyte-activating factor*** (LAF). This view changed radically when it was found that supernatants of mitogen-stimulated peripheral blood mononuclear cells promoted the long-term proliferation of T cells in the absence of antigens and mitogens. Soon afterward, it was found that this factor was produced by T cells and could be used to isolate and clonally expand functional T cell lines. This T cell-derived factor was given different names by different investigators, most notably, T cell growth factor (TCGF). Cytokines produced by lymphocytes were collectively called ***lymphokines,*** whereas those produced by monocytes and macrophages were called ***monokines.*** To complicate matters, studies of the cellular sources of lymphokines and monokines ultimately revealed that these factors were not the exclusive products of lymphocytes and monocytes/macrophages. Thus the more appropriate term *cytokine* was coined as a generic name for these glycoprotein mediators.

In 1979, an international workshop was convened to address the need to develop a consensus regarding the definition of these macrophage- and T cell-derived factors. Since they mediated signals between leukocytes, the term

Immunology: A Short Course, Fifth Edition, By Richard Coico, Geoffrey Sunshine, and Eli Benjamini
ISBN 0-471-22689-0

interleukin (IL) was coined. The macrophage-derived LAF and T cell-derived growth factors were given the names interleukin-1 (IL-1) and interleukin-2 (IL-2), respectively. Currently, numbers have been assigned to 29 interleukins, and the number will undoubtedly increase as research efforts continue to identify new members of this cytokine family.

To further illustrate the degree to which the cytokine field has outgrown the terminology established in 1979, knowledge of the functional properties of various cytokines has engendered a more liberal meaning of terms that were originally designed to define those functions. It is well known that many interleukins have important biologic effects on cell types outside of the immune system. For example, IL-2 not only acts to promote T cell proliferation but also stimulates osteoblasts, the bone-forming cells. Tumor growth factor β (TGF-β) similarly acts on many cells, including connective tissue fibroblasts as well as T cells and B cells. Thus cytokines commonly have ***pleiotropic properties,*** since they can affect the activity of many different cell types. In addition, there is a great deal of functional redundancy among cytokines, as evidenced, for example, by the ability of more than one cytokine to promote the growth, survival, and differentiation of B or T cells (e.g., IL-2 and IL-4 can both function as T cell growth factors). As we shall see later in this chapter, this redundancy is explained, in part, by the common use of cytokine receptor signaling subunits by certain groups of cytokines. Finally, cytokines rarely, if ever, act alone in vivo. Thus target cells are exposed to a milieu containing cytokines, which often exhibit ***additive, synergistic,*** or ***antagonistic properties.*** In the case of synergism, the combined effects of two cytokines is sometimes greater that the additive effects of the individual cytokines. Conversely, antagonism occurs when one cytokine inhibits the biologic activity of another.

The cytokine field has evolved rapidly since the 1970s due to the identification, functional characterization, and molecular cloning of a growing list of cytokines. The convenient nomenclature previously developed to define the sources of origin or the functional activities of certain cytokines has, in general, not held up. Nevertheless, occasionally, the field recognizes that common functional features of several glycoproteins merits the creation of yet another collective term to help define a family of cytokines. In particular, the term ***chemokines*** was adopted in 1992 to describe a family of closely related ***chemotactic cytokines*** with conserved sequences, known to be potent attractors for various leukocyte subsets, such as lymphocytes, neutrophils, and monocytes. For students of immunology, learning about the rapidly expanding list of cytokines with diverse functional characteristics may appear to be a formidable task. However, by focusing on some cytokines that deserve special mention, we hope that this will be an interesting and manageable exercise.

GENERAL PROPERTIES OF CYTOKINES

Common Functional Properties

Cytokines have several functional features in common. Some, like interferon-γ (IFNγ) and IL-2, are synthesized by cells and rapidly secreted. Others, such as tumor necrosis factor-α (TNFα) and TNFβ, may be secreted or expressed as membrane-associated proteins. Most cytokines have very ***short half-lives;*** consequently, cytokine synthesis and function typically occur in a burst.

Similar to the actions of polypeptide hormones, cytokines facilitate communication between cells and do so at very low concentrations (typically 10^{-10} to 10^{-15} M). Cytokines may act locally either on the same cell that secreted it (***autocrine***) or on other cells (***paracrine***); furthermore, like hormones, they may act systemically (***endocrine***) (Fig. 11.1). In common with other polypeptide hormones, cytokines exert their functional effects by binding to specific receptors on target cells. Thus cells regulated by specific cytokines must have the capacity to express a receptor for that factor. In turn, the activity of a responder cell may be regulated by the quantity and type of cytokines to which they are exposed or by the upregulation or downregulation of cytokine receptors, which, themselves, may be regulated by other cytokines. A good example of the latter is the ability of IL-1 to upregulate IL-2 receptors on T cells. As noted earlier, this illustrates one common feature of cytokines—namely, their ability to act in concert with one another to create synergistic effects that reinforce the other's action on a single cell.

Alternatively, some cytokines behave antagonistically toward one or more other cytokines and thus inhibit each

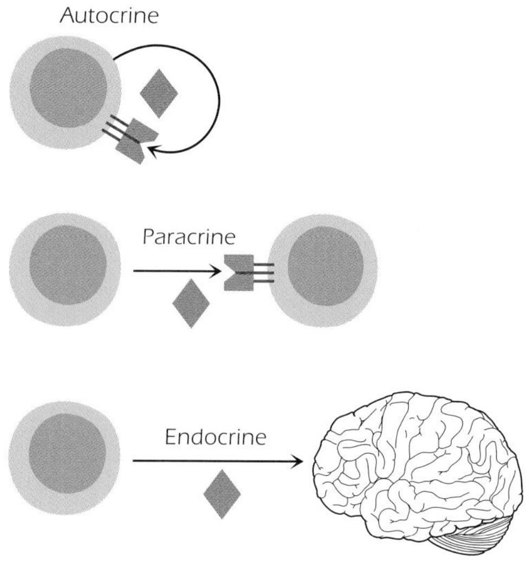

Figure 11.1. Autocrine, paracrine, and endocrine properties of cytokines. The brain is an example of an organ that responds to cytokines in an endocrine fashion.

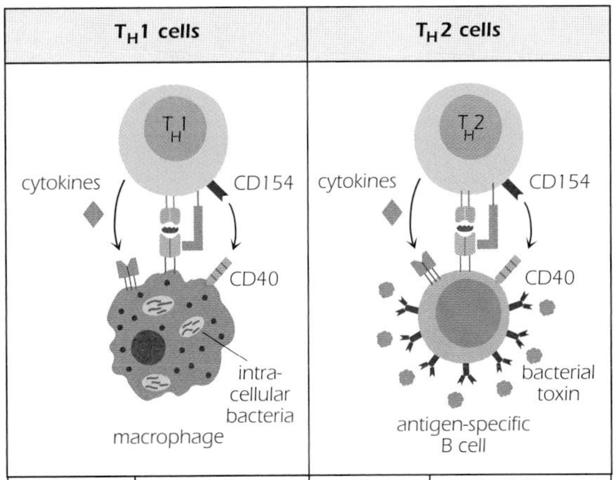

T_H1 Cytokines	Activity	T_H2 Cytokines	Activity
IFN-γ	Activates macrophages; Regulates cells	IL-4	Activates B cells
GM-CSF	Activates macrophages	IL-5	Activates B cells
TNF-α	Activates macrophages	IL-10	Inhibits macrophages
IL-3	Involved in hematopoiesis	IL-3	Involved in hematopoiesis
TNF-β	Involved in inflammatory responses	TGF-β	Inhibits monocyte activation

Figure 11.2. Cytokines produced by T_H1 and T_H2 cells.

other's action on a given cell. For example, cytokines secreted by helper T (T_H1) cells secrete IFNγ, which activates macrophages, inhibits B cells, and is directly toxic for certain cells. T_H2 cells secrete IL-4 and IL-5, which activate B cells and IL-10, which inhibits macrophage activation (Fig. 11.2).

When cells produce cytokines or chemokines in response to various stimuli (e.g., infectious agents), they establish a concentration gradient that serves to control or direct cell migration patterns, also known as ***chemotaxis*** (Fig. 11.3). As discussed in Chapter 2 and later in this chapter, cell migration (e.g., neutrophil chemotaxis) is essential to the development of inflammatory responses resulting from localized injury or other trauma. Chemokines play a key role in providing signals that upregulate expression of adhesion molecules expressed on endothelial cells to facilitate neutrophil chemotaxis and transendothelial migration.

Common Systemic Activities

Cytokines can act over both the short and the long range, with consequent systemic effects. Cytokines thus play a crucial role in the amplification of the immune response, because the release of cytokines from just a few antigen-activated cells results in the activation of multiple different cell types, which are not necessarily antigen-specific or located in the immediate area. This is apparent in a response such as delayed-type hypersensitivity (discussed in detail in Chapter 16), in which the activation of rare antigen-specific T cells is accompanied by the release of cytokines. As a consequence of cytokine effects, monocytes are recruited into the area in great numbers, dwarfing the originally activated T cell population. It is also worth noting that the production of high levels of cytokines by a powerful stimulus can trigger deleterious systemic effects, such as toxic shock syndrome, as discussed later in this chapter. Similarly, therapeutic manipulation of the immune system using recombinant cytokines or cytokine antagonists can affect multiple physiologic systems, depending on the range of biologic activity associated with a particular cytokine.

Common Cell Sources and Cascading Events

A given cell may make many different cytokines. Moreover, one cell may be the target of many cytokines, each binding to its own specific cell-surface receptor. Consequently, one cytokine may affect the action of another, which may lead to an additive, synergistic, or antagonistic effect on the target cell.

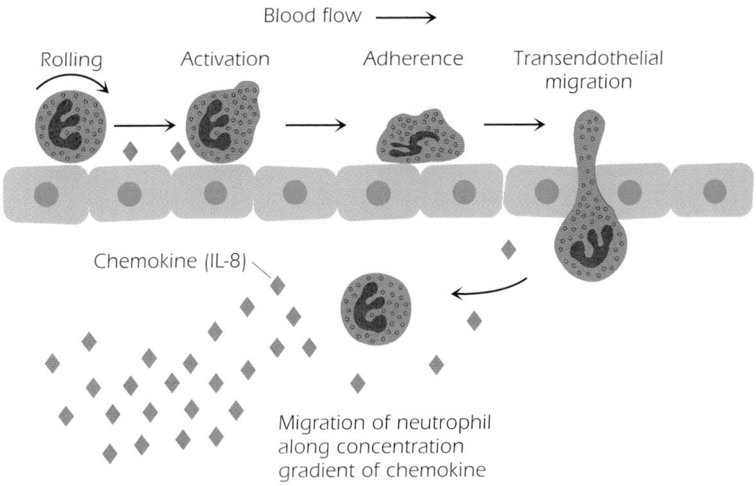

Figure 11.3. Steps involved in neutrophil chemotaxis and transendothelial migration showing reversible binding followed by activation, adherence, and movement between the endothelial cells forming the wall of the blood vessel (extravasation).

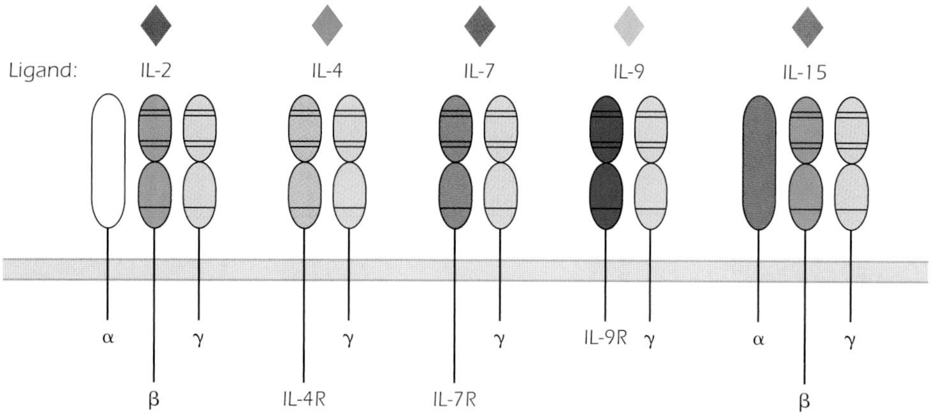

Figure 11.4. The structural features of members of the class I cytokine receptor family. The γ chain (*green*), common to all, mediates intracellular signaling.

Interactions of the multiple cytokines produced during a typical immune response are often referred to as the ***cytokine cascade.*** This cascade largely determines whether a response to an antigen will be primarily antibody-mediated (and, if so, which classes of antibodies will be made) or cell-mediated (and, if so, whether cells engaged in delayed hypersensitivity or cytotoxicity will be activated). Later in this chapter, we will discuss the cytokine-mediated control mechanisms that help determine the pattern of cytokines that develop after $CD4^+$ T cell cell activation. The antigenic stimulus appears to play a key role in the initiation of cytokine responses by these cells. Thus, depending on the nature of the antigenic signal and the cytokine milieu associated with T cell activation, naive effector $CD4^+$ T cells will generate a particular cytokine profile—one that ultimately controls the type of immune response generated (antibody versus cellular). The cytokine cascade associated with immune responses also determines what other systems are activated or suppressed as well as the level and duration of the response.

Common Receptor Molecules

As noted earlier in this chapter, it is common for cytokines to have overlapping (redundant) functions—for example, both IL-1 and IL-6 induce fever and several other common biologic phenomena. Nonetheless, these cytokines also have properties that are unique. As discussed below, several cytokines use multichain receptors to mediate their effects on target cells, and some of these receptors share at least one common receptor molecule called the ***common*** γ ***chain*** (Fig. 11.4). The common γ chain is an intracellular signaling molecule. This helps explain the functional overlap among different cytokines.

FUNCTIONAL CATEGORIES OF CYTOKINES

We will not attempt to list all of the currently well-characterized and molecularly cloned cytokines in this chapter. The major cytokines that play a role in the immune response and a brief description of their functions are listed in Table 11.1. A convenient way to begin is to classify cytokines into functional categories, discussed below, based on shared functional properties. It is important to state that this subdivision, although convenient, is somewhat arbitrary, given the pleiotropic effects of many cytokines.

Cytokines That Regulate Immune Responses

As discussed in Chapter 10, B and T cell activation in response to antigen stimulation is regulated by cytokines. Depending on the cytokines involved, regulation can be positive or negative and can affect cell proliferation, activation, and differentiation. Ultimately, cytokines regulate the intensity and duration of immune responses. A major feature of all adaptive immune responses is their antigen specificity. Given the potent immunoregulatory activities of cytokines, how does the immune system ensure that antigen-nonspecific B and T cells are not activated during an immune response? One mechanism to ensure the specificity of the immune response is through the selective expression of functional cytokine receptors only on lymphocytes that have been stimulated by antigen. As a consequence, cytokines tend to act solely on antigen-activated lymphocytes. A second mechanism that protects antigen-nonspecific lymphocytes from being activated by cytokines involves the need for cells to interact with each other through cell-to-cell contact, also known as ***cognate*** interaction. Such interactions that might occur, say, between $CD4^+$ T cells and antigen-presenting cells (APCs; e.g., dendritic cells, macrophages, B cells) generate high concentrations of cytokines at the juncture between the interacting cells. In this way, only the target cell(s) participating in the interaction are affected by the cytokines produced. Finally, since the half-life of cytokines is very short, particularly in the bloodstream and extracellular spaces, they have a very limited period to act on other target cells.

Sources and Activities of Immunoregulatory Cytokines. $CD4^+$ T cells are a major source of immunoregulatory cytokines. We have already discussed some

TABLE 11.1. Selected Cytokines and Their Functions

Cytokine	Produced By	Major Functions
Interleukin		
IL-1	Monocytes; many other cell types	Produces fever; stimulates acute-phase prtein synthesis; promotes proliferation of T_H2 cells
IL-2	T_H0 and T_H1 cells	T cell growth factor
IL-3	T_H cells; NK cells; mast cells	Growth factor for hematopoietic cells
IL-4	T_H2; $CD4^+$ T cells; mast cells	Growth factor for B cells and T_H2 $CD4^+$ T cells; promotes IgE and IgG synthesis; inhibits T_H1 $CD4^+$ T cells
IL-5	T_H2 cells; mast cells	Stimulates B cell growth and immunoglobulin secretion; growth and differentiation factor eosinophils
IL-6	T cells; many other cell types	Induces acute-phase protein synthesis, T cell activation, and IL-2 production; stimulates B cell immunoglobulin production and hematopoietic progenitor cell growth
IL-7	Bone marrow; thymic stromal cells; some T cells	Growth factor for pre-T and pre-B cells
IL-9	T cells	Mast cell activation
IL-10	T_H2 cells; macrophages	Inhibits production of T_H1 cells and macrophage function
IL-11	Fibroblasts	Stimulates megakaryocyte (platelet precursor) growth
IL-12	B cells and macrophages	Activates NK cells and promotes generation of T_H1 $CD4^+$ T cells
IL-13	T cells	Shares characteristics with IL-4 (e.g., immunoglobulin switch to IgE synthesis) but does not affect T cells; growth factor for human B cells
IL-14	T cells	Involved in the development of memory B cells
IL-15	T cells and epithelial cells	T cell growth factor; similar to IL-2
IL-16	T cells, eosinophils, mast cells	Chemotactic for T cells; proinflammatory
IL-17	T cells	Induces proinflammatory cytokine secretion; promotes hematopoietic progenitor cell differentiation
IL-18	Macrophages; monocytes; dendritic cells; many other cell types	Induces IFNγ production; enhances NK cell lytic activity
IFNγ	T_H1 cells	Activates NK cells and macrophages; inhibits T_H2 $CD4^+$ T cells; induces expression of MHC class II on many cell types
TGFβ	Lymphocytes; macrophages; platelets; mast cells	Enhances production of IgA; inhibits activation of monocyte and T-cell subsets; active in fibroblast growth and wound healing
Tumor necrosis factor		
TNFα	Macrophages; mast cells	Involved in inflammatory responses; activates endothelial cells and other cells of immune and nonimmune systems; induces fever and septic shock
TNFβ (lymphotoxin)	T cells	Involved in inflammatory responses; also plays a role in killing target cells by cytotoxic $CD8^+$ T cells
GM-CSF	T cells; monocytes	Promotes growth of granulocytes and macrophages; growth of dendritic cells in vitro
M-CSF	T cells; monocytes	Promotes macrophage growth
G-CSF	T cells; monocytes	Promotes granulocyte growth

G-CSF, granulocyte colony-stimulating factor; *GM-CSF,* granulocyte-macrophage colony-stimulating factor; *IFN,* interferon; *Ig,* immunoglobulin; *IL,* interleukin; *M-CSF,* macrophage colony-stimulating factor; *MHC,* major histocompatibility complex; *NK,* natural killer; *TGF,* transforming growth factor; T_H, helper T cell; *TNF,* tumor necrosis factor.

of the diverse functional properties of several T cell-derived cytokines, including IL-2 and IL-4 (see Chapter 10). Naive $CD4^+$ T cells differentiate into subpopulations of T_H1 and T_H2 cells, each of which possesses characteristic cytokine profiles (Fig. 11.2). During the generation of an initial immune response, antigens play a key role in determining which direction naive T_H0 cells will take in this differentiation pathway. It is important to note that the factors controlling whether CD4 T cells will differentiate into T_H1 or T_H2 cells are not fully understood. In addition to the roles played by certain cytokines in shaping the subsequent adaptive immune response (see below), the costimulators used to drive the response and the nature of the peptide-MHC interactions have an effect, as does the nature of the antigenic stimulus itself. For example, many intracellular bacteria (e.g., *Listeria*) and viruses activate dendritic cells, macrophages, and natural-killer (NK) cells to produce IL-12 and IFNγ. In the presence of these cytokines, T_H0 cells tend to develop into T_H1 cells. By contrast, other pathogens (e.g., parasitic worms) do not induce IL-12 production but instead cause release of IL-4 by other cells (e.g., mast cells). IL-4 tends to promote the development of T_H0 cells into T_H2 cells.

Another way in which antigen plays a role in determining which direction naive T_H0 cells will take in developing into T_H1 or T_H2 cells concerns the amount and nature of antigenic peptide presented to these cells during primary stimulation. Low levels of antigenic peptide bind poorly to the T cell receptor of T_H0 cells. Under these conditions, the naive T cells differentiate preferentially into T_H2 cells to produce IL-4 and IL-5. By contrast, when naive $CD4^+$ T cells are presented with a high density of ligand that binds strongly to the T cell receptor, they tend to differentiate into T_H1 cells to produce IL-2, IFNγ and TNFβ. Ultimately, the cytokines generated determine whether the response will be dominated by macrophage activation or antibody production. ***The T_H1 pathway facilitates cell-mediated immunity*** with the activation of macrophages, NK cells, and cytotoxic T lymphocyte (CTL) responses, whereas ***the T_H2 pathway is essential for humoral immunity.***

As noted earlier, T_H subsets can also regulate the growth and effector functions of each other. This phenomenon occurs as a result of the activity of cytokines produced by the subset that is being activated, and its apparent purpose is to make it difficult to shift the response to the other subset. For example, production of IL-10 and TGF-β by T_H2 cells inhibits activation and growth of T_H1 cells. Similarly, production of IFNγ by T_H1 cells inhibits proliferation of T_H2 cells. These effects permit either subset to dominate a particular immune response by inhibiting the outgrowth of the other subset.

Finally, cytokines play an important role in bringing the cells involved in an immune response back to baseline once an antigenic stimulus (e.g., an infectious pathogen) has been cleared. Therefore, cytokines provide the regulatory signals needed both to activate the immune system after antigen stimulation and then to cause the responding cells to return to a quiescent state.

Cytokines That Facilitate Innate Immune Responses and Activate Inflammatory Responses

Innate Immune Responses. Several cytokines facilitate innate immune responses stimulated by viruses and microbial pathogens. Included in this group are ***IL-1, IL-6, TNFα, IFNα,*** and ***IFNβ.*** IL-1, IL-6, and TNFα initiate a wide spectrum of biologic activities that help coordinate the host's responses to infection. They are produced largely by phagocytes (e.g., macrophages and neutrophils) and are termed ***endogenous pyrogens*** because they cause fever. Elevated body temperature is beneficial to host defenses because adaptive immune responses are more intense and most pathogens grow less efficiently at raised temperatures. Another important effect of IL-1, IL-6, and TNFα is their initiation of a response known as the acute-phase response after production of ***acute-phase proteins*** produced by hepatocytes. As discussed below, acute inflammation (e.g., in response to infections) is generally accompanied by a systemic acute-phase response. Typically, changes in acute-phase protein plasma levels occur within 2 days after infection. One of these proteins, ***C-reactive protein*** (CRP), binds to phosphorylcholine on bacterial surfaces, acts like an opsonin, and activates the classical complement pathway (Chapter 13). Another acute-phase protein with opsonin and complement-activating activity is ***mannan-binding lectin*** (MBL), which binds mannose residues accessible on many bacteria. Given these functional properties, they mimic the actions of antibodies, which opsonize bacteria and activate the complement cascade. In concert with the other members of the acute-phase protein family, CRP and MBL lead to bacterial clearance.

Another effect of the endogenous pyrogens (IL-1, IL-6, and TNFα) is to induce an increase in circulating neutrophils, which are summoned from the bone marrow and blood vessels where leukocytes attach loosely to endothelial cells. Finally, dendritic cells from peripheral tissues migrate to the lymph nodes in response to these cytokines. There, they serve as potent APCs to facilitate adaptive immune responses needed to control infections.

The term ***interferon*** was coined because they interfere with viral replication, thus blocking the spread of viruses to uninfected cells. IFNα and IFNβ are synthesized by many cell types after viral infection. They are distinguished from another glycoprotein, called IFNγ, which is produced by activated NK cells and effector T cells and thus appears after the induction of adaptive immune responses. In addition to their antiviral activities, IFNα and IFNβ induce increased MHC class I expression on most uninfected cells, enhancing their resistance to NK cells as well as making newly infected cells more susceptible to killing by $CD8^+$ cytotoxic T cells. Finally, they activate NK cells, which contribute to early host responses to viral infections.

Inflammatory Responses. Many cytokines activate the functions of inflammatory cells and are, therefore, known as ***proinflammatory cytokines.*** Examples of proinflammatory cytokines are IL-1, IL-6, and TNFα. During localized acute inflammatory responses, all three cytokines cause increased vascular permeability, which ultimately leads to the swelling and redness associated with inflammation. As inflammatory mediators, they act in concert with the chemokines to ensure the development of physiologic responses to a variety of stimuli, such as infections and tissue injury. Acute inflammatory responses develop rapidly and are of short duration. This short time course is probably related to the short half-lives of the inflammatory mediators involved as well as the regulatory influence of cytokines such as TGFβ, which limits the inflammatory response (see below). Typically, systemic responses accompany these short-lived responses and are characterized by a rapid alteration in levels of acute-phase proteins (see above). Sometimes, persistent immune activation can occur (e.g., in chronic infections), leading to chronic inflammation, which subverts the physiologic value of inflammatory responses and causes pathologic consequences.

The neutrophil plays a key role in the early stages of inflammatory responses (Fig. 11.3). Neutrophils infiltrate within a few hours into the tissue area where the inflammatory response is occurring. Their migration from the blood to the tissue site is controlled by the expression of adhesion molecules by vascular endothelial cells—a mechanism regulated by mediators of acute inflammation, including IL-1 and TNFα. After exposure to these cytokines, vascular endothelial cells increase their expression of adhesion molecules—for example, E- and P-selectin and intercellular adhesion molecule 1 (ICAM-1); see Chapter 9—which, in turn, bind to selectin ligands (e.g., sialyl Lewis moiety) expressed on the surface of neutrophils. The neutrophils attach securely to the endothelial cells and undergo a process of end-over-end rolling. Neutrophils are also activated by chemokines which induce a conformational change in their membrane integrin molecules. Figure 11.5 shows the conformational change in the heterodimeric (α and β chains) integrin molecule, LFA-1, which allows it to ligate ICAM-1. This change increases the affinity of neutrophils for the adhesion molecules on the endothelium. Finally, the neutrophil undergoes transendothelial migration, resulting in extravasation of the neutrophil, which continues its journey to the damaged or infected tissue site under the directional influence of chemokines, a process known as chemotaxis.

Lymphocytes and monocytes also undergo extravasation using the same basic steps as the neutrophil, although different combinations of adhesion molecules are involved. Other cytokines that play a significant role in inflammatory responses are IFNγ and TGFβ. In addition to its role in activating macrophages to increase their phagocytic activity, IFNγ has been shown to chemotactically attract macrophages to the site where antigen is localized. The migration of all of these cell types, including neutrophils, lymphocytes, monocytes, macrophages, eosinophils, and basophils (which are attracted to the site of tissue damage by complement activation), leads to clearance of the antigen and healing of the tissue. TGFβ plays a role in terminating the inflammatory response by promoting the accumulation and proliferation of fibroblasts and the deposition of extracellular matrix proteins required for tissue repair.

Chemokines: Cytokines That Affect Leukocyte Movement

The term ***chemokine*** is used to denote a family of closely related, low molecular weight chemotactic cytokines containing 70–80 residues with conserved sequences and known to be potent attractors for various leukocyte subsets, such as neutrophils, monocytes, and lymphocytes. Table 11.2 lists some of the important chemokines among the many (>50) that have been identified. Structurally, this large superfamily consists of four subfamilies that display one of four highly conserved NH_2-terminal cysteine amino acid residues as follows: CXC, CC, or CX3C, where *X* represents a nonconserved amino acid residue. Most chemokines fall into the CXC and CC groups. As discussed above, chemokines function in concert with inflammatory mediators to regulate the expression and conformation of cell adhesion molecules in leukocyte membranes. Some chemokines have also been shown to induce respiratory burst, enzyme

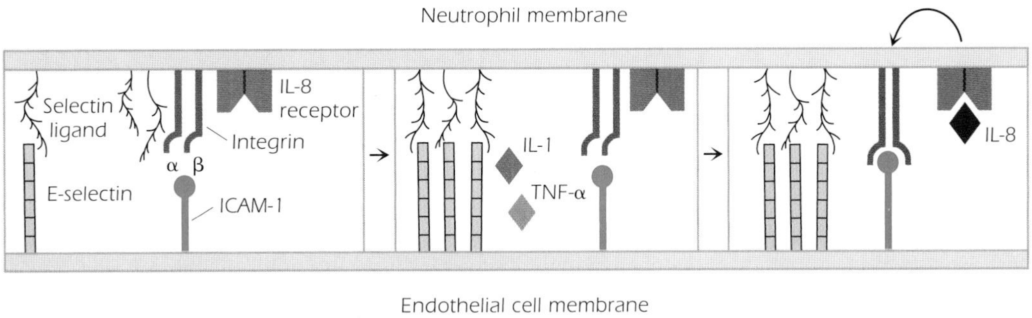

Figure 11.5. Cell-surface adhesion molecules and cytokine-activation events associated with neutrophil transendothelial migration. *Left:* Weak binding of selectin ligands on the neutrophil to E-selectin on the endothelial cells. *Middle:* Interleukin-1 (*IL-1*) and tumor necrosis factor-α (*TNFα*) upregulation of E-selectin, which facilitates stronger binding. *Right:* The activation effects of IL-8 on neutrophils cause a conformational change in the integrins (e.g., lymphocyte-activating factor 1) to allow them to bind intercellular adhesion molecule 1 (*ICAM-1*).

TABLE 11.2. Selected Chemokines and Their Functions

Chemokine	Produced By	Chemoattracted Cells	Major Functions
IL-8	Monocytes; macrophages; fibroblasts; keratinocytes; endothelial cells	Neutrophils; naive T cells	Mobilizes and activates neutrophils; promotes angiogenesis
RANTES	T cells; endothelial cells; platelets	Monocytes; NK cells; T cells; basophils; eosinophils	Degranulates basophils; activates T cells
MCP-1	Monocytes; macrophages; fibroblasts; keratinocytes	Monocytes; NK cells; T cells; basophils; dendritic cells	Activates macrophages; stimulates basophil histamine release; promotes T_H2 immunity
MIP-1α	Monocytes; macrophages; T cells; mast cells; fibroblasts	Monocytes; NK cells; T cells; basophils; dendritic cells	Promotes T_H1 immunity; competes with HIV-1
MIP-1β	Monocytes; macrophages; neutrophils; endothelial cells	Monocytes; NK cells; T cells; dendritic cells	Competes with HIV-1 for chemokine receptor binding

IL, interleukin; *MCP,* monocyte chemotactic protein; *MIP,* macrophage inflammatory protein; *NK,* natural killer; T_H, helper T cell.

release, intracellular calcium mobilization, and angiogenesis. The latter functional property of some chemokines is a biologic feature consistent with the important role these molecules play in wound healing and tissue repair. Production of chemokines may be either induced or constitutive. Those whose production is inducible or strongly upregulatable in peripheral tissues by inflammation are primarily involved in wound healing and tissue repair mechanisms. By contrast, constitutively produced chemokines fulfill housekeeping functions and may be involved in normal leukocyte traffic.

Among the >50 chemokines that have been identified to date, IL-8, a member of the CXC subfamily, is among the most well characterized. It is produced by many different cell types, including macrophages, T cells, endothelial cells, fibroblasts, and neutrophils, and plays a major role in inflammatory responses and wound healing—mainly due to its ability to attract neutrophils to sites of tissue damage. Another important function of IL-8 is its ability to activate neutrophils after their attachment to vascular endothelium (Fig. 11.5).

A noteworthy characteristic of certain CC chemokines-for example, RANTES, macrophage inflammatory protein 1α (MIP-1α), and MIP-1β—is their ability to suppress infection of T cells in vitro with M-trophic HIV strains. These strains of HIV were originally so-named because of their ability to infect macrophage cell lines in vitro, although it is now known that M-trophic HIV strains can infect dendritic cells, macrophages, and T cells in vivo (Chapter 17). Similarly, lymphocyte-trophic HIV strains infect only CD4$^+$ T cells in vitro. The different variants of HIV and the cell types they infect are largely determined by the chemokine receptor they use as a required HIV co-receptor. Dendritic cells, macrophages, and T cells express CCR5, and primary infections with M-trophic HIV variants use this chemokine receptor, which also binds to the chemokines RANTES, MIP-1α, and MIP-1β. Thus the addition of these chemokines to lymphocytes sensitive to HIV infection blocks the infection because of competition between the CC chemokines and the virus for the target cell co-receptor CCR5.

By contrast, the chemokine receptor that binds to certain members of the CXC subfamily (CXCR4) is the co-receptor responsible for entry of lymphocyte-trophic strains of HIV into target cells. The establishment of a heterotrimeric complex between the viral envelope protein gp120, CD4, and one of these chemokine receptors facilitates viral entry into cells, although the molecular mechanisms associated with this phenomenon are only beginning to be understood.

Cytokines That Stimulate Hematopoiesis

As discussed in Chapter 2, myeloid and lymphoid cells are derived from pluripotential stem cells (see Fig. 2.1). Cytokines capable of inducing growth of hematopoietic cells in vitro were initially characterized using cultures of bone marrow cells grown in soft agar and thus are referred to as ***colony-stimulating factors*** (CSF). Several biochemically distinct CSFs were identified by the particular lineage of hematopoietic cells that were stimulated to form colonies. These include ***macrophage CSF*** (M-CSF), which supports the clonal growth of macrophages; ***granulocyte CSF*** (G-CSF); which supports the clonal growth of granulocytes; and ***granulocyte-macrophage CSF*** (GM-CSF), which supports the clonal growth of both monocytes and macrophages. IL-3 is another cytokine capable of stimulating clonal growth of hematopoietic cells but, unlike the CSFs, is capable of promoting proliferation of a large number of cell populations, including granulocytes, macrophages, megakaryocytes, eosinophils, basophils, and mast calls. Moreover, in the presence of erythropoietin, a kidney-derived growth factor that has the ability to support the growth and terminal differentiation of cells of the erythroid lineage, IL-3 is also capable of stimulating development of normoblasts and red blood cells. IL-7, a cytokine produced largely by bone marrow and thymic stromal cells, induces differentiation of lymphoid stem cells into progenitor B and T cells.

Like other functional categories of cytokines, the list of factors that are involved in hematopoiesis has grown significantly in recent years. Perhaps more than any other category

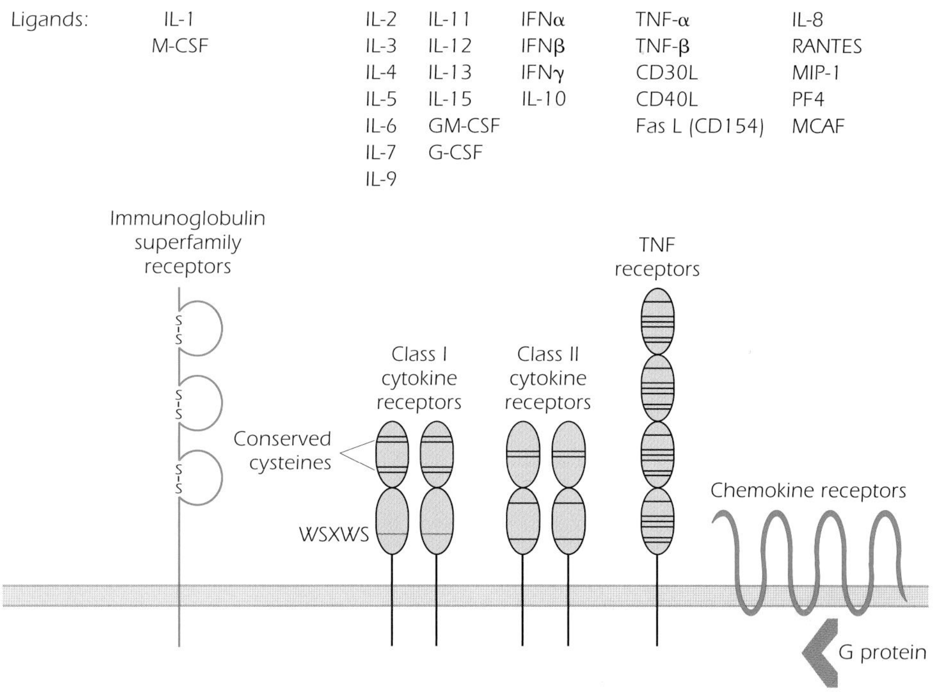

Figure 11.6. The structural features of the five types of cytokine receptors. Many contain highly conserved cysteine residues.

of cytokines, CSFs have emerged as important therapeutic agents. For example, G-CSF is used to treat patients underbreak going high-dose chemotherapy to reverse the neutropenia caused by such therapies. GM-CSF is used to treat patients undergoing bone marrow transplantation to boost clonal expansion of the granulocyte and macrophage populations.

CYTOKINE RECEPTORS

Cytokine Receptor Families

Cytokines can act only on target cells that express receptors for that cytokine. Often, cytokine receptor expression, like cytokine production itself, is highly regulated, such that resting cells either do not express a given receptor or express a low- or intermediate-affinity version of the receptor. An example of the latter is seen in the case of the IL-2 receptor, which can be expressed on the membranes of cells as either an intermediate-affinity dimer (β and γ chains) or a high-affinity trimer containing three subunit chains α, β, and γ (Fig. 11.8). IL-2 is capable of activating cells expressing the high-affinity form of the IL-2 receptor—a property unique to T cells undergoing antigen stimulation. The relative importance of these receptor subunits in binding to IL-2 and signaling the target cell is discussed later in this chapter. Suffice to say, the regulation of the receptor level expressed on the target cell membrane and/or the receptor form expressed helps ensure that only an activated target population will respond to the cytokine(s) within its local microenvironment.

Understanding how cytokines affect their target cells has been the subject of many recent studies. As discussed later in this chapter, knowledge about cytokine-cytokine receptor interactions may be useful in devising strategies to prevent the action of cytokines involved in inflammatory responses, such as rheumatoid arthritis, or in responses such as transplantation rejection.

Receptors for cytokines can be divided into five families of receptor proteins (Fig. 11.6):

- Immunoglobulin superfamily receptors.
- Class I cytokine receptor family.
- Class II cytokine receptor family.
- TNF receptor superfamily.
- Chemokine receptor family .

The ***immunoglobulin superfamily*** receptors contain shared structural features that were first defined in immunoglobulins—each having at least one immunoglobulin-like domain (see Chapter 4). Examples of cytokines whose receptors are members of the immunoglobulin superfamily include IL-1 and M-CSF. ***Class I cytokine receptors*** (also known as the *hematopoietin receptor family*) are usually composed of two types of polypeptide chains: a cytokine-specific subunit (α chain) and a signal-transducing subunit (β or γ chain). Important exceptions for the two subunit structural features of class I cytokine receptors are seen in the case of the high-affinity receptors for IL-2 and the IL-15 receptor, which are trimers. Most cytokines identified to date use the class I family of cytokine receptors.

Class II cytokine receptors are also known as the interferon receptor family because their ligands are interferons (e.g. IFNα, IFNβ, and IFNγ) or have biologic activities that overlap with those associated with some interferons (e.g., IL-10). The ***TNF receptor (TNFR) superfamily*** is divided into three divergent subgroups that are classified by motifs (or lack thereof) in their cytoplasmic tails: death receptors, decoy receptors, and activating receptors. In all cases, each of these subgroups contains similar extracellular ligand-binding domains. Activating TNFR mediate their intracellular signals through a set of adaptor proteins called ***TNF receptor-associated factors (TRAFs).*** Ligands for TNFR can be membrane-associated or secreted proteins. For example, most effector T cells express membrane forms of members of the TNFR superfamily, including TNFα and TNFβ (also known as lymphotoxin-α)—both of which can also be released as secreted proteins. Other TNFRs include Fas, which contains the "death domain" in its cytoplasmic tail, and CD40, which is involved in such functions as B cell proliferation, maturation, and class switching. In short, the TNFR and TNF superfamilies regulate the life and death of activated cells of the immune system. Finally, the chemokine receptors belong to a superfamily of serpentine ***G protein-coupled receptors***—so-called because of their unique snakelike extracellular-cytoplasmic structural configuration and their association with G proteins, which mediate signal transduction (Fig. 11.6).

A growing list of CC and CXC chemokine receptors have been cloned and some have been found to be promiscuous, since they can bind not only to chemokines but also to a diverse set of pathogens, including bacteria (e.g., *Streptococcus pneumonia,* which binds to the platelet activating-factor receptor), parasites (e.g., *Plasmodium vivax,* which binds to the chemokine receptor known as the Duffy blood group antigen), and certain viruses (e.g., T-tropic HIV-1 strains, which use the CXCR4 chemokine receptor, and M-tropic HIV-1 strains, which use the CCR5 chemokine receptor for viral entry into T cells and macrophages, respectively).

Common γ Chain

An important feature of class I cytokine receptors is that they often share common signal-transducing subunits with other members of the same family. For example, the high-affinity IL-2 receptor (IL-2R) consists of an IL-2-specific α chain (CD25) and two additional chains (β and γ) responsible for signal transduction (discussed below). As mentioned earlier, the ***common γ chain*** is used by several other cytokine receptors as the signal-transducing subunit-a structural feature that helps explain the redundancy and antagonism often exhibited by some cytokines (Fig. 11.4). The functional significance of the common γ chain is illustrated by the role it plays for the IL-2R. The IL-2R can be expressed on the membranes of cells in two forms: (1) an intermediate-affinity dimer (β and γ chains) and (2) a high-affinity trimer containing three subunit chains α, β, and γ (Fig. 11.8). IL-2 is capable of activating cells

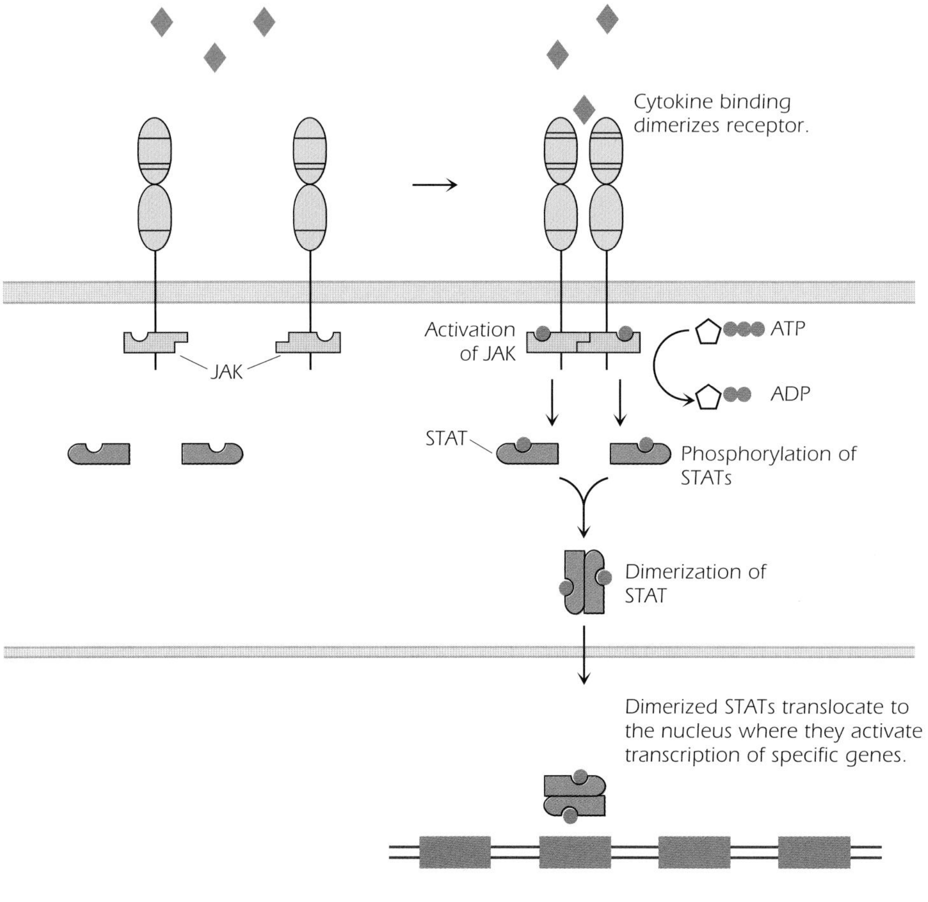
Cytokine binding dimerizes receptor.
Activation of JAK
JAK
ATP
ADP
STAT
Phosphorylation of STATs
Dimerization of STAT
Dimerized STATs translocate to the nucleus where they activate transcription of specific genes.

Figure 11.7. Model of cytokine receptor signaling using receptor-associated kinases to activate specific transcription factors. *STATS,* signal transducers and activators of transcription.

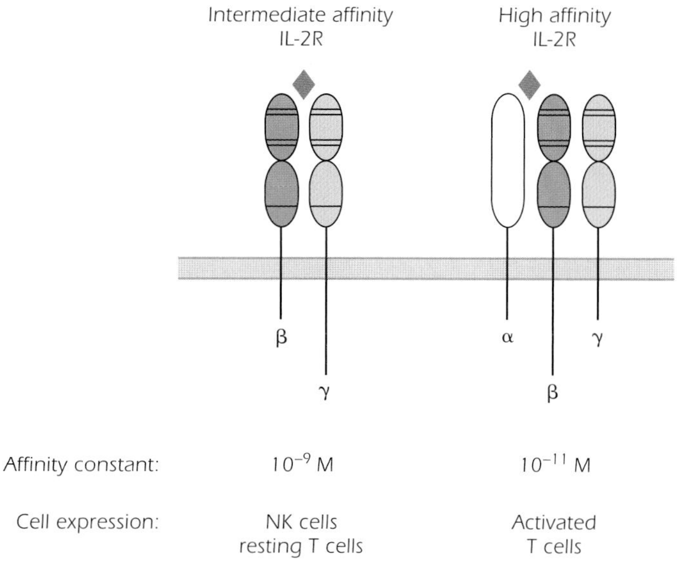

Figure 11.8. Comparison of the two forms of interleukin-2 receptors expressed on cells.

expressing the high-affinity form of the IL-2R—a property reserved for T cells undergoing antigen stimulation. A defect in the common IL-2Rγ chain has been shown to cause a profound immune deficiency in males suffering from X-linked severe combined immunodeficiency disease (Chapter 17). This defect abolishes the functional activity of multiple cytokines, owing to their shared use of the IL-2Rγ chain for normal ligation of their receptors.

CYTOKINE RECEPTOR-MEDIATED SIGNAL TRANSDUCTION

For cytokines to mediate their biologic effects on target cells, they must generate intracellular signals that result in the production of active transcription factors and, ultimately, gene expression (Fig. 11.7). Binding of a cytokine to its cellular receptor induces dimerization or polymerization of receptor polypeptides at the cell surface. The mechanism illustrated applies to most, if not all, class I and class II cytokines receptor families. It should be noted that it is not clear how signal specificity is maintained when different cytokine receptors use the same cytoplasmic signaling pathways. In the case of these two receptor families, the dimerization-polymerization of receptor subunits juxtaposes their cytoplasmic tails, thus allowing the dimeric receptor to engage the intracytoplasmic signaling machinery. Signaling is initiated by the activation of ***JAK kinases,*** a family of cytosolic protein tyrosine kinases that interact with the cytoplasmic domains of the receptor. This results in the phosphorylation of tyrosine residues present on the cytoplasmic domain of the receptor and on a family of transcription factors known as signal transducers and activators of transcription (***STATs).*** Once phosphorylated, the STAT transcription factors dimerize and subsequently translocate from the cytoplasm to the nucleus, where they bind to enhancer regions of genes induced by the cytokine.

The signaling events described above culminate in the biologic properties of the cytokine at the cellular level. However, this culmination does not terminate the signaling caused by cytokine ligation of cytokine receptors. Until recently, the mechanism(s) responsible for downregulation of cytokine-mediated signaling was poorly understood. Studies have now identified a family of intracellular proteins that plays a key role in the suppression of cytokine signaling. These ***suppressor of cytokine signaling*** (SOCS) proteins regulate signal transduction by direct interactions with cytokine receptors and signaling proteins with a generic mechanism of targeting associated proteins for degradation. Given the central contribution of cytokines to many diseases, including the ones discussed below, the deregulation of normal SOCS may play a causal role in some of these diseases. On the other hand, the manipulation of SOCS function might provide potent therapeutic options in the future.

ROLE OF CYTOKINES AND CYTOKINE RECEPTORS IN DISEASE

Given the complex regulatory properties of cytokines, it is not surprising that overexpression or underexpression of cytokines or cytokine receptors has been implicated in many diseases. Here we discuss some examples of diseases with cytokine-associated pathophysiology.

Toxic Shock Syndrome

Toxic shock syndrome is initiated by the release of ***superantigen*** (enterotoxin) from certain microorganisms. For example, the toxins derived from *Staphylococcus aureus* or *Streptococcus pyogenes* cause a burst of cytokine production by T cells. The toxin does this by activating large numbers of $CD4^+$ T cells, which use certain V_β segments as part of their

T cell receptor (TCR). The toxin cross-links the V_β segment of the TCR with an MHC class II molecule expressed on APCs (see Fig. 9.8). It has been estimated that one in every five T cells can be activated by superantigens. Superantigen-activated T cells results in excessive production of cytokines that ultimately cause dysregulation of the cytokine network, leading to extremely high levels of IL-1 and TNFα. These cytokines induce systemic reactions, including fever, blood clotting, diarrhea, a drop in blood pressure, and shock. Sometimes these reactions are fatal.

Bacterial Septic Shock

Overproduction of cytokines is also associated with infections caused by certain gram-negative bacteria, including *Escherichia coli, Klebsiella pneumonia, Enterobacter aerogenes, Pseudomonas aeruginosa,* and *Neisseria meningitidis.* Endotoxins produced by these bacteria stimulate macrophages to overproduce IL-1 and TNFα, causing an often fatal form of bacterial septic shock.

Cancers

Several lymphoid and myeloid cancers have been shown to be associated with abnormally high levels of cytokines and/or cytokine receptor expression. Perhaps the best example of an association between malignancy and overproduction of both a cytokine and its receptor is seen in patients with adult T cell leukemia disease, which is strongly associated with human T cell leukemia virus 1 (HTLV-1). T cells infected with HTLV-1 constitutively produce IL-2 and express the high-affinity IL-2R in the absence of activation by antigen. This results in autocrine stimulation of infected T cells, leading to their uncontrolled growth. Other examples of malignancies associated with overproduction of cytokines include myelomas (neoplastic B cells), which produce large amounts of the autocrine IL-6, and Hodgkin's disease, a lymphoma in which the reactive milieu is the result of abundant cytokine production, particularly IL-5 (see Chapter 17).

Autoimmunity and Other Immune-Based Diseases

Much evidence suggests that T cells exert a controlling influence on the generation of autoantibodies and on the regulation of autoimmunity (see Chapter 12). It is likely that some of the observed phenomena are manifestations of the actions of T_H subset-derived cytokines, including IL-10, IFNγ, and IL-4. Several cytokine and cytokine receptor abnormalities have been shown to be associated with systemic autoimmune diseases. Some occur late in illness and are probably not causal, while others may be involved in dysregulation of immune responses and may help promote autoreactivity. The autoimmune disease systemic lupus erythematosus (SLE) has been shown to be associated with elevated levels of IL-10. Recent studies of cytokines involved in autoimmune diseases have examined whether skewing of the T_H cell subset phenotype contributes to disease initiation or disease progression. Although most of this work has been performed using experimental animal models of autoimmune disease, the importance of T_H2 cells in promoting systemic autoimmunity has been reported. Futher studies are needed to clearly elucidate the disease-related roles played by cytokines, cytokine receptors, and T_H subsets in autoimmunity.

Cytokines also play an important role in the pathophysiology of other immune-based diseases, including allergy, asthma, and inflammatory diseases (e.g., rheumatoid arthritis). Thus it is not surprising that many clinical features associated with these diseases are the result of cytokine receptor-mediated signaling and the biologic effects of such signaling (e.g., cell activation, cell death). Our understanding of the roles played by cytokines and cytokine receptors in disease manifestation continues to expand. Below, we discuss some of the fruits of such knowledge that have given rise to the development of antagonists used to treat patients with some of these diseases.

THERAPEUTIC AND DIAGNOSTIC EXPLOITATION OF CYTOKINES AND CYTOKINE RECEPTORS

Knowledge of the cellular and molecular components of immune responses to infectious microbes and, specifically, the roles played by cytokines in regulation and homeostasis of hematopoietic cells has opened opportunities for new forms of therapeutics. The many opportunities for clinical uses of cytokines, soluble cytokine receptors (antagonists), cytokine analogs, and anticytokine or anticytokine receptor antibody therapies have sparked a great deal of commercial interest in cytokines. These biologic therapeutics have shown promise in several ways.

Cytokine Inhibitors/Antagonists

Several naturally occurring soluble cytokine receptors have been identified in the bloodstream and extracellular fluids. These act, in vivo, as ***cytokine inhibitors,*** or ***antagonists,*** and are released from the cell surface as a result of enzymatic cleavage of the extracellular domain of the cytokine receptor. Circulating soluble cytokine receptors maintain their ability to bind to the cytokine for which the receptor is specific, thus neutralizing their activity. Examples of such inhibitors are those that bind to IL-2, IL-4, IL-6, IL-7, IFNγ, and TNF. Experimental use of soluble TNF receptors has led to the development of a new class of biologic response modifier drugs called ***TNF inhibitors.*** TNF inhibitors have shown significant clinical utility in the treatment of rheumatoid arthritis (RA). Patients with RA have increased levels of TNF and IL-1 in

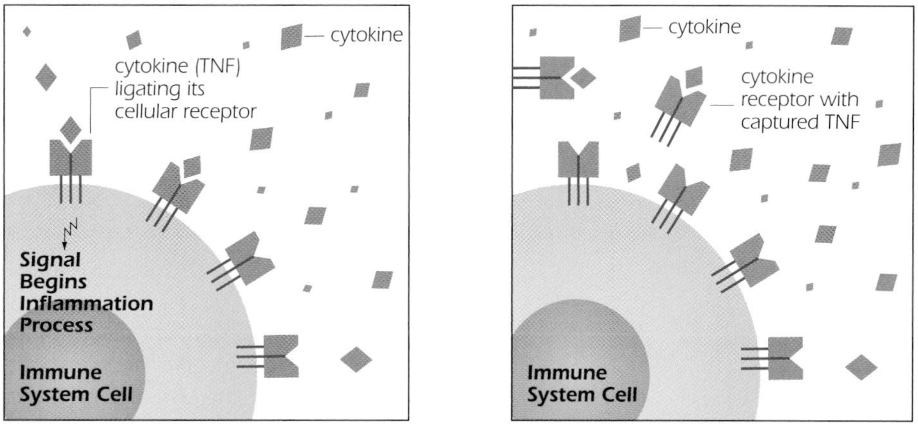

Figure 11.9. Soluble tumor necrosis factor (TNF) receptors can interfere with inflammatory properties of TNF.

their joints—a phenomenon that leads to RA-associated pain, swelling, stiffness, and other symptoms. TNF inhibitors (***soluble TNF receptor molecules***) compete with endogenously produced TNF for binding to TNF receptors (Fig. 11.9). Most RA patients treated with TNF inhibitors show significant improvement of their symptoms, although ~30% are nonresponsive to this treatment.

The soluble IL-2R has also been studied extensively. It is formed by the proteolytic release of a 45-kDa portion of the IL-2α chain (CD25) of the IL-2R. Chronic T cell activation is associated with very high bloodstream levels of soluble IL-2R. Thus it has been used as a clinical marker for chronic T cell activation in patients with certain autoimmune diseases and those undergoing transplant rejection.

Another well-characterized cytokine antagonist is the naturally occurring ***IL-1 receptor antagonist*** (IL-1Ra). This protein also plays a role in regulating the intensity of inflammatory responses by binding to the IL-1 receptor on $CD4^+$ T cells, thus preventing their activation. Binding of IL-1Ra to the IL-1 receptor does not mediate cell signaling through this receptor. IL-1Ra has been cloned and is currently under clinical investigation to determine whether it can be used as a therapeutic agent for chronic inflammatory diseases.

Reversing Cellular Deficiencies

Cytokines have been used to treat acute events such as cellular deficiencies arising from chemotherapy or radiotherapy by administration of growth factors (e.g., G-CSF or GM-CSF). As discussed earlier in this chapter, treatment with these hematopoietic growth factors escalates the rate of natural reconstitution of desired hematopoietic cell lineages.

Treatment of Immunodeficiencies

Cytokines have also been used to treat patients with immunodeficiency diseases, many of which are discussed in Chapter 17 . For example, patients with X-linked agammaglobulinemia have been treated successfully with G-CSF to reverse their disease-associated neutropenia. Patients suffering from a form of severe combined immunodeficiency disease (SCID) due to adenosine deaminase (ADA) deficiency—a disease that is often associated with a profound IL-2 deficiency—have been treated with recombinant human IL-2. Finally, several leukocyte adhesion deficiency diseases characterized by recurrent or progressive soft tissue infection, periodontitis, poor wound healing, and leukocytosis have been successfully treated with recombinant IFNγ to reduce the severity and frequency of infections, probably by increasing nonoxidative antimicrobial activity

Treatment of Cancer and Transplant Patients

Patients with cancer have also benefited from the use of cytokines in passive cellular immunotherapies that use ***lymphokine-activated killer*** (LAK) cells (Chapter 19). Culturing populations of NK cells or cytotoxic T cells in the presence of high concentrations of IL-2 generates effector cells with potent antitumor activities. The availability of recombinant IL-2 in large quantities has made the LAK cell plus IL-2 therapy feasible, and some melanoma and renal carcinoma patients have shown objective responses. Another variation of passive cellular immunotherapy is the concurrent use of IFNγ, which enhances the expression of MHC class II molecules and tumor-associated antigens on tumor cells, thereby augmenting the killing of tumor cells by the infused effector cells.

Cytokine receptor-specific antibodies have also proven useful in the treatment of certain cancers. The relative accessibility of particular cytokine receptor-positive leukemic cells has encouraged numerous trials with native as well as toxin-conjugated antibodies. In one subset of leukemia called adult T cell leukemia/lymphoma (ATLL), in which leukemic cells constitutively express the IL-2R α chain (CD25), antibodies to CD25 (also known as anti-Tac antibodies) have been shown to induce therapeutic responses in approximately one third of the patients treated.

Anti-CD25 therapy has also been used as part of a regimen of immunosuppressive therapy to treat patients receiving organ transplants. The rationale for such treatment is based on the chronic activation of alloreactive T cells caused by their exposure to alloantigens expressed by the grafted tissue. Such activation induces the expression of CD25 by these cells. Anti-CD25 therapy is often used together with other immunosuppressive drugs to dampen the host's immune response to the alloantigens, thus reducing the incidence of graft rejection. Chapter 18 contains additional information related to immunotherapies used to treat patients who have received organ transplants.

Treatment of Allergies and Asthma

Our current understanding of the functional properties of T_H2 cells and the roles played by specific cytokines they produce (e.g., IL-4, IL-13) in IgE production suggests that therapies that target these cytokines or their receptors may prove to be effective in the treatment of allergies and asthma (Chapter 14). Given the cross-antagonistic effects of T_H1 and T_H2 cells, it may be possible to skew the production of antibody away from IgE in response to a given allergen using strategies that selectively silence the undesired T_H2 subset. At present, this remains an experimental goal, which is being aggressively investigated in animal models. Promising results have emerged from clinical trials using a related strategy that specifically targets IL-4, the major cytokine responsible for promoting B cell isotype class switching to IgE (see Chapters 10 and 14). Injection of antibodies specific for IL-4 has been shown to dramatically decrease IL-4 production in mice. Another related strategy to treat asthma and allergic diseases involves the use of soluble IL-4 receptors, again, with promising, although preliminary results reported to date. The clinical applications of such research cannot be underestimated given the enormous number of individuals who suffer from allergies worldwide. Chapter 14 discusses other cytokine-based treatment strategies used in patients with allergies and asthma.

SUMMARY

1. Cytokines are low molecular weight antigen-nonspecific proteins that mediate cellular interactions involving immune, inflammatory, and hematopoietic systems.
2. Cytokines exhibit properties of pleiotropy and redundancy and often display synergism or antagonism with other cytokines.
3. Cytokines are short lived and may act locally either on the same cell that secreted it (autocrine) or on other cells (paracrine). Like hormones, they may act systemically (endocrine).
4. Cytokines have a wide variety of functional activities as illustrated by their ability to (1) regulate specific immune responses, (2) facilitate innate immune responses, (3) activate inflammatory responses, (4) affect leukocyte movement, and (5) stimulate hematopoiesis.
5. Subsets of $CD4^+$ T_H cells have been defined by the range of cytokines they produce. T_H1 cells secrete IL-2 and IFNγ (as well as several other cytokines) but not IL-4 or IL-5. Cytokines produced by these cells also activate other T cells, NK cells, and macrophages (cell-mediated immune responses). By contrast, T_H2 cells secrete IL-4 and IL-5 (as well as other cytokines), but not IL-2 or IFNγ and predominantly affect antibody responses.
6. Cytokines can act only on target cells that express receptors for that cytokine. Cytokine receptor expression is highly regulated, so that resting cells either do not express a given receptor or express a low- or intermediate-affinity version of that receptor. Increased levels of cytokine receptor expression or expression of high-affinity forms of a given receptor predispose target cells to respond to a cytokine.
7. The common γ chain is a cytokine receptor subunit used by several cytokine receptors as the signal transducing subunit, including IL-2, IL-4, IL-7, IL-9, and IL-15. This structural feature helps explain the redundancy and antagonism often exhibited by some cytokines.
8. Ligation of cytokine receptors by cytokines generates intracellular signals that result in the production of active transcription factors and, ultimately, gene expression. Binding of a cytokine to its cellular receptor often induces dimerization or polymerization of receptor polypeptides at the cell surface and permits association of JAK kinases with the receptor cytoplasmic domain. This association activates the kinases and causes phosphorylation of tyrosine residues in STATs. Once phosphorylated, the STAT transcription factors dimerize and subsequently translocate from the cytoplasm to the nucleus, where they bind to enhancer regions of genes induced by the cytokine. Suppression of cytokine signaling proteins downregulate signal transduction and helps terminate cytokine responses.
9. Overexpression or underexpression of cytokines or cytokine receptors has been implicated in several diseases, including bacterial toxic shock, bacterial sepsis, certain lymphoid and myeloid cancers, and autoimmunity.

10. Cytokine-related therapies offer promise for the treatment of certain immunodeficiencies, in preventing graft rejection, and in treating certain cancers. The use of cytokine-related therapies is best seen in (1) hematopoietic growth factors (G-CSF, GM-CSF) to reverse certain cellular deficiencies associated with chemotherapy or radiotherapy, (2) anti-IL-2R therapy to help reduce graft rejection, and (3) IL-2 to generate LAK cells (NK and cytotoxic T cells) employed in the treatment of patients with certain cancers.

REFERENCES

Alexander WS (2002): Suppressor of cytokine signaling (SOCS) in the immune system. *Nature Reviews, Immunology* 2:410.

Campbell JJ, Butcher EC (2000): Chemokines in tissue-specific and microenvironment-specific lymphocyte homing. *Curr Opin Immunol* 12:336.

Cocchi RI, DeVico AL, Garzino-Demo A, Arya SK, Gallo RC, Lusso P (1995): Identification of RANTES,MIP-1α and MIP-1β as the major HIV-suppressive factors produced by CD8$^+$ T cells. *Science* 270:1811.

DeVries ME, Kelvin DJ (1999): On the edge: the physiological and pathophysiological role of chemokines during inflammatory and immunological responses. *Semin Immunol* 11:95.

Dong C, Flavell RA (2001): T_H1 and T_H2 cells. *Curr Opin Hematol* 8:47.

Fernandez-Botran R, Crespo FA, Sun X (2000): Soluble cytokine receptors in biological therapy. *Expert Opin Biol Ther* 2:585.

Ihle JN (1995): Cytokine receptor signaling. *Nature* 377:591.

Kisseleva T, Bhattacharya S, Braunstein J, Schindler CW (2000): Signaling through the JAK/STAT pathway, recent advances and future challenges. *Gene* 20:1.

Leonard WJ (2001): Cytokines and immunodeficiency diseases. *Nat Rev Immunol* 1:200.

Minami Y, Kono T, Miyazaki T, Taniguchi T. (1993): The IL-2 receptor complex: its structure, function, and target genes. *Ann Rev Immunol* 11:245.

Rubinstein M, Dinarello CA, Oppenheim JJ, Hertzhog P (1999): Recent advances in cytokines, cytokine receptors, and signal transduction. *Cytokine Growth Factor Rev* 9:175.

Waldman H, Gililand LK, Cobbold SP, Lane G (1999): Immunotherapy. In Paul WE (ed): Fundamental Immunology, 4th ed. New York: Lipincott-Raven.

Ward SG, Bacon K, Westwick J (1998): Chemokines and T lymphocytes: more than an attraction. *Immunity* 9:1.

REVIEW QUESTIONS

For each question, choose the ONE BEST answer or completion.

1. Once a T_H1 or T_H2 response has been generated, it is perpetuated by cytokines that downregulate the opposing response. If a humoral response has been stimulated, which cytokines will maintain that response?

A) IL-4 and IL-10
B) IL-4 and IL-5
C) IL-4 and TNFβ
D) IL-1 and IL-6

2. A patient with active rheumatoid arthritis feels systemically ill with low-grade fever, malaise, morning stiffness, and fatigue. The protein(s) or cytokine(s) most likely to be responsible for these symptoms are

A) rheumatoid factor.
B) TNF and IL-1.
C) IL-4 and IL-10.
D) Complement components 1–9
E) altered γ-globulin

3. When IL-2 is secreted by antigen-specific T cells activated due to presentation of antigen by APCs, what happens to naive antigen-nonspecific T cells in the vicinity?

A) They proliferate due to their exposure to IL-2.
B) They often undergo apoptosis.
C) They begin to express IL-2R.
D) They secrete cytokines associated with their T_H phenotype.
E) Nothing happens.

4. IL-1, IL-6, and TNFα are proinflammatory cytokines that are known to

A) cause increased vascular permeability.
B) act in concert with chemokines to promote migration of inflammatory cells to sites of infection.
C) initiate acute-phase responses.
D) have endogenous pyrogen properties.
E) All of the above.

5. Which of the following cytokines plays a role in terminating inflammatory responses?

A) IL-2
B) IL-4
C) TGFβ
D) IFNα
E) IL-3

6. Assuming there were no other compensatory mechanisms to replace IL-8 function, which of the following would be preserved as a functional activity in an IL-8 knockout mouse strain?

A) activation of neutrophils
B) attraction of neutrophils to sites of tissue damage
C) wound healing
D) extravasation of neutrophils
E) reduction of cytokine production by T_H1 cells

7. Superantigens cause a burst of cytokine production by T cells due to their ability to cross-link

A) the V_β segments of T cell receptors with MHC class II molecules on APCs.
B) the V_α segments of T cell receptors with MHC class II molecules on APCs.
C) T cell receptors and CD3.
D) multiple cytokine receptors on a large population of T cells.
E) CD3.

CASE STUDY

A 7-year-old boy with an infected wound on his leg is admitted to the emergency department. His mother states that a high fever with diarrhea occurred during the last 12 hours. Within the last 2 hours he had become very lethargic, was unable to stand, and was very disoriented. The attending physician observes that his blood pressure is dangerously low and suspects that the boy is suffering from bacterial septic shock caused by the wound infection. Discuss the etiology of bacterial septic shock as well as the roll of cytokines in the pathogenesis of this disease. Speculate on future therapeutic strategies that might be employed by using monoclonal antibodies or other biologic agents to treat this disease.

ANSWERS TO REVIEW QUESTIONS

1. ***A*** Humoral immune responses are facilitated by cytokines produced by T_H2 cells, which produce IL-4 and IL-10, among other cytokines. IL-4 activates B cells together with IL-5, which is also produced by T_H2 cells. IL-10 inhibits T_H1 cells, thereby inhibiting macrophage activation.

2. ***B*** Patients with rheumatoid arthritis have elevated levels of proinflammatory cytokines TNF and IL-1 in their joints, which plays a key role in the pain, swelling, stiffness, and other symptoms associated with this disease.

3. ***E*** Cytokines secreted by antigen-activated T cells regulate only the activities of other cells involved in that immune response by binding to cytokine receptors (e.g., high-affinity IL-2R) expressed by these cells. Such cytokine receptors are upregulated on only antigen-activated T cells that bear the appropriate T cell receptor for that antigen; they are not upregulated on antigen-nonspecific T cells in the vicinity; thus these cells will not be activated by IL-2.

4. ***E***

5. ***C*** Among the cytokines listed, TGFβ plays a role in terminating inflammatory responses by promoting the accumulation and proliferation of fibroblasts and the deposition of extracellular matrix proteins required for tissue repair.

6. ***E*** IL-8 plays no role in regulation of cytokine production by T_H1 cells-a biologic property ascribed to IL-10 produced by T_H2 cells. Therefore, functional integrity of T_H1 would be predicted in IL-8 knockout mice. IL-8 chemotactically attracts and activates neutrophils and induces their adherence to vascular endothelium and extravasation (activities that should be deficient in IL-8 knockouts). Because these activities are important for wound healing, this phenomenon would also be predicted to be deficient in such mice.

7. ***A*** Superantigens bind simultaneously to MHC class II molecules and to the V_β domain of the T cell receptor activating all T cells bearing a particular V_β domain. Thus they activate large numbers of T cells (5–25%), regardless of their antigen specificity, causing them to release harmful quantities of cytokines.

ANSWER TO CASE STUDY

Bacterial septic shock is a condition that can develop within a few hours following infection by certain gram-negative bacteria, including *Escherichia coli, Klebsiella pneumonia, Pseudomonas aeruginosa, Enterobacter aerogenes,* and *Neisseria meningitidis.* The symptoms are often fatal and include a drop in blood pressure, fever, diarrhea, and widespread blood clotting in various organs. It develops when bacterial cell wall endotoxins stimulate macrophages to overproduce IL-1 and TNF-α. Therapeutic strategies using monoclonal antibodies capable of neutralizing the effects of IL-1 and TNF-α or antagonists such as IL-1 receptor antagonist (IL-1Ra) may offer hope for the treatment of bacterial septic shock in humans.

12

TOLERANCE AND AUTOIMMUNITY

The immune system functions to protect the host from invasion by foreign organisms. However, this protective response can cause damage to the host if it is directed to the individual's own antigens often referred to as ***self antigens.*** Therefore, the immune system has developed a series of checks and balances that enable it to distinguish dangerous from harmless signals and allow it to respond to foreign but not self antigens. Both innate and adaptive responses have evolved to engage in this endeavor. This chapter focuses on the adaptive immune responses that are the basis for tolerance to self antigens.

One of the earliest experiments that demonstrated tolerance was performed by Ray Owens in 1945. He showed that dizygotic cattle twins, which shared a common vascular system in utero, were mutually tolerant of skin grafts from one another as adults. Thus "foreign" antigens expressed by cells of the other twin had produced long-lasting tolerance. These observations provided the basis for classic experiments by Peter Medawar and co-workers in the 1950s, which resulted in their receiving the Nobel Prize. Medawar first showed that adult mice of strain A rejected skin grafts from mice of strain B that differed in expression of MHC molecules. However, if mice of strain A were injected within 24 h after birth with bone marrow stem cells from strain B, they would not reject skin grafts from the donor B strain when they grew to adulthood. This phenomenon came to be known as ***neonatal tolerance.*** The basis for neonatal tolerance is that the recipient mouse becomes chimeric with T cells and APCs derived from both the host and the donor stem cells. Mature T cells become tolerant to the MHC antigens of the donor cells because the developing T cells in these mice are negatively selected on APCs from the host and donor.

CENTRAL TOLERANCE

Tolerance is defined as a state of unresponsiveness to antigen. It occurs when the interaction of an antigen with antigen-specific lymphocytes results in signals that either do not activate or inactivate the cell. Only cells with antigen-specific receptors—that is, lymphocytes—can be tolerized. As a consequence of the tolerizing interaction, the cell or the individual exposed to the antigen is said to be tolerant. Tolerance induced during the early stages of lymphocyte development is referred to as ***central tolerance,*** whereas tolerance induced in mature lymphocytes is referred to as ***peripheral tolerance.*** Central tolerance occurs in the primary lymphoid organs, namely, the bone marrow for B cells and the thymus for T cells.

The process of generating diversity in B cell receptors (BCRs) and T cell receptors (TCRs) inevitably generates receptors that can recognize self antigens. B and T cells with receptors for self antigen are referred to as ***autoreactive.*** Germline-encoded autoreactive B cells are generally tolerized in the bone marrow where they arise, and germline-encoded autoreactive T cells are tolerized in the thymus as part of a process known as ***negative selection*** (Chapter 8).

Contributed by Linda Spatz and Betty Diamond

Immunology: A Short Course, Fifth Edition, By Richard Coico, Geoffrey Sunshine, and Eli Benjamini
ISBN 0-471-22689-0

Negative selection ensures that the majority of B and T cells that emerge into the periphery react only with foreign antigens.

Mechanisms for Maintaining Self Tolerance

The immune system has developed several mechanisms for maintaining central tolerance in the B and T cell compartments. They include anergy, deletion, and clonal ignorance. In addition, receptor editing has been demonstrated to be an important mechanism for maintaining tolerance in naive B cells. Which mechanism of tolerance is employed and under what conditions it is implemented are explored below.

Anergy, Receptor Editing, Deletion, and Clonal Ignorance

Anergy is defined as the functional inactivation of a cell, resulting in nonresponsiveness upon contact with self antigen. Anergic B cells cannot be activated to proliferate and differentiate into antibody-secreting cells upon engagement of their BCRs with antigen. Likewise, ligation of the TCRs of anergic T cells does not activate them to proliferate and differentiate into functional T cells that produce cytokines and cytokine receptors. Evidence for B cell anergy was first observed by Nossal and Pike in 1980, who demonstrated that when immature IgM^+ B cells were exposed to an antibody specific for IgM that cross-linked the IgM, the cells lost their ability to differentiate and secrete antibody. B cell anergy has been shown more recently in transgenic mouse systems in which anti-self B cells are generated by introducing rearranged immunoglobulin genes into the germline of mice.

In the late 1960s Bretscher and Cohn hypothesized that B cells specific for T-dependent antigens require two signals to be activated; the first signal provided by antigen and the second signal provided by T cells. They also hypothesized that in the absence of the second signal B cells would be rendered unresponsive. We now know that this second signal can be provided by the engagement of CD40 ligand (CD40L) on the surface of a T cell with CD40 expressed on a B cell. Studies using transgenic mouse models confirm that B cells exposed to self antigen in the absence of T cell help may undergo anergy induction (Fig. 12.1). Anergic B cells cannot successfully compete with B cells specific for foreign antigen in order to gain entry into B cell follicles in the spleen and lymph nodes. Therefore, the self reactive B cells remain excluded from the follicles and eventually die by apoptosis.

T cells also require two signals to be activated (Chapter 10). Signal one is provided by the MHC–peptide complex. A second signal is provided by an interaction between costimulatory molecules expressed by professional antigen-presenting cells (APCs), such as mature dendritic cells and B cells and their ligands on T cells. A major costimulatory signal is provided by ligation of B7-1 (CD80) and/or B7-2 (CD86) expressed on the APCs with CD28 expressed on the T cell. Delivery of the first signal leads to the induction of several transcription factors, one of which binds to the promoter region of the interleukin 2 (IL-2) gene, allowing for its transcription in the T cell. As a result of the B7–CD28 interaction, the half-life of mRNA specific for IL-2 is increased, and IL-2 protein is synthesized. If the first signal is not accompanied by the costimulatory B7–CD28 interaction, however, the IL-2 mRNA is rapidly degraded, and IL-2 protein is not made. Thus in the absence of costimulation, as occurs when cells that do not express costimulatory molecules present antigen, the activation process is aborted and the T cell is anergized (Fig. 12.2).

Receptor editing is the process whereby a rearranged immunoglobulin variable H or L chain gene undergoes a secondary rearrangement such that an upstream V region replaces it, thereby altering (editing) the receptor specificity (see Chapters 6 and 7). This is preceded by reexpression of *RAG-1* and *RAG-2* genes. It has been postulated that receptor editing has evolved as a mechanism for averting autoreactivity, since it leads to a BCR or a TCR with a new specificity that often lacks autoreactivity. Evidence for B cell receptor editing was first observed in the bone marrow of mice transgenic for an antibody to double-stranded DNA (dsDNA) and

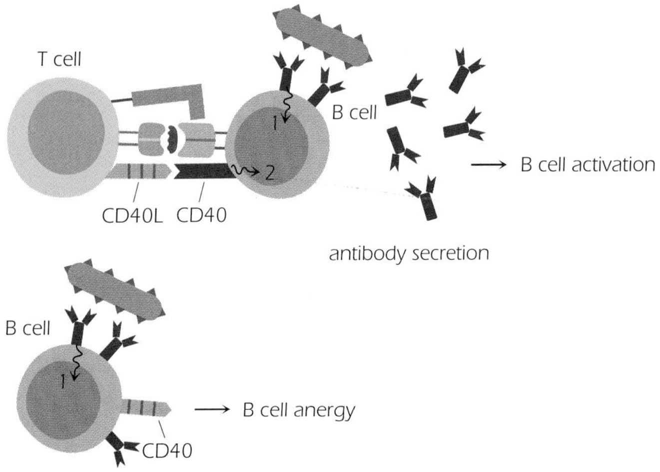

Figure 12.1. Lack of co-stimulation leads to B cell anergy. Two signals are required for B cell activation by a T-dependent antigen. Signal 1 is provided by antigen binding to and cross-linking the BCR. Signal 2 is provided by the interaction of CD40L expressed on the T cell with CD40 on the B cell. In the absence of this second costimulatory signal, B cells fail to be activated and are anergized.

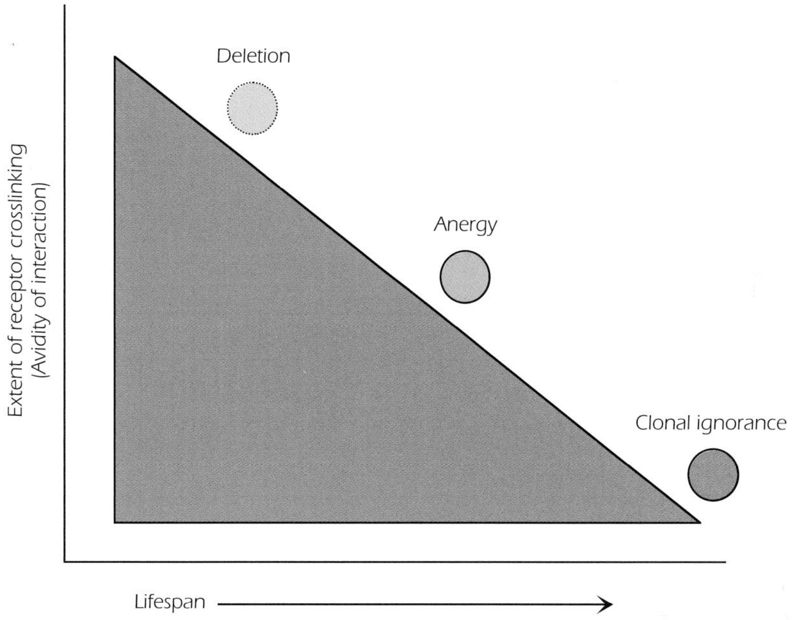

Figure 12.2. The life span of an autoreactive B cells is directly related to the extent of receptor cross-linking, which depends on the avidity of interaction between the immunoglobulin receptor and the autoantigen.

in mice transgenic for an antibody to an endogenous MHC class I antigen. BCR editing has also been observed in immature B cells in the spleen. More recently, receptor editing has been observed at the V_{α} locus of double positive T cells undergoing negative selection in the thymus.

Deletion is the mechanism by which autoreactive B and T cells are eliminated from the repertoire. Apoptosis (programmed cell death) is the basis for much of the negative selection of developing T and B cells in the thymus and bone marrow, respectively. Double positive T cells that bind with high affinity to antigens plus MHC in the thymus have been shown to undergo rapid deletion. Likewise, immature B cells that bind with strong affinity to self antigen in the bone marrow undergo deletion.

Clonal ignorance refers to a state whereby autoreactive lymphocytes are neither anergized, deleted, nor receptor edited. Instead, they co-exist with antigen and remain in an unactivated state because of their weak affinity for the autoantigen or a low concentration of autoantigen. Unlike anergic cells, clonally ignorant cells are not inherently unresponsive to antigen. In fact, they can be activated under certain conditions; therefore, their presence poses a potential threat to the host. For instance, if B cells with a low affinity for a self antigen undergo somatic mutation and acquire a higher affinity for self antigen, they can subsequently be activated by the self antigen. In addition, clonally ignorant T cells exposed to a low level of self peptide can be activated if the concentration of the self peptide is increased.

Immature B or T cells are more easily tolerized than mature lymphocytes. The strength or avididty of interaction of the BCR or TCR with its autoantigen determines whether the autoreactive cell is anergized or deleted. For B cells, avidity depends on affinity of interaction between the immunoglobulin receptor and its antigen, density of the receptors on the surface of the B cell, and the nature and concentration of the autoantigen. The higher the affinity of the antibody for its antigen and the more immunoglobulin receptor that is expressed on the B cell membrane, the greater the avidity of the antigen–antibody interaction. This directly correlates with the extent of immunoglobulin receptor cross-linking. B cells with a high avidity for an autoantigen are targeted for deletion, while those with a more moderate avidity are targeted for anergy (Fig. 12.3). B cells with a weak avidity for autoantigen become clonally ignorant. The nature of the autoantigen determines its ability

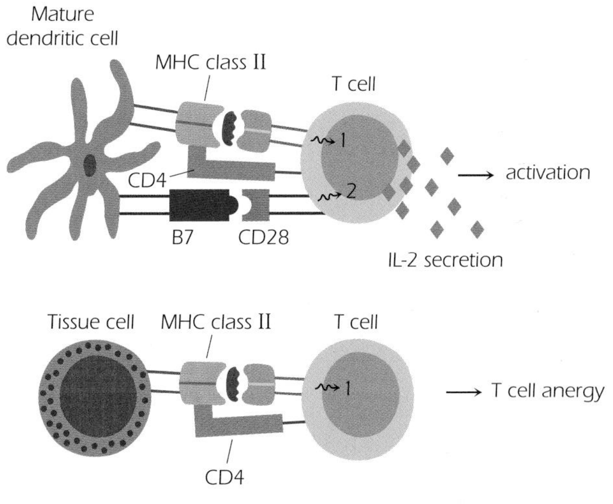

Figure 12.3. Antigen recognition in the absence of costimulation leads to T cell anergy. Two signals are required for T cell activation. Signal 1 is provided by the recognition of peptide plus MHC. Signal 2 is provided by the interaction of a costimulatory molecule (B7) expressed on the surface of an APC (mature dendritic cell) with a receptor (CD28) on the surface of a T cell. If a T cell receives signal 1 in the absence of signal 2, it is anergized.

to induce BCR cross-linking. For instance, multivalent and membrane-bound antigens mediate more extensive receptor cross-linking than monovalent or soluble antigens. B cells that encounter membrane-bound autoantigen are more likely to be deleted, and those that encounter soluble antigen are anergized.

In the thymus, the affinity of the TCR for peptide plus MHC, the level of TCR on the surface of the T cell, and the level of MHC molecules expressed on the surface of the APC determine avidity and influence T cell selection. All T cells that recognize peptide plus MHC expressed on epithelial cells in the cortex are first positively selected. Then at the corticomedullary junction T cells with a high avidity for peptide plus MHC are negatively selected and are either deleted or receptor edited.

Finally, the microenvironment in which the autoreactive lymphocyte encounters autoantigen seems to influence cell fate. Recent studies suggest that other cells that come in contact with autoreactive B cells may provide signals that determine whether the B cell is deleted or edited. In mice a population of bone marrow stromal cells has been identified and shown to protect immature autoreactive B cells from undergoing apoptosis upon BCR cross-linking by autoantigen. These cells express a marker that is also found on natural-killer (NK) cells, and they induce the reexpression of *RAG* genes, enabling autoreactive B cells to undergo receptor editing. The depletion of these stromal cells from the bone marrow results in deletion of immature autoreactive B cells rather than receptor editing. Studies of the thymus suggest that cortical epithelial cells that present peptide plus MHC to double positive thymocytes tend to facilitate receptor editing rather than apoptosis; by contrast, presentation of peptide plus MHC by bone marrow–derived APCs favors apoptosis. This may be because cortical epithelial cells lack the signals that may be required for thymocyte apoptosis.

PERIPHERAL TOLERANCE

Occasionally autoreactive B and T cells escape negative selection and enter the periphery. In addition, B cells undergo somatic mutation in the periphery and sometimes the mutations result in the acquisition of autoreactive specificities. Therefore, peripheral tolerance has evolved as a safety net to catch autoreactive B and T cells that escape to or arise in the periphery. Mechanisms of peripheral tolerance include not only anergy and deletion but also activation-induced cell death and the induction of regulatory T cells. Although receptor editing has been shown to occur in the periphery, it is not yet clear whether the objective of peripheral editing is to avert autoreactivity.

T cell anergy is believed to be a major mechanism for inducing unresponsiveness to self antigen that is encountered in the periphery. Cells from tissues such as the pancreas kidney, liver, and other organs do not normally express costimulatory molecules. Thus antigens presented by these cells are likely to induce anergy rather than activation. Similarly, B cells encountering antigen in the periphery but lacking T cell help will undergo anergy induction. Deletion also occurs in the periphery.

Fas–Fas L INTERACTIONS

Fas-mediated apoptosis is thought to play a critical role in the removal of mature autoreactive B and T lymphocytes. Fas is a monomer expressed by activated lymphocytes and is a member of the tumor necrosis factor (TNF) receptor family. The ligation of Fas by Fas ligand (Fas L), a member of the TNF family of membrane proteins, delivers an apoptotic signal to the cell expressing Fas. Fas L is expressed by several cell types, including activated T cells and certain epithelial cells. Fas L is a trimer; when it binds to Fas, it causes it to trimerize. This then activates a "death" domain in Fas that interacts with the death domains of several cytosolic adaptor proteins, the major one being Fas-associated death domain (FADD). This then triggers the activation of a series of cysteine proteases, known as caspases, resulting in apoptosis of the cell (Fig. 12.4).

The importance of Fas–Fas L interactions was initially shown by studying mouse strains with an autoimmune condition that causes them to accumulate enormous numbers of T cells in the spleen and lymph nodes. The defects in these mice, strains known as *lpr* (for lymphoproliferative) and *gld* (for generalized lymphoproliferative disease), are shown to be mutations in Fas and Fas L, respectively. These mutations prevent the mice from deleting autoreactive B and T cells, resulting in an elevated lymphocyte population. People with a mutated Fas have also been described; they have an autoimmune condition known as ***autoimmune lymphoproliferative syndrome*** (ALPS), with characteristics similar to those described for the mutant mice. Fas–Fas L mediated apoptosis has been shown to play a role in eliminating autoreactive T cells in the periphery, and recent studies suggest that it may be involved in mediating negative selection of thymocytes as well. Anergized B cells are also susceptible to Fas-mediated apoptosis.

REGULATORY/SUPPRESSOR T CELLS

In the early 1970s, experiments suggested that a specialized population of T cells suppressed the responses of other lymphocytes. However, the inability to isolate and clone a suppressor T cell population led to skepticism about whether this population really existed. Renewed interest in ***T suppressor cells*** emerged in the 1990s when a population of $CD4^+$ T cells with the ability to downregulate T cell function was identified. These T suppressor or regulatory T cells (T_{reg}) as they are often called, were observed to express CD25, the IL-2 receptor α chain and are therefore ***$CD4^+$ $CD25^+$***. CD25 is not unique to suppressor T cells and is also expressed on

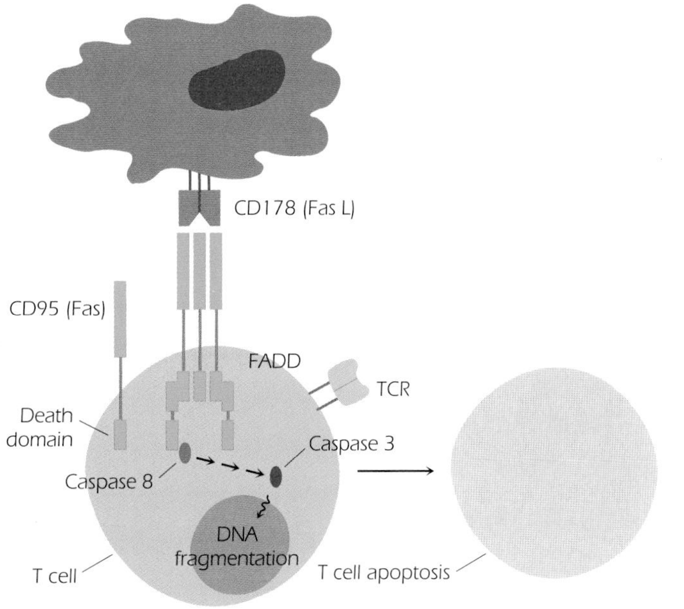

Figure 12.4. Fas mediated apoptosis of T cells. The ligation of FasL to Fas causes Fas to trimerize. This activates the death domain in Fas, which then interacts with the death domain in FADD. This induces the activation of a caspase cascade, which ultimately leads to apoptosis of the Fas-expressing cell.

activated, effector $CD4^+$ T cells. This has made it difficult to isolate a pure suppressor T cell subset for functional studies.

$CD4^+CD25^+$ suppressor T cells constitute approximately 10% of peripheral $CD4^+$ cells. When athymic nude mice (*nu/nu*), which are deficient in all T cells (Chapter 5), were reconstituted with $CD4^+$ T cells that were depleted of this $CD4^+CD25^+$ T suppressor population, they developed autoimmune diseases, such as thyroiditis, gastritis, insulitis, and glomerulonephritis. However, disease could be prevented if $CD4^+CD25^+$ T suppressor cells were inoculated into these mice along with $CD4^+CD25^-$ T cells, thus demonstrating the role of $CD25^+$ T cells in maintaining tolerance. $CD4^+CD25^+$ T suppressor cells have also been shown to suppress graft versus host disease (discussed in Chapter 18) induced by $CD4^+CD25^-$ T cells as well as the development of diabetes in mice genetically predisposed to diabetes (nonobese diabetic, NOD, mice).

$CD4^+CD25^+$ T suppressor cells were initially discovered in mice but have since been found in humans as well. They appear to be derived from a unique lineage of $CD4^+$ T cells that is selected during T cell development in the thymus. *They produce either no or very low levels of IL-2.* Some may produce the immunosuppressive cytokine tumor growth factor (TGFβ), but this is not a requirement for their suppressive activity. They express the chemokine receptors CCR4 and CCR8, which aid in their migration to inflamed organs and draining lymph nodes. They constitutively express CTLA-4, although the significance of this is not yet known.

$CD4^+CD25^+$ T suppressor cells require specific TCR engagement to be activated but do not proliferate in response to TCR-mediated stimulation. Once they are activated, their *suppressive function is antigen-nonspecific* and requires contact with responder T cells (Fig. 12.5). They inhibit the proliferation and activation of $CD4^+$ and $CD8^+$ T cells and prevent the transcription of IL-2 in these responder T cells.

$CD4^+CD25^+$ T suppressor cells may be clinically relevant. Enhancement of these T cells may be important for treating autoimmune diseases and for suppression of allograft rejection. Depletion of these T cells may enhance immune responses to tumor vaccines and vaccines for infectious agents such as HIV.

Two other types of T cells that have suppressive activity have been identified within the $CD4^+$ T cell subset. These are known as ***type 1 T regulatory cells*** (Tr1) and ***T_H3 cells.*** These suppressor T cells appear to be either $CD25^-$ or $CD25^{low}$ and are distinguished by their cytokine profiles. Tr1 cells produce high levels of IL-10, and TGF-β and mediate suppression via these cytokines. They produce very little or no IL-2 and IL-4. Tr1 cells seem to be involved in mediating protection against inflammatory bowel disease in mice and autoimmune diabetes in rats. Studies suggest that these T cells can arise when $CD4^+$ T cells are activated in the presence of IL-10. T_H3 cells have been identified in oral tolerance studies (see below). They are distinct from T_H1 and T_H2 subsets of $CD4^+$ T cells. They primarily produce TGF-β and mediate suppression via secretion of this cytokine. They also produce variable amounts of IL-10 and IL-4, which are responsible for their differentiation. The similarity and differences between $CD4^+CD25^+$, Tr1, and T_H3 regulatory/suppressor T cells and their possible relationship to one another are currently under intense investigation.

ORAL TOLERANCE

Oral tolerance is defined as the lack of a humoral or cellular immune response to ingested food antigens. It is

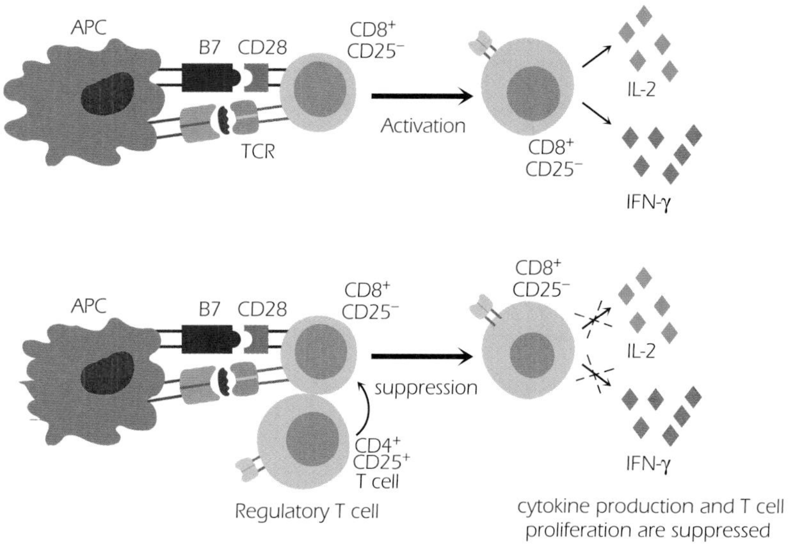

Figure 12.5. T cell suppression. Regulatory $CD4^+CD25^+$ T cell induces cell contact mediated suppression of the $CD8^+CD25^-$ responder T cell.

mediated by T cells, and the mechanisms for maintaining it depend on the dose of ingested antigen. Low-dose antigen induces T_H3 suppressor T cells, whereas high-dose antigen induces T cell anergy or deletion. Oral tolerance is first initiated when orally administered antigen encounters gut-associated lymphoid tissue (GALT), including the epithelial cells of the villi, intraepithelial lymphocytes, lamina propria lymphocytes, and lymphoid nodules of the Peyer's patches (PP). Dendritic cells (DCs) are the major APCs in GALT and thus process and present most ingested antigens, although other APCs such as macrophages, B cells, and epithelial cells are also present. When large doses of food antigen are administered, not all is degraded by the time it reaches the small intestine; consequently, some food antigens get absorbed intact into the systemic circulation. The antigen is then processed and presented by peripheral APCs in the absence of co-stimulatory interactions, which results in unresponsiveness of T_H1 cells.

Low-dose tolerance is induced locally, in the gut. The cytokine milieu of the GALT contains elevated levels of IL-4, IL-10, and TGFβ, which promotes differentiation into T_H2 and T_H3 cells and inhibits differentiation into T_H1 cells. T_H3 cells, as previously discussed, mediate suppression via secretion of TGFβ. Triggering of T_H3 cells is antigen specific, but their suppression is antigen nonspecific.

Several laboratory studies have demonstrated that low doses of oral antigen can suppress models of autoimmune diseases in animals. ***Experimental autoimmune encephalomyelitis*** (EAE) is an animal model for ***multiple sclerosis*** (MS). Rats or mice immunized with myelin basic protein (MBP) or proteolipid protein (PLP) in complete Freund's adjuvant (CFA) develop cellular infiltration in the myelin sheaths of the central nervous system, leading to demyelination and eventual paralysis. These symptoms mimic those observed in MS patients. Mice fed low doses of MBP before injection with MBP are protected from developing EAE by regulatory T_H3 cells, which are induced. Similarly, oral administration of type II collagen suppresses collagen-induced arthritis in susceptible rodent strains, and oral administration of thyroglobulin suppresses autoimmune thyroiditis in mice.

Studies using orally administered antigen to treat patients with autoimmune diseases have met with limited success. The cytokine environment and the presence of certain co-stimulatory molecules may influence the response to oral antigen. It has been reported that the cytokine milieu in the human gut may differ from that in the mouse and may favor a T_H1 response rather than a T_H2 response. These differences will have to be characterized more carefully before oral tolerance can be used as an effective therapy for autoimmune diseases.

IMMUNE PRIVILEGE

There are several sites in the body that do not develop immune responses to pathogens, tumor cells, and histoincompatible tissue transplants. These sites, known as ***immune privileged sites,*** include the ***eye, testis, brain, ovary,*** and ***placenta.*** The eye most clearly exemplifies an immune privileged site. This is illustrated by the fact that corneal transplants in humans do not require tissue matching or immunosuppressive therapy in order to be accepted. It was previously thought that immune protection in privileged sites was due to lack of lymphatic drainage and the blood barrier that prevented inflammatory cells from reaching antigens in these sites. However, it is now known that other factors, such as immunosuppressive cytokines and the expression of Fas L, play a predominant role in establishing immune privilege. Studies have demonstrated that Fas L is expressed on several types of cells found in immune privileged sites and the interaction of these Fas L-expressing cells with infiltrating Fas-expressing inflammatory T cells leads to apoptosis of these T cells. Human retinal pigment epithelial cells and corneal endothelial cells have been observed to express Fas L and to induce apoptosis of inflammatory T cells. The success of corneal transplants in mice has been shown to be due to expression of Fas L by cells of the graft, which then eliminate infiltrating Fas^+ T cells, thereby preventing inflammatory damage to the graft. When corneas from mice lacking functional Fas L (*gld* mice) are transplanted into allogeneic recipients, the grafts are rejected because infiltrating Fas^+ lymphocytes can no longer be eliminated by Fas L-mediated apoptosis.

AUTOIMMUNITY AND DISEASE

Tolerance to self is an evolutionary phenomenon that must remain intact for normal growth, development, and species survival. When something occurs to destroy the integrity of self-tolerance (and there are various exogenous and endogenous influences that can precipitate such an event), an immune response to self, ***autoimmunity,*** may develop.

The consequences of autoimmunity may vary from minimal to catastrophic, depending on the extent to which the integrity of self-tolerance has been affected. Thus a distinction should be made between autoimmune responses and autoimmune disease, in which recognition of self antigen evokes pathologic consequences that can involve antibody, complement, immune complexes, and cell-mediated immunity.

We now discuss some of the more common and better-understood autoimmune diseases, together with their pathophysiology (mechanisms of disease). Several issues need to be addressed before we discuss specific autoimmune diseases. One concerns the definition of autoimmune diseases. A growing number of diseases are suspected of having an autoimmune basis, but the evidence for their autoimmune origin may not be straightforward. The criteria used to redefine an idiopathic disease (i.e., a disease with unknown origin) to one that has an autoimmune basis are discussed.

A second issue involves the cause of those diseases. Most infectious diseases can be ascribed to a single agent; some genetic diseases are due to a defect in a single gene. In contrast, it is much more difficult to attribute the agent or agents responsible for autoimmune diseases. The most notable quality of autoimmune disease is that the cause is multifactorial, involving both genetic and environmental influences.

A third issue is that some autoimmune phenomena may occur ***secondary*** to a disease, and although significantly contributing to the pathology, the disease should not be considered a primary autoimmune disease.

Criteria for Autoimmune Disease

Guidelines have been established for classifying specific diseases as having an autoimmune cause using three types of evidence, as discussed below.

Transferring autoantibody or self-reactive lymphocytes to a host and reproducing the disease is the most definitive ***direct proof.*** For ethical reasons, this criterion has been achieved in only a few circumstances in humans. It can occur when pathogenic antibody is transmitted transplacentally from mother to fetus, in conditions such as ***neonatal myasthenia gravis, Graves disease,*** and ***polychondritis.*** To provide an approach to establishing the pathogenic potential of a T cell population, severe combined immunodeficiency disease (SCID) mice, which lack an immune system, can be used as a living "tissue culture flask" for human cells. For example, peripheral blood lymphocytes from patients with ***systemic lupus erythematosus*** (SLE) transferred into these immunologically depleted mice have already been shown to induce immune complex lesions in the kidney of the mice, mimicking human lupus nephritis.

Indirect evidence must be used because of the difficulty in providing direct proof for autoimmune mechanisms. One strategy is *to identify the target antigen in humans, isolate the homologous antigen in an animal model, and reproduce the disease in the experimental animal* by administering the offending antigen. Among the examples in which this approach has succeeded are the induction of ***autoimmune thyroiditis*** with thyroglobulin, ***myasthenia gravis*** with acetylcholine receptor, ***autoimmune uveitis*** with uveal S antigen, and ***autoimmune orchitis*** with sperm. Problems arise, however, for human diseases for which a suitable experimental animal model has not been found, when multifactorial events must occur before the disease arises, when several autoantigens are involved, and when the pathogenic antigen is not known.

Another line of indirect evidence that has been used is to study ***genetically determined animal models.*** New Zealand black mice (NZB) spontaneously develop autoimmune hemolytic anemia, whereas New Zealand white mice (NZW) do not. $(NZB \times NZW)F_1$ animals develop high levels of anti-nuclear antibodies and have been used as a model for human SLE.

The third type of indirect evidence is based on *isolating self-reactive antibodies or T cells from the target organs.* As examples, antierythrocyte antibodies can be eluted from erythrocytes in patients with ***autoimmune hemolytic anemia,*** anti-DNA antibodies can be isolated from patients with ***SLE,*** and cytotoxic T cells have been found in the thyroid of patients with ***Graves disease.*** However, the pathologic significance of these antibodies or T cells has not been easy to establish.

Circumstantial evidence for autoimmunity is based on clinical clues, including familial tendency, lymphocyte infiltration, MHC association, and most important, clinical improvement with immunosuppressive agents. For most human diseases, the latter criterion is used most often to define the disease as an autoimmune one.

Causes of Autoimmune Disease

Genetic Susceptibility. The most common evidence for the existence of a ***genetic predisposition*** to autoimmune disease is in the higher incidence of the disease in monozygotic twins, with a lower but still increased incidence in dizygotic twins and family members compared to an unrelated population. Although familial tendencies occur, the pattern of inheritance is generally complex and indicates that disease is polygenic. This means that no individual gene is sufficient to elicit the disease and many genes may interact with one another.

Many autoimmune diseases are genetically heterogeneous—i.e., the same clinical disease may result from the combined effect of different genes. The fact that predisposing genes are usually common in the general population adds to the difficulty in studying genetic susceptibility.

One gene family that is associated with autoimmune disease and has been extensively studied is the ***HLA complex,*** the human MHC. Considering the importance of HLA molecules in shaping the TCR repertoire and their role in recognition by the TCR, this association is not surprising Specific autoimmune diseases associated with HLA alleles will be discussed later in this chapter (Table 12.1). While susceptibility to an autoimmune disease may be linked to a specific MHC allele, eliciting the disease may require other genes or certain environmental triggers.

Studies in mice have shown that alterations in the expression of a variety of non-HLA genes can interfere with many different pathways of cellular function and contribute to autoimmunity. Over expression or underexpression of genes involved in apoptosis and cell survival, cytokines, BCR signaling pathways, costimulatory interactions, and immune clearance of apoptotic cells and immune complexes have been shown to lead to an autoimmune phenotype in mice. A deficiency in proapoptotic molecules (e.g., Fas or Fas L) or overexpression of antiapoptotic molecules (e.g., bcl-2) lead to diminished apoptosis and result in an increased number of autoreactive B and T cells and increased autoantibody production, especially the production of antinuclear antibodies. T cell autoreactivity is often the consequence of overexpression of proinflammatory cytokines (such as IL-10), excessive costimulation due to overexpression of costimulatory molecules (such as B7 and CD28), or a deficiency of inhibitors of costimulatory interactions (such as CTLA-4 and PD-1). An alteration in the strength of the signal transduced by the B cell receptor due to underexpression of signaling molecules, such as CD22 or Lyn, or overexpression of molecules such as CD19 is associated with autoantibody production in mice. Enhanced T cell help, such as occurs with enhanced expression of CD40 or CD40L, similarly leads to autoantibody production. Finally, underexpression of proteins such as serum amyloid protein (SAP) that are involved in clearance of apoptotic particles or decreased clearance of immune complexes owing to a deficiency of an early component of the classical pathway of complement (either C1q, C2, C3, or C4) leads to autoantibody production. Target organ damage in autoimmune disease may also be genetically determined. Murine models of autoimmune myocarditis reveal that disease susceptibility and cardiac damage depend on strain-specific cardiac myosin antigen accessibility.

Environmental Susceptibility. In addition to genetic predisposition, several environmental factors, either infectious or noninfectious, can trigger autoimmunity by inducing the release of ***sequestered antigens*** or ***molecular mimicry*** or by ***polyclonal activation.***

TABLE 12.1. Autoimmune Diseases

Autoimmune Disease	MHC Association	Allele	Strength of Association
Class I			
Ankylosing spondylitis	B27	B*2702, −04, −05	Strong
Reiter syndrome	B27		Strong
Acute anterior uveitis	B27		Strong
Hyperthyroidism (Graves)	B8		Weak
Psoriasis vulgaris	Cw6		Intermediate
Class II			
Rheumatoid arthritis	DR4	DRB1*0401, −04, −05	Strong
Sjogren syndrome	DR3		Intermediate
Systemic lupus erythematosus			
Caucasian	DR3		Weak
Japanese	DR2		Intermediate
Celiac disease	DR3	DQA1*0501	Strong
Pemphigus vulgaris	DR4, DR6		Strong
Type I diabetes mellitus	DR4	DQB1*0302	Strong
	DR3		Intermediate
Multiple sclerosis	DR2	DRB1*1501	Intermediate
Myasthenia gravis	DR3		Weak
Goodpasture syndrome	DR2		Intermediate

As described earlier in this chapter, a few autoantigens are protected (*sequestered*) from the immune system. Thus, even if some individuals possess autoreactive T and B cells, these cells will not be activated to initiate autoimmunity because they never come in contact with the autoantigen. The chondrocyte antigens in cartilage and some neuronal and cardiac antigens are considered to be examples of sequestered antigens. When they are exposed to the immune system—by some ***physical accident*** or ***due to infection***—an autoimmune response may result. ***Autoimmune myocarditis*** has been observed to arise in some cases following a ***cardiac ischemic attack.*** It is believed that autoreactivity to cardiac antigens develops as a consequence of exposure of sequestered antigens upon heart damage.

Autoimmunity may also arise when an antibody or T cell specific for a ***microbial antigen*** cross-reacts with a self antigen (due to an epitope in the microbial antigen that is highly homologous to an epitope present on the self antigen). This is referred to as ***molecular mimicry.*** Generally, a T-dependent self antigen does not elicit an autoantibody response from a B cell because there are no autoreactive T helper cells available to provide help, since they have been either deleted or anergized. However, a foreign antigen that contains an epitope that is similar to an epitope on a self antigen can elicit an autoantibody response if it contains a T cell epitope that is distinct from that of the self antigen (Fig. 12.6A). This is because the foreign epitope activates T cells that have not been tolerized, and these T cells can then provide help to the autoreactive B cells. ***Molecular mimicry*** is believed to play a role in the onset of ***rheumatic fever,*** which sometimes follows a ***streptococcal infection.*** Autoantibodies to cardiac myosin are believed to be elicited by cross-reactivity with a streptococcal antigen. ***Viral infections*** can sometimes trigger autoimmunity because of T cell cross-reactivity. A T cell specific for a viral peptide can cross-react with a peptide derived from an autoantigen. In autoimmune diabetes, a T cell that recognizes a peptide from glutamic acid decarboxylase (an antigen in β-islet cells) has been shown to cross-react with a peptide derived from coxsackievirus. Thus molecular mimicry can initiate autoimmune disease following a microbial infection.

Microbial antigens can also induce autoimmunity by ***polyclonal activation.*** Polyclonal activators may nonspecifically trigger many B cell or T cell clones (including the autoreactive ones). Many bacterial and viral antigens act as ***superantigens,*** which can activate several different clones of T cells, regardless of their specificicity, due to their binding to V_β gene domains that lie outside of the peptide-binding domains (see Fig. 9.8). Conserved molecular structures on a large group of microorganisms (pathogen-associated molecular patterns; PAMPs) have been observed to act as polyclonal activators of B cells (Fig. 12.6B). Receptors, known as pattern-recognition molecules, that bind these PAMPs have been found on all B cells as well as other APCs. Lipopolysaccharide is a cell wall component of gram-negative bacteria that can polyclonally activate mouse B cells. Other common PAMPs, such as microbial lipoproteins and hypomethylated bacterial DNA, can induce polyclonal activation of human B cells as well.

Triggers for Autoimmunity. Noninfectious triggers of autoimmunity include hormones, drugs, and the loss of T suppressor cells. The influence of hormones is illustrated by gender-specific factors that help trigger autoimmune diseases—for example, SLE is 10 times more common in women than in men and may be exacerbated by estrogen. Certain drugs can chemically alter the T cell carrier epitope of a self antigen to render it immunogenic. Finally, inhibition or loss of T suppressor cells can contribute to autoimmunity. T suppressor cells normally suppress the activation of $CD4^+$ and $CD8^+$ T cells. Loss of such cells seems to favor an increase in cell-mediated activity, which can lead to T cell–mediated autoimmunity. Patients with diabetes and inflammatory bowel disease often have reduced numbers of T suppressor cells.

Examples of Autoimmune Disease

Traditionally, autoimmune diseases have been classified as B cell– or T cell–mediated diseases. We now know that most B cell responses are T cell dependent and that B cells may be important APCs for T cell activation. Thus the distinction no longer seems useful. Alternatively, autoimmune diseases were classified as systemic or organ specific. Again, the classification no longer seems useful. In some diseases, the autoantigen is ubiquitous, but the damage is limited to a single tissue. Other autoimmune diseases previously thought to be due to pathogenic manifestations of organ-specific immune responses are now recognized as diseases that involve multiple organs. We have, therefore, classified diseases by the effector mechanism that appears most responsible for organ damage: antibody, complement, or T cells. This also is not a perfect system, because all mechanisms are operative in many diseases. Table 12.2 lists many autoimmune diseases, their target autoantigen, and the effector cells that mediate them.

Autoimmune Diseases in Which Antibodies Play the Predominant Role in Mediating Organ Damage

Autoimmune Hemolytic Anemia. Hemolytic anemia is autoimmune when antibodies react with self ***red blood cells*** (RBCs). In this condition, the number of RBCs in the circulation is decreased because antibody directed against an antigen on the surface of the blood cell destroys or removes the cells. The destruction of the RBCs can be attributed to two mechanisms. One involves the activation of the complement cascade and eventual lysis of the cells. The resultant release of hemoglobin may lead to its appearance in the urine—that is, ***hemoglobinuria.*** The second is by the opsonization of

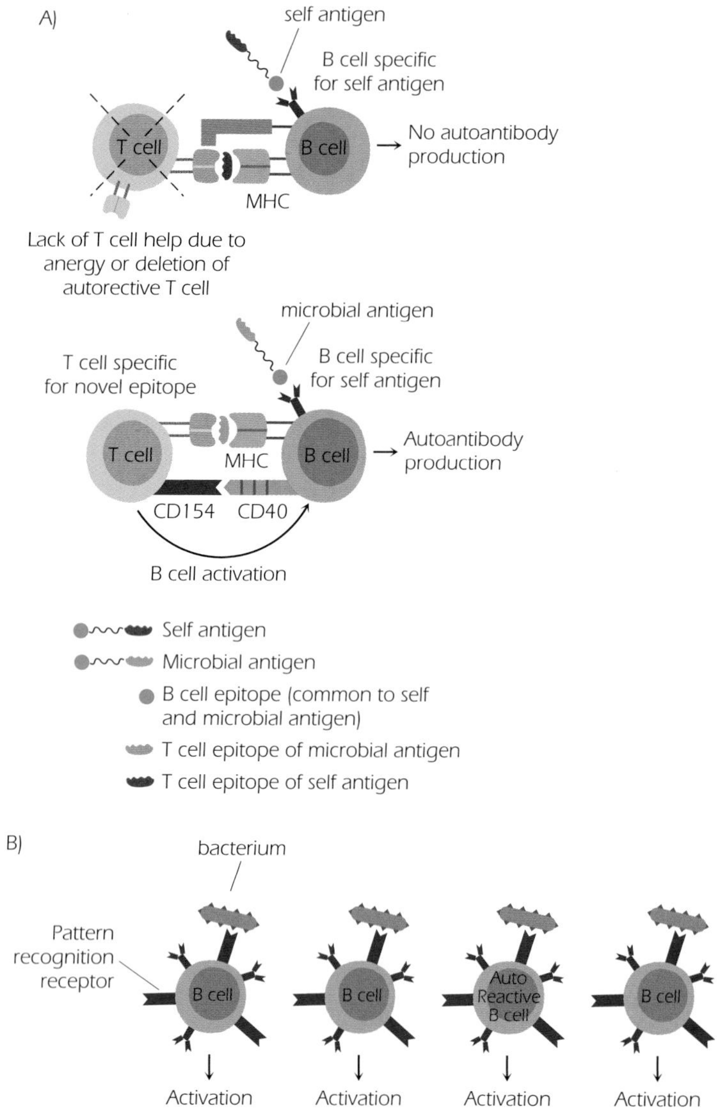

Figure 12.6. Possible mechanisms for the induction of autoimmunity. **(A)** In molecular mimicry, a B cell specific for a self antigen fails to be activated in the absence of T cell help (left) however, it can be activated by a microbial antigen that contains a crossreactive epitope that is shared by the self antigen and a carrier epitope that is distinct. A T cell specific for this non-self carrier can provide help for activation of the autoreactive B cell (right). **(B)** In polyclonal B cell activation; all mouse B cells, including some that are autoreactive, may be activated nonspecifically by a polyclonal activator that binds to a receptor.

RBCs facilitated by antibody and the C3b components of complement (see Chapter 13). In the latter case, the RBCs are bound to and engulfed by macrophages whose receptors for Fc and C3b attach to the antibody-coated RBCs.

It is customary to divide the antibodies responsible for autoimmune hemolytic anemia into two groups on the basis of their physical properties. The first group consists of the ***warm autoantibodies,*** so-called since they react optimally with RBCs at 37°C. The warm autoantibodies belong primarily to the ***IgG class,*** and some react with rhesus (Rh) antigens on the surface of the blood cells. Because activation of the complement cascade requires the close alignment of at least two molecules of IgG and Rh antigens sparsely distributed on the surface of the erythrocyte, complement-mediated lysis does not occur. On the other hand, IgG antibodies to these antigens are effective in inducing immune adherence and phagocytosis. Individuals with autoimmune hemolytic anemia can be identified by a ***Coombs test*** (see Chapter 5), which is designed to detect bound IgG on the surface of RBCs.

A second kind of antibody, the ***cold agglutinins,*** attaches to RBCs only when the temperature is below 37°C and dissociates from the cells when the temperature rises above 37°C. Cold agglutinins belong primarily to the ***IgM class*** and are specific for I or i antigens present on the surface of RBCs. Since the cold agglutinins belong to the IgM class, they are highly efficient at activating the complement cascade and causing lysis of the erythrocytes to which they attach. Nevertheless, hemolysis is not severe in patients with autoimmune hemolytic anemia due to cold agglutinins, as long as their body temperature is maintained at 37°C. When arms, legs, or skin are exposed to cold and the temperature of the circulating blood is allowed to drop, severe attacks of hemolysis may occur.

TABLE 12.2. Autoimmune Diseases, Target Autoantigens, and Effector Cells

Autoimmune Diseases	Autoantigen	Effector cells
Graves disease	TSH receptor	B cells/autoantibody
Myasthenia gravis	Acetylcholine receptor	B cells/autoantibody
Pernicious anemia	Gastric parietal cells; intrinsic factor	B cells/autoantibody
ANCA-associated vasculitis	Myeloperoxidase; serine proteinase	B cells/autoantibody
Autoimmune hemolytic anemia	Rh blood group antigens	B cells/autoantibody
Idiopathic thrombocytopenic purpura	Platelet membrane protein, integrin	B cells/autoantibody
SLE	dsDNA; histones; ribonucleo proteins (snRNPs)	B cells/autoantibody
Sjogren syndrome	Salivary duct antigens; SS-A, SS-B nucleoproteins	B cells/autoantibody
Scleroderma	Centromeric proteins in fibroblasts; nucleolar antigens; IgG; Scl-70	Unknown
Pemphigus vulgaris	Desmoglein 3	B cells; autoantibody
Goodpasture syndrome	Renal and lung basement membrane collagen type IV	B cells; autoantibody
Rheumatoid arthritis	Unknown cartilage antigen, IgG	$CD4^+$ T cells; CTLs; B cells/autoantibody
Hashimoto thyroiditis	Thyroid proteins (thyroglobulin, microsomal antigens, thyroid peroxidase)	$CD4^+$ T cells; B cells/autoantibody
Insulin-dependent diabetes mellitus	Pancreatic β-islet cell antigen	$CD4^+$ T cells; CTLs; B cells/autoantibody
Multiple sclerosis	Myelin basic protein	$CD4^+$ T cells

Although the cause of autoantibody formation is often not known, some clues are offered by drug-induced anemia. A drug like penicillin, which behaves as a hapten, may bind to some protein on the surface of the RBCs, and this entire complex may then act as an antigen eliciting antibodies to the surface of the cell, causing lysis or phagocytosis. In such cases, however, the disease is self-limited and disappears when drug use is discontinued.

Another example of drug-induced anemia occurs in a small minority of patients using α-methyldopa, an antihypertensive drug. It leads to a disorder that is almost identical to that characterized by warm autoantibodies. Sometimes, cold agglutinins appear after infection by *Mycoplasma pneumoniae* or viruses, implicating a role of an infectious disease trigger in genetically susceptible individuals.

Myasthenia Gravis. Another autoimmune disease in which antibodies to a well-defined target antigen are implicated is myasthenia gravis. The target self antigen in this disease is the ***acetylcholine receptor*** at neuromuscular junctions. The autoantibody acts as an antagonist that blocks the binding of acetylcholine (ACh) to the receptor. This inhibits the nerve impulse from being transmitted across the neuromuscular junction, resulting in severe muscle weakness, manifested by difficulty in chewing, swallowing, and breathing, and eventually death from respiratory failure (Fig. 12.7). It affects individuals of any age, but the peak incidence is women in their late 20s and men in their 50s and 60s. The female to male ratio is approximately 3:2. Some babies of myasthenic mothers have transient muscle weakness, presumably because they received sufficient amounts of pathogenic IgG by transplacental passage.

The disease can be experimentally induced in animals by immunization with ACh receptors purified from torpedo fish or electric eel, which demonstrate significant cross-reactivity with mammalian receptors. In the experimental disease, resulting from the formation of antibodies against the foreign receptors, the antibodies bind to the mammalian receptors and mimic almost exactly the natural form of the disease. The disease may be passively transferred with antibody.

The development of myasthenia gravis appears to be linked to the thymus, since many patients have concurrent thymoma, or hypertrophy of the thymus, and removal of the thymus sometimes leads to regression of the disease. Molecules cross-reacting with the ACh receptor have been found on various cells in the thymus, such as thymocytes and epithelial cells, but whether these molecules are the primary stimulus for the development of the disease is unknown. There is a genetic component to the disease as myasthenia gravis is associated with HLA-DR3 alleles.

Graves Disease. One of the main manifestations of Graves disease is a hyperactive thyroid gland (***hyperthyroidism***). This aspect of the disease serves as an example in which antibodies directed against a hormone receptor may activate the receptor rather than interfere with its activity.

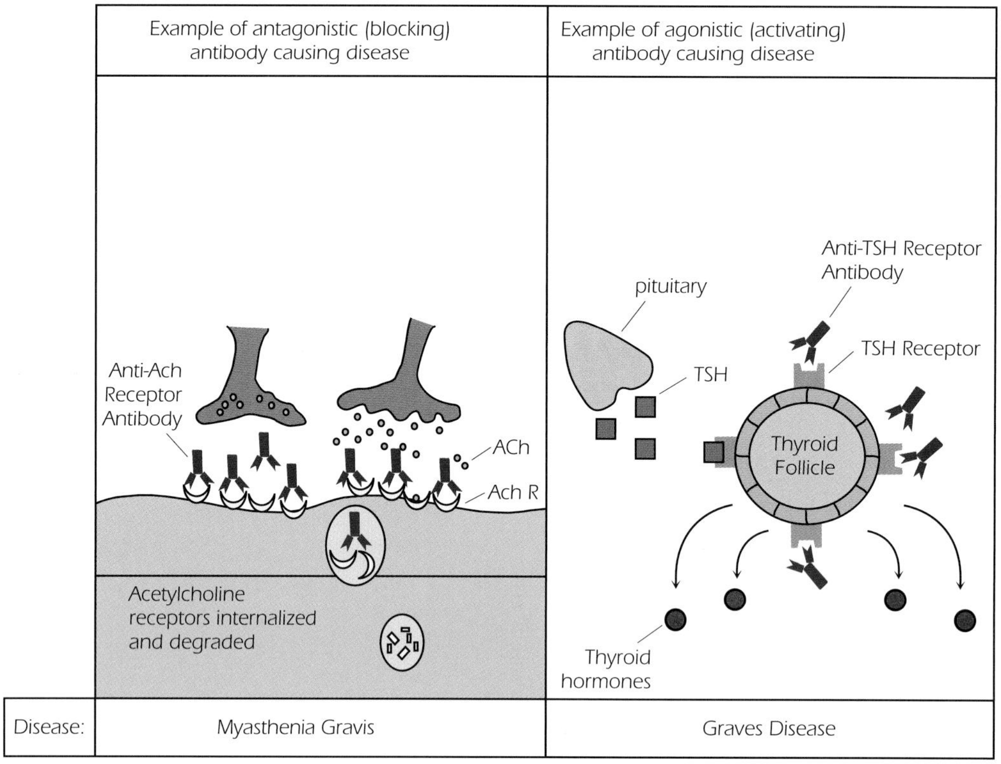

Figure 12.7. Autoantibodies specific for cell-surface receptors can be either receptor agonists or antagonists. The antibody to the acetylcholine receptor in myasthenia gravis acts as a an antagonist that blocks binding of ACh to the receptor and prevents transmission of the nerve impulse across the neuromuscular junction. The antibody to the TSH receptor in Graves disease acts as a receptor agonist and induces chronic stimulation of the thyroid to release thyroid hormones.

For reasons not yet understood, in Graves disease, patients develop autoantibodies against thyroid cell-surface ***receptors for thyroid-stimulating hormone*** (TSH). The interaction of these antibodies with the receptor activates the cell in a manner similar to the activation by TSH. Hence the autoantibody behaves as an agonist (Fig. 12.7). The long-lasting stimulation by these antibodies causes hyperthyroidism due to the continuous stimulation of the thyroid gland.

The indirect evidence that Graves disease is autoimmune includes familial predisposition, genetic association with HLA class II genes, and correlation of antibody titer to TSH receptors with disease severity. However, the best evidence is the transmission of thyroid-stimulating antibodies from a thyrotoxic mother across the placenta, causing ***transient neonatal hyperthyroidism*** until the maternal IgG is catabolized. The disease most commonly affects women in their 30s and 40s. In nongoitrous areas, the female to male ratio is about 7:1. Genetic factors play a role with a linkage to MHC class II genes, and a familial predisposition. Recently, the International Consortium for the Genetics of Autoimmune Thyroid Disease found a new Graves disease susceptibility gene on chromosome 20 (20q11.2).

Systemic Lupus Erythematosus. SLE gets its name (literally, "red wolf") from a reddish facial rash on the cheeks, which is a frequent early symptom. However, the distribution of the rash resembles the wings of a butterfly rather than the face of a wolf (Fig. 12.8). The designation wolf-like is thus far-fetched, but the term *systemic* is quite appropriate since the disease attacks many organs of the body and causes fever, joint pain, and damage to the central nervous system, heart, and kidneys. The pathophysiology of the kidney lesions, which cause the most mortality from SLE, is the most clearly understood.

Despite the mystery concerning the origin of this disease, details of the immunologic mechanisms responsible for the pathology are partially known. Patients with SLE produce antibody against several nuclear components of the body (antinuclear antibodies; ANA), notably against native dsDNA. Occasionally, antibodies are also produced against denatured, single-stranded DNA and against nucleohistones; but clinically, the presence of anti-double-stranded DNA correlates best with the pathology of renal involvement in SLE (see below). Antibodies to single-stranded DNA are produced in normal individuals, but they are generally low-affinity IgM antibodies. They can, however, undergo isotype switching

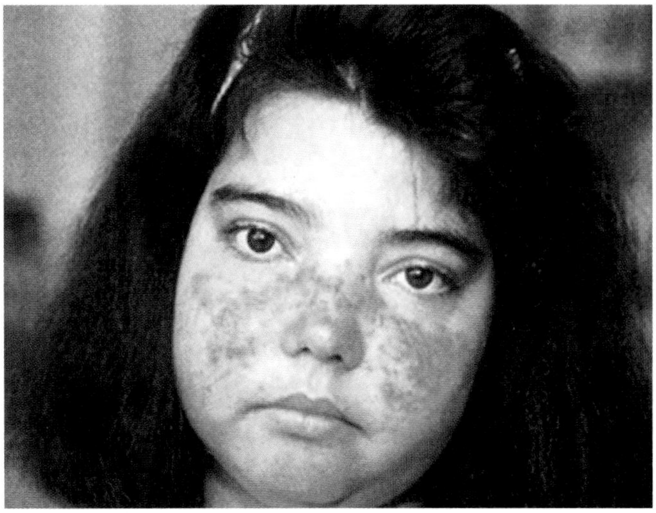

Figure 12.8. Typical reddish, butterfly or malar rash on the face of a young girl with SLE. (Courtesy of L. Steinman, Department of Pathology, Stanford University School of Medicine.)

and somatic mutation to result in the production of high-affinity IgG antibodies to both single- and double-stranded DNA, provided the B cells are given appropriate T cell help.

Double-Stranded DNA may become trapped in the glomerular basement membrane through electrostatic interactions with a constituent of the membrane such as collagen, fibronectin, or laminin. The bound dsDNA may then trap circulating IgG anti-dsDNA antibodies and lead to the formation of immune complexes. These complexes may activate the complement cascade and attract granulocytes. Alternatively, anti-dsDNA antibodies may cross-react with glomerular antigens. Deposition of IgG antibodies in the kidney of lupus patients can be demonstrated by immunostaining a tissue section from the kidney with a fluorescently labeled antibody to human IgG (Fig. 12.9). In the kidney, the extent of the inflammatory reaction forms the basis of classifying kidney pathology. The resulting damage to the kidneys (glomerulonephritis) leads to leakage of protein (proteinuria) and sometimes hemorrhage (hematuria), with symptoms waxing and waning as the rate of formation of immune complexes rises and falls. As the condition becomes chronic, inflammatory $CD4^+$ T_H1 cells enter the site and attract monocytes, which further contribute to the pathologic lesions.

Although the antigen that initiates production of these antibodies is unknown, infectious agents have been proposed. SLE may be the result of an immune response made by only a few genetically disposed individuals to some common environmental organism. Other environmental factors include ultraviolet light that exacerbates the disease, the influence of hormones, and the induction of SLE-like symptoms by drugs, such as penicillamine. Evidence for genetic predisposition include the increased risk of developing SLE among family members, the higher rate of concordance (25%) in monozygotic twins compared to dizygotic twins ($<3\%$), linkage with HLA class II genes, and the presence of an inherited deficiency of an early complement component in 6% of SLE patients.

Autoimmune Diseases in Which T Cells Play a Predominant Role in Organ Damage

Multiple Sclerosis. Multiple Sclerosis (MS) involves *demyelinization of central nervous system tissue* and is characterized by either a relapsing–remitting or a chronic progressive paralytic course. It is considered to be a ***T cell–mediated*** autoimmune disease. The lesions resemble the cellular infiltrates associated with T_H1 cells, reminiscent of delayed-type hypersensitivity (see Chapter 16).

It is not clear whether the autoimmune response is due to failure of clonal deletion, from neuroantigen sensitization, or from ***molecular mimicry to a neuroepitope*** following a virus infection. The evidence that MS is an autoimmune disease is indirect and has relied on the EAE rodents, described earlier

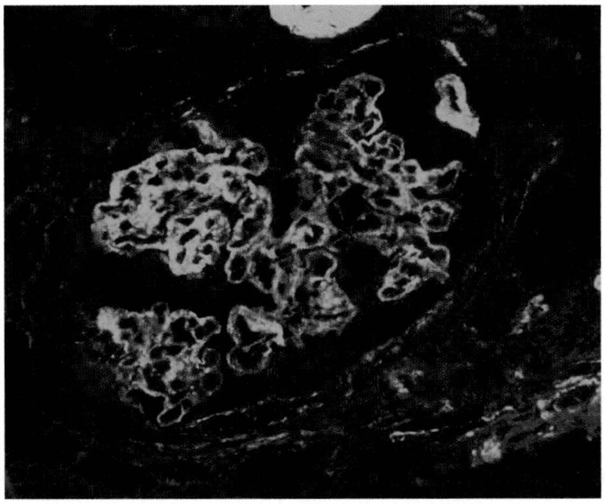

Figure 12.9. Antibody deposition in the kidney of a patient with SLE. Fluorescent-labeled antibody to human IgG, used to immunostain a kidney section, shows deposits of IgG antibody in glomeruli. (Courtesy of H. Rennke, Department of Pathology, Brigham and Women's Hospital, Boston.)

in this chapter. Animals with EAE develop many of the same characteristics as patients with MS. $CD4^+$ T cell clones specific for myelin basic protein and many other central nervous system antigens can transfer the EAE disease. Circumstantial evidence for the autoimmune nature of MS includes the HLA class II association with the disease susceptibility and the finding of a higher T cell response to myelin components in cerebral spinal fluid of MS patients than in control subjects.

One area of study has established the ability of activated T cells to penetrate the blood–brain barrier, which ordinarily prevents cells and macromolecules from entering the central nervous system. In activated T cells, integrins are unregulated that may allow the T cells to adhere to the vessels near the brain. Activated T cells can produce metalloproteinases, which disrupt the collagen in the basal lamina, allowing T cells to accumulate into the central nervous system. Once there, the T cells must undergo antigenic stimulation (perhaps via microglia, the macrophage-like APC present in the brain) to persist in the brain. Chemokines are produced that attract additional inflammatory cells. This results in the accumulation not only of $CD4^+$ T cells but also of macrophage and microglia; all these cells contribute to tissue injury. The inflammatory process induces Fas expression to be upregulated on oligodendrocytes, making them targets for T cells and microglia, which express Fas L; consequently, programmed cell death is induced in the oligodendrocytes.

Familial aggregations occur in MS with a higher concordance rate among identical twins (25–30%) than in dizygotic twins (2–5%). It is twice as common in females than in males, and its peak incidence is at age 35. Recent genetic studies suggest that approximately 12 regions of the human genome may be important for susceptibility to MS. Identifying these genes and determining how they relate to the immune system will aid in understanding the underlying defect and immunopathogenesis of MS.

Type 1 Insulin-Dependent Diabetes Mellitus. Insulin-dependent diabetes mellitus (IDDM) is a form of diabetes that involves chronic *inflammatory destruction of the insulin-producing β-islet cells* of the pancreas. In IDDM, the major contributors to β cell destruction are ***cytotoxic T cells*** and cytokines followed by autoantibodies. Genetic factors include several genes in the MHC class II regions, the insulin gene on chromosome 11, and at least 11 other non-HLA linked diabetes susceptibility genes. Some HLA class II haplotypes predispose for the disease, and others are protective. For example, approximately 50% of IDDM

(A)

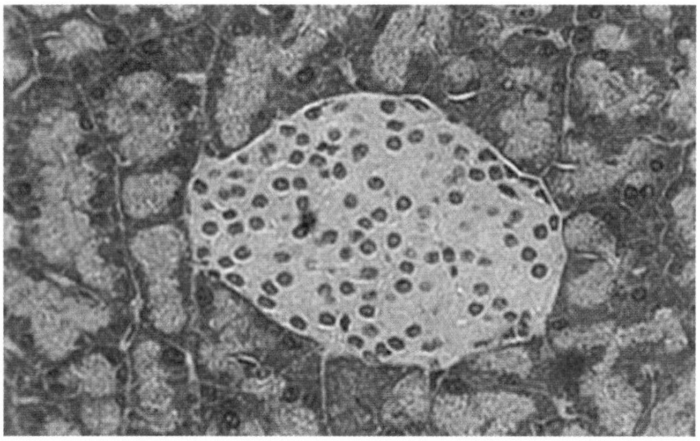

(B)

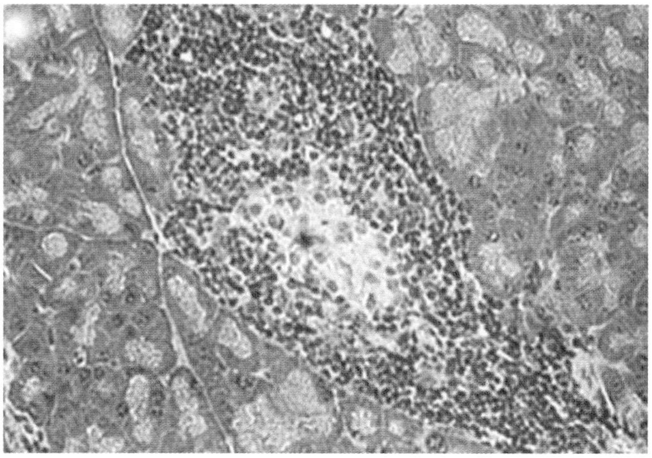

Figure 12.10. Light micrograph of islets of Langerhans. (**A**) Pancreas of a normal mouse. (**B**) Pancreas of an NOD mouse with IDDM-like disease revealing the infiltration of lymphocytes in the islets of Langerhans (insulitis). (Courtesy of M. Atkinson, Department of Pathology, University of Florida College of Medicine, Gainsville.)

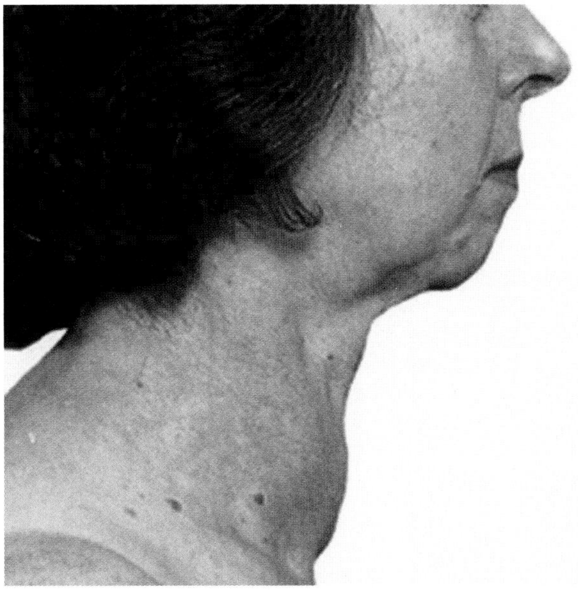

Figure 12.11. Formation of a goiter in a patient with Hashimoto thyroiditis. (From Roitt Im; Brostoff J, Malem DK (eds) (1989): Immunology; 2nd ed. New York: Grower Medical, with permission.)

patients are HLA-DR3/DR4 heterozygotes in contrast to 5% of the normal population. On the other hand, individuals with HLA-DQB1*0602 rarely develop the disease.

An experimental animal model, the NOD mouse, shares many key features with the human disease, including the destruction of pancreatic β-islet cells by infiltrating lymphocytes (Fig. 12.10), the association with MHC susceptibility genes, and the transmission by T cells. At least 14 genes contribute to diabetes found in NOD mice. There are, however, notable differences between the human disease and the mouse model. These include the predominance of T cells in NOD mice compared to IDDM in humans and a greater bias to incidence of disease in female mice than female patients.

Hashimoto's Thyroiditis. Hashimoto's thyroiditis is a disease of the thyroid most commonly found in middle-aged women that leads to the initial formation of a ***goiter*** (Fig. 12.11) and eventual atrophy of the thyroid gland, which results in hypothyroidism and destruction of thyroid function. There is a greater incidence of other autoimmune diseases in family members of patients with Hashimoto's thyroiditis than in the normal population. The disease is mediated primarily by T cells, but antibodies may contribute to the disease process.

Several target antigens are involved in this disease process, including ***thyroglobulin,*** the major hormone produced by the thyroid. ***Microsomal antigens*** from thyroid epithelial cells also have been implicated, and antibodies to both these types of antigen have been found in Hashimoto's disease patients. Histologic findings show that there is an infiltration of predominantly mononuclear cells into the thyroid follicles (Fig. 12.12). The mononuclear infiltrates contain large numbers of B cells, T cells, and macrophages. Progressive destruction of thyroid follicles accompanies the presence of these infiltrates, and the gland attempts to regenerate and becomes enlarged. When destruction of follicles reaches a certain level, the output of thyroid hormone declines and the symptoms of hypothyroidism appear: dry skin, puffy face, brittle hair and nails, and a feeling of being continuously cold.

Evidence implicating T cell–mediated responses comes from a study of experimental autoimmune thyroiditis, which may be induced in animals either by immunization with thyroglobulin in complete Freund's adjuvant or by passively transferring clones of $CD4^+$ T_H1 cells specific for thyroglobulin. An important distinction between the experimental and the naturally occurring autoimmune disease is that the former is acute and nonrecurring, whereas the latter has a chronic, recurrent course. Thus the precipitating event in the naturally occurring autoimmune disease is probably some ongoing process, rather than a single immunizing event.

Rheumatoid Arthritis. Rheumatoid arthritis (RA) is characterized by ***chronically inflamed synovium,*** densely crowded with lymphocytes, which results in the destruction of cartilage and bone. The inflamed synovial membrane, usually one cell thick, becomes so cellular that it mimics lymphoid tissue and forms new blood vessels. The synovium is densely packed with dendritic cells, macrophages, T, B, and NK cells, and clumps of plasma cells; in some cases, the synovium develops secondary follicles. The pathology in its most intense form is probably the consequence of a mixture of immunopathologic mechanisms, specifically, antigen–antibody complexes, complement, polymorphonuclear neutrophils, inflammatory $CD4^+$ T cells, $CD8^+$ cytotoxic T cells, activated macrophages, and NK cells. This "angry mix" releases a variety of cytokines (of which TNFα and IL-1 are among the earliest), degradative enzymes, and mediators that destroy the integrity of the cartilage. Chondrocytes, the cells of the cartilage, become exposed to the immune

(A)

(B)

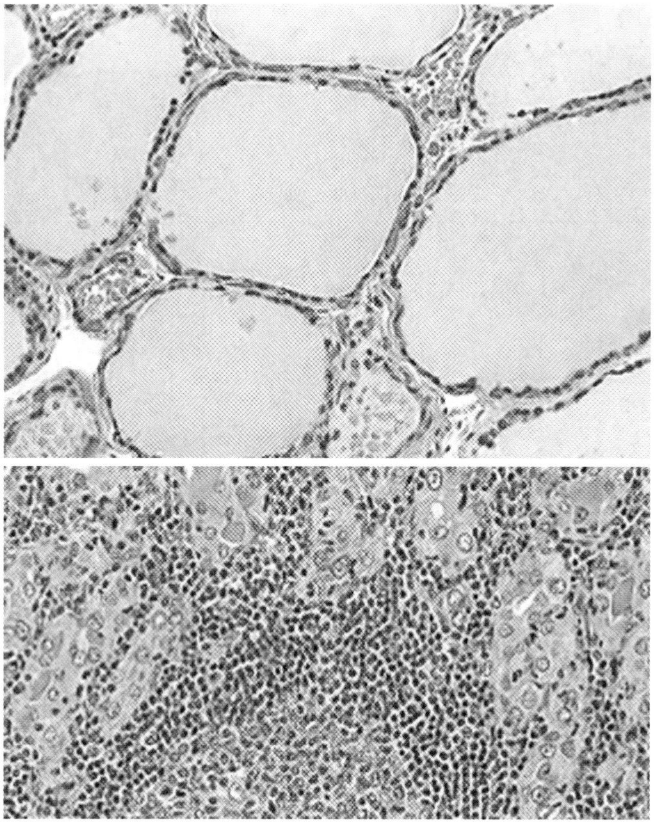

Figure 12.12. Thyroid glands. (**A**) Light micrograph of a normal thyroid gland showing follicular epithelial cells lining a follicle. (**B**) Thyroid gland from a patient with Hashmoto thyroiditis in which the normal architecture of the thyroid has been replaced by intense lymphocyte proliferation. (From Goldsby RA, Kindt TJ, Osborne BA (eds) (2000): *Kuby Immunology*, 4th ed. New York: Freeman, with permission.)

system and perpetuate the damage not only by serving as potential targets but also by releasing cytokines and growth factors. Synovial fluid often accumulates in the joints of RA patients and contains large numbers of polymorphonuclear neutrophils. After repeated bouts of inflammatory insults, ***fibrin is deposited,*** cartilage is replaced by fibrous tissue, and the joint fuses (***ankylosis***).

It has been suggested that inflammatory processes are initiated by abnormally produced antibody, generally ***IgM***—called ***rheumatoid factor*** (RF)—*which is specific for a determinant on the Fc portion of the patient's own IgG molecules.* However, it is unlikely that RF is the common initiator of the disease, since 30% of RA patients do not have detectable levels of the factor. The group of patients with RF tends to develop a more aggressive disease. RF serves as a useful marker of disease activity, since reduced levels of serum RF are found during remission. The presence of RF contributes to the pathology of RA but probably does not account for the T cell response.

The initial insulting trigger may be diverse. A high proportion of RA patients have elevated numbers of B cells infected with Epstein-Barr virus; $\gamma\delta$ T cells from RA patients recognize heat-shock proteins; and bacteria have been associated with RA.

Women are affected three times more often than men, and the age of onset is usually during the 4th and 5th decades of life. The association of various genes has been examined in family studies in RA for many different populations. In many, the association of HLA-DR4 alleles and RA has been confirmed although the subtype varies. For example, the HLA-DRB1 association for North American Whites is *0401 and *0404, whereas for Israelis, it is *0102 and *0405, and for Yakima Indians, it is *1402. In others, there is no association with DR4 genes. DNA sequencing of all these MHC class II molecules show that they share a segment of the outermost domain of the HLA-DR β-chain, called the ***shared epitope.*** Individuals with two different HLA-DRB1 that share the β-chain epitope have the highest risk for developing RA and express the most severe form of the disease. Other genes strongly associated with RA include TNF and heat shock proteins.

Autoimmune Diseases Arising from Deficiency in Components of Complement

Many patients with deficiencies in the early components of complement develop autoimmune diseases such as SLE (see Chapter 17). In addition, specific alleles of some complement components predispose individuals to the development of autoimmunity. Both the classical and alternative complement pathways inhibit the formation of large immune complexes. C1, C4, and C2 from the classical pathway appear to directly affect the size of immune complexes; whereas C3b plays a key role in both pathways. Incorporation of C3b solubilizes immune complexes. C3b reduces the lattice size of the complex, perhaps by disrupting the capacity of the antibody to bind to the antigens. The addition of C3b to the antigen–antibody complex promotes the binding to C3b receptor on many cell types, including phagocytic cells and RBCs. The complexes bound to erythrocytes are rapidly transported to the liver and spleen, and those taken up by phagocytes are degraded.

The inappropriate deposition of immune complexes leading to disease can occur under several different circumstances. For example, excessive immune complex formation may overwhelm complement clearance mechanisms as in serum sickness (see Chapter 15). In addition, inherited deficiencies of components of the classical complement pathway may also cause this to occur (see Chapter 17). A defect in the C1, C4, or C2 complement components prevents the activation of the classical pathway, and deficiency of C4b and C3b results in failure to clear immune complexes by macrophages. SLE occurs in $>80\%$ of individuals with complete deficiency of C1, C4, or C2. Finally, abnormalities in complement or Fc receptors on cells also lead to inefficient clearance of immune complexes.

Therapeutic Strategies

For many years, the major approach to the treatment of most autoimmune disease has been to eliminate autoreactive cells. Because it is not routinely possible to distinguish an autoreactive B or T cell from one that will protect against microbial infection, broadly ablative therapies have been used. Therapeutic agents are often ***cytotoxic drugs,*** such as ***cyclophosphamide*** and ***azathioprine,*** that interfere with DNA replication and indiscriminately destroy the body's white blood cells. In addition, drugs like ***cyclosporin A*** and ***FK506*** block intracellular signaling pathways and prevent cellular activation (see Chapter 18).

More recently, ***anticytokine therapies*** have proven to be very successful in several diseases. Blockade of ***TNFα*** by antibody or soluble receptor is an important therapeutic option in rheumatoid arthritis and inflammatory bowel disease. Inhibition of ***IL-1β*** by soluble receptor also seems a useful strategy in rheumatoid arthritis. These immunomodulatory agents prevent an inflammatory response. While they appear to curtail the disease process, they also render the host immunosuppressed. Thus infections represent a major complication of the treatment of many autoimmune diseases. Some autoimmune diseases may be treated by removing or administering a cytokine—for example, interferon-β (INFβ) is used in the treatment of multiple sclerosis. How the cytokine exerts a therapeutic effect is not understood.

Recently, more targeted approaches to therapy have been explored. A nondepleting ***monoclonal antibody to CD3*** is being tested in new-onset autoimmune diabetes. Costimulatory blockade, to prevent the interaction of B7 molecules with CD28, appears promising in RA and psoriasis. These new approaches have demonstrated efficacy, but it is likely that they will interfere with protective as well as pathogenic immune responses and thus be immunosuppressive. Additional information about the mechanisms of action of these and other immunosuppressive drugs is presented in Chapter 18.

There are some antigen-specific approaches to therapy that may eliminate autoreactivity without causing global immunosuppression. Altered peptide ligands, peptides that bind to the MHC groove but are not capable of activating a given T cell, have been used to induce tolerance in rodent models of disease but have not demonstrated efficiency in humans. Oral antigen has also been used to induce tolerance in animal models, but clinical trials with oral collagen and myelin basic protein in RA and MS, respectively, have not demonstrated efficacy. T cell receptors have been administered to patients as an immunogen in an effort to raise clonotype-specific cytolytic T cells. These studies are ongoing.

The recent recognition of multiple populations of regulatory T cells has led to yet another therapeutic strategy. Several studies suggest an absence or a decrease in numbers of T suppressor cells in autoimmune individuals. Investigators are beginning to learn how to generate regulatory cells in autoimmune individuals. There are as yet no clinical trials that are attempting to activate suppressor cells, but in mice this strategy appears quite effective.

SUMMARY

1. Tolerance is the state of lymphocyte unresponsiveness to antigen. There are several mechanisms for inducing B and T cell tolerance to self antigen; anergy (functional inactivation of the cell), deletion, receptor editing, and T cell suppression.
2. Tolerance can be induced in both immature and mature lymphocytes. To be tolerized, a cell must express an antigen-specific receptor (BCR or TCR).
3. The avidity of interaction of the BCR or the TCR for an autoantigen and the microenvironment in which the autoreactive lymphocytes encounter self antigen influence cell fate.
4. Lack of costimulatory interactions can induce T and/or B cell anergy.
5. T cell suppression is mediated by $CD4^+CD25^+$ regulatory T cells.

6. Low-dose tolerance to food antigen induces T cell suppression, whereas high-dose tolerance induces T cell anergy or deletion.

7. The expression of Fas L and the production of immunosuppressive cytokines by certain cell types play a role in establishing immune privileged sites.

8. Autoimmunity is a condition in which the body mounts an immune response to one or more of its own constituents.

9. Establishing a disease as autoimmune rests on several types of evidence: (1) direct proof made by transferring autoantibodies or self-reactive lymphocytes and reproducing the disease in an otherwise healthy individual; (2) indirect proof, which requires finding an experimental animal model to mimic the disease; and (3) circumstantial evidence based on familial tendency, involvement of immune cells and antibodies, and clinical improvement with immunosuppressive drugs.

10. Initiation of autoimmune diseases usually requires a combination of genetic and environmental events. It is believed that many autoreactive clones of T and B cells exist normally but are held in check by homeostatic mechanisms. It is the breakdown of these controls, by various mechanisms, that leads to the activation of autoreactive clones and autoimmune disease.

11. Many organs and tissues are involved in autoimmune disease, and the effector mechanisms of tissue damage may involve antibody, complement, T cells, and macrophages.

REFERENCES

Bretscher PA, Cohn M (1968): Minimal model for the mechanism of antibody induction and paralysis by antigen. *Nature* 166:444.

Davidson A, Diamond B (2001): Autoimmune diseases. *New Engl J Med* 345:340.

Frank MM, Austen KF, Claman HN, Unanue ER (eds) (1995): Samter's Immunologic Diseases, 5th ed. Boston: Little, Brown.

Fulcher DA, Lyons AB, Korn SL, Cook MC, Koleda C, Parish C, Fazekas de St Groth B, Basten A (1996): The fate of self-reactive B cells depends primarily on the degree of antigen receptor engagement and availability of T cell help. *J Exp Med* 183:2313.

Gay D, Saunders T, Camper S, Weigert M (1993): Receptor editing: an approach by autoreactive B cells to escape tolerance. *J Exp Med* 177:999.

Green DR, Ferguson TA (2001): The role of Fas ligand in immune privilege. *Nature Rev Mol Cell Biol* 2:917.

Hahn BV (1998) Mechanisms of disease: antibodies to DNA. *N Engl J Med* 338:1333.

Hartley SB, Crosbie J, Brink R, Kantor AB, Basten A, Goodnow C (1991): Elimination from peripheral lymphoid tissues of self-reactive B lymphocytes recognizing membrane-bound antigens. *Nature* 353:765.

Kishimoto H, Sprent J (2000): The thymus and negative selection. *Immunol Res* 21:315.

Levings MK, Sangregorio R, Sartirana C, Moschin AL, Battaglia M, Orban PC, Roncarolo M-G (2002): Human $CD25^+CD4^+$ T suppressor cell clones produce transforming growth factor-β, but not interleukin-10, and are distinct from type 1 T regulatory cells. *J Exp Med* 196:1335.

Nagler-Anderson C, Shi HN (2001): Peripheral nonresponsiveness to orally administered soluble protein antigens. *Crit Rev Immunol* 21:121.

Nossal GJ, Pike BL (1980): Clonal anergy: persistence in tolerant mice of antigen-binding B lymphocytes incapable of responding to antigen or mitogen. *Proc Natl Acad Sci USA* 77: 1602.

O'Dell JR (1999): Anticytokine therapy—a new era in the treatment of rheumatoid arthritis? *New Engl J of Med* 340:310.

Powell JD, Ragheb JA, Kitagawa-Sakakida S, Schwartz RH (1998): Molecular regulation of interleukin-2 expression by CD28 co-stimulation and anergy. *Immunol Rev* 165:287.

Rose NR (1998): The role of infection in the pathogenesis of autoimmune disease. *Semin Immunol* 10:5.

Rozzo SJ, Allard JD, Choubey D, Vyse TJ, Izui S, Peltz G, Kotzin BL (2001): Evidence for an interferon-inducible gene, Ifi202, in the susceptibility to systemic lupus. *Immunity* 15:435.

Sandel PC, Monroe JG (1999): Negative selection of immature B cells by receptor editing or deletion is determined by site of antigen encounter. *Immunity* 10:289.

Shevach EM (2002): $CD4^+CD25^+$ suppressor T cells: more questions than answers. *Nature Rev Immunol* 2:389.

Sorensen TL, Ransohogg RM (1998): Etiology and pathogenesis of multiple sclerosis. *Semin Neurol* 18:287.

Tiegs SL, Russell DM, Nemazee D (1993): Receptor editing in self-reactive bone marrow B cells. *J Exp Med* 177: 1009.

Weiner H (2001): Oral tolerance: immune mechanisms and the generation of Th3-type TGF-beta-secreting regulatory cells. *Microbes Infect* 3:947.

REVIEW QUESTIONS

For each question, choose the ONE BEST answer or completion.

1. An individual normally does not make an immune response to a self-protein because
A) self-proteins cannot be processed into peptides.
B) peptides from self-proteins cannot bind to MHC class I molecules.
C) peptides from self-proteins cannot bind to MHC class II molecules.
D) lymphocytes that express a receptor reactive to a self-protein are inactivated by deletion, anergy, or receptor editing.
E) developing lymphocytes cannot rearrange V genes required to produce a receptor for self-proteins.

2. Which of the following autoimmune diseases has been proven to be due to a single gene defect?
A) Systemic lupus erythematosus
B) Autoimmune lymphoproliferative syndrome
C) Multiple sclerosis
D) Rheumatoid arthritis
E) Hashimoto thyroiditis

3. Rheumatoid factor, found in synovial fluid of patients with rheumatoid arthritis, is most frequently found to be
A) IgM reacting with L chains of IgG.
B) IgM reacting with H chain determinants of IgG.
C) IgE reacting with bacterial antigens.
D) antibody to collagen.
E) antibody to DNA.

4. In which of the following diseases do T_H1 $CD4^+$ cells, cytotoxic $CD8^+$ T cells, and autoantibody all contribute to the pathology?
A) Myasthenia gravis
B) Systemic lupus erythematosus
C) Graves disease
D) Autoimmune hemolytic anemia
E) Insulin-dependent diabetes mellitus

5. Systemic lupus erythematosus
A) is due to a mutation in double-stranded DNA.
B) is a classic example of a T cell–mediated autoimmune disease.
C) has multiple symptoms and affects many organs.
D) results from antibodies specific to thyroid tissue.
E) affects only skin epithelial cells.

6. Blocking any of the following processes can result in peripheral tolerance in mature T cells except which?
A) the interaction of costimulatory molecules on T cells with their ligands on APC
B) intracellular signal transduction mechanisms
C) negative selection of thymocytes
D) activation of the IL-2 gene
E) the binding of antigen with MHC molecules

7. Which of the following is least likely to lead to autoimmunity?
A) loss of suppressor T cells
B) release of sequestered self antigen
C) genetic predisposition
D) polyclonal activation
E) increased clearance of immune complexes

CASE STUDY

A 31-year-old woman developed a red, malar rash on her face after she was out in the sun at a family picnic. At first, she thought it was a bad sunburn, but no one else at the picnic had gotten burned. She noted that she was feeling rather tired over the past couple of months and that her hair was thinning, which prompted her to see a physician. Upon questioning, she acknowledged that her joints hurt intermittently over the past several months. She also noticed that her fingers and toes turned purple when she was cold or stressed (Raynaud syndrome). A blood test revealed she was mildly anemic. What is a likely diagnosis and what tests should be ordered to confirm this? Why might the skin rash flare during sun exposure?

ANSWERS TO REVIEW QUESTIONS

1. ***D*** Negative selection generally ensures that a lymphocyte expressing a receptor reactive to a self-protein is inactivated by deletion or anergy or receptor editing in the case of an autoreactive B cell.

2. ***B*** ALPS has been shown to arise as a direct consequence of a mutated Fas gene, which leads to impaired Fas-mediated apoptosis of lymphocytes. Most other autoimmune diseases (such as SLE, MS, RA and Hashimoto thyroiditis) are multigenic in origin; environmental triggers may play a role as well.

3. ***B*** Rheumatoid factor is generally an IgM antibody that reacts with determinants on the Fc portion of IgG.

4. ***E*** Autoantibody has been implicated in myasthenia gravis, Graves disease, SLE, and autoimmune hemolytic anemia. Type I insulin-dependent diabetes is mediated by effector T cells and autoantibodies.

5. *C* Lupus erythematosus affects the skin, kidneys, heart, and joints. DNA may be involved as an antigen, but mutation plays no role, and the disease is initiated primarily by antibodies and is not considered a classic T cell disease.

6. *C* Interfering with negative selection of thymocytes disrupts central rather than peripheral T cell tolerance.

7. *E* A decrease (not an increase) in the clearance of immune complexes, as observed in certain complement deficiencies, would predispose the individual to autoimmune disease.

ANSWERS TO CASE STUDY

The most likely diagnosis is systemic lupus erythematosus (SLE). Common symptoms of this autoimmune disease include rashes, painful joints (arthritis), sun sensitivity, unusual loss of hair, and fatigue. However, SLE can cause serious damage to almost any organ, particularly the kidney. No single test can determine whether a person has lupus, but several tests aid in the diagnosis. The antinuclear antibody (ANA) test is commonly done to test for the presence of antinuclear antibodies in a patient's serum. Most SLE patients test positive for ANA. There are also blood tests that can be performed to detect specific autoantibodies, such as antibodies to double-standed DNA and antibodies to ribonuclear proteins. blood test that measures the level of complement is also useful, as patients with lupus often have low levels of complement, especially during flares. In addition, a biopsy of the skin or kidney may be performed if these organs are affected.

Many lupus patients observe that their symptoms, especially skin rashes worsen when they are exposed to the sun. One theory that has gained much support is that the damage done to the skin by UV light exposure induces increased apoptosis. Blebs on the surface of apoptotic cells have been found to contain autoantigens, such as nucleosomes, which may elicit autoantibody production.

13

COMPLEMENT

INTRODUCTION

The complement system, made up of approximately 30 circulating and membrane-expressed proteins, is an important effector arm of both the innate and antibody-mediated acquired immune responses. Named from some of the earliest observations of its activity—a heat-sensitive material in serum that "complemented" the ability of antibody to kill bacteria—we now know that complement plays a major role in defense against many infectious organisms. The most important of these functions are (1) the production of ***opsonins,*** molecules that enhance the ability of macrophages and neutrophils to phagocytose material (see Fig. 2.1); (2) the production of ***anaphylatoxins,*** peptides that induce local and systemic inflammatory responses; and (3) direct killing of organisms.

We have also learned that complement has other important functions, including enhancing antigen-specific immune responses and maintaining ***homeostasis*** (the maintenance of stability within the body) by removing immune complexes and dead or dying cells. We also know that if complement activation is not tightly regulated, the host can be damaged.

Complement components are synthesized in the liver and by cells involved in the inflammatory response. In the circulation, the concentration of all complement proteins is about 3 mg/mL. (For comparison, circulating IgG levels are approximately 12 mg/mL; see Table 4.2). Some complement components are found at high concentrations (e.g., C3 at about 1 mg/mL), while others (such as factor D and C2) are found in only trace amounts.

In this chapter we will describe how complement is activated, how it is regulated, its most important functions, and clinical conditions that result from either inappropriate activation of complement or complement deficiency.

COMPLEMENT ACTIVATION PATHWAYS

The early steps in complement activation involve a sequential activation—a cascade—of successive components. In this part of the activation pathway, the activation of one component induces enzymatic function that triggers the activation of the next component in the sequence. Because one active enzyme molecule can cleave multiple substrate molecules, this cascade of reactions amplifies a relatively small initiating signal. These cascade properties of the complement system are similar to those of other serum cascades that are a feature of the clotting pathways and those required to generate kinins, the vascular mediators of inflammation described in Chapter 2.

Upon activation, individual components are split into fragments, designated by lower-case letters. The smaller of the cleaved fragments is generally designated with a lower-case *a*, and the larger fragment with a lower-case *b*; for historical reasons, however, the larger cleavage fragment of C2 is usually referred to as C2a and the smaller fragment C2b. (In some texts and articles, though, the fragments of complement component C2 are designated in the reverse way.)

Immunology: A Short Course, Fifth Edition, By Richard Coico, Geoffrey Sunshine, and Eli Benjamini
ISBN 0-471-22689-0 © 2003 John Wiley & Sons, Inc.

Further cleavage fragments are designated with additional lower-case letters, such as C3d.

Three pathways of complement activation are known: the ***classical, lectin,*** and ***alternative pathways.*** The initiation of each pathway involves distinct recognition events and components, but the later stages of all three pathways use the same components. The characteristics of each pathway and the agents that activate it are discussed in the following paragraphs.

The Classical Pathway

The classical pathway was so named because it was the first complement pathway to be worked out. The component proteins are designated C1, C2,... C9. (The numbers designate the order in which the components were discovered, rather than their position in the activation sequence.) ***Antigen–antibody complexes*** are the predominant activators of the classical pathway; thus this pathway is a major effector pathway of the humoral adaptive immune response. Other activators include some viruses, necrotic cells and subcellular membranes (e.g., from mitochondria), aggregated immunoglobulins, and β-amyloid, found in Alzheimer's disease plaques. ***C-reactive protein***—an acute-phase protein that is a component of the inflammatory response—binds to the polysaccharide phosphocholine expressed on the surface of many bacteria (such as *Streptococcus pneumoniae*) and also activates the classical pathway.

The classical pathway is initiated when C1 binds to the antibody in an antigen–antibody complex; for example, antibody bound to an antigen expressed on the surface of a bacterium (Fig. 13.1). C1 is a complex of three different proteins: C1q (made up of six identical subunits) combined with two molecules each of C1r and C1s. To activate C1, the globular head regions of C1q subunits bind to C1q-specific receptors on the Fc regions of either one IgM or two closely spaced IgG molecules bound to the antigen (IgG binding is shown in Fig. 13.1.) Thus IgM and IgG are efficient complement-activating antibodies. Among the human immunoglobulins, the ability to bind and activate C1 is, in decreasing order, IgM > IgG3 > IgG1 ≫ IgG2. IgG4, IgD, IgA, and IgE do not have C1q receptors; these antibodies do not bind or activate C1 and thus do not activate the classical complement pathway.

As a consequence of C1 binding to the antigen–antibody complex, C1s becomes enzymatically active. This enzymatically active form, known as ***C1s esterase,*** cleaves the next component in the classical pathway, C4, into two pieces, C4a and C4b. C4a, the smaller piece, remains in the fluid phase, but C4b binds covalently to the surface of the bacterium or other activating substance. The C4b bound to the cell surface then binds C2, which is cleaved by C1s. Cleavage of C2 generates the fragments C2b, which remains in the fluid phase, and C2a. C2a binds to C4b on the surface of the cell to form a complex, C4b2a. The C4b2a complex is known as the ***classical pathway C3 convertase,*** because, as we shall describe subsequently, this enzyme cleaves the next component in the pathway, C3.

The Lectin Pathway

The lectin pathway is activated by terminal mannose residues of proteins and polysaccharides found on the surface of bacteria. These terminal mannose residues are not found on the surface of mammalian cells, and so the lectin pathway of complement activation may be thought of as discriminating between self and non-self. Because this pathway is activated in the absence of antibody, it is part of the innate immune defenses.

Figure 13.1 shows that bacterial mannose residues bind to a circulating complex of ***mannose-binding lectin*** (MBL; structurally homologous to that of C1q in the classical pathway) and two associated proteases, known as ***mannose-associated serine protease 1*** (MASP-1) and ***2*** (MASP-2). Binding activates MASP-1 to sequentially cleave the classical complement pathway components C4 and C2 to form C4b2a, the classical pathway C3 convertase, on the surface of the bacterium. MASP-2 appears to be able to cleave C3 directly. Thus the lectin pathway converges with the classical pathway at the activation of C3.

The Alternative Pathway

The alternative pathway of complement activation is triggered by almost any foreign substance. The most widely studied include lipopolysaccharide (LPS; also referred to as endotoxin, from the cell walls of gram-negative bacteria), the cell walls of some yeasts, and a protein present in cobra venom, known as cobra venom factor. Some agents that activate the classical pathway—viruses, aggregated immunoglobulins, and necrotic cells—also trigger the alternative pathway. Activation of the alternative pathway occurs in the absence of specific antibody. Thus the alternative pathway of complement activation is an effector arm of the innate immune defenses. Some of the components of the alternative pathway are unique (the ***serum factors B and D*** and ***properdin,*** also known as ***factor P***), and others (C3, C3b, C5, C6, C7, C8, and C9) are common to those used in the classical pathway.

C3b is generated in the circulation in small amounts by the spontaneous cleavage of a reactive thiol group in C3. This "preformed" C3b can bind to hydroxyl groups of proteins and carbohydrates expressed on cell surfaces (Fig. 13.1). The deposition of C3b on the cell surface initiates the alternative pathway. C3b deposition can occur on either foreign or host cells, so in a sense the alternative pathway is always "on." However, as we shall describe in more detail below, host cells regulate the progression of the alternative pathway, whereas foreign cells lack these regulators and cannot prevent the development of the subsequent steps in the alternative pathway.

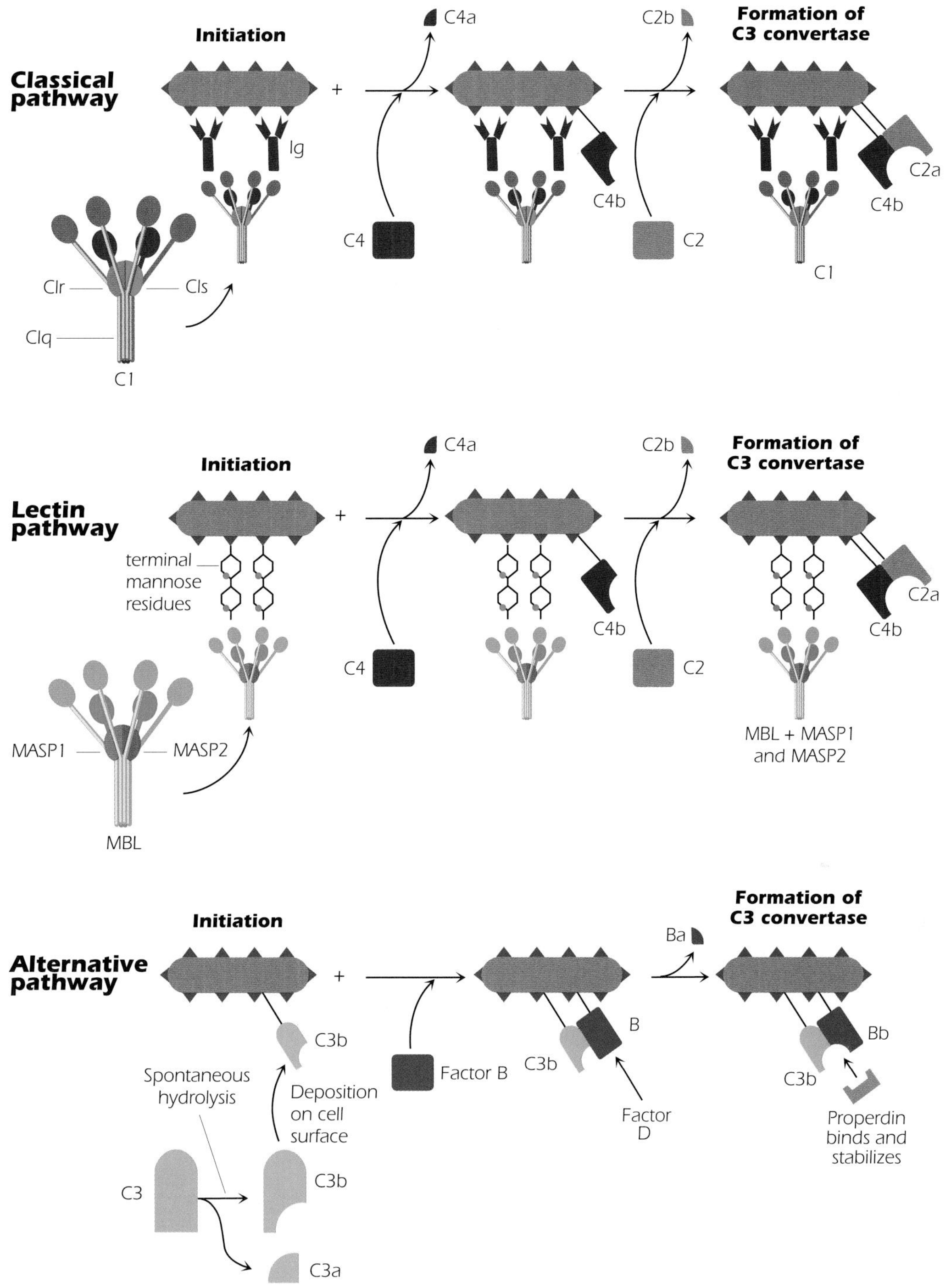

Figure 13.1. Activation of the classical, lectin, and alternative complement pathways, showing how each pathway is initiated and how the C3 convertase is formed.

The next step in the alternative pathway is that the serum protein, ***factor B,*** combines with C3b on the cell surface to form a complex, C3bB. ***Factor D*** then cleaves factor B in the cell-surface-associated C3bB, generating the fragments, Ba, which is released into the fluid phase, and Bb, which remains attached to C3b. This C3bBb is the ***alternative pathway C3 convertase,*** which cleaves C3 into C3a and C3b.

C3bBb normally dissociates rapidly but can be stabilized by binding ***properdin*** (Fig. 13.1). As a result, the properdin-stabilized C3bBb is able to bind and cleave high levels of C3 in a short time. Deposition on the cell surface of these rapidly produced and increased levels of C3b results in an almost explosive triggering of the alternative pathway. In this way, properdin binding to C3bBb creates an ***amplification loop*** in

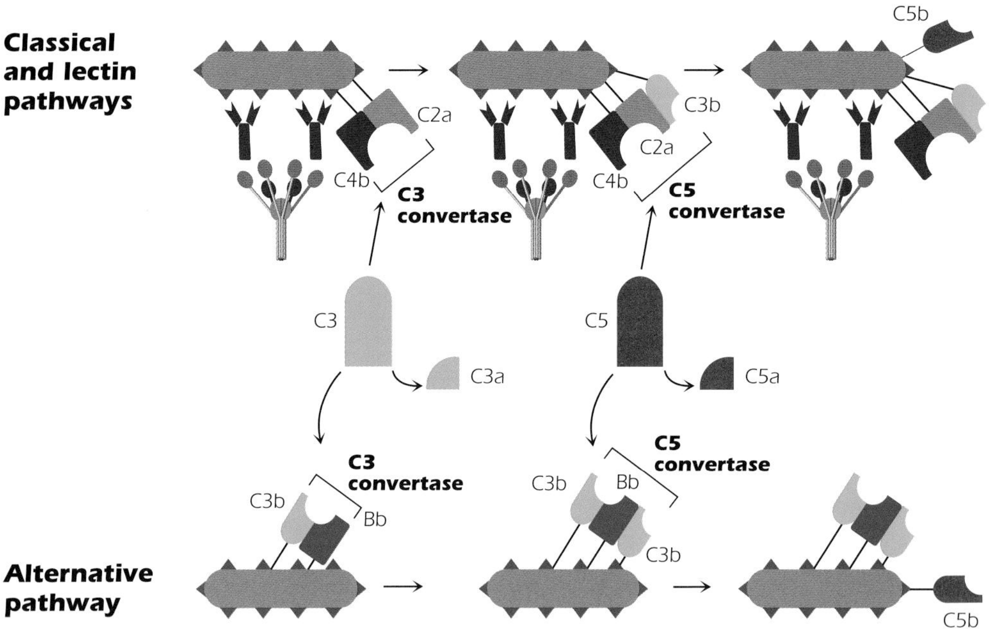

Figure 13.2. The cleavage of C3 by C3 convertase and C5 by C5 convertase in the classical and lectin pathways (top) and alternative pathway (bottom). In all the pathways, C3 is cleaved into C3b, which deposits on the cell surface, and C3a, released into the fluid phase. Similarly, C5 is cleaved into C5b, which deposits on the cell surface, and C5a, released into the fluid phase.

the alternative pathway. As we shall describe below, properdin's ability to activate this amplification loop is balanced by negative regulatory proteins. Consequently, the alternative pathway is not continually activated.

Activation of C3 and C5

C3 cleavage is a critical step in all three complement pathways. Figure 13.2 shows that the C3 convertases of the classical and alternate pathways (C4b2a and C3bBb, respectively) cleave C3 into two fragments: the smaller, C3a, is a fluid-phase ***anaphylatoxin***—that is, it activates cells involved in the inflammatory response. The larger fragment, C3b, continues the complement activation cascade by binding to the cell surface around the site of complement activation. As we shall describe below, C3b is also involved in host defense, inflammation, and immune regulation.

C3b binding to either the classical or alternative pathway C3 convertases allows the next component in the sequence, C5, to bind and be cleaved (Fig. 13.2). For this reason, the C3 convertases with bound C3b are referred to as ***C5 convertases*** (C4b2a3b in the classical pathway; C3bBb3b in the alternative pathway.) The cleavage of C5 produces two fragments: C5a is released into the fluid phase and is a potent anaphylatoxin. C5b binds to the cell surface and forms the nucleus for the binding of the terminal complement components, described in the next section.

The Terminal Pathway

The terminal components of the complement cascades—C5b, C6, C7, C8, and C9—are common to all the complement activation pathways. These components bind to each other and form a ***membrane attack complex*** (MAC) that results in cell lysis (Fig. 13.3).

The first step in MAC formation is C6 binding to C5b on a cell surface. C7 then binds to C5b and C6 and inserts into the outer membrane of the cell. The subsequent binding of C8 to C5b67 results in the complex penetrating deeper into the cell's membrane. C5b–C8 on the cell membrane acts as a receptor for C9, a perforin-like molecule (see Chapter 10) that binds to C8. Additional C9 molecules interact with the C9

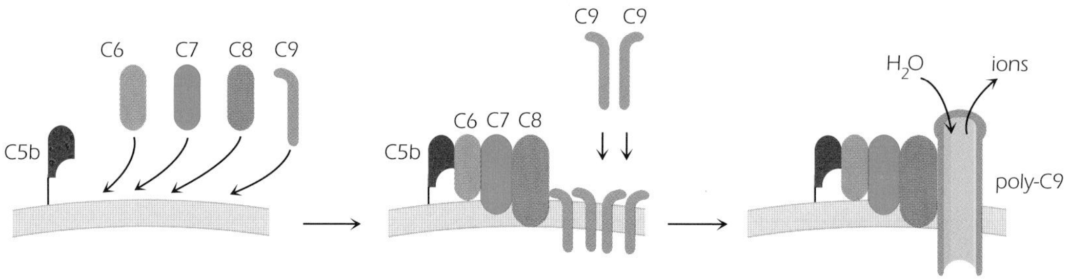

Figure 13.3. Formation of the membrane attack complex. Late stage complement components C5b-C9 bind sequentially to form a complex on the cell surface. Multiple C9 components bind to this complex and polymerize to form poly-C9, creating a channel that disrupts the cell membrane.

molecule in the complex to form polymerized C9 (poly-C9). This poly-C9 forms a transmembrane channel that disturbs the cell's osmotic equilibrium: Ions pass through the channel, and water enters the cell. The cell swells, and the membrane becomes permeable to macromolecules, which then escape from the cell. The result is cell lysis.

REGULATION OF COMPLEMENT ACTIVITY

Uncontrolled complement activation can rapidly deplete complement components, leaving the host unable to remove infectious agents. In addition, as we shall describe later in the chapter, complement activation generates activated fragments (especially the cleavage products of C3, C4, and C5) that induce potent inflammatory responses to remove infectious agents. However, the very potency of these responses may damage the host. Indeed, complement activation is believed to play an adverse role in conditions such as Alzheimer's disease (we previously referred to the activation of the classical pathway by β-amyloid), in the presence of autoantibodies, and in heart attack, which are described later in the chapter.

Normally, inappropriate activation of complement does not occur, because many steps in the complement pathways are negatively regulated by specific inhibitors. The importance of these complement regulators is underscored by the clinical conditions, described at the end of this chapter, that arise when regulatory molecules are lacking: The individual may be either damaged by inflammatory responses or become susceptible to infectious diseases.

Many of the molecules that regulate complement activation are expressed on the surface of mammalian but not microbial cells. Consequently, the regulators of complement activity limit damage to the individual, while allowing activated complement components to focus on removing microbial pathogens. The most important regulators of complement activation are described below.

The first step in the activation of the classical complement pathway is inhibited by ***C1 esterase inhibitor*** (C1INH), which binds to C1r and C1s, causing them to dissociate from C1q and preventing complement activation. Recent evidence indicates that C1INH also regulates the alternative pathway, by inhibiting the function of C3bBb, and the lectin pathway, by inhibiting MASP-1 and MASP-2. As we shall describe below, C1INH also inhibits the function of enzymes in other serum cascades, particularly those involved in clotting and in the formation of kinins, potent mediators of vascular effects.

Figure 13.4A shows that several proteins regulate the classical pathway C3 convertase, C4b2a, by binding to C4b and displacing C2a—the activated enzyme component—from the complex. These regulators are a serum protein known as ***C4b-binding protein*** (C4BP), the widely

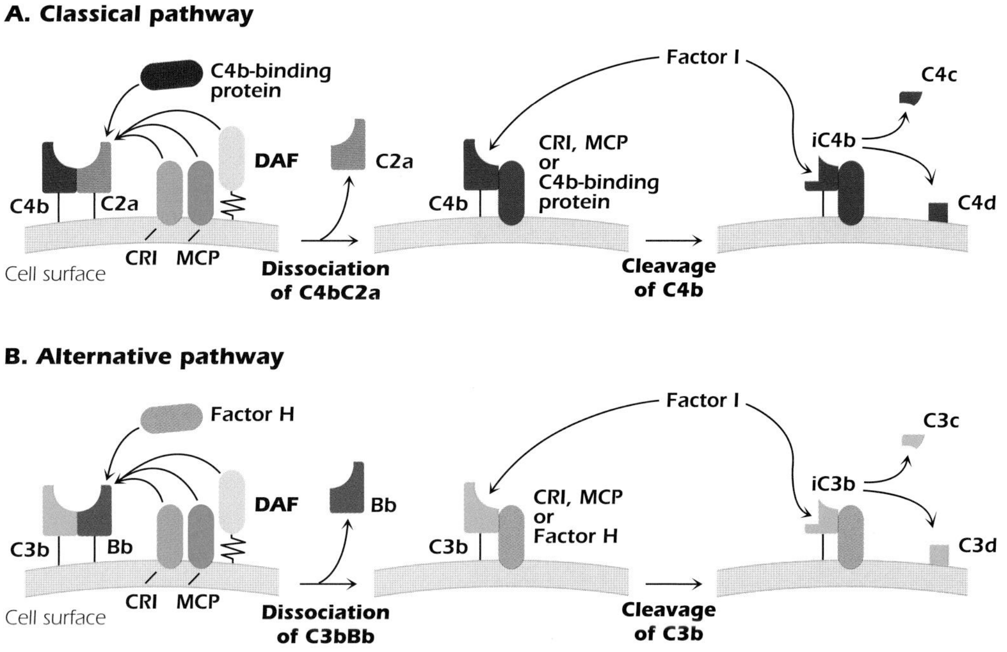

Figure 13.4. Fluid-phase and cell-surface regulators of the C3 convertases in the classical (top) and alternative (bottom) pathways. Regulators may dissociate the convertase, cleave the complement component remaining on the cell surface, or act as a cofactor for this cleavage. C4b binding protein exclusively regulates the classical pathway and Factor H the alternative pathway. Factor I, DAF, CR1, and MCP regulate both pathways.

distributed cell-surface molecules ***decay-accelerating factor (DAF; CD55)*** and ***membrane cofactor protein (MCP; CD46);*** and the cell surface component ***complement receptor 1 (CR1) (CD35)***. Figure 13.4A also illustrates that another serum protein, ***factor I,*** cleaves C4b on the cell surface after C2a has been displaced. C4BP, MCP, and CR1 are referred to as ***cofactors*** for factor I–mediated cleavage because factor I cleavage of C4b requires the presence of one or more of these molecules. (Note that DAF dissociates the C4b2a complex but does not act as a cofactor for factor I.) Factor I cleaves C4b into two fragments: C4c, released into the fluid phase, and C4d, which remains attached to the cell surface. C4c and C4d do not continue the complement cascade and have no known biologic activity.

Activation of the alternative pathway is also regulated. The serum protein ***factor H*** has two important regulatory functions in the alternative pathway. First, factor H competes with the previously described factor B for binding to C3b on a cell surface (Fig. 13.1). Factor B binding to C3b continues the alternative pathway, but if factor H binds to C3b, the pathway does not progress. The nature of the surface to which the C3b is bound is important in determining which factor binds to C3b: The sialic acid coating of mammalian cells favors the binding of factor H, whereas bacterial cells—which lack sialic acid—favor the binding of factor B to C3b. As a result, mammalian cells are protected by the regulatory function of factor H, but bacterial cells are targeted for further activation of the complement pathway.

Figure 13.4B demonstrates factor H's second function: It binds to C3b in the alternative pathway C3 convertase C3bBb and displaces Bb, preventing further activation of the complement cascade. Once factor H has bound to C3b, the previously described factor I cleaves C3b; thus factor H is a cofactor for factor I–mediated cleavage of both C3b and C4b. C3b is cleaved stepwise, first to ***iC3b*** and then to two additional fragments, ***C3c,*** which is released into the fluid phase and lacks biologic function, and ***C3d,*** which remains attached to the cell surface. The breakdown products iC3b, C3c, and C3d do not continue the complement cascade—but, as we shall describe below, iC3b and C3d have important biologic functions. Figure 13.4B also shows that the alternative pathway convertase C3bBb is regulated by the same cell-surface regulatory molecules (DAF, MCP, and CR1) that inhibit the function of the classical pathway C3 convertase, C4b2a.

The terminal pathway of complement activation and the formation of the MAC are also regulated. Because the association of C5b with cell membranes is relatively nonspecific, the association of the terminal pathway components C6–C9 with C5b on cell surfaces would form a MAC that could damage or lyse "innocent bystander" cells. Both membrane-associated and fluid-phase proteins prevent this from occurring. ***CD59,*** a widely distributed membrane protein, prevents lysis by binding to C5b-8 on the cell surface and preventing C9 polymerization. ***S protein*** (vitronectin) and **SP-40,40** (clusterin) are fluid-phase proteins that bind to the hydrophobic regions of C5b6, C5b67, C5b678, and C5b6789 and prevent interaction with membranes.

BIOLOGIC ACTIVITIES OF COMPLEMENT

The major functions of the complement system are summarized below and shown in Figures 13.5 and 13.6.

Production of Opsonins

Complement's most important host defense response is generally considered to be the generation of fragments with opsonic activity that deposit on the surface of pathogens. C3b and C4b are the major opsonins generated, but iC3b, a fragment of C3b that does not activate complement, also has opsonic activity (Fig. 13.5). Bacteria coated by opsonins are rapidly taken up and destroyed by phagocytic cells, such as macrophages and neutrophils. These cells express the receptors CR1, CR3, and CR4, which have broad specificities for complement pathway–generated opsonins and for other complement components. The role of CR1 in regulating complement activation was described earlier in the chapter. Table 13.1 lists the names, functions, and cellular pattern of expression of these and other receptors specific for complement components. The table illustrates the wide range of cells with which complement components interact.

Production of Anaphylatoxins

The complement components C3a, C4a, and C5a are known as ***anaphylatoxins.*** They are small peptides that participate in the inflammatory response, which forms part of the body's defenses in removing an infectious agent that has penetrated the tissues. C5a is the most potent, followed by C3a, with C4a much less potent. The name derives from the earliest recognition of their function: The ability to induce the shock-like characteristics of the systemic allergic or *anaphylactic* response (see Chapter 14).

The anaphylatoxins interact with receptors expressed on many different cell types (Table 13.1). They activate vascular endothelial cells (lining the walls of blood vessels), increasing the permeability of blood vessels, and leading to local accumulation of fluid (edema) in the tissue (Fig. 13.5). The influx into the tissue of fluid, which contains phagocytic cells (macrophages and neutrophils), antibodies, and complement components, enhances the response to the pathogen. The anaphylatoxins are also ***chemotactic*** for neutrophils—that is, the cells migrate from an area of lesser concentration to an area of higher concentration. As a result, neutrophils circulating in the blood are activated, leave the circulation at the tissue site of inflammation, and destroy the foreign material. The

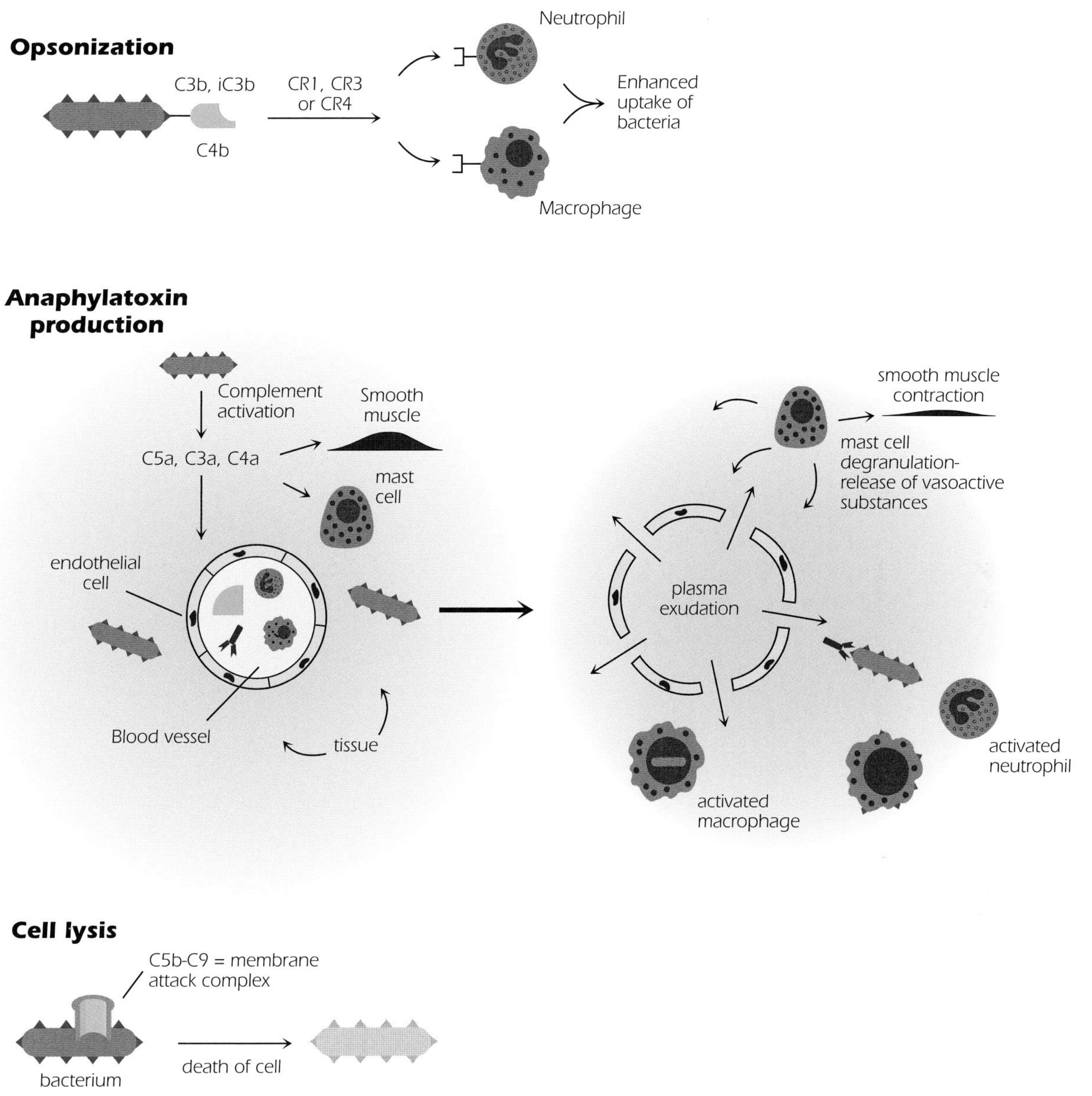

Figure 13.5. Major functions of complement (1): production of opsonins and anaphylatoxins, and cell lysis.

anaphylatoxins also induce smooth muscle contraction. Interaction of the anaphylatoxins with basophils or mast cells in tissues results in the release of many inflammatory mediators, including histamine. The effects of histamine and the anaphylatoxins on vascular permeability and smooth muscle contraction are similar.

Lysis of Cells

The final stage in all three complement activation pathways is the formation of a MAC on the surface of a cell. This results in the lysis of cells, particularly microbial pathogens (Fig. 13.5).

Enhancing B Cell Responses to Antigens

Antibodies are important effector molecules in removing pathogens. Complement components enhance antibody responses in several ways and thus facilitate the removal of microorganisms (Fig. 13.6). (1) Interactions of the complement fragment C3d and CR2 with a microbial antigen enhance the B cell response to the antigen. Antigen bound to IgM on the B cell surface can bind to C3d generated as a consequence of any one of the complement activation pathways. C3d can also bind to the B cell surface molecule CR2 (CD21), which with CD19 and CD81 forms part of a coreceptor signaling complex associated with the B cell receptor for antigen (discussed in

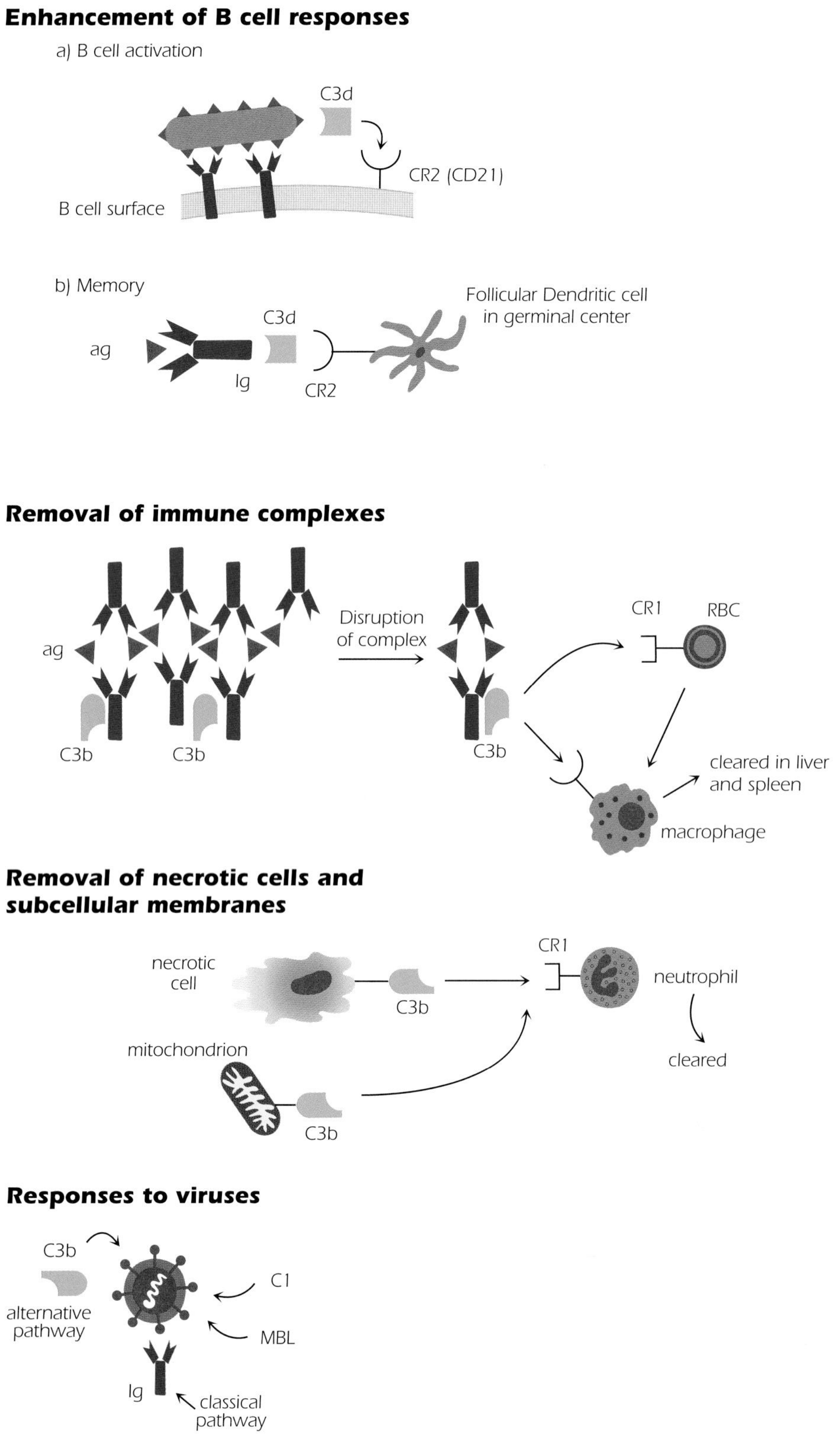

Figure 13.6. Major functions of complement (2): enhancement of B cell responses, removal of immune complexes, removal of necrotic cells and subcellular membranes, and responses to viruses.

TABLE 13.1. Complement Receptors

Complement Receptor	Cell Distribution	Complement Components Bound	Receptor Function
CR1 (CD35)	Erythrocytes, monocytes, macrophages, eosinophils, neutrophils, B cells, some T cells, follicular dendritic cells, and mast cells	C3b, iC3b, C3c, and C4b	Enhances phagocytosis; regulates complement activation pathways
CR2 (CD21)	Late precursor and mature B lymphocytes, some T cells (including thymocytes), and follicular dendritic cells	C3b, iC3b, and C3d	Enhances activation of B cells by bacteria
CR3 (CD11b/CD18, also known as Mac-1)	Monocytes, macrophages, natural killer cells, and granulocytes	iC3b (and many noncomplement components, including bacterial lipopolysaccharide and other surface molecules, zymosan, and fibrinogen)	Enhances phagocytosis
CR4 (CD11c/CD18)	Myeloid cells, dendritic cells, activated B cells, natural killer cells, some cytotoxic lymphocytes, and platelets	iC3b (and many noncomplement ligands, similar to CR3)	Enhances phagocytosis
C3a receptor	Platelets, mast cells, macrophages, neutrophils, basophils, eosinophils, monocytes, and endothelial cells	C3a	Mediates anaphylatoxic response
C5a receptor (CD88)	Granulocytes, platelets, mast cells, liver parenchymal cells, lung vascular smooth muscle, endothelium, astrocytes, and microglial cells in the brain	C5a	Mediates anaphylatoxic response

Chapter 10.) Thus the cross-linking of antigen via IgM and via C3d on the B cell surface delivers simultaneous signals to the B cell. Studies indicate that this C3d pathway lowers the threshold for antigen activation of the B cell—that is, far less antigen is required to trigger the B cell than in the absence of C3d. (2) B cell processing of T-dependent (TD) antigens is more rapid when the antigen is bound to C3d than when it is not; presumably the binding of C3d to CR2 on the B cell surface enhances uptake and processing of the antigen. This may be one way in which complement enhances B cell responses to TD antigens. (3) Complement also plays a role in the induction of memory responses: C3d covalently bound to antigen in immune complexes is taken up by germinal center follicular dendritic cells that express CR2 (see Fig. 13.6 and Chapter 7). This provides a long-lasting deposit of antigen.

Controlling the Formation and Clearance of Immune Complexes

When antibodies bind to multivalent antigens, cross-linking between the molecules tends to produce large antigen–antibody complexes that increase in size until they become insoluble. Although this precipitation of complexes has proved useful for identifying antigens and antibodies in vitro (see Chapter 5), the formation of large insoluble complexes in vivo can be detrimental to the host. As we describe in the final section of the chapter, people deficient in early components of the classical pathway components may show large insoluble immune complexes in tissues such as the skin and kidneys, inducing inflammation and damaging surrounding cells.

Deposition of C3b on large antigen–antibody complexes interferes with the bonds that keep the complex together (Fig. 13.6). As a result, the complex breaks up into smaller pieces that can be cleared by macrophages. Deposition of C3b on the antigen–antibody complex also allows binding to erythrocytes, which express the receptor CR1 on their surface. Erythrocytes clear the complexes from the circulation by transporting them through the circulation to the liver and spleen. In these organs, the complexes are transferred from the erythrocyte CR1 to macrophage CR3 and Fc receptors. Macrophages phagocytose the complexes and destroy them.

Removing Dead or Dying Cells

Cells dying by necrosis can activate complement, leading to C4b and C3b deposition on the cell surface. The cell is then cleared by interacting with CR1 or CR3 on phagocytic cells (Fig. 13.6). Subcellular membranes, from organelles such as mitochondria and endoplasmic reticulum, also directly activate both classical and alternative pathways and are cleared similarly. C-reactive protein, the acute-phase protein and component of the inflammatory response that we referred to earlier in the chapter, also binds to damaged and necrotic cells and activates the classical complement pathway. The same structure that C-reactive protein binds to on the surface of bacterial cells, the polysaccharide phosphocholine, is also exposed on damaged and necrotic cells. Recent evidence indicates that cells dying as a result of apoptosis may also trigger complement. In all these situations, complement removes dead or dying cells from the tissues and contributes to homeostasis.

In some conditions, however, complement activation by dead or dying cells may have clinical consequences. Notable examples are when complement is activated by ***ischemia*** and in ***reperfusion.*** In ischemia, an area of tissue dies after blood and oxygen supplies have been cut (important examples are in cardiac tissue after a heart attack or in the brain after a stroke), and reperfusion is the attempt to restore blood supply to the tissue. Inflammatory responses that damage healthy tissue are associated with both these states, and complement activation is considered a major contributor to these conditions. Complement-based therapies are currently being tested to reduce the deleterious effects of the inflammatory response in these conditions.

Responses to Viruses

Complement plays a role in defense against viral infection (Fig. 13.6). C1 can bind directly to and become activated by the surface of several viruses, including the type C retroviruses, lentiviruses, HIV-1, and human T lymphotropic virus 1 (HTLV-1). In addition, MBL of the lectin pathway binds and is activated by mannose residues on the surfaces of HIV-1, HIV-2, and influenza virus. Antibodies generated in the response against these viruses mediate further binding and activation of the classical pathway on the surface of the virus. Repeating subunits on the viral capsid or membrane surfaces also activate the alternative pathway. Binding of complement proteins leads to opsonization of the virus and lysis of the virion. Complement binding also interferes with the virus's ability to interact with the membrane of its target cells and thus blocks viral entry into the cell.

Many viruses have evolved to subvert the action of complement proteins. For example, some viruses produce proteins that mimic complement inhibitors of function: The herpes viruses make proteins that have DAF- and/or MCP-like activities and others that block C5b-9 formation. In addition, vaccinia virus produces a protein that binds to C3b and C4b and inhibits complement activation: The protein has both decay-accelerating activity and acts as a cofactor for factor I. HIV-1, HTLV-1, simian immunodeficiency virus (SIV), and cytomegalovirus (CMV) capture the complement control proteins DAF, MCP, and CD59 when the virions bud from host cell membranes. As a consequence, the viruses are protected from complement-mediated lysis in the same way that host cells are protected.

Some viruses also bind to complement receptors and thus gain entry into cells. One of the most studied interactions is the Epstein-Barr virus (EBV) infection of human B lymphocytes: The virus's membrane glycoprotein, gp350/220, binds to CR2 (CD21) expressed on the B cell surface, allowing the virus to be taken into the cell. Some viruses activate complement and use the C3b deposited on them to bind to host cell complement receptors; in this way, HIV-1 uses CR1, CR2, and CR3 to infect T cells, B cells, and monocytes. Other viruses bind to membrane-expressed complement regulators: Paramyxovirus (measles virus) uses MCP, and viruses of the picornavirus family use DAF to infect epithelial cells.

COMPLEMENT DEFICIENCIES

As we have described above, the complement system plays an important role in defending the host against microorganisms. It is particularly important in defending against what are known as ***pyogenic*** (pus-forming) bacteria, which include *Neisseria* species (the bacteria responsible for meningitis and some sexually transmitted diseases), *Streptococcus pneumoniae, Haemophilus influenzae,* and *Staphylococcus aureus.* The major pathways of defense against these organisms appear to be the production of IgG antibody that binds to the bacteria, accompanied by opsonization, complement activation, phagocytosis, and intracellular killing. Thus, a situation in which any one of these activities is diminished, resulting from either genetic deficiencies or acquired conditions, renders a person particularly susceptible to these organisms. In addition, we have described how complement is important in removing immune complexes from the circulation; we shall describe in this section how deficiencies of certain complement components can result in immune complexes depositing in tissues, leading to inflammatory, autoimmune conditions.

The conditions associated with deficiencies of complement components, complement regulatory proteins, and complement receptors are shown in Table 13.2. Individuals genetically deficient in specific complement components are relatively rare (approximately 1 in 10,000 people), and deficiencies are not always associated with disease.

Deficiencies in any of the classical pathway components C1, C4, or C2 are associated with increased susceptibility to autoimmune diseases such as systemic lupus erythematosus (SLE; see Chapter 12). This predisposition for SLE in these individuals appears to be the result of an impaired ability to process and clear immune complexes. Typically in SLE, large insoluble immune complexes accumulate along the basement membrane in the kidney. Individuals deficient in C1, C4, or C2 also have an increased risk of infection with pyogenic bacteria. Individuals deficient in alternative pathway or late components, however, have an even higher risk of infection with pyogenic bacteria. This suggests that activation of the classical complement pathway may not be as important as the alternative pathway in defense against these bacteria.

C3 deficiency is rare, but can be severe and even life threatening because C3 is central to all the complement pathways. C3-deficient individuals are susceptible to recurrent pyogenic infection. They may also develop inflammatory disorders associated with circulating immune complexes, such as ***membranoproliferative glomerulonephritis*** (inflammation of the capillary loops in the glomeruli of the kidney,

TABLE 13.2. Complement Deficiencies

Deficient Complement Component	Effect on Complement Function	Clinical Condition
C1, C4, or C2	No activation of classical pathway	Autoimmune conditions (SLE) and pyogenic infections
C3	C3b and other opsonic fragments not produced, terminal components not activated	Severe pyogenic infections and inflammatory conditions (glomerulonephritis)
Properdin, factor B, or factor D	Inability to form membrane attack complex	Severe pyogenic infections
Mannose binding lectin	No activation of lectin pathway	Recurrent bacterial infections
C5, C6, C7, C8, or C9	Inability to form membrane attack complex	Recurrent neisserial infections
C1 inhibitor (C1INH)	Unregulated activation of classical pathway	Angioedema
CD59, DAF	Membrane attack complex damages host cells	Paroxysmal nocturnal hemoglobulinemia (hemolysis and thrombosis)
Factor H, factor I	Unregulated activation of C3	Glomerulonephritis, hemolytic-uremic syndrome
Complement receptor 3 (CR3)	Impaired adhesion and migration of leukocytes	Recurrent bacterial infections

characterized by increased cell number and thickening of capillary walls).

Deficiency of the alternative pathway component properdin or of factor B or D is associated with pyogenic, particularly neisserial, infections. Deficiency of mannose-binding lectin can be a major problem in early life, manifesting as severe recurrent bacterial infections. Individuals lacking components of the membrane attack complex C5b-C9 tend to get recurrent neisserial infections.

Deficiencies or disorders of either complement receptors or complement regulatory proteins may also have serious consequences. Patients with a defect in CR3 may have a rare disorder known as Leukocyte Adhesion Deficiency 1 (described in more detail in Chapter 17) in which adhesion and migration of all leukocytes is impaired. These patients suffer from recurrent pyogenic bacterial infections, but pus is not formed. Deficiency of factor H or I results in uncontrolled activation of the alternative pathway, leading to depletion of C3. The outcomes are similar to those seen in individuals with C3 deficiency described above: enhanced susceptibility to infection by pyogenic organisms and to immune complex diseases. Factor H deficiency is also associated with ***hemolytic-uremic syndrome,*** characterized by destruction of red blood cells, damage to endothelial cells, and (in severe cases) kidney failure.

Deficiency of the regulatory protein C1INH, the only control protein for the classical pathway components C1r and C1s, results in uncontrolled cleavage of C2 and C4. Genetic deficiency of C1INH results in ***hereditary angioedema*** (HAE). The condition is characterized by localized edemas in the skin and mucosa resulting from dilatation and increased permeability of the capillaries. The symptoms are recurrent attacks of swollen tissues, such as the face and limbs, pain in the abdomen, and swelling of the larynx, which can compromise breathing. C1INH also inhibits enzymes in serum cascades other than complement activation. One of these serum cascades forms kinins, including bradykinin, which are potent vasodilators and inducers of vascular permeability and smooth muscle contraction. Deficiency of C1INH is thought to lead to increased production of these vascular mediators.

Paroxysmal nocturnal hemoglobinuria (PNH) is a rare acquired disorder that also involves complement regulatory proteins. The condition occurs primarily in young adults and is characterized by chronic destruction of red blood cells and thrombus formation (an aggregate of platelets and blood factors that causes vascular blockage), hemolytic anemia and the presence of hemoglobin in urine, predominantly at night. The condition results from a somatic mutation in the gene that controls the production of the glycosylphosphatidylinositol (GPI) anchor that attaches many membrane proteins to the cell surface (see Chapter 6). In PNH, the anchor is not made properly and the proteins do not attach to the cell surface; they are secreted from the cell into the fluid phase. Several proteins are affected, including the complement regulatory proteins DAF and CD59. The absence of these molecules makes the red cell membrane particularly sensitive to complement-mediated lysis.

In other acquired conditions, C3 may become depleted to an extent that immune complexes are not cleared or an individual becomes susceptible to infection. This can occur in some people who produce an autoantibody known as ***C3 nephritic factor:*** The antibody stabilizes the alternative pathway C3 convertase (C3bBb), generating a highly efficient and long-lived fluid-phase enzyme that cleaves C3. C3 nephritic factor has been described in some individuals with SLE and a rare disease known as partial lypodistrophy, involving the loss of fat from the upper part of the body. These conditions are also characterized by a glomerulonephritis. The connection of complement with partial lypodistrophy is that fat cells, particularly those in the upper part of the body, produce factor D, which cleaves C3bBb. The loss of fat cells in the condition may result from localized complement-mediated cell lysis.

SUMMARY

1. Complement consists of serum- and membrane-expressed proteins that play a key effector role in innate immunity and antibody-mediated adaptive responses to microbial pathogens.
2. Complement activation is a cascade that sequentially generates biologically active molecules—enzymes, opsonins, and anaphylatoxins.
3. Complement can be initiated by three distinct pathways: (1) the classical pathway, predominantly by the binding of antigen-antibody complexes to C1q; (2) the lectin pathway, by terminal carbohydrate residues on the surface of bacteria interacting with mannose-binding lectin; and (3) the alternative pathway, by many agents, including the cell walls of some bacteria and yeasts, and requiring C3b, serum factors B and D, and properdin.
4. The final stages of the complement pathways converge in forming a membrane attack complex, comprising components C5b through C9.
5. The activity of complement and its components is tightly regulated by several proteins. These are found in the fluid phase (factors H and I, C1inhibitor, C4b-binding protein) and on the surface of many cells (DAF, MCP, and CR1). Complement regulator proteins are not expressed on the surface of microbial cells.
6. Complement components interact with specific receptors expressed on multiple cell types.
7. The major functions of complement are (1) production of opsonins (particularly C3b and C4b), (2) production of anaphylatoxins (C5a, C3a, C4a); (3) lysis of cells (C5b through C9), (4) enhancing B lymphocyte responses to antigens (C3d and CR2), (5) controlling the formation and clearance of immune complexes (C3b, C4b), (6) removal of dead and dying cells (C3b, C4b), and (7) interactions with viruses (multiple components).
8. Deficiencies of complement components, regulators of complement pathways, or receptors for complement components may result in increased susceptibility to infection or the development of inflammatory conditions.

REFERENCES

Barilla-LaBarca ML, Liszewski MK, Lambris JD, Hourcade D, Atkinson JP (2002): Role of membrane cofactor protein (CD46) in regulation of C4b and C3b deposited on cells. *J Immunol* 168:6298.

Fearon DT (1998): The complement system and adaptive immunity. *Semin Immunol* 10:355.

Fishelson Z, Attali G, Mevorach D (2001): Complement and apoptosis. *Mol Immunol* 38:207.

Monsinjon T, Richard V, Fontaine M (2001): Complement and its implications in cardiac ischemia/reperfusion: strategies to inhibit complement. *Fundam Clin Pharmacol* 15:293.

Sturfelt G (2002): The complement system in systemic lupus erythematosus. *Scand J Rheumatol* 31:129.

Sullivan KE (1998): Complement deficiency and autoimmunity. *Curr Opin Pediatr* 10:600.

Volanakis JE, Frank MM (1998): The human complement system in health and disease. New York: Marcel Dekker.

Walport MJ (2001): Complement. *N Engl J Med* 344:1058, 1140.

REVIEW QUESTIONS

For each question, choose the ONE BEST answer or completion.

1. A patient is admitted with multiple bacterial infections and is found to have a complete absence of C3. Which complement-mediated function would remain intact in such a patient?
   A) lysis of bacteria
   B) opsonization of bacteria
   C) generation of anaphylatoxins
   D) generation of neutrophil chemotactic factors
   E) None of the above.

2. Complement is required for
   A) lysis of erythrocytes by the enzyme lecithinase.
   B) NK-mediated lysis of tumor cells.
   C) phagocytosis.
   D) antibody-mediated lysis of bacteria.
   E) All of the above.

3. Which of the following is associated with the development of systemic lupus erythematosus (SLE)?
   A) deficiencies in C1, C4, or C2
   B) deficiencies in C5, C6, or C7
   C) deficiencies in the late components of complement
   D) increases in the serum C3 level
   E) increases in the levels of C1, C4, or C2

4. Activated fragments of C5 can lead to all of the following, *except*
   A) contraction of smooth muscle.
   B) vasodilation.
   C) attraction of leukocytes to a site of infection.
   D) attachment of lymphocytes to macrophages.
   E) initiation of formation of the membrane attack complex

5. The alternative pathway of complement activation is characterized by all of the following *except*
   A) activation of complement components beyond C3 in the cascade.
   B) participation of properdin.
   C) generation of anaphylatoxins.
   D) activation of C4.

6. Decay-accelerating factor (DAF) regulates the complement system to prevent complement-mediated lysis of cells. This involves
   A) dissociation of the C3 convertase complex.
   B) blocking the binding of the C3 convertase to the surface of bacterial cells.
   C) inhibiting the membrane attack complex from binding to bacterial membranes.
   D) acting as a cofactor for the cleavage of C3b.
   E) causing dissociation of C5 convertase.

7. The following activate(s) the alternative pathway of complement:
   A) lipopolysaccharides
   B) some viruses and virus-infected cells
   C) fungal and yeast cell walls
   D) many strains of gram-positive bacteria
   E) all of the above.

ANSWERS TO REVIEW QUESTIONS

1. *E* All these functions are mediated by complement components that are generated later in the complement activation sequence than C3. Thus, all these functions are disrupted in the absence of C3.

2. *D* Complement is required for lysis of bacteria by IgM or IgG (classical pathway). Complement is not required for lysis of erythrocytes by lecithinase, nor for phagocytosis. However, opsonins such as C3b that are generated during complement activation can enhance phagocytosis. Although some tumor cells can initiate the alternate pathway of complement activation, complement plays no role in NK-mediated lysis of these cells.

3. *A* Inherited homozygous deficiency of one of the early proteins of the classical complement pathway (C1, C4, or C2) is strongly associated with the development of systemic lupus erythematosus (SLE). Such deficiencies probably result in abnormal processing of immune complexes in the absence of a functional classical pathway of complement fixation. Serum levels of C3 and C4 decrease in SLE due to the large number of immune complexes that bind to them. Deficiencies in the late components are associated with recurrent infections with pyogenic organisms.

4. *D* C5a is an anaphylatoxin, which induces degranulation of mast cells, resulting in the release of histamine, causing vasodilation and contraction of smooth muscles. C5a is also chemotactic, attracting leukocytes to the area of its release where an antigen is reacting with antibodies and activates the complement system; this is a part of the inflammatory response to an infection. C5b deposits on membranes and initiates the formation of the terminal membrane attack complex. Neither C5a nor C5b promotes the attachment of lymphocytes to macrophages.

5. *D* The alternative pathway of complement activation connects with the classical pathway at the activation of C3. Thus, it does not require C1, C4, or C2. Properdin is essential for the activation through the alternative pathway, since it stabilizes the complex formed between C3b and activated serum factor B, C3bBb, which acts as a C3 convertase and activates C3. During the activation of the alternative pathway both C3a and C5a are generated; both are anaphylatoxins and cause degranulation of mast cells.

6. *A* DAF is a cell surface regulator of complement activation that destabilizes the C3 convertases of the alternate and classical pathways (C3bBb and C4b2a, respectively). Like other regulators of complement activation—including CR1, factor H, and C4bBP—these proteins accelerate decay (dissociation) of the C3 convertase, releasing the component with enzymatic activity (Bb or C2a) from the component bound to the cell membrane (C3b or C4b).

7. *E* Each of these pathogens and particles of microbial origin can initiate the alternate pathway of complement activation. Teichoic acid from the cell walls of gram-positive organisms, as well as parasites such as trypanosomes, can also activate complement via this pathway.

14

HYPERSENSITIVITY REACTIONS: ANTIBODY-MEDIATED (TYPE I) REACTIONS

INTRODUCTION

Under some circumstances, immune responses produce damaging and sometimes fatal results. Such deleterious reactions are known collectively as ***hypersensitivity.*** It should be remembered that hypersensitivity reactions differ from protective immune reactions only in that they are exaggerated or inappropriate and damaging to the host. The cellular and molecular mechanisms of the two types of reaction are virtually identical.

Coombs-Gell Hypersensitivity Designations

In the early 1960s, hypersensitivity reactions were divided into four types, designated I to IV by Coombs and Gell.

- **Type I.** IgE-mediated reactions are stimulated by the binding of IgE (via its Fc region) to high-affinity IgE-specific Fc receptors (FcεRI) expressed on mast cells and basophils. When cross-linked by antigens, the IgE antibodies trigger the mast cells and basophils to release inflammatory mediators that lead to clinical manifestations (***allergic reactions***), including rhinitis, asthma, and, in severe cases, anaphylaxis (from the Greek *ana,* which means "away from," and *phylaxis,* which means "protection"). Reactions are rapid, occurring within minutes after challenge—that is re-exposure to antigen. Thus allergic reactions are also called ***immediate hypersensitivity.*** In recent years, the term ***allergy*** has also become synonymous with type I hypersensitivity. Henceforth, we will generally use this term in lieu of "type I hypersensitivity."
- **Type II.** Cytolytic or cytotoxic reactions occur when IgM or IgG antibodies bind to antigen on the surface of cells and activate the complement cascade, culminating in destruction of the cells.
- **Type III.** Immune complex reactions occur when complexes of antigen and IgM or IgG antibody accumulate in the circulation or in tissue and activate the complement cascade. Granulocytes are attracted to the site of activation, and damage results from the release of lytic enzymes from their granules. Reactions occur within hours of challenge with antigen.
- **Type IV.** Cell-mediated immunity (CMI) reactions—commonly called delayed-type hypersensitivity (DTH)—is mediated by T cell-dependent effector mechanisms involving both $CD4^+$ T_H1 cells and $CD8^+$ cytotoxic T cells. Antibodies do not play a role in type IV hypersensitivity reactions. On activation, the T_H1 cells release cytokines that cause accumulation and activation of macrophages, which, in turn, cause local damage. This type of reaction has a delayed onset that may occur days or weeks after challenge with antigen.

This chapter deals with type I hypersensitivity, also known as allergic reactions. Hypersensitivity types II and III are discussed in Chapter 15, and type IV hypersensitivity is discussed in Chapter 16.

Immunology: A Short Course, Fifth Edition, By Richard Coico, Geoffrey Sunshine, and Eli Benjamini
ISBN 0-471-22689-0

GENERAL CHARACTERISTICS OF ALLERGIC REACTIONS

The sequence of events involved in the development of allergic reactions can be divided into several phases: (1) the ***sensitization phase,*** during which IgE antibody is produced in response to an antigenic stimulus and binds to specific receptors on mast cells and basophils; (2) the ***activation phase,*** during which re-exposure, or challenge to antigen triggers the mast cells and basophils to respond by release of the contents of their granules; and (3) the ***effector phase,*** during which a complex response occurs as a result of the effects of the many inflammatory mediators released by the mast cells and basophils. The clinical manifestations of these effector mechanisms include ***eczema, asthma,*** and ***rhinitis.***

SENSITIZATION PHASE

The immunoglobulin responsible for allergic reactions is ***IgE.*** All normal individuals can make IgE antibody specific for a variety of antigens when antigen is introduced parenterally in the appropriate manner. However, some individuals are genetically predisposed to certain allergies, as will be discussed below. It is important to note that allergic reactions can be elicited not only upon re-exposure to the same antigen that initiated IgE synthesis in the first place but also to ones that share common epitopes with that antigen. Sensitization to ***allergens*** can occur through any means of contact, including skin contact, ingestion, injection, and inhalation. Approximately 50% of the population generates an IgE response to airborne antigens that are encountered only on mucosal surfaces, such as the lining of the nose and lungs and the conjunctiva of the eyes. However, after repeated exposure to a plethora of these airborne allergens—such as plant pollens, mold spores, house dust mites, and animal dander—approximately 20% of the general population develops clinical symptoms, resulting in seasonal or perennial allergic rhinitis. An outdated, yet commonly used term used to describe the clinical symptoms induced by airborne allergens is ***hay fever.***

The term ***atopy*** (from the Greek word *atopos,* meaning "out of place") is frequently used to refer to IgE-mediated hypersensitivity and the term ***atopic,*** to describe affected patients. Children of atopic individuals often suffer from allergies themselves, indicating that ***familial tendencies*** are common. Evidence suggests that IgE responses are genetically controlled by MHC-linked genes located on chromosome 6. Recently, other IgE regulatory genes have been implicated, including the high-affinity ***FcεRI gene*** on chromosome 11 and the ***T_H2 interleukin 4 (IL-4) gene cluster*** on chromosome 5, which contains gene for IL-3, IL-4, IL-5, IL-9, and IL-13.

IgE Antibody Production Is T_H2 Cell Dependent

Several lines of evidence have demonstrated the T_H2 cell dependency of IgE responses. The mechanism by which these cells promote B cell isotype switching has not been fully elucidated, although it is clear that certain cytokines produced by these cells, most notably IL-4 and IL-13, play a pivotal role. The administration of neutralizing antibodies to IL-4 in mice inhibits IgE production. In addition, IL-4 knockout mice cannot produce IgE following infection with *Nippostrongylus brasiliensis*—a nematode that induces high IgE responses in normal mice. A comparison of IL-4 levels in allergic versus nonallergic people has shown that IL-4 levels are significantly higher in the allergic population. Consistent with this observation is the fact that IgE levels are approximately 10-fold higher in allergic individuals compared to normal subjects. In normal individuals, the concentration of serum IgE is the lowest of all immunoglobulins. It has been suggested that the low levels of IgE antibody in nonallergic individuals are maintained by suppressor effects mediated by interferon (IFN-γ) produced by T_H1 cells that downregulate IgE production. Thus, in normal individuals, a balance is maintained between T_H2-derived cytokines that upregulate IgE responses and T_H1-derived cytokines that downregulate IgE responses. Natural events such as infections with certain pathogens may disturb this balance and stimulate IgE-producing B cells. Therefore, allergic sensitization may result from failure of a control mechanism leading to overproduction of IL-4 by T_H2 cells and, ultimately, increased IgE production by B cells. Once adequate exposure to the allergen has been achieved by repeated mucosal contact, ingestion, or parenteral injection, and IgE antibody has been produced, an individual is considered to be ***sensitized.*** Once IgE antibody is made and secreted by allergen-stimulated B cells, it rapidly attaches to ***mast cells*** and ***basophils*** as it circulates past them.

Mast cells, the main effector cells responsible for allergic reactions, are a ubiquitous family of cells generally found around blood vessels in the connective tissue, in the lining of the gut, and in the lungs. They are large mononuclear cells, heavily granulated and deeply stained by basic dyes (Fig. 14.1). Mast cells are derived from progenitor cells that migrate to the tissue, where they differentiate into mature mast cells. In some species, including humans, circulating basophils also take part in allergic responses and function in much the same way as the tissue-based mast cells. Unlike the mast cells, they mature in the bone marrow and are present in the circulation in their differentiated form. One of the most important features that mast cells and basophils have in common is that they both have receptors (FcεRI) on their cell membranes that bind with high affinity to the Fc region of IgE. Once bound, the IgE molecules persist at the cell surface for weeks, that cell will remain sensitized as long as enough antibody remains attached, and it will trigger the activation of the cell when it comes into contact with antigen.

Sensitization may also be achieved passively by transfer of serum that contains IgE antibody to a specific antigen. A procedure of historical interest only, known as the Prausnitz-Kustner (P-K) test, used to be performed as a test for the antibodies responsible for anaphylactic reactions. In

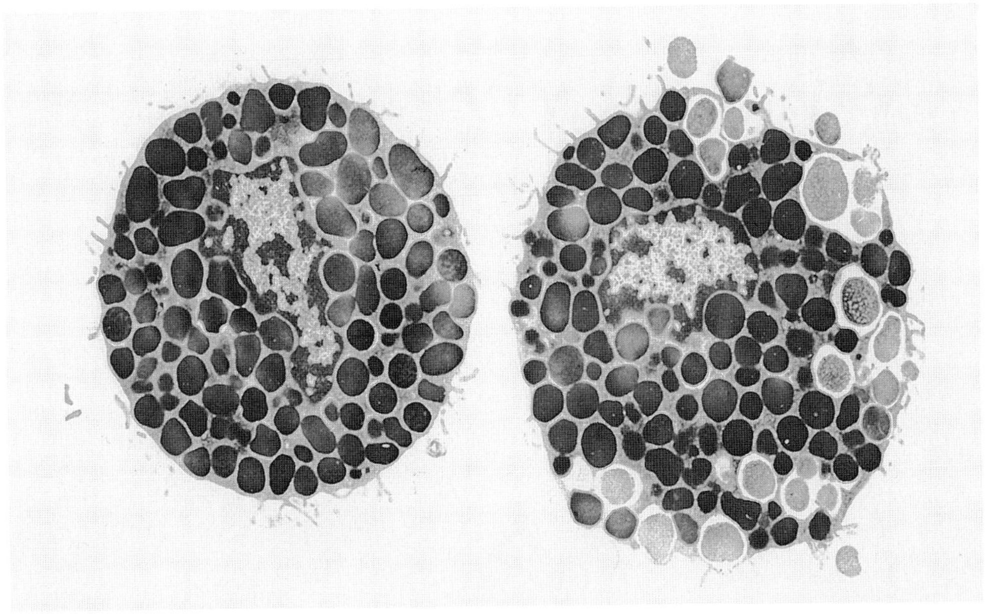

Figure 14.1. Electron micrograph of a normal mast cell showing the large monocyte-like nucleus and the electron-dense granules. On the right, a mast cell has been triggered and is beginning to release the contents of its granules, as seen by their decrease in opacity and the formation of vacuoles connecting with the exterior. (Courtesy of T. Theoharides, Tufts Medical School.)

the P-K test, serum from an allergic individual was injected into the skin of a nonallergic person. After 1–2 days, during which the locally injected antibody diffused toward neighboring mast cells and became bound to them, the site of injection was said to be sensitized and would respond with an ***urticarial reaction*** (hives) when injected with that antigen to which the donor was allergic. Such a reaction in passively sensitized animals is called ***passive cutaneous anaphylaxis*** (PCA).

ACTIVATION PHASE

The activation phase of allergic reactions begins with the triggering of the mast cell to release its granules and their inflammatory mediators. It requires that at least two of the receptors for the Fc region of the IgE molecules be bridged together in a stable configuration. In the simplest and immunologically most relevant manner, this linkage is accomplished by a multivalent antigen that can bind a different molecule of IgE to each of several epitopes on its surface, thus cross-linking them and effectively triggering the cell to respond by degranulating (Fig. 14.2). The physiologic consequences of IgE-mediated mast cell degranulation depend on the dose of antigen and route of entry. Mast cells that degranulate within the ***gastrointestinal track*** cause increased fluid secretion and peristasis, which, in turn, can result in diarrhea and vomiting. In contrast, degranulation of mast cells in the ***lung*** causes a decrease in airway diameters and increased mucus secretion. These events lead to congestion and blockage of the airways (coughing, wheezing, phlegm) and to swelling and mucus secretion in nasal passages. Finally, degranulation of mast cells present in the ***blood vessels*** causes increased blood flow and vascular permeability, resulting in increased fluid in tissues. This, in turn, causes increased flow of lymph from the local lymph nodes, leading to increased cells and protein in tissue, all of which contribute to the inflammatory response.

Cross-linking of FcεRI receptors may also be accomplished in other experimentally useful ways, such as by addition of an antibody that is specific for IgE molecules (anti-IgE or anti-idiotype antibodies); or for the IgE receptor molecules on the surface of mast cells, exposure to sugar-binding lectins; or even by use of chemical cross-linkers (Fig. 14.3). As expected, dimers or aggregates of IgE will also cross-link these Fc receptors and activate mast cells to degranulate. Finally, activation of mast cells can also be achieved using calcium ionophores, which induce a rapid influx of calcium ions into the cell, triggering the signaling cascade leading to degranulation.

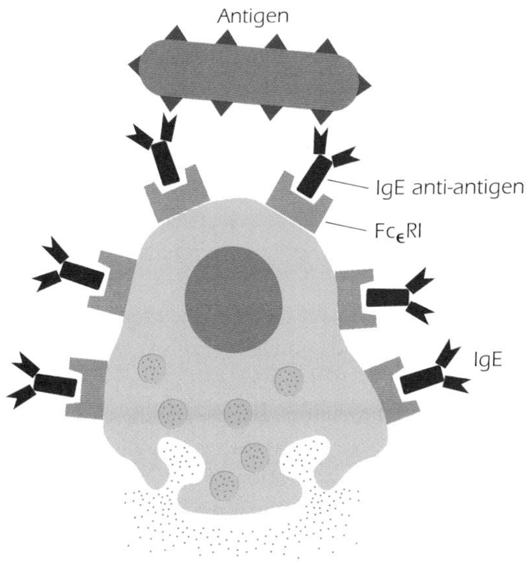

Figure 14.2. Mast cell degranulation mediated by antigen cross-linking of IgE bound to IgE Fc receptors (FcεRI).

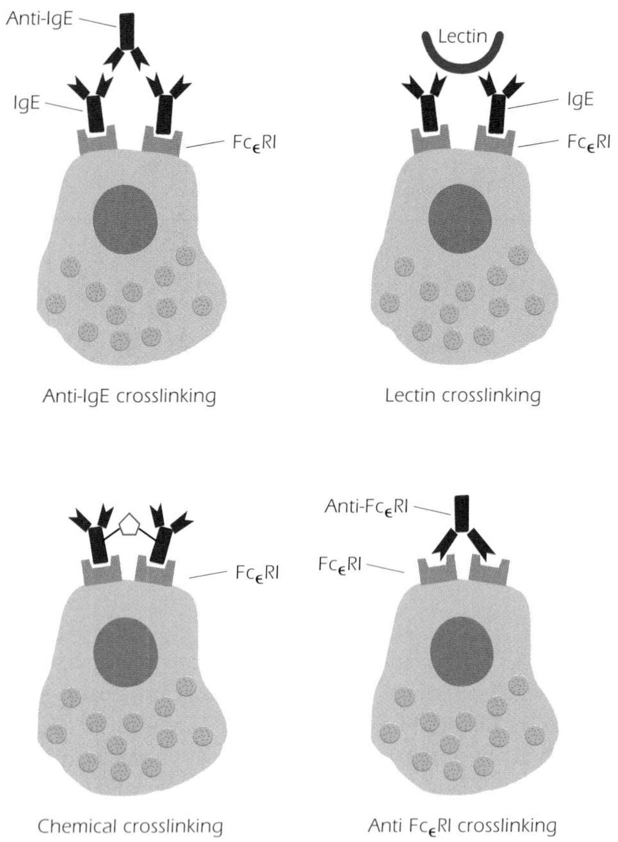

Figure 14.3. Alternate ways in which mast cells can be induced to undergo degranulation.

Mast cells may also be activated through mechanisms other than IgE Fc receptor cross-linking. The ***anaphylatoxins*** C3a and C5a, products of complement activation (see Chapter 13), and various drugs (such as codeine, morphine, and iodinated radiocontrast dyes) produce anaphylactoid reactions. Physical factors such as heat, cold, or pressure can also activate mast cells, as seen, for example, in cold-induced urticaria (an anaphylactic rash induced in certain individuals by chilling an area of skin). Finally, as noted above, certain lectins (sugar-binding molecules) can also cross-link IgE Fc receptors (Fig. 14.3). High concentrations of lectins are found in certain foods (e.g., strawberries). This might explain the urticaria induced in some individuals after eating these foods.

The triggering of a mast cell by the bridging of its receptors initiates a rapid and complex series of events culminating in the degranulation of the mast cell and the release of potent inflammatory mediators. Because of the ease with which its outcome can be measured, the mast cell has served as a model for the study of activation of cells in general. Among the rapid events known to occur are receptor aggregation and changes in membrane fluidity, which result from methylation of phospholipids, leading to transient increase in intracellular levels of cyclic adenosine monophosphate (cAMP) followed by an influx of Ca^{++} ions. The intracellular levels of cAMP and cyclic guanosine monophosphate (cGMP) are known to affect subsequent events and are important in the regulation of those events. In general, a sustained increase in intracellular cAMP at this stage will slow, or even stop, the process of degranulation. Thus activation of adenylate cyclase, the enzyme that converts adenosine triphosphate (ATP) to cAMP, provides an important mechanism for controlling anaphylactic events.

As noted earlier, allergic reactions are often called immediate hypersensitivity. This term is appropriate in light of the very rapid consequences of IgE Fc receptor cross-linking, beginning with movement of mast cell granules by microfilaments to the cell surface. Once at the cell surface, granule membranes fuse with the cell membrane, and the contents are released to the exterior in a process known as exocytosis (Fig. 14.1). Depending on the extent of cross-linking on the cell surface, any cell can release some or all of its granules. Furthermore, this explosive release of granules is physiologic and does not imply lysis or death of the cell. In fact, the degranulated cells regenerate and, once the contents of the granules have been synthesized, the cells are ready to resume their function.

EFFECTOR PHASE

The symptoms of allergic reactions are entirely attributable to the inflammatory mediators released by the activated mast cells. It is helpful to consider these mediators in two major categories (Fig. 14.4). One category consists of basic ***preformed mediators,*** which are stored in the granules by electrostatic attraction to a matrix protein and are released as a result of the influx of ions, primarily Na^+. Cytokines released from mast cells undergoing degranulation, including IL-3, IL-4, IL-5, IL-8, IL-9, TNFα, and granulocyte-macrophage colony-stimulating factor (GM-CSF), also play a role in attracting and activating inflammatory cells to the site. Inflammatory cells participate in the so-called late-phase reactions (described later in this chapter) of allergic reactions in concert with the second category of mast cell mediators—those synthesized *de novo*. ***Newly formed mast cell mediators*** consist of substances synthesized, in part, from membrane lipids. Many potent substances are released during degranulation; however, only the most important members of each category are considered here.

Preformed Mediators

Histamine. Histamine is formed in the cell by decarboxylation of the amino acid histidine and is stored bound by electrostatic interaction to an acid matrix protein called heparin. When released, histamine binds rapidly to a variety of cells via two major types of receptors, H1 and H2, which have different distributions in tissue and which

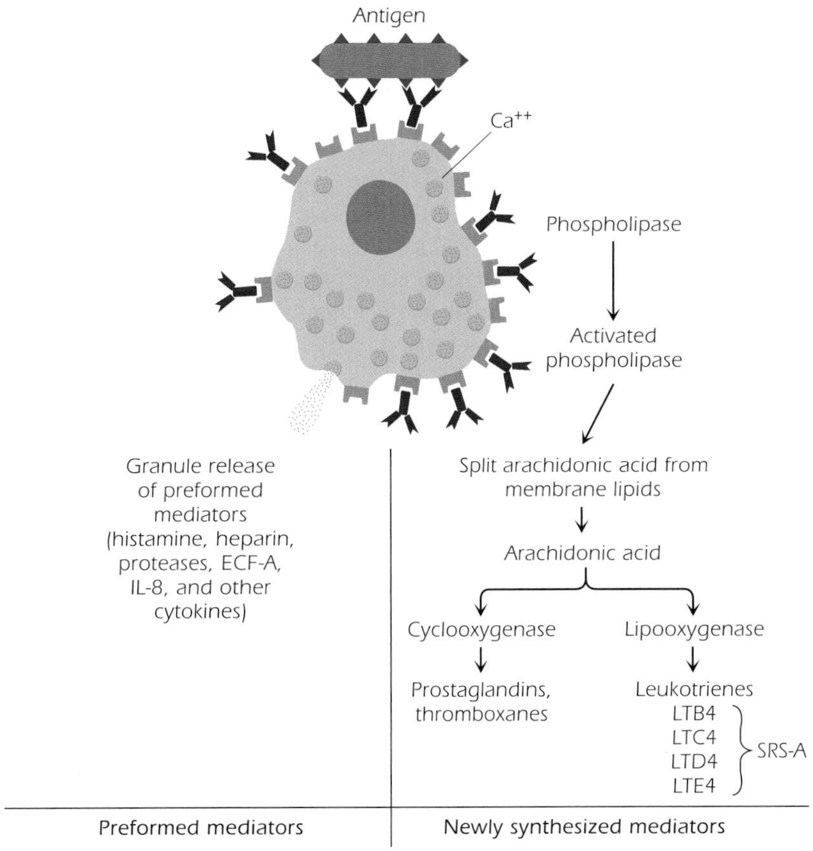

Figure 14.4. **Mediators released during activation of mast cells.**

mediate different effects. When histamine binds to H1 receptors on smooth muscles, it causes constriction; when it binds to H1 receptors on endothelial cells, it causes separation at their junctions, resulting in vascular permeability. H2 receptors are those involved in mucus secretion and increased vascular permeability as well as in the release of acid from stomach mucosa. All these effects are responsible for some of the major signs in systemic anaphylaxis: difficulty in breathing (asthma) or asphyxiation, due to constriction of smooth muscle around the bronchi in the lung, and a drop in blood pressure that results from extravasation of fluid into tissue spaces as the permeability of blood vessels increases. H1 receptors are blocked by antihistamines, such as Benadryl, by direct competition; and when these drugs are given soon enough, they can counteract the effects of histamine. Blockage of H2 receptors requires other drugs, such as cimetidine. However, some time after the introduction of antihistamines, it was noted that they were ineffective in controlling constriction of smooth muscles that was slower in onset and more persistent than that produced by histamine. This observation led to the discovery of the ***slow-reacting substance of anaphylaxis*** (SRS-A), now known to consist of a group of ***leukotrienes*** (see below).

Serotonin. Serotonin is present in the mast cells of only certain species, such as rodents. Its effects are similar to those of histamine, in that it causes constriction of smooth muscle and increases vascular permeability.

Cytokines and Chemotactic Factors. A variety of cytokines and chemotactic factors are released after degranulation of mast cells. These include such cytokines, as GM-CSF, IL-5, and TNFα. A set of low molecular weight peptides called ***eosinophilic chemotactic factors*** (ECFs) are also released. These produce a chemotactic gradient capable of attracting eosinophils to the site. In addition, the late-phase mediators ***platelet activating factor*** (PAF) and ***leukotrienes*** (see below) also participate in the chemotaxis of inflammatory cells to the site. Another important inflammatory cell attracted to the site is the neutrophil. Chemotaxis of these polymorphonuclear granulocytes occurs in response to IL-8 released by activated mast cells. As we shall see later, granulocytes are important in the late phase of IgE-mediated hypersensitivity. Other cells attracted to the site in response to mast cell–derived chemotactic factors include basophils, macrophages, platelets, and lymphocytes.

In allergic reactions, ***eosinophils*** appear to serve as a late indicator of the presence of IgE-mediated reactions, especially the late-phase reaction discussed later; they may also release arylsulfatase and histaminase, which destroy several mediators of the hypersensitivity reaction, thus serving as one of the mechanisms to limit the reaction. Eosinophils have an additional function in parasitic worm infections, also discussed later in this chapter.

Heparin. Heparin is an acidic proteoglycan that constitutes the matrix of the granule and to which basic mediators, such as histamine and serotonin, are bound. Its acidic nature accounts for the metachromatic (high-staining) properties of the mast cell when basic dyes, such as toluidine blue, are applied to it. Release of heparin causes inhibition of coagulation, which may be of some use in the subsequent recovery of the mast cell or further introduction of antigen into the reaction area; however, it is not directly involved in the symptoms of anaphylaxis.

Newly Synthesized Mediators

Leukotrienes. When a preparation of smooth muscle, such as a guinea pig uterine horn, is treated with histamine, rapid contraction occurs. As noted above, this phenomenon was originally said to be due to SRS-A. SRS-A is now known to consist of a set of peptides that are coupled to a metabolite of ***arachidonic acid*** and are collectively called ***leukotrienes*** (LTs). The leukotrienes have been named LTB4, LTC4, LTD4, and LTE4; in minute amounts, they cause prolonged constriction of smooth muscle. They are considered to be the cause of much antihistamine-resistant asthma in humans.

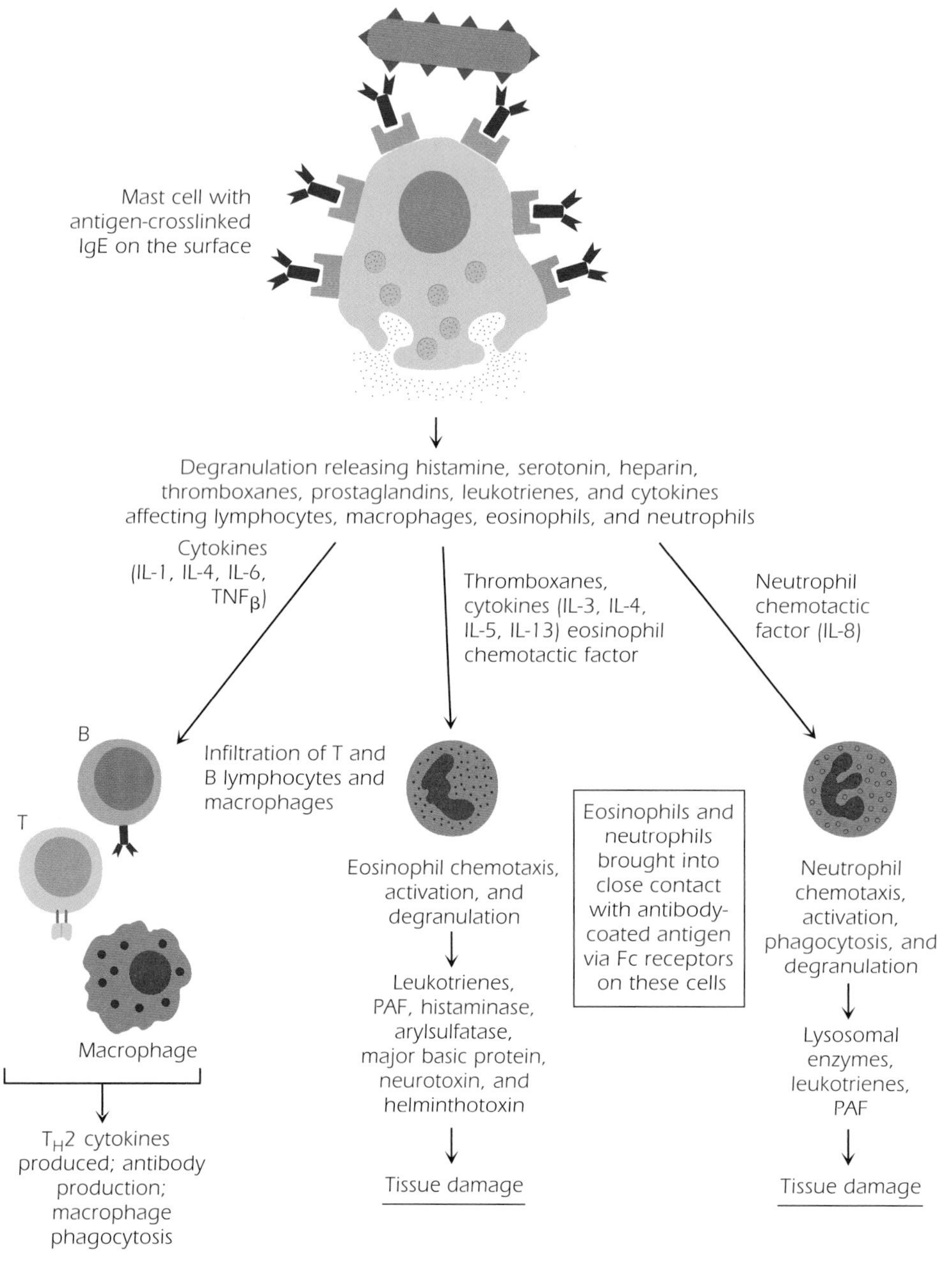

Figure 14.5. A late-phase reaction of type I IgE-mediated hypersensitivity with some of the mediators involved.

Thromboxanes and Prostaglandins. Leukotrienes are only a small part of the complex series of products produced from arachidonic acid released from cell membrane lipids by phospholipases during mast cell triggering. Arachidonic acid is a polyunsaturated, long-chain hydrocarbon that can be oxygenated in two separate pathways (Fig. 14.4): by lipoxygenase to give the above-mentioned leukotrienes and by cyclooxygenase to give ***prostaglandins*** and ***thromboxanes.*** Many of these latter compounds are vasoactive, causing bronchoconstriction, and are chemotactic for a variety of white cells, such as neutrophils, eosinophils, basophils, and monocytes.

Platelet-Activating Factor. PAF induces platelets to aggregate and release their contents of mediators, which include ***histamine*** and, in some species, ***serotonin.*** Activation of platelets may also induce release of metabolites of arachidonic acid, thus augmenting effects generated by mast cells. PAF itself is one of the most potent causes of bronchoconstriction and vasodilation known, producing shock-like symptoms rapidly in very small doses.

Late-Phase Reaction

As mentioned above, many of the substances released during mast-cell activation and degranulation are responsible for the initiation of a profound inflammatory response with infiltration and accumulation of eosinophils, neutrophils, basophils, lymphocytes, and macrophages. Most important, and constituting a large percentage of the cells, are eosinophils and neutrophils that become activated and exacerbate the inflammation. This response often occurs within 48 h and may persist for several days. This is referred to as the ***late-phase reaction*** and is shown in Figure 14.5. The mast cell, degranulated by cross-linking of IgE on its surface by antigen, releases eosinophil chemotactic factor A (ECF-A), which recruits eosinophils to the reaction area. Their passage, as well as the passage of other leukocytes from the circulation to the tissue, is facilitated by the increased vascular permeability caused by histamine and other mediators. Various cytokines, including GM-CSF, IL-3, IL-4, IL-5, and IL-13 play an important role in eosinophil growth and differentiation and cell adhesion of certain cell types. Together, these inflammatory mediators generate a second, albeit milder wave of smooth muscle contraction than the immediate response, and they produce sustained edema. In the case of individuals suffering from allergic asthma, the late-phase reaction also promotes the development of one of the cardinal features of this form of asthma—namely, the airway hyperreactivity to nonspecific bronchoconstrictor stimuli, such as histamine and methacholine.

Eosinophils can also bind to IgE by virtue of their expression of the low-affinity IgE Fc receptor (FcεRII or CD23). They also express Fc receptors to the Fc region of IgG. Thus both IgE- and IgG-bound antigen will bind to their respective Fc receptors on eosinophils, causing these cells to be activated. Like mast cells, once these receptors are triggered, they degranulate, releasing leukotrienes that cause muscle contraction. They also release PAF and ***major basic protein*** (MBP). MBP has the ability to destroy various parasites (such as schistosomes) by affecting their mobility and damaging their surface. Also, MBP is toxic to mammalian epithelium of the respiratory tract. Finally, the eosinophilic degranulation releases ***eosinophilic cationic protein*** (ECP), a potent neurotoxin and helminthotoxin. All these biologically active substances, while directed toward foreign invaders, can cause tissue damage.

Neutrophils recruited to the site in response to chemotactic factors come into close contact with antibody-coated antigen via IgG Fc receptors, which are normally expressed on these cells. Consequently, these cells become activated to phagocytose the antigen-antibody immune complexes. In addition, they release their powerful lysosomal enzymes, which cause tissue damage. Like degranulation products of eosinophils, degranulation products of neutrophils also include leukotrienes and PAF. Lymphocytes (both T and B) as well as macrophages enter the area, further defending the host against the offending antigen or microorganism.

Figure 14.6 illustrates the general mechanism underlying allergic reactions. This dramatic series of events triggered and mediated by IgE is involved in the elimination of parasites, as described later in this chapter. Unfortunately,the same events take place in certain individuals when the antigen is a harmless substance such as pollen, animal dander, or the common dust mite, resulting in tissue damage.

CLINICAL ASPECTS OF ALLERGIC REACTIONS

The clinical consequences of allergic reactions can range from localized reactions, including allergic rhinitis, asthma, atopic dermatitis, and food allergies to severe, life-threatening systemic reactions, such as anaphylaxis. It is important to note, however, that, although defined as localized anaphylaxis, asthmatic reactions can also be fatal. Mast cell degranulation is the central mechanism in each of these reactions.

Allergic Rhinitis

Allergic rhinitis (commonly known as ***hay fever***) is the most common atopic disorder worldwide. It is caused by airborne allergens that react with IgE-sensitized mast cells in the nasal passages and conjunctiva. Mediators released from mast cells increase capillary permeability and cause localized vasodilation, leading to the typical symptoms, which include sneezing and coughing.

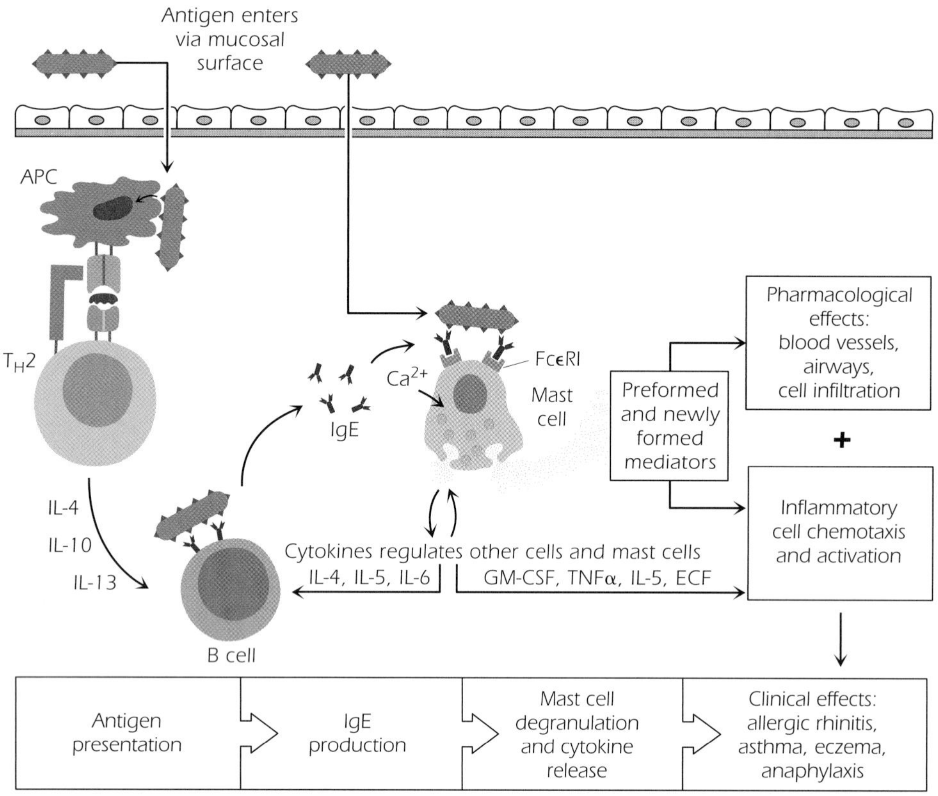

Figure 14.6. Overview of induction and effector mechanisms in type I hypersensitivity.

Food Allergies

Food allergies, another common atopic disorder, are caused by the intake of certain foods (e.g., peanuts, rice, eggs). When susceptible individuals ingest foods to which they are allergic, it can trigger the cross-linking of allergen-specific IgE on mast cells located in the upper and lower gastrointestinal tract. Mast cell degranulation and mediator release leads to localized smooth muscle contraction and vasodilation, often causing vomiting and diarrhea. In some cases, the allergen is absorbed into the bloodstream as a consequence of increased permeability of mucous membranes. Food allergens can then be transported to encounter mast cells present in skin, causing ***wheal and flare reactions*** (atopic urticaria; Fig. 14.7) commonly known as ***hives***.

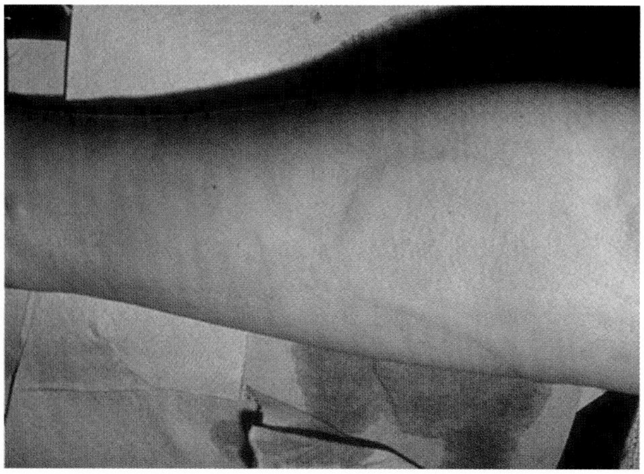

Figure 14.7. The wheal and flare reaction (atopic urticaria).

Atopic Dermatitis

A form of allergic reactions most frequently seen in young children is ***allergic dermatitis***. This clinical disorder is caused by the development of inflammatory skin lesions induced by mast cell cytokines released following degranulation. These potent inflammatory cytokines released near the site of allergen contact stimulate chemotaxis of large numbers of inflammatory cells—especially eosinophils. The skin eruptions that develop are erythematous and pus-(white cell) filled.

Asthma

Asthma is another common form of localized anaphylaxis. Asthma is a chronic obstructive disease of the lower airways characterized by episodic exacerbations of at least partially reversible airflow limitation. The clinical manifestations of asthma are believed to be the result of three basic pathophysiologic events within the airways: (1) reversible obstruction, (2) augmented bronchial responsiveness to a variety of physical and chemical stimuli (airways hyperreactivity), and (3) inflammation. In recent years, the incidence and the severity of asthma have increased dramatically in the United States. Mortality rates have been highest in children living in inner cities. Epidemiologic studies have suggested that the cockroach calyx is a major asthma-inducing allergen in these children.

Many other allergens, including airborne pollens, dust, viral antigens, and various chemicals can induce allergic asthma. Alternatively, asthma may be induced by such things as exercise or exposure to cold temperatures independent of allergen exposure, a phenomenon known as *intrinsic asthma*.

Airway inflammation is believed to play a major role in the pathogenesis of this disorder and is therefore a major target for pharmacological intervention. Cytokine-induced recruitment of large numbers of inflammatory cells, particularly eosinophils, ultimately causes significant tissue injury. Tissue damage is mediated by the many toxic substances released by these inflammatory cells, including oxygen radicals, nitric oxide, and cytokines. These events lead to the development of mucus, buildup of proteins and fluids (edema), and sloughing-off of epithelium, all of which combine to cause occlusion of the bronchial lumen. Adhesion molecules play a key role in the early events after inflammatory cell recruitment. Various cytokines released by T_H2 cells and by mast cells (e.g., IL-4, IL-13, TNFα) upregulate the expression of leukocyte and endothelial adhesion molecules, including intercellular adhesion molecule 1 (ICAM-1), E selectin, vascular cell adhesion molecule 1 (VCAM-1), and leukocyte function-associated antigen 1 (LFA-1). Once upregulated, eosinophil–endothelial cell adhesion increases, thereby facilitating transendothelial migration and prolonged survival within the lung tissue. Experimental adhesion molecule antagonists (e.g., anti-ICAM-1 monoclonal antibodies) are being investigated as candidate therapies for the treatment of asthma. Promising results using such immuotherapeutic reagents in animal models have stimulated interest in the development of antagonists that can be safely administered to humans.

CLINICAL TESTS FOR ALLERGIES AND CLINICAL INTERVENTION

Detection

In a clinical setting, the degree of sensitivity to a particular allergen is usually determined by the patient's complaints and by the extent of skin test reactions. To avoid serious consequences from intradermal challenge in patients who may be extremely sensitive to certain allergens, a ***skin-prick test*** that introduces minute amounts of antigen is given first. A positive response to intradermal challenge, called ***wheal and flare,*** is characterized by ***erythema*** (redness due to dilation of blood vessels) and ***edema*** (swelling produced by release of serum into tissue) (Fig. 14.7). The reaction is the most rapid of all hypersensitivity reactions and reaches its peak within 10–15 min, after which it fades without leaving any residual damage.

The size of the local skin reaction observed when an allergic patient is tested or challenged by intradermal injection of a battery of potential allergens is roughly indicative of the degree of sensitivity to that particular substance. In addition, if the clinical history of symptoms correlates well with the time of contact with the antigen, then the cutaneous anaphylactic response may be taken as evidence that the symptoms (e.g., sneezing, itchy eyes) are attributable to the allergens of that particular plant pollen or animal dander that engendered the skin response. Other, more quantitative, tests are used as well.

More quantitative assays that correlate, albeit not 100%, with clinical symptoms, are available in the laboratory. One assay, known as the ***radioallergosorbent test*** (RAST), involves covalent coupling of the allergen to an insoluble matrix, such as paper disks or beads. The antigen-coated matrix is then dipped into a sample of the patient's serum and allowed to bind any antibody that is specific for the allergen. After the disk is washed, a radiolabeled antibody specific for IgE is added. The amount of radioactivity bound is a measure of the amount of specific IgE antibody in the serum sample. More commonly, assays to quantitate allergen-specific serum IgE use an approach similar to RAST, except that fluorescent or ***enzyme-linked immunoadsorbent assays*** (*ELISAs*) in which enzyme-linked anti-IgE is used for the detection of allergen-specific IgE in patient's serum in lieu of radiolabeled antibody.

Intervention

Environmental Intervention. In some cases, the easiest way for individuals to control their allergies is to ***avoid exposure*** to known allergens, advice followed infrequently. If some pollens are the cause of the reaction, it may be possible for the patient to go to pollen-free areas during the season when the offending plant is pollinating. ***Masks*** and ***air filters*** also have a useful role to play, but usually avoidance is difficult for the general allergic population.

Pharmacological Intervention. Modern pharmaceutical chemistry has provided a host of drugs that are more or less effective at various stages in the evolution of the allergic reactions. Many of these are bronchodilators used to treat patients with obstructive pulmonary diseases, such as asthma. Bronchodilators are agents that cause expansion of the air passages of the lungs. This allows the patient to breathe more easily to help overcome acute bronchospasms. They are also employed as adjuncts in prophylactic and symptomatic treatment of other obstructive pulmonary diseases, such bronchitis, and emphysema. Table 14.1 provides a list of the major pharmacological agents used to treat allergies and obstructive pulmonary diseases.

Immunologic Intervention. For many years, clinical immunologists have practiced a form of immunotherapy, called ***hyposensitization,*** whereby patients are injected, over an extended period, with increasing doses of the antigen to which they are sensitive. The improvement in symptoms noted in some patients has been ascribed to several different factors. The most popular rationale is based on the observation by some groups of investigators that such injections

TABLE 14.1. Pharmacologic Agents Used in the Treatment of Allergies and Obstructive Pulmonary Diseases

Pharmacological Category	Agent(s)	Pharmacological Activity	Clinical Use
β-agonists (bronchodilators)	Albuterol	Relaxes contractions of the smooth muscle of the bronchioles; expands air passages of the lungs; short acting (rescue therapy)	Asthma, bronchitis, and emphysema; prevention of exercise-induced bronchospasm
	Salmeterol	Similar to albuteral, except cannot be used for rescue therapy	Same as albuterol
	Epinephrine	Antagonist of histamine; relaxes smooth muscle and decreases vascular permeability	Acute attacks of bronchospasms associated with emphysema, bronchitis, or anaphylaxis
	Metaproterenol	Adrenergic agent that has primary β_2-activity; main effect is to relax the bronchioles	Same indications as epinephrine; may also be used for the prevention of bronchospasms associated with chronic obstructive pulmonary diseases
	Isoproterenol	Adrenergic agent has primary β_2-activity	Asthma, bronchitis, emphysema, and mild bronchospasms
Xanthine derivatives (bronchodilators)	Aminophylline	Directly relaxes smooth muscle of the bronchi and pulmonary blood vessels	Prevents severe attacks of bronchial asthma; used in the treatment of apnea and bradycardia of prematurity in infants
	Theophylline	Directly relaxes smooth muscle of the bronchi and pulmonary blood vessels; inhibits mast cell degranulation	Similar to aminophylline
Mast cell membrane stabilizers	Cromolyn sodium	Decreases or prevents mast cell degranulation; prevents Ca^{++} influx	Used to treat or prevent mild bronchospasms associated with asthma; allergic rhinitis
Leukotriene modifiers	Zafirlukast	Binds to leukotriene receptors thereby preventing airway edema, smooth muscle constriction, and altered inflammatory processes	Asthma
	Ziluton	Inhibits the formation of leukotrienes to prevent bronchoconstriction	Asthma
Antihistamines	Many are available, including fexofenadine (Allegra), loratidine (Claritin), and cetirizine (Zyrtec)	Primarily act by blocking the H1 receptors; inhibits smooth muscle (lung and gut) contraction, dilatation of small blood vessels, and mucus production	Allergic rhinitis, atopic dermatitis, hives, some rashes
Corticosteroids	Many are available, including hydrocortisone, methylprednisolone, prednisolone, prednisone, budesonide, flunisolide, and fluticasone propionate	Potent anti-inflammatory drugs with immunosuppressive activity when used in high doses; effects are numerous and widespread; immunomudulatory effects mainly act through inhibition of gene transcription (e.g., inhibition of COX-2 synthesis)	Asthma, allergic rhinitis, urticaria, eczema

serve to increase the synthesis of IgG antibody specific for the allergen. Such antibody in the circulation presumably binds to and removes the allergen before it has a chance to reach and react with the IgE antibody on the surface of mast cells. Thus the term ***blocking antibody*** has become associated with this IgG, and there is a rough correlation between titers of this IgG antibody generated and clinical improvement.

Other findings associated with hyposensitization include an initial increase in levels of IgE antibody, followed by a prolonged decrease on continued therapy. This decrease has

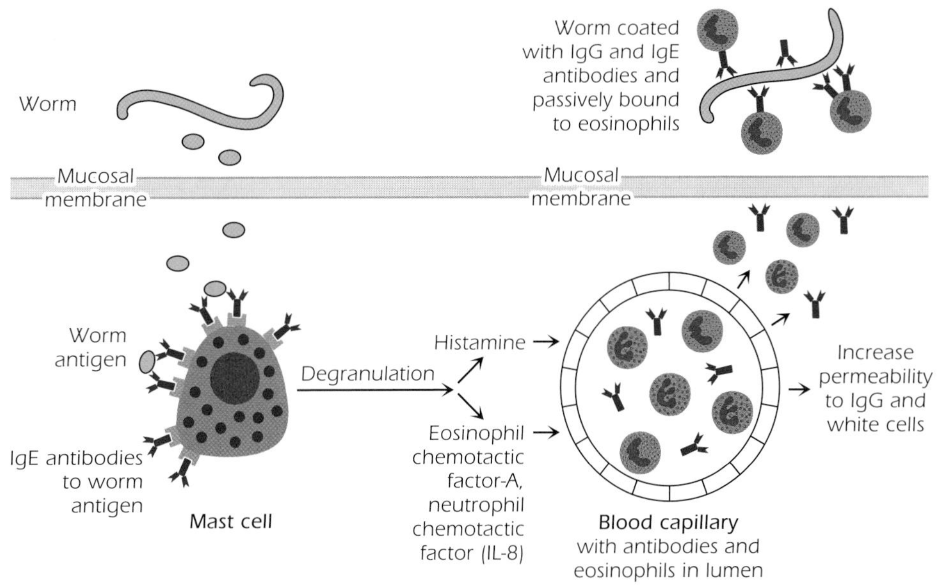

Figure 14.8. The destruction of a worm by eosinophils that have migrated to the area and been activated after IgE- and antigen-mediated mast cell degranulation.

been linked to a decrease in intensity of symptoms and is attributed either to induction of tolerance or to a switch from T_H2 to T_H1 T cells. After repeated subclinical doses of the antigen, there is also a progressive decrease in the sensitivity of mast cells and basophils to triggering by antigen. It is likely that the explanation for the apparent benefits of this immunologic therapy encompasses more than one of these demonstrable effects. Whatever the reason, this form of therapy is generally more successful in dealing with allergens that enter the circulation directly, such as bee-sting venom, than for those allergens contacted via mucosal surfaces, such as pollen, where IgG antibody is unlikely to be effective.

Potentially promising experimental immunotherapies for the treatment of IgE-mediated hypersensitivity are being investigated. A promising therapy for the treatment of patients with asthma and allergic rhinitis employs the use of humanized anti-IgE monoclonal antibody (see Chapter 5) engineered such that it does not cross-link IgE bound to mast cells and basophils. The use of plasmid DNAs encoding a specific antigen (used to induce hyporesponsiveness); cytokines, such as IL-12 and IL-10 (used to cause a shift from T_H2 to T_H1 responses); anti-cytokines, such as anti-IL-4 (used to inhibit IL-4 production); and cytokine receptor antagonists are also under investigation.

Other immunologic intervention approaches have been attempted in experimental animals. For example, it has been demonstrated that administration of a chemically altered allergen (e.g., ragweed pollen denatured by urea or coupled to polyethylene glycol) suppresses a primary or established IgE response. The mechanism may involve the induction of suppressor T cells that are both antigen-specific and isotype-specific. The modified allergens do not combine with preexisting IgE antibodies and, therefore, do not trigger anaphylactic responses. Use of such modified allergens seems to offer a promising approach to treatment of allergy. Another experimental approach involves efforts to skew the T_H2 responses in the direction of T_H1 responses. The rationale for this approach is based on the knowledge that T_H2 cells play a key role in allergic reactions by producing cytokines, such as IL4, that induce IgE class switching in B cells.

THE PROTECTIVE ROLE OF IgE

The protective effects of allergic reactions may be seen in situations where the sensitizing antigen is derived from one of many parasitic worms such as helminths. The immune response to these worms favors the induction of IgE. As a consequence of antigens from the worm cross-linking IgE on the surface of mast cells (and eosinophils), histamine, and other mediators associated with the anaphylactic response are released. The effects of increased permeability due to histamine release serve to bring serum components, which include IgG antibody, to the site of worm infestation. The IgG antibody binds to the surface of the worm and attracts the eosinophils, which have migrated to the area as a result of the chemotactic effects of ECF-A. The eosinophils then bind to the IgG-coated worm, by virtue of their membrane receptors for Fc, and release the contents of their granules (Figs. 14.8 and 14.9). As noted earlier,eosinophils also express the low-affinity Fc receptor for IgE, which facilitates the binding of these cells to IgE-coated worms. The major constituent of the contents of the granules released by eosinophils is an MBP, referred to previously, which coats the surface of the worm and leads, in some unknown way, to the death of the worm and its eventual expulsion. Thus all components of the type I reaction combine to perform this protective function. This beneficial effect of the anaphylactic response in many animals suggests that responses involving IgE may have evolved to play a role in dealing with worm parasitism.

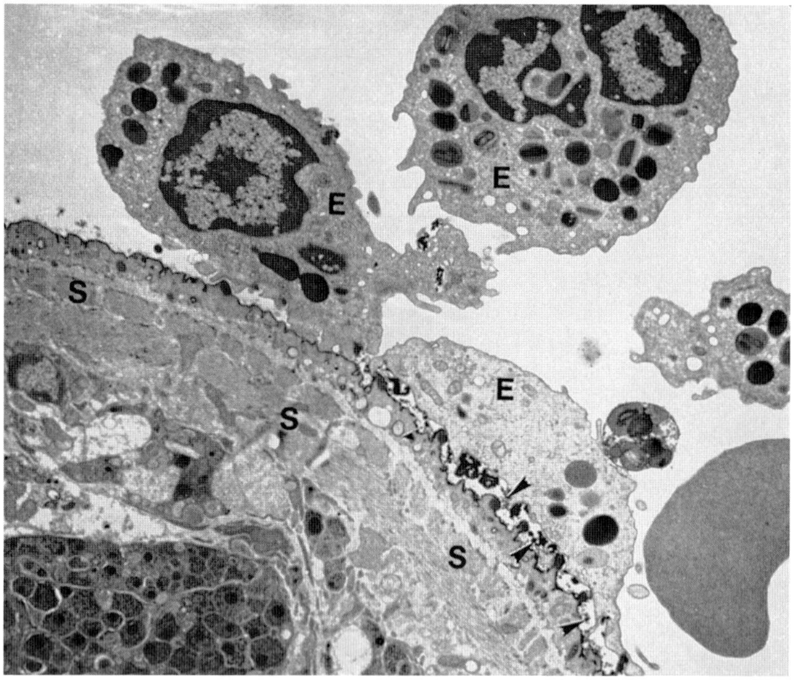

Figure 14.9. Electron micrograph (×6,000) of eosinophils (*E*) adhering to an antibody-coated schistosomulum (*S*). The cell on the left has not yet degranulated, but the one on the right has discharged-electron-dense material (*arrows*), which can be seen between the cell and the worm. (Courtesy of J. Caulfield, Harvard Medical School.)

SUMMARY

1. Allergic reactions are mediated by IgE antibodies, which bind to receptors specific for IgE Fc (FcεR) on the surface of mast cells and basophils. When these receptors are cross-linked by contact with specific antigen, the cell is triggered to respond by releasing its granules and their inflammatory mediators, as well as synthesizing other products from its membrane.

2. IgE responses are T cell-dependent. Allergens stimulate the induction of T_H2 cells, which release cytokines (IL-4, IL-13) that stimulate B cell class switching to produce IgE.

3. Following antigen cross-linking of IgE on mast cells, the inflammation caused by the inflammatory mediators released by these cells can be divided into early and late stages, the latter of which may persist for several days.

4. The symptoms of allergic reactions are entirely attributable to the inflammatory mediators released by the activated mast cells. These produce the immediate symptoms typical of these responses, including increased vascular permeability, constriction of smooth muscles, and influx of eosinophils.

5. The early stage of allergic reactions (immediate reaction) is characterized by preformed or rapidly synthesized short-lived mediators, such as histamine and prostaglandins, that cause a rapid increase in vascular permeability and contraction of smooth muscle.

6. Late-phase allergic reactions are caused by induced synthesis and release of mediators, including leukotrienes, cytokines, and chemokines released by activated mast cells. These recruit other leukocytes, including eosinophils and T_H2 cells, to the site of inflammation. These produce a milder form of smooth muscle contraction than the immediate response, sustained edema, and—in the case of individuals suffering from asthma—airway hyperreactivity to nonspecific bronchoconstrictor stimuli, such as histamine and methacholine.

7. Clinical manifestations of allergic reactions include localized reactions, such as allergic rhinitis; atopic dermatitis; food allergies; and obstructive pulmonary diseases, such as asthma, bronchitis, and emphysema.

8. Systemic reactions can lead to life-threatening anaphylaxis.

9. Despite the dangerous systematic reactions produced by type I hypersensitivity reactions mediated by IgE, its value probably lies in the ability of IgE to provide immunity to parasitic infections.

10. Common therapeutic agents used to treat allergic reactions include bronchodilators (β-agonists and xanthine derivatives), corticosteroids, cromolyn sodium, antihistamines, and leukotriene modifiers.

REFERENCES

Bacharier LB, Geha RS (2000): Molecular mechanisms of IgE regulation. *J Allergy Clin Immunol* 105:S547.

Bames PJ (1999): Therapeutic strategies for allergic diseases. *Nature* 402:B31.

Bevan MA, Metzger H (1993): Signal transduction by Fc receptors: the FcεRI case. *Immunol Today* 14:222.

Cookson W (1999): The alliance of genes and environment in asthma and allergy. *Nature* 402:B5.

Coombs RRA, Gell PGH (1963): The classification of allergic reactions underlying disease. In Gell PGH, Coombs RRA (eds): Clinical Aspects of Immunology. Oxford, UK: Blackwell.

Galli SJ (2000) Allergy. *Curr Biol* 10:R93.

Galli SJ, Lantz CS (1998): Allergy. In Paul WE (ed): Fundamental Immunology, 4th ed. New York: Lippincott-Raven.

Hamawy MM, Mergenhagen SE, Siraganian RS (1994): Adhesion molecules as regulators of mast cell and basophil function. *Immunol Today* 15:62.

Heusser C, Jardieu P (1997): Therapeutic potential of anti-IgE antibodies. *Curr Opin Immunol* 9:805.

Lichenstein LM (1993): Allergy and the immune system. *Sci Am* Sept, 126.

Marone G (1998): Asthma: recent advances. *Immunol Today* 19:5.

Mygid N (1986): Essential Allergy. Oxford, UK: Blackwell.

Naclerio R, Solomon W (1997): Rhinitis and inhalant allergins. *J Am Med Assoc* 278:1842.

Pearlman DS (1999): Pathophysiology of the inflammatory response. *J Allergy Clin Immunol* 104:S132.

Ray A, Cohen L (1999): T_H2 cells and GATA-3 in asthma: new insights into the regulation of airway inflammation. *J Clin Invest* 104:985.

Terr AI (1994): The atopic diseases. In Stites DP, Terr AI, Parslow TG (eds): Basic and Clinical Immunology, 8th ed. East Norwalk, CT: Appleton & Lange.

REVIEW QUESTIONS

For each question, choose the ONE BEST answer or completion.

1. A 26-year-old male, with significant cat allergies, visits a home with multiple cats. He arrives at an urgent care center 2 h later with a severe exacerbation of asthma. He is treated with a short-acting bronchodilator and epinephrine. Initially, after treatment, his symptoms resolved; however, 8 h later he is forced to go the emergency room with another exacerbation. What is the most likely cause of his symptoms?

A) Additional IgE cross-linking on mast cells, leading to lipid mediator and cytokine release
B) $CD4^+$ T_H1 cell production of IFN-γ
C) complement activation, leading to mast cell degranulation by C5a and C3a
D) eosinophil and basophil infiltration, leading to the release of proinflammatory mediators
E) neutrophil recruitment and the release of cytoplasmic granule components

2. A 24-year-old male who is allergic to cat dander wore a facial mask to reduce his contact with the allergen when exposed to a friend's cat. Several hours later, he is wheezing and coughing. Which of the following best explains the allergic reaction seen in this individual?

A) Mast cells in his gastrointestinal track degranulated following the cross-linking of allergen-specific IgE on their surface, and the inflammatory mediators traveled to his lung.
B) Mast cells in his blood vessels degranulated following the cross-linking of allergen-specific IgE on their surface, causing a systemic inflammatory response.
C) Mast cells in his lung degranulated following the cross-linking of allergen-specific IgE on their surface.
D) Mast cells in his skin degranulated following the cross-linking of allergen-specific IgE on their surface, causing a systemic inflammatory response.

3. The usual sequence of events in an allergic reaction is as follows:

A) The allergen combines with circulating IgE and then the IgE–allergen complex binds to mast cells.
B) The allergen binds to IgE fixed to mast cells.
C) The allergen is processed by antigen-presenting cells (APCs) and then binds to histamine receptors.
D) The allergen is processed by antigen-presenting cells and then binds to mast cells.
E) The allergen combines with IgG.

4. Epinephrine

A) causes bronchodilation.
B) is effective even after anaphylactic symptoms commence.
C) relaxes smooth muscle.
D) decreases vascular permeability.
E) All of the above.

5. A human volunteer agrees to be passively sensitized with IgE specific for a ragweed antigen (allergen). When challenged with the allergen intradermally, he displayed a typical skin reaction due to an immediate hypersensitivity reaction. If the injection with sensitizing IgE was preceded by an injection (at the same site) of Fc fragments of human IgE, followed by intradermal injection with allergen, which of the following outcomes would you predict?

A) No reaction would occur because the Fc fragments would interact with the allergen and prevent it from gaining access to the sensitized mast cells.

B) No reaction would occur because the Fc fragments would interact with the IgE antibodies, making their antigen-binding sites unavailable for binding to antigen.
C) No reaction would occur because the Fc fragments would interact with FcεR receptors on mast cells.
D) The reaction would be exacerbated due to the increased local concentration of IgE Fc fragments.
E) The reaction would be exacerbated due to the activation of complement.

6. Which of the following mechanism(s) may be involved in the clinical efficacy of desensitization therapy to treat patients with allergies to known allergens?
A) enhanced production of IgG, which binds allergen before it reaches mast cells
B) skewing of T cell responses from T_H2 to T_H1
C) decreased sensitivity of mast cells and basophils to degranulation by allergen
D) decreased production of IgE antibody
E) all of the above

7. Antihistamines
A) block H1 receptors and inhibit smooth muscle contraction, dilatation of small blood vessels, and mucus production.
B) directly bind to histamine, thereby blocking its inflammatory effect.
C) influence the activity of leukotrienes.
D) inhibit binding of IgE to mast cells.
E) are adrenergic agents that mainly relax the bronchioles.

8. In the RAST assay for ragweed pollen
A) the patient's serum is first mixed with a radiolabeled anti-IgE.
B) only IgE anti-ragweed antibodies are detected.
C) the patient's serum competitively inhibits binding of the anti-IgE.
D) monovalent IgE is used.
E) complement is used.

9. Anaphylactic reactions
A) develop within minutes and abate within 30 min.
B) may be followed by inflammatory sequelae hours later.
C) are the consequences of released pharmacological agents.
D) may involve components of the mast cell granule matrix.
E) all of the above

CASE STUDY

While playing tennis on a warm day, a young man felt a wasp on his arm and brushed it off but still received a mild sting, which he ignored. Ten minutes later he felt dizzy and began to itch under his arms and on his scalp. When he broke out in hives and felt a tightness in his chest, he headed for the hospital. On the way, he felt cold and clammy and collapsed on the seat of the taxi. In the emergency unit, his pulse was barely detectable. What happened, and why?

ANSWERS TO REVIEW QUESTIONS

1. *D* The timing of the symptoms exhibited in this individual are characteristic of late-phase allergic reactions in which eosinophil infiltration occurs. This recruitment of eosinophils as well as the passage of other leukocytes from the circulation to the tissue, is facilitated by the increased vascular permeability caused by proinflammatory cytokines and histamine.

2. *C* Despite the use of protective barriers, such as facial masks, to prevent an individual's inhalation of allergens, small amounts of airborne antigens such as cat dander can enter by this route and cause degranulation of IgE-sensitized mast cells in the lung. The other choices are all incorrect.

3. *B* Allergic individuals have already made IgE responses to specific allergens. IgE binds passively to cells expressing high-affinity Fc receptors for IgE (e.g., mast cells) and interacts with the allergen when present. This results in cross-linking of the high-affinity FcεR, resulting in mast cell degranulation. The allergen does not need to be processed by APCs in order to bind to IgE.

4. *E* All are effects of epinephrine and make it useful for treatment of acute anaphylactic symptoms.

5. *C* Since the IgE Fc fragments would bind to the high-affinity FcεR expressed on the surface of mast cells, the allergen-specific IgE would not have access to these receptors and, therefore, would not bind to these cells. When the allergen is introduced intradermally, while it would bind to the allergen-specific IgE at the site, this would not result in cross-linking of FcεRs, which are saturated with soluble IgE Fc fragments. Hence no immediate hypersensitivity reaction would take place.

6. *E* All are considered to be involved to varying degrees in injection therapy.

7. *A* Antihistamines act by blocking H1 histamine receptors *not* the histamine itself. They do not act by influencing the activity of leukotrienes or by binding to IgE on mast cells and are not andrenergic agents.

8. *B* The RAST assay measures IgE antibody that is allowed to bind to allergen coupled to an insoluble matrix. It detects IgE antiragweed antibodies. It does not use monovalent IgE, and complement is not used in the test

9. *E* All are true. A and C are true of the classic wheal and flare type response, while B and D describe features of the late-phase response, which is a complication of some anaphylactic reactions.

ANSWER TO CASE STUDY

This is a classic case of systemic anaphylaxis. In the emergency room, epinephrine was promptly administered, and the symptoms due to vascular permeability (hives, low blood pressure) and smooth muscle constriction (difficulty in breathing) were reversed. When he revived sufficiently, he revealed that he had been stung by similar-looking insects in the past, the last time 3 months ago, but without any noticeable effects. These stings were apparently the sensitizing *immunizations* building up sufficient levels of IgE antibody to sensitize his mast cells and basophils. Thus the last sting, despite the fact that little venom was injected, was sufficient to precipitate a systemic reaction. A careful skin test, involving intradermal injection of very dilute wasp venom, should show an immediate "wheal and flare" response, confirming this sensitivity. The young man should be advised to (1) avoid wasps, (2) carry an emergency vial of injectable epinephrine, and (3) undergo desensitization therapy aimed at hyposensitization to the wasp venom antigen.

15

HYPERSENSITIVITY REACTIONS: ANTIBODY-MEDIATED (TYPE II) CYTOTOXIC REACTIONS AND IMMUNE COMPLEX (TYPE III) REACTIONS

INTRODUCTION

Hypersensitivity reactions characterized as type II and type III reactions are mediated by antibodies belonging to the IgG, IgM, and—in some cases—IgA or IgE isotypes. It is now clear that these reactions share certain effector mechanisms. The distinction between these two forms of hypersensitivity lies in the type and location of antigen involved and the way in which antigen is brought together with antibody. It is important to understand that in many cases, the target antigens involved in such hypersensitivity reactions are self-antigens. Cytotoxic type II hypersensitivity reactions are stimulated by the binding of antibody directly to an antigen on the surface of a cell. Type III reactions are stimulated by antigen–antibody immune complexes. The immune mechanisms that manifest the clinical outcomes of such hypersensitivity reactions are the subject of this chapter.

Cytotoxic Reactions: Type II Hypersensitivity

As illustrated in the examples of clinically important type II hypersensitivity reactions discussed below, many of these cytotoxic reactions are manifestations of antibody-mediated autoimmunity. Mechanisms associated with the generation of autoantibodies were discussed in Chapter 12. The antibodies involved in these hypersensitivity reactions are either directed against normal self-antigens (e.g., cross-reactive antibodies elicited following an infection) or modified self-antigens (e.g., drug-induced autoantibodies elicited following the binding of drugs to certain cell membranes). The targeted cell is either damaged or destroyed through a variety of mechanisms. Three different antibody-mediated mechanisms are involved in these cytotoxic reactions.

Complement-Mediated Reactions

In complement-mediated hypersensitivity reactions, antibodies react with a cell membrane component, leading to complement fixation. This activates the complement cascade (discussed in Chapter 13) and leads either to ***lysis*** of the cell or ***opsonization*** mediated by receptors for Fc or C3b (Fig. 15.1A). Opsonization culminates in the phagocytosis and destruction of the cell by macrophages and neutrophils expressing surface receptors for Fc or C3b. Blood cells are most commonly affected by this mechanism. Interestingly, IgG Fc receptor knockout mice fail to mount type II (and type III) hypersensitivity reactions—a finding that underscores the pivotal role played by IgG Fc receptors in initiating these reaction cascades.

Antibody-Dependent Cell-Mediated Cytotoxicity

Antibody-dependent cell-mediated cytotoxicity (ADCC) uses Fc receptors expressed on many cell types (e.g., natural killer cells, macrophages, neutrophils, eosinophils) as a means of bringing these cells into contact with antibody-coated target cells (Fig. 15.1B). Lysis of these target cells

Immunology: A Short Course, Fifth Edition, By Richard Coico, Geoffrey Sunshine, and Eli Benjamini
ISBN 0-471-22689-0

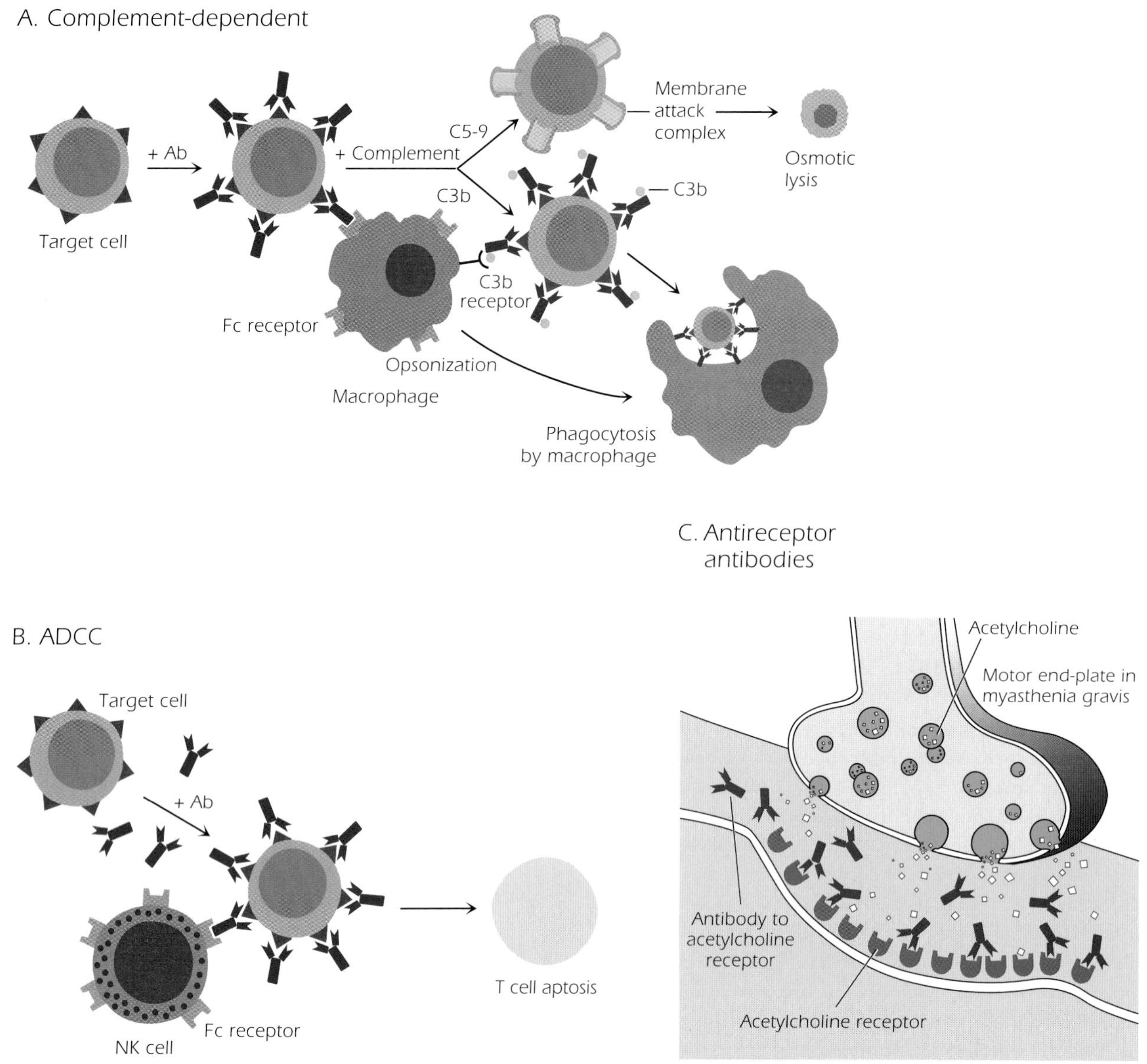

Figure 15.1. Three different mechanisms of antibody-mediated injury in type II hypersensitivity. **(A)** Complement-dependent reactions that lead to lysis of cells or render them susceptible to phagocytosis. **(B)** In ADCC, IgG-coated target cells are killed by cells that bear Fc receptors for IgG (e.g., such as natural killer (NK) cells and macrophages). **(C)** Antireceptor antibodies disturb the normal function of receptors. In this example, acetylcholine receptor antibodies impair neuromuscular transmission in myasthenia gravis.

requires contact but does not involve phagocytosis or complement fixation. Instead, ADCC lysis of target cells is analogous to that of cytotoxic T cells and involves the release of cytoplasmic granules (modified lysosomes) containing ***perforin*** and ***granzymes.*** Once released from the lytic granules, perforins insert into the target cell membrane and polymerize to form pores In contrast, granzymes, which consist of at least three serine proteases, enter the cytoplasm of the target cell and activate events leading to apoptosis.

ADCC reactions involve IgG and IgG Fc receptors (FcγIII, also known as CD16). Specifically, IgG subclasses IgG_1 and IgG_3 are capable of eliciting ADCC reactions since their Fc regions can bind to CD16. However, IgE antibodies can also be involved in ADCC. In this situation, the low-affinity IgE Fc receptor (FcεRII) expressed on certain cells, including eosinophils as discussed in the previous chapter, binds to the Fc region of IgE antibodies bound to target antigens (e.g., parasites, see Fig. 14.7).

Antibody-Mediated Cellular Dysfunction

Cell surface receptors can also serve as target antigens in type II hypersensitivity reactions. When autoantibodies bind to such receptors, they impair or dysregulate function without causing cell injury or inflammation.

In the following section, we provide several examples of clinically important antibody-mediated cytotoxic hypersensitivity reactions.

EXAMPLES OF CYTOTOXIC HYPERSENSITIVITY REACTIONS

Transfusion Reactions

Transfusion of ***ABO-incompatible blood*** results in complement-mediated cytotoxic reactions. As an example, people with type O blood have in their circulation, for reasons that are still not completely clear, IgM anti-A and anti-B antibodies (***isohemagglutinins***), which react with the A and B blood-group substances, respectively. If such a person were to be transfused with type A red blood cells (RBCs), the immediate consequences could be disastrous. Since there is a considerable amount of IgM anti-A antibody in this person's circulation, all the transfused type A RBCs would bind some antibody. Because of the efficiency of IgM antibody in activating complement (a single IgM molecule is sufficient to activate many complement molecules; see Chapter 13) and because of the absence of repair mechanisms, RBCs would be lysed intravascularly by the destructive action of complement on their membranes. Not only does this nullify the desirable effects of the transfusion but the individual would be faced with the risk of kidney damage from blockage by large quantities of red blood cell membrane plus the possible toxic effects from the release of the heme complex.

Drug-Induced Reactions

In some people, certain drugs act as ***haptens*** and combine with cells or with other circulating blood constituents and induce antibody formation. When antibody combines with cells coated with the drug, cytotoxic damage results. The type of pathologic injury depends on the type of cell that binds the drug. For example, some drugs can bind to platelets, causing them to become immunogenic. The antibody responses generated cause lysis of the platelets and resulting thrombocytopenia (low blood platelet count). This disorder, in turn, can give rise to purpura (hemorrhage into the skin, mucous membranes, and internal organs), which is the main problem in drug-induced thrombocytopenia purpura. Withdrawal of the offending drug leads to a cessation of symptoms. Other drugs, such as chloramphenicol (an antibiotic), may bind to white blood cells (WBCs); phenacetin (an analgesic) and chlorpromazine (a tranquilizer) may bind to red blood cells. The consequences of an immune response to these drugs can lead to an agranulocytosis (decrease in granulocytes) in the case of WBCs and a hemolytic anemia in the case of RBCs. Damage to the target cell in these examples may be mediated by either of the two mechanisms described above: by cytolysis via the complement pathway or by destruction of cells by phagocytosis mediated by receptors for Fc or C3b.

Rhesus-Incompatibility Reactions

A somewhat similar mechanism is exemplified by the rhesus (Rh) incompatibility reaction seen in infants born of parents with Rh-incompatible blood groups. Rh antigens are so-named because rabbit antisera raised against rhesus monkey RBCs agglutinate the erythrocytes from approximately 85% of humans tested. RBCs from such individuals are therefore said to be Rh^+, whereas cells from the remaining 15% of the population are Rh^-. Rh^- mothers can become sensitized to Rh antigens during their first pregnancy with a child whose RBCs are Rh^+. This occurs as a result of the release of some of the baby's red blood cells into the mother's circulation during birth. If the mother is thereby sufficiently immunized to produce anti-Rh antibody of the IgG isotype, subsequent Rh^+ fetuses will be at risk, since, as we saw in Chapter 4, IgG antibody is capable of crossing the placenta. Thus in second or subsequent pregnancies, when the anti-Rh IgG antibodies have crossed the placenta, they bind to the Rh antigen on the RBCs of the fetus. Because the density of Rh antigen on the surface of RBCs is low, these antibodies usually fail to agglutinate or lyse the cells directly. However, the antibody-coated cells are readily destroyed by the opsonic effect of the Fc regions of the IgG, which interact with the receptors for Fc on the phagocytic cells of the reticuloendothelial system. The result is progressive destruction of the fetal or newborn red blood cells, with the pathologic consequences that come from decreased transport of oxygen and result in jaundice from the products of the breakdown of hemoglobin—a condition known as ***hemolytic disease of the newborn*** (***erythroblastosis fetalis***). Prevention of this Rh incompatibility reaction can be achieved with the administration of anti-Rh antibodies to the mother within 72 h of parturition to effectively block the sensitization phase. This also causes a rapid clearance of Rh^+ cells from the mother's circulation. One widely used preparation of anti-Rh antibodies involves the use of antibodies (***Rhogam***) against the D antigen, now known to be the strongest immunogen and the most important of all the Rh antigens.

Autoimmune Reactions Involving Cell Membrane Receptors

An example of antibody-mediated cellular dysfunction due to reactivity with a cell receptor is seen in the autoimmune disease ***myasthenia gravis.*** Antagonistic autoantibodies reactive with ***acetylcholine receptors*** in the motor end plates of skeletal muscles impair neuromuscular transmission, causing muscle weakness (Fig. 15.1C). Conversely, autoantibodies can serve as agonists in some cases, causing stimulation of the target cells. An example of this is seen in ***Graves's disease*** in which antibodies directed against thyroid-stimulating hormone (TSH) receptor on thyroid epithelial cells stimulate the cells, resulting in hyperthyroidism. These disorders are discussed in more detail in Chapter 12.

Autoimmune Reactions Involving Other Cell Membrane Determinants

As a consequence of certain infectious diseases or for other, still unknown, reasons, some people produce an antibody reactive against their own blood cells (***autoimmune hemolytic anemia***). When RBCs are the target, binding of ***anti-RBC autoantibody*** shortens their life span or destroys them altogether by mechanisms that involve hemolysis or phagocytosis via receptors for Fc and C3b. This may lead to progressive anemia if the production of new red blood cells cannot keep pace with destruction. Occasionally, the antibody binds effectively only at lower temperatures (cold agglutinin), in which case lowering of body temperature, particularly the lower temperature of the arms and legs, leads to effective antibody binding and destruction of the RBCs.

Another example of cell destruction by autoantibodies is ***idiopathic thrombocytopenia purpura.*** In this condition, antibodies directed to platelets as a result of drug-induced reactions (see above) or other autoimmune mechanism, result in platelet destruction by complement or phagocytic cells with Fc or C3b receptors. Decrease in platelet numbers may lead to bleeding (purpura). Similarly, autoantibodies directed against granulocytes can induce agranulocytosis predisposing individuals to various infections. Finally, antibodies may form against other tissue components such as basement membrane collagen, causing ***Goodpasture syndrome*** (see Chapter 12), and desmosomes, resulting in ***pemphigus vulgaris.***

It should be pointed out that whereas the preceding discussion emphasizes type II reactions induced by drugs, hypersensitivity to drugs may also induce IgE-mediated immediate hypersensitivity reactions (type I), delayed-type hypersensitivity reactions (type IV; see Chapter 16), and the immune complex–mediated reactions (type III), discussed below. Some reactions are induced by a drug acting as a hapten conjugated to some body components; as discussed in the next chapter, other reactions can be induced by the drug acting as a contact sensitizer.

IMMUNE COMPLEX REACTIONS: TYPE III HYPERSENSITIVITY

Under normal conditions, circulating immune complexes are removed by phagocytic cells—a phenomenon involving the binding of such complexes to IgG Fc receptors expressed on these cells. In addition, RBCs that have C3b receptors may bind complexes that have fixed complement and transport them to the liver, where the complexes are removed by phagocytic Kupffer cells. When large quantities of immune complexes of a certain size are formed in the circulation, they can get deposited in the tissues and trigger a variety of systemic pathogenic events known as ***type III hypersensitivity reactions.*** These reactions can be ***systemic*** or ***localized*** and are mediated by the inadvertent deposition of ***immune complexes*** in the tissues, especially the kidneys, skin, joints, choroid plexus, and ciliary artery of the eye. The formation of immune complexes can be initiated by exogenous antigens such as bacteria and viruses or, as in the case of the Arthus reaction (described below), by intradermal or intrapulmonary exposure to large amounts of foreign protein. Alternatively, endogenous antigens, such as DNA, can serve as a target for autoantibodies as seen in ***systemic lupus erythematosus*** (SLE). In the latter case, the clinical outcome is more accurately defined as an autoimmune phenomenon (see Chapter 12). Patients with SLE often have both systemic (multiorgan) and localized manifestations of immune complex disease. Localized tissue injury occurs as a result of antigen–antibody complexes forming at extravascular sites as in situ immune complexes (e.g., in the glomeruli of the kidneys). This also occurs in a variety of ***glomerular diseases*** in which immune complexes are formed in situ on the glomerular basement membrane.

The mechanism of injury seen in immune complex–mediated disease is the same regardless of which pattern of immune complex deposition is seen (i.e., systemic vs. local). Central to the pathogenesis of tissue injury is the fixation of complement by the immune complexes, activation of the complement cascade, and release of biologically active fragments (e.g., anaphylotoxins C3a and C5a; see Chapter 13). Complement activation results in increased vascular permeability and stimulates the recruitment of polymorphonuclear phagocytes that release lysosomal enzymes (e.g., neutral proteases) that can damage the glomerular basement membrane.

The immunoglobulin isotype involved in type III hypersensitivity reactions is usually IgG, but IgM can also be involved. As with type II hypersensitivity reactions, IgG Fc receptors (CD16) expressed on leukocytes play a pivotal role in initiating type III reaction cascades. The antibody–antigen complexes may fix complement and/or activate effector cells (the main cell type being the neutrophil) that cause tissue damage. C3a and C5a generated by complement activation induce mast cells and basophils to release arachidonic acid metabolites and chemokines that attract additional basophils, eosinophils, macrophages and neutrophils into the area. The polymorphs release their lysosomal enzymes at the surface of the affected tissues. Macrophages are stimulated to release tumor necrosis factor-α (TNFα) and interleukin-1 (IL-1), while platelets form microthrombi and contribute to cellular proliferation by releasing platelet-derived growth factor (PDGF).

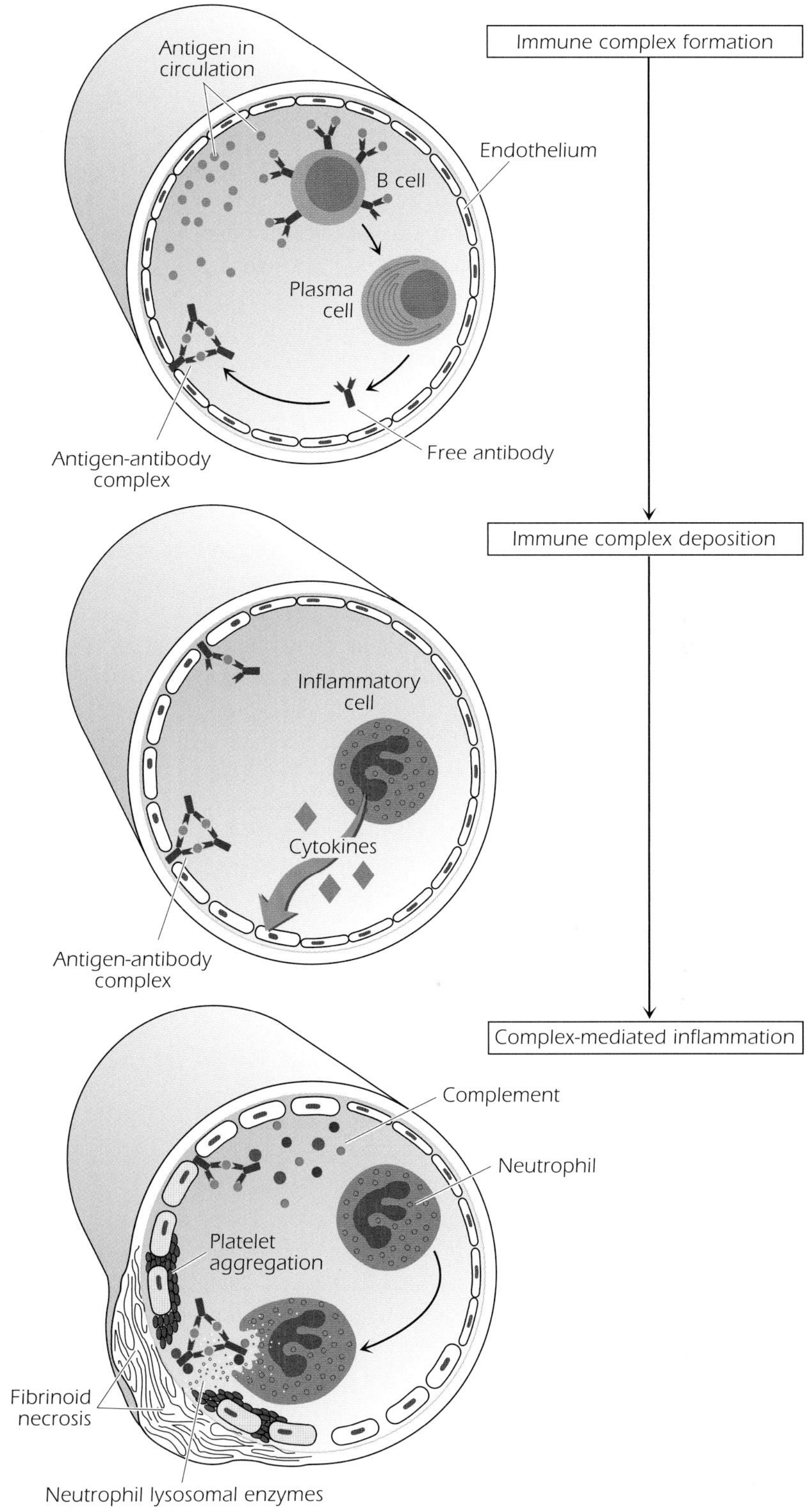

Figure 15.2. The three sequential phases in the induction of systemic type III (immune complex) hypersensitivity.

Systemic Immune Complex Disease

The pathogenesis of systemic immune complex disease can be divided into three phases. In the first phase, antigen–antibody immune complexes form in the circulation. This is followed by deposition of immune complexes in various tissues, which initiates the third phase, in which inflammatory reactions in various tissues occur (Fig. 15.2). Several factors help determine whether immune complex formation will lead to tissue deposition and disease. The size of the complexes appears to be important. Very large complexes formed under conditions of antibody excess are rapidly removed from the circulation by phagocytic cells and, therefore, are harmless. Small or intermediate complexes circulate for longer periods of time and bind less avidly to IgG Fc receptors expressed on phagocytic cells. Therefore, small to intermediate immune complexes tend to be more pathogenic than large complexes. A second factor that can influence the development of systemic immune complex disease is the integrity of the mononuclear phagocytic system. An intrinsic dysfunction of this system increases the probability of persistence of immune complexes in the circulation. As expected, overloading this phagocytic system with large quantities of immune complexes also compromises its ability to mediate clearance of such complexes from the circulation. For reasons that are not well understood, the favored sites of immune complex deposition are the kidneys, joints, skin, heart, and small vessels. Localization in the kidney can be explained, in part, by the filtration function of the glomeruli.

Serum Sickness. The prototype of systemic immune complex disease is ***serum sickness.*** This term derives from observations made at the turn of the twentieth century by von Pirquet and Schick of the consequences of the treatment of certain infectious diseases, such as diphtheria and tetanus, with antisera made in horses. It was well known that the pathologic consequences of infection by both the *Corynebacterium* and the *Clostridium* organisms were due to the secretion of exotoxins that are extremely damaging to host cells (Chapter 20). The bacteria themselves are relatively noninvasive and of little consequence. Hence the strategy that evolved to treat these diseases was to neutralize the toxins rapidly, before quantities large enough to kill the host became fixed in tissues. Since active immunization required several weeks before useful levels of antibody were produced, it was necessary to protect the individual through passive immunization by injecting large amounts of a preformed antitoxin antibody as soon as the disease was diagnosed, to prevent death by toxin. Horses, which were readily available, easily immunized, and capable of yielding large quantities of useful antisera, were the animals of choice for the production of antitoxin. Today, we know that the administration of large quantities of heterologous serum from another species causes the recipient to synthesize antibodies to the foreign immunoglobulin, leading to the formation of antigen–antibody complexes that result in the clinical symptoms associated with serum sickness. Serum sickness can also occur in patients as a secondary reaction to the administration of nonprotein drugs. The classic clinical manifestations consist of fever, arthralgia, lymphadenopathy, and skin eruption. In addition, the potential development of serum sickness is becoming an important consideration in patients being treated for malignancy, graft rejection, or autoimmune disease with monoclonal antibodies made in rodents.

Infection-Associated Immune Complex Disease. Perhaps the best example of infection-associated immune complex diseases is ***rheumatic fever.*** In susceptible individuals, this disease is associated with infections (e.g., throat) caused by ***group A streptococci,*** and it involves inflammation and damage to heart, joints, and kidneys. A variety of antigens in the cell walls and membranes of streptococci have been shown to be cross-reactive with antigens present in human heart muscle, cartilage, and glomerular basement membrane. It is presumed that antibody to the streptococcal antigens binds to these components of normal tissue and induces inflammatory reactions via a pathway similar to that described above. In rheumatoid arthritis, there is evidence for the production of rheumatoid factor, an IgM autoantibody that binds to the Fc region of normal IgG. These immune complexes participate in causing inflammation of joints and the damage characteristic of this disease.

In a variety of other infections some individuals produce antibodies that cross-react with some constituent of normal tissue. For example, individuals predisposed to ***Goodpasture syndrome*** (see Chapter 12) sometimes develop this disease after viral respiratory infections. The pulmonary hemorrhage and glomerulonephritis seen in these patients are due to antibodies that bind directly to basement membrane in the lung and kidney, activate complement, and cause membrane damage as a consequence of accumulation of neutrophils and release of degradative enzymes. Goodpasture syndrome is sometimes considered to be a type II hypersensitivity reaction, since it also involves an antibody-mediated cytotoxic effect on normal cells. The distinction between this infection-associated antibody-mediated disease and the immune complex disease of serum sickness is that microscopic examination of the lesions reveals a linear, ribbonlike deposit along the basement membrane (see Fig. 15.3), as would be expected if an even carpet of antibody were bound to surface antigens. By contrast, in serum sickness the pile up of preformed immune complexes on the basement membrane leads to lumpy-bumpy deposits (Fig. 15.4).

In a number of infectious diseases (malaria, leprosy, dengue) there may be times during the course of the infection when large amounts of antigen and antibody exist

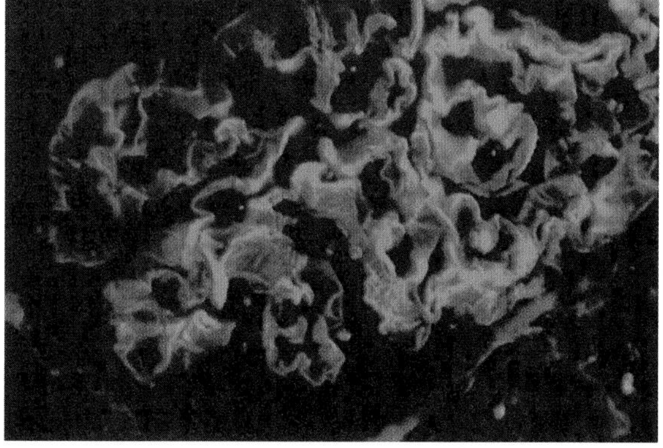

Figure 15.3. Ribbon-like deposit of antibody along the basement membrane revealed by fluorescent antibodies to human immunoglobulin. (Courtesy of A. Ucci, Tufts University Medical School.)

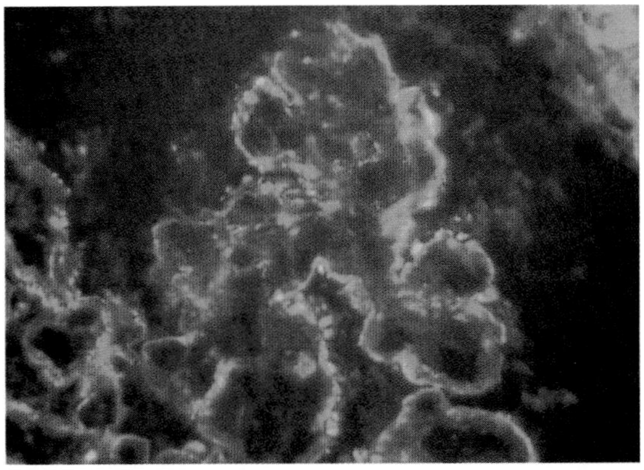

Figure 15.4. Lumpy-bumpy staining pattern of fluorescent antibody specific for human immunoglobulin: immune complex deposits in glomerular basement membrane. (Courtesy of A. Ucci, Tufts University School of Medicine.)

simultaneously and cause the formation of immune aggregates that are deposited in a variety of locations. Thus the complex of symptoms in any of these diseases may include a component attributable to a type III hypersensitivity reaction.

Complement Deficiency. As noted above, most immune complexes do not cause damage because they are removed from circulation before they become lodged in the tissues. Complexes that contain C3b bind to erythrocytes bearing CR1. The erythrocytes deliver the complexes to mononuclear phagocytes within the liver and spleen for removal by phagocytosis. The components of the classical complement pathway reduce the number of antigen epitopes that antibodies can bind by intercalating into the lattice of the complex, resulting in smaller, soluble complexes. It is these small, soluble complexes that bind most readily to the erythrocytes. In patients with complement deficiencies affecting C1, C2, and C4 (see Chapters 13 and 16), the complexes remain large and bind poorly to the erythrocytes. These non-erythrocyte-bound complexes are taken up rapidly by the liver and then released to be deposited in tissues such as skin, kidney and muscle, where they can set up inflammatory reactions.

Localized Immune Complex Disease

In 1903, a French scientist named Arthus immunized rabbits with horse serum by repeated intradermal injection. After several weeks, he noted that each succeeding injection produced an increasingly severe reaction at the site of inoculation. At first, a mild erythema (redness) and edema (accumulation of fluid) were noticed within 24 h of injection. These reactions subsided without consequence by the following day, but subsequent injections produced larger edematous responses, and by the fifth or sixth inoculations the lesions became hemorrhagic with necrosis and were slow to heal. This phenomenon, known as the ***Arthus reaction,*** is the prototype of localized immune complex reactions. As with systemic immune complex hypersensitivity reactions, localized reactions involve soluble antigens. The local inflammatory responses generated occur after reactivity of antigen with already formed, antigen-specific IgG antibody. When such preformed antibodies come in contact with antigen at the appropriate concentrations (antibody excess), in or near vessel walls (venules), insoluble immune complexes form and accumulate as they would on a gel-diffusion plate (see Chapter 5). The subsequent pathophysiologic events are very similar to those described in the systemic pattern (Fig. 15.2). The end result is rupture of the vessel wall and hemorrhage, accompanied by necrosis of local tissue (Fig. 15.5).

A clinical example of Arthus-type hypersensitivity reactions is seen in a disease called ***farmer's lung.*** This is an intrapulmonary III hypersensitivity reaction that occurs in patients with ***extrinsic allergic alveolitis.*** As its name implies, the disease sometimes occurs in individuals involved in farming—thus it is classified as an occupational disease. In sensitive individuals, exposure to moldy hay leads, within 6–8 h, to severe respiratory distress or pneumonitis. It has been shown that affected individuals have made large amounts of IgG antibody specific for the spores of thermophilic actinomycetes that grow on rotting hay. Inhalation of the bacterial spores

A

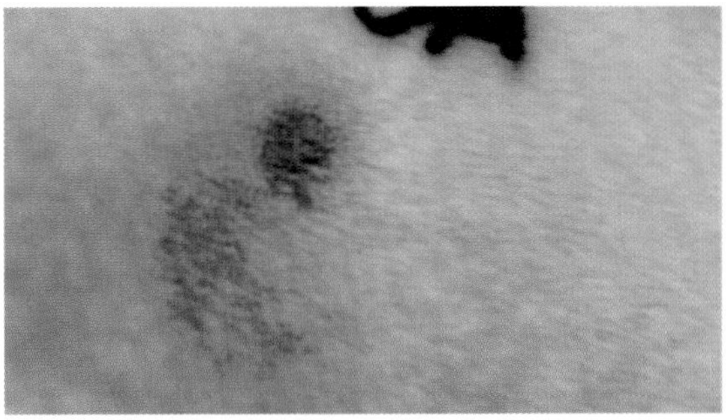

B

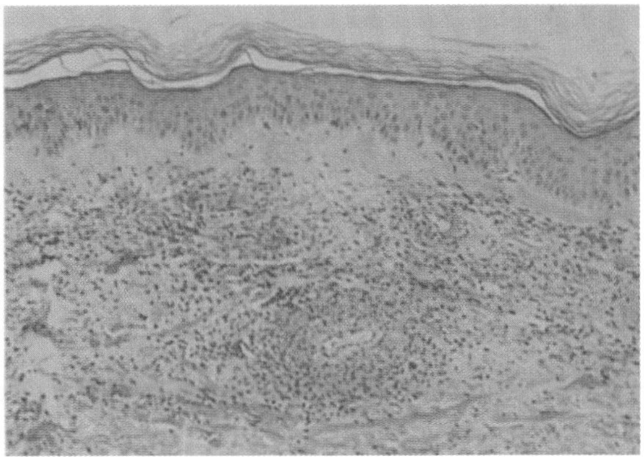

Figure 15.5. Type III hypersensitivity Arthus reaction. **(A)** Gross views of hemorrhagic appearance (purpura). **(B)** Histologic features of Arthus reaction showing neutrophil infiltrate. (Courtesy of M. Stadecker, Tufts University Medical School.)

leads to a reaction in the lungs that resembles the Arthus reaction seen in skin—namely, the formation of antigen–antibody aggregates and consequent inflammation.

There are many similar pulmonary type III reactions that bear names related to the occupation or causative agent, such as pigeon breeder's disease, cheese washer's disease, bagassosis (bagasse refers to sugarcane fiber), maple bark stripper's disease, paprika worker's disease, and the increasingly rare thatched roof worker's lung. Dirty work environments, involving massive exposure to potentially antigenic material, obviously lend themselves to the development of this form of occupational disease.

SUMMARY

1. Type II hypersensitivity reactions involve damage to target cells and are mediated by antibody through three major pathways. (1) In the first pathway, antibody (usually IgM, but also IgG) activates the entire complement sequence and causes cell lysis. (2) In the second pathway, antibody (usually IgG) serves to engage receptors for Fc on phagocytic cells and C3b engages receptors on phagocytic cells, with C3b receptors, causing destruction of the antibody and/or C3b-coated target through ADCC. These reactions usually involve circulating blood cells, such as RBCs, WBCs, and platelets, and the consequences are those that would be expected from destruction of the particular type of cell. (3) The third pathway leads to dysfunctional cellular consequences caused by the binding of disease-causing antagonistic or agonistic autoantibodies to cell surface receptors (e.g., myasthenia gravis and Graves disease, respectively).

2. Type III immune complex reactions involve the formation of antigen–antibody complexes that can activate the complement cascade and induce acute inflammatory responses. Release of certain products of complement (C3a and C5a) causes a local increase in vessel permeability and permits the release of serum (edema) and the chemotactic attraction of neutrophils. The neutrophils, in the process of ingesting the immune complexes, release degradative lysosomal enzymes that produce the tissue damage characteristic of these reactions.

3. If the site of a type III reaction is a vessel wall, the outcome is hemorrhage and necrosis; if the site is a glomerular basement membrane, loss of integrity and release of protein and RBCs into the urine results; and if the site is a joint meniscus, destruction of synovial membranes and cartilage occurs.

4. Multiple forms of type III hypersensitivity reactions exist, ranging from localized to systemic reactions, depending on the type and location of antigen and the way in which it is brought together with antibody. In all cases, however, the outcome depends on complement and granulocytes as mediators of tissue injury.

REFERENCES

Birmingham DJ, Rovin BH, Yu CY, Hebert LA (2001): Of mice and men: the relevance of the mouse to the study of human SLE. *Immunol Res* 24:211.

Cotran RS, Kumar V, Robbins SL (1989): The Kidney in Pathologic Basis of Disease. Philadelphia: Saunders.

Cuellar ML (2002): Drug-induced vasculitis. *Curr Rheumatol Rep* 4:55.

Dixon FJ, Cochrane CC, Theofilopoulus AN (1988): Immune complex injury. In Samter M, Talmage DW, Frank MM, Austen KF, Claman HN (eds): Immunological Diseases, 4th ed. Boston: Little, Brown.

Fye KH, Sack KE (1994): Rheumatic diseases. In Stites DP, Terr AI, Parslow TG (eds): Basic and Clinical Immunology, 8th ed. East Norwalk, CT: Appleton & Lange.

Hopken UE, Lu B, Gerard NP, Gerard C (1997): Impaired inflammatory responses in the reverse Arthus reaction through genetic deletion of the C5a receptor. *J Exp Med* 29:749.

Kumar V, Cotran RS, Robbins SL (ed) (1997): Disorders of the immune system. In: Basic Pathology, 6th ed. Philadelphia: Saunders.

Lawley TJ, Frank MM (1980): Immune complexes and immune complex diseases. In Parker CW (ed): Clinical Immunology, Vol 1. Philadelphia: Saunders.

Ravetch JV, Bolland S (2001): IgG Fc receptors. *Annu Rev Immunol* 19:275.

Taki T (1996): Multiple loss of effector cell functions in FcR gamma-deficient mice. *Int Rev Immunol* 13:396.

Terr AI (1994): Immune complex disease. In Stites DP, Terr AI, Parslow TG (eds): Basic and Clinical Immunology, 8th ed. East Norwalk, CT: Appleton & Lange.

Theofilopoulos AN, Dixon FJ (1979): The biology and detection of immune complexes. *Adv Immunol* 28:89.

REVIEW QUESTIONS

For each question, choose the ONE BEST answer or completion.

1. The development of which of the following diseases in predisposed individuals is most likely to involve a reaction to a hapten in its etiology?

A) Goodpasture's syndrome following a viral respiratory infection
B) hemolytic anemia following treatment with penicillin
C) rheumatoid arthritis following a parasitic infection
D) farmer's lung following exposure to moldy hay

2. In an experimental mouse model for the study of autoimmune hemolytic anemia, intravenous administration of a monoclonal mouse IgA antibody specific for a RBC antigen did not cause anemia to occur. The best explanation for this observation is that

A) the IgA would localize in the gastrointestinal tract.
B) the Fc region of the IgA antibody does not bind receptors for Fc receptors on phagocytic cells.
C) IgA cannot activate complement beyond the splitting of C2.
D) the IgA used has a low affinity for the RBC antigen.
E) the IgA used requires secretory component to work.

3. The glomerular lesions in immune complex disease can be visualized microscopically with a fluorescent antibody against

A) IgG H chains.
B) κ light chains.
C) C1.
D) C3.
E) all of the above.

4. Immune complexes are involved in the pathogenesis of which of the following rheumatic fever–associated diseases?

A) post-streptococcal glomerulonephritis
B) pigeon breeder's disease
C) serum sickness
D) autoimmune hemolytic anemia

5. The final damage to vessels in immune complex-mediated arthritis is due to

A) cytokines produced by T cells
B) histamine and SRS-A
C) the C5, C6, C7, C8, C9 membrane attack complex
D) lysosomal enzymes of polymorphonuclear leukocytes
E) cytotoxic T cells

6. Serum sickness is characterized by

A) deposition of immune complexes in blood vessel walls when there is a moderate excess of antigen.
B) phagocytosis of complexes by granulocytes.
C) consumption of complement.
D) appearance of symptoms before free antibody can be detected in the circulation.
E) all of the above.

7. Type II hypersensitivity

A) is antibody-independent.
B) is complement-independent.
C) is mediated by $CD8^+$ T cells.
D) requires immune complex formation.
E) involves antibody-mediated destruction of cells.

8. A patient is suspected of having farmer's lung. A provocation test involving the inhalation of an extract of moldy hay is performed. A sharp drop in respiratory function is noted within 10 min and returns to normal in 2 h, only to fall again in another 2 h. The most likely explanation is that

A) the patient has existing T cell-mediated hypersensitivity.
B) this is a normal pattern for farmer's lung.
C) the patient developed a secondary response after the inhalation of antigen.
D) the symptoms of farmer's lung are complicated by an IgE-mediated reactivity to the same antigen.
E) All of the above.

CASE STUDY

A technician in a snake venom–producing farm got careless one day and was bitten by a rare lethal Egyptian cobra. He was rushed to the emergency department and a call went out immediately for antivenom serum. Fortunately, some was located and within 5 hr he was given 15 mL intravenously. The next day, he received another 10 mL, the last available. Within days he was well on the way to recovery and left the hospital a week later. He returned 10 days after leaving the hospital complaining of joint pain, fever, and recurrent itchy hives on his trunk, arms, and legs. What do you suspect is happening, and how would you confirm it?

ANSWERS TO REVIEW QUESTIONS

1. ***B*** Penicillin can function as a hapten, binding to RBCs and inducing a hemolytic anemia. A, C, and D are examples of immune complex (type III) reactions requiring complement and neutrophils for pathologic effects.

2. ***B*** Since phagocytic cells have Fc receptors for IgG, bound IgA would not cause engulfment and damage. Thus A, C, D, and E are false.

3. ***E*** The lesions in immune complex disease depend on the presence of antigen, antibody, and complement. Hence all can be demonstrated by immunofluorescence at a lesion: A and B, because they are parts of IgG; C and D, because they are the early components of complement activated by the immune aggregates.

4. ***A*** Rheumatic fever is a disease associated with infections caused by group A streptococci. It involves the development of anti-streptococci antibodies that are cross-reactive with antigens present in human heart muscle, cartilage, and glomerular basement membrane.

5. ***D*** Neither T cells nor mast cells are responsible for the final tissue damage in immune complex disease. Therefore A, B, and E are eliminated. The final lytic complex of complement is similarly not involved, since complement activation up to C5 is sufficient to bring in the polymorphonuclear leukocytes, whose lysosomal enzymes cause the tissue damage.

6. ***E*** All are characteristics of serum sickness.

7. ***E*** Type II hypersensitivity reactions occur after development of antibodies against target antigens expressed on normal cells or cells with altered membrane determinants. Antibodies bind to the surface of these cells and mediate damage or destruction by one or more mechanisms, including complement-mediated reactions. $CD8^+$ cytotoxic T cells and immune complexes are not involved in these reactions.

8. ***D*** Type III hypersensitivity reactions in farmer's lung and similar occupational diseases have an onset of symptoms that usually occur several hours after exposure to the causal antigen. The appearance of breathing difficulties within minutes would create a strong suspicion that a type I anaphylactic response is also present. Presumably the patient made both IgE and IgG antibodies to the actinomycete antigens. A positive wheal and flare reaction on skin testing would provide further confirmation.

ANSWER TO CASE STUDY

Most antivenoms of exotic species such as snake, spider, and scorpion would be made in horses. The horse antiserum neutralized the toxin and saved the patient's life. However, being a foreign protein, it induced an immune response with resultant formation of antigen–antibody complexes and the symptoms of type III hypersensitivity, serum sickness. The localization of these complexes in joints and the activation of complement to give anaphylatoxins were responsible for the joint pain, hives, and itching he experienced. It is possible that he could subseqently develop symptoms of glomerulonephritis as well. Treatment would consist of corticosteroid administration for its general anti-inflammatory effects, Confirmatory studies of your diagnosis might include looking for depressed levels of serum C3 and C4 as a result of activation in tissue by the antigen–antibody aggregates. In the convalescent stage, one might also find antibody to horse immunoglobulin as a final definitive proof of your diagnosis.

16

HYPERSENSITIVITY REACTIONS: T CELL–MEDIATED (TYPE IV) DELAYED-TYPE HYPERSENSITIVITY

INTRODUCTION

In contrast to antibody-mediated hypersensitivity reactions discussed in the previous two chapters, T cell–mediated hypersensitivity—also known as ***delayed-type hypersensitivity*** (DTH) or ***type IV hypersensitivity***—involves immune responses initiated primarily by antigen-specific T cells. Thus, unlike antibody-mediated hypersensitivity reactions, which can be transferred from an immunized or sensitized individual to a nonimmune individual via serum, experimental animal models have demonstrated that type IV hypersensitivity reactions can be transferred only with T cells. Similar to antibody-mediated hypersensitivity, T cell–mediated hypersensitivity reactions are sometimes damaging to the host. Thus, when activated by contact with an antigen presented by an antigen-presenting cell (APC), the responding T cells release inappropriately large amounts of cytokines, some of which attract and activate other mononuclear cells that are not antigen specific such as monocytes and macrophages. The recruitment and activation of these antigen-nonspecific mononuclear cells are mainly responsible for the eventual deleterious outcome of the reactions. Antigens eliciting this type of response may be foreign tissue (as in allograft reactions), intracellular parasites (e.g., viruses, mycobacteria, or fungi), soluble proteins, or one of many chemicals capable of penetrating skin and coupling to body proteins that serve as carriers.

GENERAL CHARACTERISTICS AND PATHOPHYSIOLOGY OF DTH

The clinical features of type IV hypersensitivity reactions vary, depending on the sensitizing antigen and the route of antigen exposure. These variants include contact hypersensitivity, tuberculin-type hypersensitivity, and granulomatous hypersensitivity (see next section). In general, however, common pathophysiologic mechanisms account for each of these variants. The major events leading to these reactions involve the following three steps: (1) activation of antigen-specific inflammatory T_H1 cells in a previously sensitized individual, (2) elaboration of proinflammatory cytokines by the antigen-specific T_H1 cells, and (3) recruitment and activation of antigen-nonspecific inflammatory leukocytes. These events typically occur over a period of several days (24–72 h)—hence the term *delayed-type hypersensitivity*. This time course characteristically distinguishes DTH from antibody-mediated reactions, which appear much more quickly (see Chapters 14 and 15).

Mechanisms of DTH

The mechanisms involved in the sensitization to DTH and the elucidation of the reaction following antigenic challenge are now well understood. It is important to underscore that, as with antibody-mediated hypersensitivity reactions,

Immunology: A Short Course, Fifth Edition, By Richard Coico, Geoffrey Sunshine, and Eli Benjamini
ISBN 0-471-22689-0

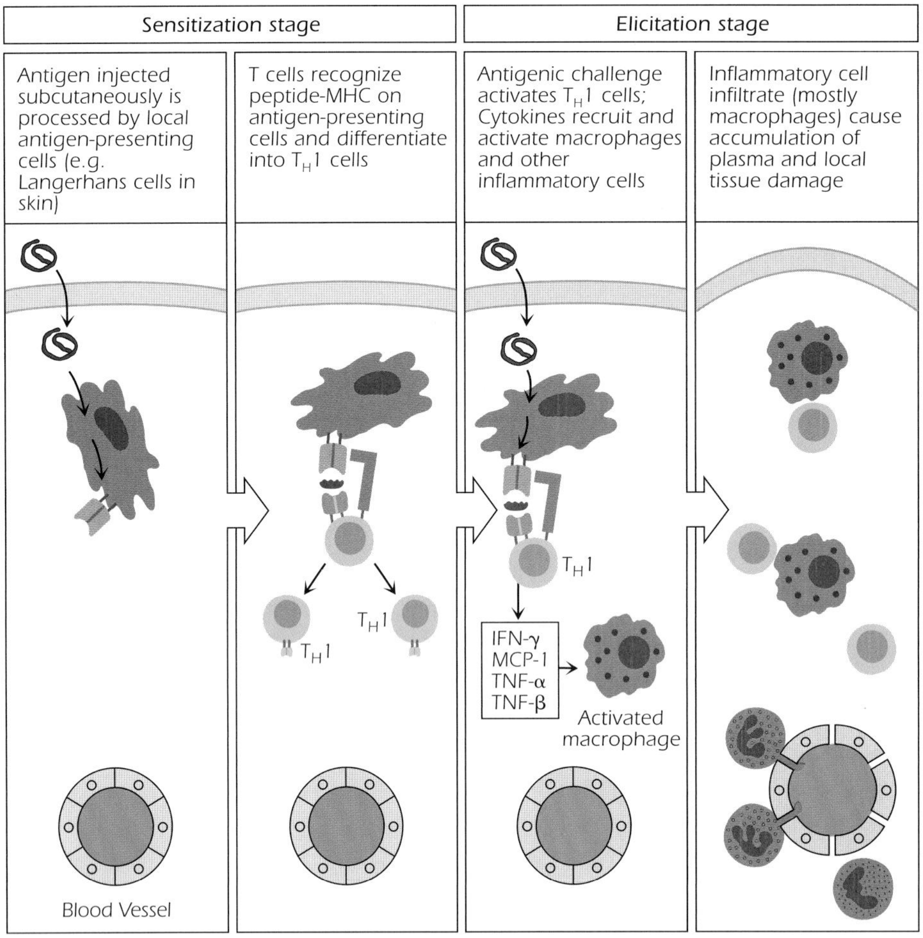

Figure 16.1. The DTH reaction. Stage of sensitization by antigen involves presentation of antigen to T cells by APCs, leading to the release of cytokines and differentiation of T cells to T_H1 cells. Challenge with antigen involves antigen presentation to T_H1 cells by APCs, leading to T_H1 activation, release of cytokines, and recruitment and activation of macrophages. *MCP,* membrane cofactor protein; *TNF,* tumor necrosis factor.

previous exposure to the antigen is required to generate DTH. Such exposure (the ***sensitization stage***) activates and expands the number of antigen-specific memory T_H1 cells that, when subsequently challenged with the same antigen, respond to produce a DTH reaction (the ***elicitation stage***). These stages are shown in Figure 16.1. The sensitization stage typically occurs over a 1 to 2-week period, during which normal mechanisms of T cell activation occur (see Chapter 10). In contrast, the elicitation stage requires approximately 24–72 h from time of antigenic challenge to recruit and activate these cells—a period that culminates in the histologic and clinical features of DTH. The clinical manifestations of DTH can last for several weeks or, in some cases, can be chronic (e.g., DTH occurring in certain autoimmune diseases).

The antigen-challenged T_H1 cells, produce several cytokines during the elicitation stage, most notably, chemokines and interferon-γ (IFN-γ), which cause chemotaxis and activation of macrophages (Fig. 16.2). The recruitment and activation of antigen-nonspecific cells by antigen-specific T_H1 cells demonstrate the interaction between acquired and innate immunity, discussed in Chapter 2. Another cytokine produced by these cells is interleukin-12 (IL-12). IL-12 suppresses the T_H2 subpopulation and promotes the expansion of the T_H1 subpopulation, thereby driving the response to produce more T_H1-synthesized cytokines that activate macrophages. Thus IL-12 plays an important role in DTH. Table 16.1 summarizes the important cytokines involved in DTH reactions.

DTH reactions also involve $CD8^+$ T cells, which are first activated and expanded during the sensitization stage of the response. These cells can damage tissues by cell-mediated cytotoxicity (see Chapter 10). Activation of $CD8^+$ T cells occurs as a consequence of the ability of many lipid-soluble chemicals capable of inducing DTH reactions to cross the cell membrane (e.g., pentadecacatechol—the chemical that induces ***poison ivy***). Within the cell, these chemicals react with cytosolic proteins to generate modified peptides that are translocated to the endoplasmic reticulum and then delivered to the cell surface in the context of MHC class I molecules. Cells presenting such modified self-proteins are subsequently damaged or killed by $CD8^+$ T cells.

Consequences of DTH

It should be apparent from the preceding discussion that many of the effector functions in DTH are performed by activated macrophages. In the most favorable circumstances, DTH results in destruction of an infectious organism (see below)

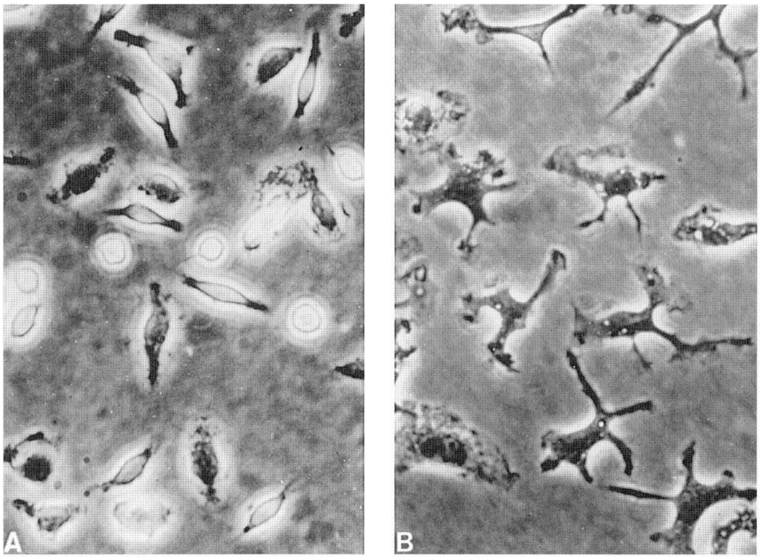

Figure 16.2. The effect of IFN-γ on peritoneal macrophages. **(A)** Normal macrophages in culture as they are just beginning to adhere. **(B)** Macrophages that after activation with IFN-γ have adhered, spread out with development of numerous pseudopodia, and grown larger. More lysosomal granules are also visible. (Courtesy of M. Stadecker, Tufts University Medical School).

that may have elicited the response in the first place. This destruction is believed to result predominantly from ingestion of the organism by ***macrophages,*** their activation by ***IFN-γ,*** followed by degradation by lysosomal enzymes as well as by the by-products of the burst of respiratory activity, such as peroxide and superoxide radicals (Chapter 2). Foreign tissues, tumor tissue, and soluble or conjugated antigens are dealt with in a similar manner.

EXAMPLES OF DTH

Several known variants of classical DTH have the same basic mechanisms but have additional features, which are described in this section.

Contact Sensitivity

Contact sensitivity (sometimes called ***contact dermatitis***) is a form of DTH in which the target organ is the skin, and the inflammatory response is produced as the result of contact with sensitizing substances on the surface of the skin. Thus it is primarily an epidermal reaction characterized by ***eczema*** at the site of contact with the allergen, which typically peaks 48–72 h after contact. The prototype for this form of DTH is ***poison ivy dermatitis*** (Fig. 16.3A). The offending substance is contained in an oil secreted by the leaves of the poison-ivy vine and other related plants. These oils contain a mixture of catechols (dihydroxyphenols) with long hydrocarbon side chains. These features allow it to penetrate the skin by virtue of its lipophilicity (which gives it the ability to dissolve in skin oils) and its ability to couple covalently (by formation of quinones) to cell-associated proteins (e.g., carrier molecules on cell surfaces). Other contact sensitizers are generally also lipid-soluble haptens. They have a variety of chemical forms, but all have in common the ability to penetrate skin and form hapten-carrier conjugates. Chemicals such as 2,4-dinitrochlorobenzene (DNCB) are used to induce contact sensitivity. Since virtually every normal individual is capable of developing contact hypersensitivity to a test dose of this compound, it is frequently used to assess a patients potential for T cell reactivity (cell-mediated immunity). Various metals, such as nickel and chromium, which are present in jewelry and clasps of undergarments, are also capable of inducing contact sensitivity, presumably by way of chelation (ionic interaction) by skin proteins.

The induction of contact sensitivity is thought to proceed via presentation of the offending allergen by ***Langerhans cells*** (antigen-presenting cells in the skin). It is not yet resolved whether the sensitizer couples directly to components on the cell surface of the Langerhans cell or whether it couples first to proteins in serum or tissue that are then taken up by the Langerhans cells. The initial contact results in expansion of the clones of T_H1 cells capable of recognizing the specific contact sensitizer. Subsequent contact (challenge) with the sensitizing antigen triggers the elicitation stage of

TABLE 16.1. Cytokines Involved in DTH Reactions

Cytokine[a]	Functional effects[b]
IFN-γ	Activates macrophages to release inflammatory mediators
Chemokines MCP-1 RANTES	Recruit macrophages and monocytes to the site
MIP-1α	
MIP-1β	
TNFα	Causes local tissue damage
TNFβ	Increases expression of adhesion molecules on blood vessels

[a] *MCP,* membrane co-factor protein; *MIP,* macrophage inflammatory protein; *TNF,* tumor necrosis factor.
[b] Additional functional effects are described in Chapter 11.

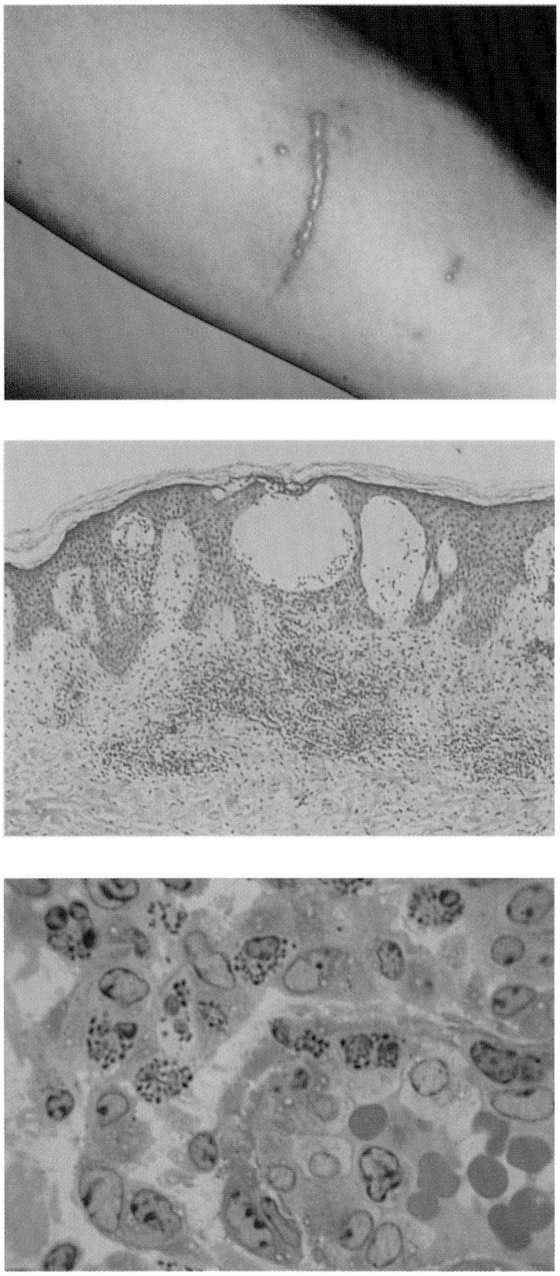

A

B

C

Figure 16.3. **(A)** Type IV contact sensitivity reaction—gross appearance of reaction to poison ivy. **(B)** Type IV contact hypersensitivity reaction—histologic appearance showing intraepithelial blister formation and mononuclear infiltrate in the dermis. **(C)** Cutaneous basophil reaction showing basophils and some mononuclear cells 24 h after skin test. (All panels courtesy of M. Stadecker, Tufts University Medical School.)

DTH discussed earlier. The histologic appearance of this variant of DTH shows intraepithelial ***blister formation*** and mononuclear infiltrates in the dermis (Fig. 16.3B) that manifests as the separation of epidermal cells, spongiosis (an inflammatory intercellular edema of the epidermis), and blister formation (Fig. 16.3A).

In many cases, enough of the sensitizing antigen remains at the site of the initial contact so that in approximately 1 week, when sufficient T cell expansion has taken place, the antigen that persists serves as the challenging antigen and a reaction in this area will flare up. Therefore, the elicitation phase can occur without new contact with the sensitizing antigen.

The commonly performed procedure for testing for the presence of contact sensitivity is the patch test in which a solution of the suspected antigen is spread on the skin and covered by an occlusive dressing. The appearance, within 3 days, of an area of ***induration*** and ***erythema,*** indicates sensitivity.

Granulomatous Hypersensitivity

In circumstances, such as those associated with contact dermatitis, in which the antigen is readily disposed of, the lesion resolves slowly, with little tissue damage. Sometimes, however, the antigen may be protected and very persistent; for example, schistosomal eggs and lipid-encapsulated mycobacteria are resistant to enzymatic degradation. In these cases, the response can be prolonged and destructive to the host. Continuous accumulation of macrophages leads to clusters of epithelioid cells, which fuse to form giant cells in ***granulomas.*** The maximal reaction time for the development of a granuloma is 21–28 days. The pathologic changes result from the inability of macrophages to destroy phagocytized pathogens (e.g., *Mycobacterium leprae*) or to degrade large inert antigens. Granulomas can be destructive because of their displacement of normal tissue and can result in caseous (cheesy) necrosis. This is typical in such diseases as tuberculosis caused by infections with *M. tuberculosis,* in which a cuff of lymphocytes surrounds the core, and there may be considerable fibrosis.

The disease process may then be attributable not so much to the effects of the invading organisms as to the persistent attempts of the host to isolate and contain the parasite by the mechanisms of DTH. In diseases such as smallpox, measles, and herpes, the characteristic exanthems (skin rashes) seen are partly attributable to DTH responses to the virus, with additional destruction attributable to the attack by cytotoxic $CD8^+$ T cells on the virally infected epithelial cells.

Tuberculin-Type Hypersensitivity

Tuberculin-type reactions are ***cutaneous inflammatory reactions*** characterized by an area of firm red swelling of the skin that is maximal at 48–72 h after challenge. The term *tuberculin-type* derives from the prototype DTH reaction in which a lipoprotein antigen isolated from *M. tuberculosis* called *tuberculin* was used to test for evidence of exposure to the causative agent of tuberculosis (TB). It's important to note, however, that soluble antigens from other organisms (including *M. leprae* and *Leishmania tropica*) induce similar tuberculin-type DTH reactions. Today, TB tests are performed by intradermal injecting a more purified lipoprotein

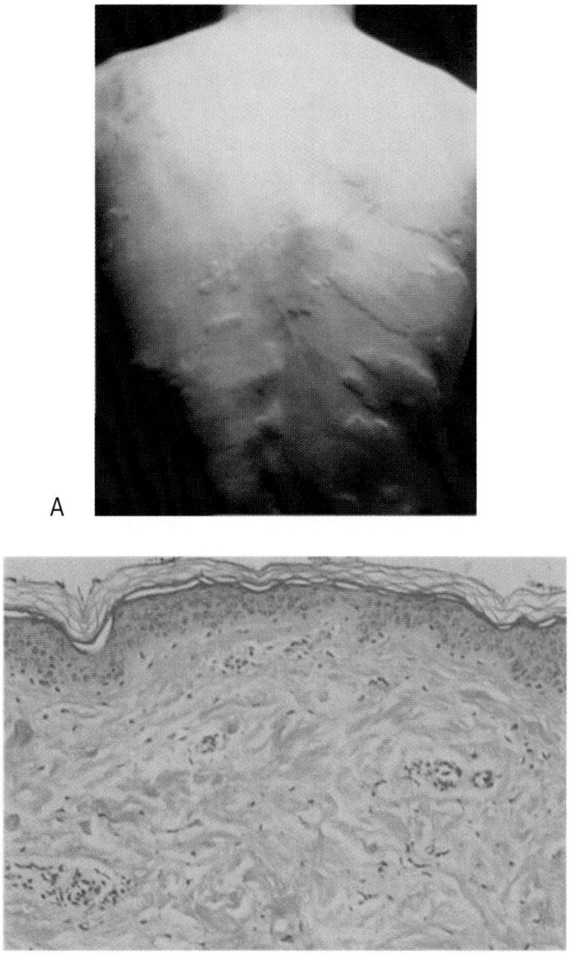

Figure 16.4. **(A)** Type IV DTH reaction (tuberculin reaction)—gross appearance showing induration and erythema 48 h after tuberculin test. (Courtesy of A. Gottlieb, Tulane University Medical School.) **(B)** Type IV DTH reaction—histologic picture showing dermal mononuclear cell infiltrate and perivascular cuffing. (Courtesy of M. Stadecker, Tufts University Medical School.)

extract isolated from *M. tuberculosis* called ***purified protein derivative*** (PPD). The PPD test (also called the Mantoux test) is extremely useful for public health surveillance of TB. If an individual has been previously sensitized to antigens expressed by *M. tuberculosis* as a consequence of infection with this organism, the characteristic tuberculin-type lesion will appear at the site of injection within 48–72 h. Evidence of ***erythema*** (redness) and ***induration*** (raised thickening) appear, reaching maximal levels 72 h after the challenge (Fig. 16.4A). The induration can easily be distinguished from edema (fluid) by absence of pitting when pressure is applied. These reactions, even when severe, rarely lead to necrotic damage, and they resolve slowly. A biopsy taken early in the reaction reveals primarily mononuclear cells of the monocyte–macrophage series with a few scattered lymphocytes. Characteristically, the mononuclear infiltrates appear as a perivascular cuff before extensively invading the site of deposition of antigen (Fig. 16.4B). Neutrophils are not a prominent feature of the initial reaction. In more severe cases, tuberculin-type hypersensitivity reactions may progress toward granulomatous hypersensitivity (discussed above). Biopsies of tissue in which this is evident show a more complex pattern, with the arrival of B cells and the formation of granulomas in persistent lesions. The hardness or induration is attributable to the deposition of fibrin in the lesion.

While the PPD test is usually very reliable, false-negative and false-positive reactions may be seen in some situations. Immunosuppressed individuals (e.g., those infected with HIV and some individuals on high-dose chemotherapy) may have false-negative PPD reactions due to the inability of antigen-specific T cells to respond (anergy; see Chapter 12).

In contrast, when PPD is used to test individuals to determine whether they have been previously exposed to *M. tuberculosis,* individuals who have been vaccinated with a nonpathogenic attenuated strain of the organism that causes TB in cattle—namely *M. bovis* bacillus Calmette-Guerin (BCG)—generate false-positive reactions. The efficacy of the BCG vaccine against human pulmonary TB varies enormously in different populations. The prevailing hypothesis attributes this variation to interactions between the vaccine and the mycobacteria common in the environment, but the precise mechanism has not yet been clarified. Routine BCG vaccination is not performed in many countries, including the United States, because of its questionable efficacy and the impact such a practice would have on our ability to confirm whether individuals have been exposed to *M. tuberculosis.*

Allograft Rejection

As we shall discuss in more detail in Chapter 18, if an individual receives grafts of cells, tissues, or organs taken from an allogeneic donor (a genetically different individual of the same species), it will usually become vascularized and be initially accepted. However, if the genetic difference is at any of the histocompatibility genes, especially genes in the MHC, a T cell–mediated rejection process ensues, the duration and intensity of which is related to the degree of incompatibility between donor and recipient. After vascularization, there is an initial invasion of the graft by a mixed population of antigen-specific T cells and antigen-nonspecific monocytes through the blood vessel walls. This inflammatory reaction soon leads to destruction of the vessels; this deprivation of nutrients is quickly followed by necrosis and breakdown of the grafted tissue.

Additional Examples of DTH

An unusual form of delayed reaction has been observed in humans following repeated intradermal injections of antigen. The response is delayed in onset (usually by about 24 h) but consists entirely of erythema, without the induration typical of classic delayed-hypersensitivity reactions. When this condition was studied experimentally, it was found that the erythema was attended by a cellular infiltrate but that the predominant cell type was the basophil. Studies in guinea pigs showed that the response was primarily mediated by T cells and was subject to the same MHC restrictions as classic T cell–mediated responses. When classic delayed hypersensitivity was present, however, infiltrates of basophils were not seen. Thus cutaneous basophil hypersensitivity seemed to be a variant of T cell–mediated responses, but its exact mechanism was unknown. The picture was complicated still further when it was shown that passive transfer of serum could, under some circumstances, evoke a basophil response.

The physiologic significance of cutaneous basophil hypersensitivity remained a mystery until it was shown that guinea pigs bitten by certain ticks had severe cutaneous basophil hypersensitivity reactions at the site of attachment of the tick. The infiltration of basophils and, presumably, the release of inflammatory mediators from their granules resulted in death of the tick and its eventual detachment. Thus cutaneous basophil hypersensitivity may have an important role in certain forms of immunity to parasites. More recently, basophil infiltrates were also found in cases of contact dermatitis with allergens such as poison ivy, in cases of rejection of renal grafts, and in some forms of conjunctivitis. These observations indicate that basophils may also play a role in some types of delayed hypersensitivity disease.

Other examples of DTH include reactions to self-antigens in certain autoimmune diseases (see Chapter 12). As with persistent infections that can cause chronic DTH reactions, these reactions are often chronic, resulting from the continuous clonal activation of autoreactive T_H1 cells. Examples of autoimmune diseases in which DTH reactions are involved are rheumatoid arthritis, type 1 diabetes, and multiple sclerosis.

TREATMENT OF DTH

Therapies to treat T cell–mediated hypersensitivity vary in accordance with the variant of DTH. In most cases, DTH reactions, such as contact dermatitis and tuberculin-type reactions, resolve after a period of days to weeks after removal of the antigen. Corticosteroids, applied either topically or systemically, constitute a very effective treatment for these forms of DTH. In more severe variants of DTH, such as pathogen-induced granulomatous hypersensitivity, allograft rejection, and those seen in certain autoimmune diseases, more aggressive forms of immunosuppressive therapy are commonly used, including treatment with drugs such as azathioprine or cyclosporine (see Chapter 18 for additional discussion of immunosuppressive therapies).

SUMMARY

1. The normal events associated with cell-mediated immunity are a crucial mode of immunologic reactivity for protection against intracellular parasites, such as viruses, many bacteria, and fungi. However, the nature of the reaction and its mediators also cause DTH reactions.
2. DTH reactions are T cell–mediated responses classified as type IV hypersensitivity by Coombs and Gell.
3. The major events leading to these reactions involve three steps: (1) activation of antigen-specific inflammatory T_H1 cells in a previously sensitized individual, (2) elaboration of proinflammatory cytokines (especially IFN-γ, which activates macrophages) by the antigen-specific T_H1 cells, and (3) recruitment and activation of antigen-nonspecific inflammatory leukocytes
4. There are several varieties of DTH, including (1) contact hypersensitivity characterized by eczema, which peaks 48–72 h after allergen contact; (2) granulomatous hypersensitivity characterized by a granuloma that is maximal 21–28 days after antigen is introduced; and (3) tuberculin-type hypersensitivity characterized by an area of firm red erythema (redness) and induration (raised thickening) that is maximal 48–72 h after challenge. Other variants include reactions occurring in certain T cell–mediated autoimmune diseases and in some individuals who have received allografts.
5. Cytotoxic $CD8^+$ T cells can also participate in the damage associated with DTH reactions.
6. Phagocytic macrophages are the major histologic feature of DTH and account for the protective outcome of this form of hypersensitivity when pathogens are involved.
7. In situations in which macrophages are unable to destroy the pathogen, a granuloma is induced (granulomatous hypersensitivity). Granulomas can also develop following phagocytosis of inert substances. Granulomas are characterized histologically by the presence of macrophages, epithelioid cells, giant cells, and $CD4^+$ and $CD8^+$ lymphocytes.

REFERENCES

Brandt L, Feino CJ, Weinreich OA, Chilima B, Hirsch P, Appelberg R, Andersen P (2002): Failure of the *Mycobacterium bovis* BCG vaccine: some species of environmental mycobacteria block multiplication of BCG and induction of protective immunity to tuberculosis. *Infect Immun* 70:672.

Burger D, Dayer JM (2002): Cytokines, acute-phase proteins, and hormones: IL-1 and TNF-alpha production in contact-mediated activation of monocytes by T lymphocytes. *Ann N Y Acad Sci* 966:464.

Celada A, Nathan C (1994): Macrophage activation revisited. *Immunol Today* 15:100.

Grabbe S, Schwartz T (1998): Immunoregulatory mechanisms involved in elicitation of allergic contact hypersensitivity. *Immunol Today* 19:37.

Kobayashi K, Kaneda K, Kasama T (2001): Immunopathogenesis of delayed-type hypersensitivity. *Microsc Res Tech* 15:241.

Rosenberg H, Gallin JI (2003): Inflammation. In Paul WE (ed): Fundamental Immunology, 5th ed. New York: Lippincott-Raven.

Terr AI (1994): Cell-mediated hypersensitivity disease. In Stites DP, Terr AI, Parslow TG (eds): Basic and Clinical Immunology, 8th ed. East Norwalk, CT: Appleton & Lange.

Turk JL (1980): Delayed Hypersensitivity, 3rd ed. Amsterdam: Elsevier.

REVIEW QUESTIONS

For each question, choose the ONE BEST answer or completion.

1. Which of the following does not involve cell-mediated immunity?
- A) contact sensitivity to lipstick
- B) rejection of an allograft
- C) serum sickness
- D) the Mantoux test
- E) immunity to chickenpox

2. A positive delayed-type hypersensitivity skin reaction involves the interaction of
- A) antigen, complement, and cytokines.
- B) antigen, antigen-sensitive T cells, and macrophages.
- C) antigen–antibody complexes, complement, and neutrophils.
- D) IgE antibody, antigen, and mast cells.
- E) antigen, macrophages, and complement.

3. Cell-mediated immune responses are
- A) enhanced by depletion of complement.
- B) suppressed by corticosteroids.
- C) enhanced by depletion of T cells.
- D) suppressed by antihistamine.
- E) enhanced by depletion of macrophages.

4. Delayed skin reactions to an intradermal injection of antigen may be markedly decreased by
- A) exposure to a high dose of X-irradiation.
- B) treatment with antihistamines.
- C) treatment with an antineutrophil serum.
- D) removal of the spleen.
- E) decreasing levels of complement.

5. Which of the following statements is characteristic of contact sensitivity?
- A) The best therapy is oral administration of the antigen.
- B) Patch testing with the allergen is useless for diagnosis.
- C) Sensitization can be passively transferred with serum from an allergic individual.
- D) Some chemicals acting as haptens induce sensitivity by covalently binding to host proteins acting as carriers.
- E) Antihistamines constitute the treatment of choice.

6. Positive skin tests for delayed-type hypersensitivity to intradermally injected antigens indicate that
- A) a humoral immune response has occurred.
- B) a cell-mediated immune response has occurred.
- C) both T cell and B cell systems are functional.
- D) the individual has previously made IgE responses to the antigen.
- E) immune complexes have been formed at the injection site.

7. T cell–mediated immune responses can result in
- A) formation of granulomas.
- B) induration at the reaction site.
- C) rejection of a heart transplant.
- D) eczema of the skin in the area of prolonged contact with a rubberized undergarment.
- E) All of the above.

8. Which one of the following statements about the PPD skin test is true?
- A) It is specific for *Mycobacterium tuberculosis.*
- B) It can be positive in an individual who was previously immunized with BCG.
- C) It does not distinguish a present or past infection of tuberculosis.
- D) It can vary in the extent of induration so that a positive test depends on the underlying immune status of the patient tested.
- E) B, C, and D are all true.

CASE STUDY

As a member of an anthropologic research team, you have occasion to visit a primitive tribe in the remote reaches of the Amazon jungle. During your visit, the natives conduct a ceremony celebrating the rites of passage for young males. This consists, among other things, of covering their bodies with elaborate patterns of stripes and circles using a variety of colors extracted from local plants. On your return 3 weeks later, you are asked to look at a young male who has developed alarmingly itchy and *weepy* red areas of skin that run in sharply demarcated stripes across his back and on one arm. Remembering your introductory course in immunology, you make an educated guess as to the cause. How, under such primitive conditions, could you confirm your diagnosis?

ANSWERS TO REVIEW QUESTIONS

1. ***C*** Serum sickness is an example of those reactions mediated by an antibody–antigen complex that involves components of the complement system and neutrophils. All others involve cell-mediated immunity to a significant extent.

2. ***B*** Cell-mediated reactions result from the triggering of T cells by antigen with recruitment of macrophages. Antibody, complement, and mast cells do not play roles in this process, although they do play a role in immediate hypersensitivity responses.

3. ***B*** Corticosteroids have a general anti-inflammatory effect and also induce apoptosis in some T cells. Complement plays no role, and antihistamines have little effect on this type of response. Depletion of T cells or macrophages would suppress, not enhance, this type of response, since the response depends on these cells.

4. ***A*** High doses of X-irradiation will destroy T cells, which are responsible for initiating the response. Histamine, neutrophils, the spleen, and complement do not play a role, and any treatment that affects them would not affect a DTH response.

5. ***D*** Patch testing consists of application of the offending allergen under an occlusive dressing, and a positive DTH response after 24–48 h is considered evidence of sensitivity; thus B is wrong. The allergens involved are those capable of penetrating skin and binding to host carrier proteins; thus D is correct. Oral ingestion of antigen, which, in certain experimental situations, was shown to induce suppression after subsequent induction of contact sensitivity, has not yet been shown to be an effective therapeutic maneuver in humans; thus A is wrong. Corticosteroids, not antihistamines, constitute the treatment of choice for contact sensitivity; thus E is also incorrect. Passive transfer of cell-mediated immune responses is accomplished with T cells, not with serum, thus C is wrong.

6. ***B*** A DTH reaction, evidenced by erythema and induration within 24–72 h of antigen injection, indicates that a cell-mediated reaction has occurred. Such reactions do not involve antibody produced by B cells, thus A, C, D, and E are incorrect.

7. ***E*** All of these effects are manifestations of cell-mediated immunity. Induration usually takes place at the reaction site. Formation of granulomas is characteristic of a chronic DTH reaction. Rejection of the heart is an example of an allograft response. Some of the chemicals contained in rubberized undergarments can induce contact sensitivity after prolonged exposure of the skin to them.

8. ***E*** Each of the statements except for statement A are true. Positive PPD tests occur in immunocompetent individuals who have been infected with *M. tuberculosis*. However, positive reactions to PPD tests will also occur in individuals previously vaccinated with *M. bovis* BCG.

ANSWER TO CASE STUDY

The appearance of the skin lesion and its sharp demarcations and *weepy,* itchy nature all suggest contact sensitivity. One of the dyes used to paint the body is most likely the sensitizer and, since it persisted on the skin, was also able to provoke a T cell–mediated reaction after the initial expansion of the specific clones. In the absence of sophisticated testing equipment, a simple patch test using samples of the various dyes applied to healthy areas of skin should show a localized contact reaction 24–48 hr later at the site to which the causative dye was applied. (In the laboratory one might also look for an in vitro proliferative response of the patient's peripheral blood lymphocytes to added dye. A biopsy of the lesion should reveal an intense infiltrate of mononuclear cells.)

17

IMMUNODEFICIENCY DISORDERS AND NEOPLASIAS OF THE LYMPHOID SYSTEM

INTRODUCTION

At first glance, the connection between immunodeficiency disorders and neoplasias of the lymphoid system is not apparent, raising the question of why they should be discussed in the same chapter. Immunodeficiency syndromes are characterized by *absences* or deficiencies, whereas neoplasias reflect *excesses* or uncontrolled proliferations. Their relationship, however, demonstrates how finely tuned and interwoven the immune system is. As described in this chapter, deficiencies, particularly in a single arm of the immune system, affect the ability of the remaining elements to control their growth. For this reason, immunodeficiencies are fertile ground for the development of neoplasia. This does not apply to defects in precursor or early stem cells that result in more global impairment of immune function. Autoimmune phenomena are further manifestations of the loss of immune regulation that frequently accompanies immunodeficiency. Thus three seemingly disparate disease states—***immunodeficiency, autoimmunity,*** and ***lymphoid neoplasia***—often co-exist in one organism. Primary autoimmune diseases were discussed in Chapter 12; autoimmune reactions resulting from immunodeficiency or leading to lymphoid malignancy will be highlighted throughout this chapter.

As we have seen in previous chapters, the immune response is mediated by T and B lymphocytes, natural killer (NK) cells, myeloid/monocytic lineage cells, and complement. The interactions among these cells, their soluble mediators (antibodies and cytokines), and complement are tightly controlled. Disorders in the development and differentiation of the cells, synthesis of their products, or interactions among them may lead to immune deficiencies that range in clinical severity from mild to fatal. Noticeably absent from clinical detection, however, are deficiencies in which the immune system shows *redundancy,* such as in parts of the cytokine network, in which the function of one component can be replaced by another.

Although inborn immunodeficiency diseases (conditions people are born with) are generally rare, early descriptions of these "experiments of nature" shed light on the functioning of the immune system. Animal models that mimicked different types of human immunodeficiencies helped show the cellular subdivisions of specific immunity into T and B lymphocytes—that is, cell-mediated versus humoral immunity. Today, these rare immunodeficiency syndromes and lymphoid neoplasias are analyzed at the molecular level. The information gained from studying these diseases is applied to their treatment and to the development of immunotherapies for autoimmune diseases and nonlymphoid malignancies. Thus the chapter begins with a description of inborn and acquired immune deficiency syndromes and concludes with neoplasias of the immune system.

This chapter was contributed by Dr. Susan Gottesman, Department of Pathology, State University of New York Downstate Medical Center, New York.

Immunology: A Short Course, Fifth Edition, By Richard Coico, Geoffrey Sunshine, and Eli Benjamini
ISBN 0-471-22689-0

IMMUNE DEFICIENCY SYNDROMES

Immune deficiencies are divided into two major categories: ***primary,*** which may be hereditary or acquired, in which the deficiency is the cause of disease, and ***secondary,*** in which the immune deficiency is a result of other disease(s) or conditions.

Primary immune deficiencies can be categorized based on clinical presentation. This roughly corresponds to the arm of the immune system malfunctioning: (1) ***T cell,*** or cell-mediated immunity; (2) ***B cell,*** or antibody-mediated immunity; (3) both B and T cell immunity; (4) nonspecific immunity mediated by ***phagocytic cells*** and/or ***NK cells;*** and (5) ***complement*** activation. This classification organizes the broad spectrum of immune disorders.

Abnormalities of cytokine and cytokine receptors—the means by which cells communicate and function—do not form a separate category but are incorporated into the first four groups. Since an expressed immune response is often the result of interactions among several cell types, a deficiency of, for example, antibody production and B cell function may actually be caused by an underlying problem in T cells or in T–B cell interaction. Classification based on the apparent *expressed* defect and not necessarily on its underlying cause (which may be unknown) is a useful framework for diagnosing new patients. This classification also allows correlation with animal models in which the fundamental immune defect may be identified.

Immune deficiency should always be suspected in a patient with recurrent infections. As shown in Table 17.1, the types of infections found can often facilitate diagnosis of the underlying problem. For example, recurrent bacterial otitis media (ear infection) and bacterial pneumonia are common in individuals with B cell and antibody deficiency. Increased susceptibility to fungal, protozoan, and viral infections is seen with T cell and cell-mediated immune deficiency. Systemic infections with bacteria, normally of low virulence, superficial skin infections, or infections with ***pyogenic*** (pus-producing) organisms suggest deficiencies in phagocytic cells; and recurrent infections with pyogenic organisms are associated with complement deficiencies. Of particular significance is the occurrence of ***opportunistic infections,*** diseases caused by microorganisms present in the environment and nonpathogenic in immunocompetent individuals. *Pneumocystis carinii,* cytomegalovirus (CMV), toxoplasmosis, *Mycobacterium avium,* and *Candida* are among the most common organisms involved and are most often associated with deficiencies in cell-mediated immunity.

Primary Immunodeficiency Syndromes

With the exception of IgA deficiency (discussed later in this chapter), the frequency of primary immune deficiency syndromes is very low—on the order of about 1 in 10,000. Approximately 50% of all cases are antibody deficiencies, 20% are combined deficiencies in antibody and cell-mediated immunity, 18% are phagocytic disorders, 10% are disorders of cell-mediated immunity alone, and 2% are complement deficiencies. Figure 17.1 shows that in general the earlier the genetic defect or block occurs in development, the more arms of the immune system are affected and the more severe the disease.

Severe Combined Immunodeficiency Diseases. Severe combined immunodeficiency disease (SCID) comprises a heterogeneous group of diseases in which both cell-mediated immunity and antibody production are defective (Fig. 17.1). Originally called Swiss-type agammaglobulinemia, *individuals with SCID are susceptible to virtually every type of microbial infection* (viral, bacterial, fungal, and

TABLE 17.1. Major Clinical Manifestations of Immune Disorders

Disorder	Associated Disease
Deficiency	
B lymphocyte deficiency—deficiency in antibody-mediated immunity	Recurrent bacterial infections—e.g., otitis media, recurrent pneumonia
T lymphocyte deficiency—deficiency in cell-mediated immunity	Increased susceptibility to viral, fungal, and protozoal infections
T and B lymphocyte deficiency—combined deficiency of antibody- and cell-mediated immunity	Acute and chronic infections with viral, bacterial, fungal, and protozoal organisms
Phagocytic cell deficiency	Systemic infections with bacteria of usually low virulence; infections with pyogenic bacteria; impaired pus formation and wound healing
NK cell deficiency	Viral infections, associated with several T cell disorders and X-linked lymphoproliferative syndromes
Complement component deficiency	Bacterial infections; autoimmunity
Unregulated excess	
B lymphocytes	Monoclonal gammopathies; other B cell malignancies
T lymphocytes	T cell malignancies
Complement components	Angioneurotic edema due to absence of C1 esterase inhibitor

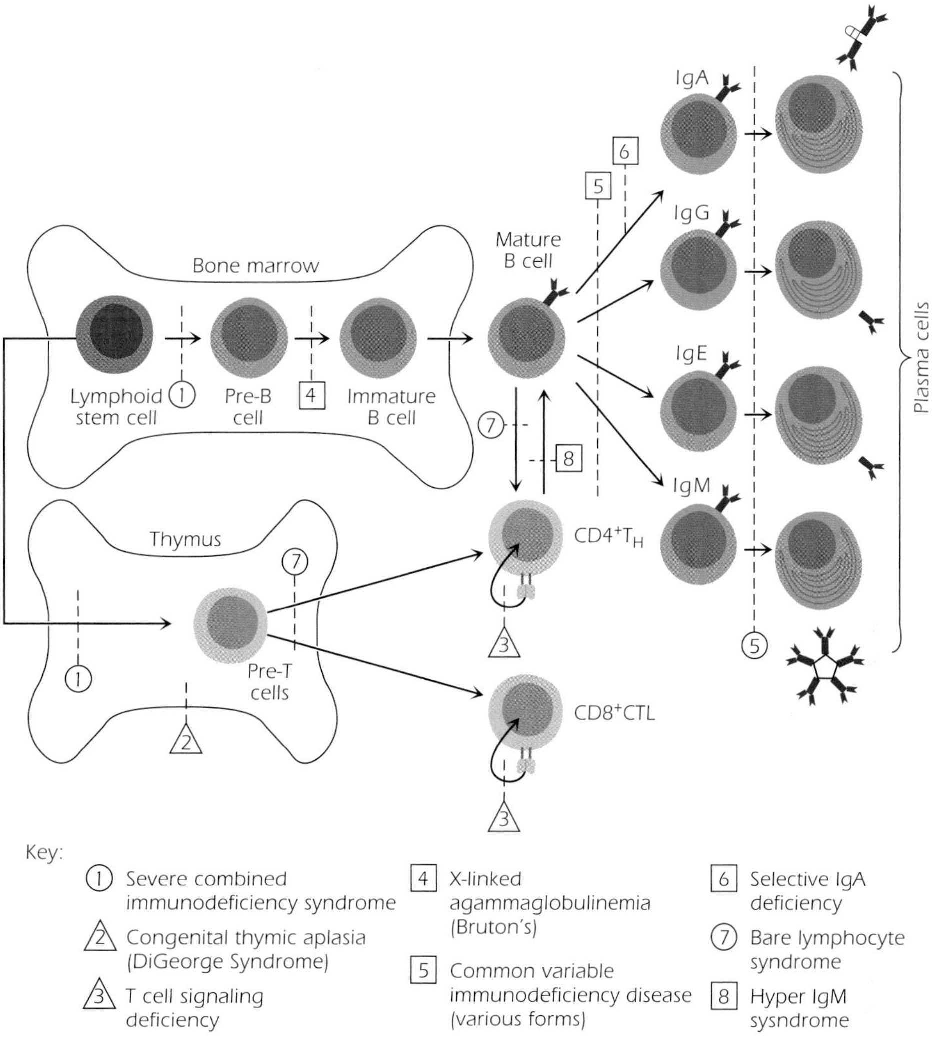

Figure 17.1. Sites of defective lymphopoietic development associated with primary immunodeficiency syndromes. *Circles*, lesions presenting as combined immunodeficiencies; *triangles*, lesion presenting as T cell disorders; *squares*, lesions presenting as *predominantly* B cell or humoral immune deficiencies .

protozoal), most notably CMV, *Pneumocystis carinii, and Candida.* Vaccination with attenuated live virus could prove fatal in such infants.

Patients can be subclassified at initial evaluation according to the lymphocyte subsets present in their blood (Table 17.2). One group designated T^-B^+ has essentially absent T cells and normal or increased numbers of nonfunctioning B cells. This group of patients may also lack NK cells. A second group, T^-B^-, has severe lymphopenia due to the absence of both T and B cells. A few patients are T^+B^+ and rare patients are T^+B^-. The preferred treatment for all SCID patients is a T cell–depleted bone marrow transplant from an HLA-matched sibling donor.

T^-B^+ Subgroup

X-LINKED SCID. Patients with X-linked SCID constitute 40–50% of SCID cases, with the majority showing T^-B^+ lymphopenia. Mutations have been found in the gene located on the X chromosome that codes for the γ-chain that is common to the receptors for the cytokines interleukin 2 (IL-2), IL-4, IL-7, IL-9, and IL-15 (see Chapter 11). Thus the mutation impairs responses to a multitude of cytokines (Fig. 17.2A).

Animal models with targeted defects have proven very instructive in delineating the human deficiencies. In mouse gene knockout models (see Chapter 5), γ-chain knockouts, like SCID patients, have defective development of both T and B cell lineages. IL-7 and IL-7R knockouts also resemble SCID patients, suggesting that IL-7 is crucial for T/NK cell development and that its functions are not compensated for by other cytokines. In contrast, IL-2 knockouts show only some immune dysfunction, with normal T and B cell development and without a SCID phenotype.

AUTOSOMAL RECESSIVE SCID. A small subgroup of patients characterized by T^-B^+ lymphopenia show an autosomal recessive rather than an X-linked pattern of inheritance. These individuals have an identical phenotype to the X-linked SCID group and cannot be distinguished clinically. Mutations are localized in the gene for ***JAK3 tyrosine kinase,*** (Fig. 17.2B) the intracellular molecule responsible for transmitting signals from the γ-chain of the receptors

TABLE 17.2. Severe Combined Immunodeficiency Diseases

Disorder	Underlying Deficiency[a]	Mode of Inheritance[a]
T^-B^+ Subgroup		
X-linked SCID	Mutated γ-chain of cytokine receptors	X-linked
Autosomal recessive SCID	Mutated JAK3 tyrosine kinase	AR
T^-B^- Subgroup		
ADA deficiency	ADA enzyme	AR
PNP deficiency	PNP enzyme	AR
Recombinase deficiency	*RAG* 1 or *RAG* 2 enzyme	AR
T^+B^- Subgroup		
Omenn syndrome	Partial *RAG* deficiency	AR
T^+B^+ Subgroup		
Bare lymphocyte syndrome	MHC class II transcription activator (4 proteins)	AR
ZAP-70 deficiency	Kinase domain of the TCR-associated PTK, ZAP-70	AR
Multisystem Disorders		
Wiskott-Aldrich syndrome	WASP	X-linked
Ataxia telangectasia	ATM protein for DNA repair	AR

[a] *PTK*, protein tyrosine kinase; *AR*, autosomal recessive.

(see Chapter 11). Expression of JAK3 is normally restricted to hematopoietic cells.

T^-B^- Subgroup

Adenosine Deaminase Deficiency. Adenosine deaminase (ADA), an enzyme in the purine salvage pathway, is a ubiquitously expressed housekeeping enzyme (i.e., used in the everyday function of cells.) Individuals lacking this enzyme account for approximately 20% of SCID patients and show an autosomal recessive pattern of inheritance. The deficiency results in buildup of toxic wastes, causing symptom progression over time and making early detection and treatment particularly critical in this group.

ADA deficiency has greatest impact on the immune system, resulting in failure of both T and B lymphocyte development. Many patients have an associated characteristic skeletal abnormality. Why these patients do not have more multisystem problems is not completely understood. Investigation of this rare genetic disease has shown the particular importance of the salvage pathway in lymphocyte development and differentiation and has led to the development of antileukemic drugs to prevent the growth of malignant lymphocyte precursors. ADA-deficient patients lacking a matched sibling marrow donor have been the first group to be treated with gene therapy, by infecting a functional gene for ADA. However, even after years of development, this experimental

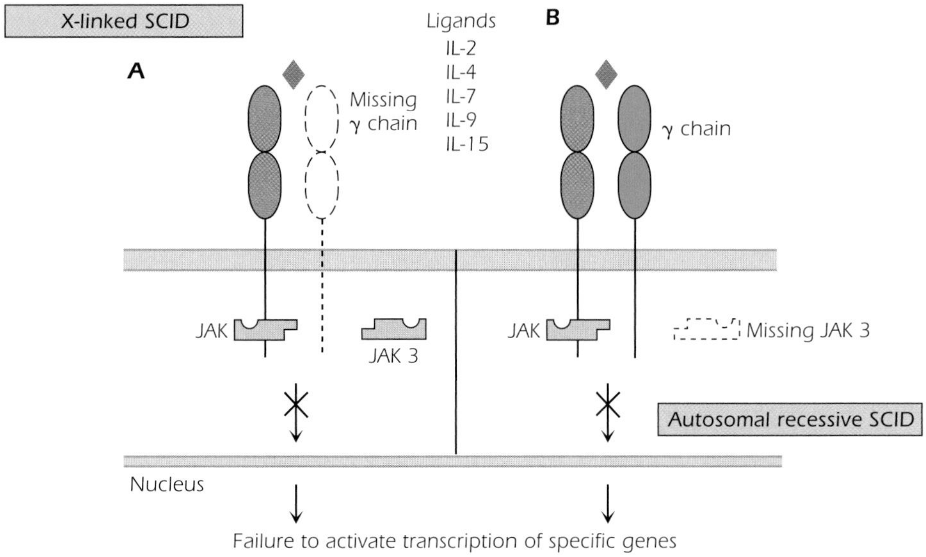

Figure 17.2. **(A)** Cytokine receptors that share the common γ-chain fail to generate intracellular signals following ligand binding when this chain is missing. **(B)** Cytokine receptor signalling mediated by the common γ-chain is defective when JAK3 tyrosine kinase is missing. Both result in SCID.

approach remains fraught with difficulties. Continuous enzyme supplementation is an alternative treatment.

PURINE NUCLEOSIDE PHOSPHORYLASE DEFICIENCY. A mutation in another enzyme in the purine salvage pathway, purine nucleoside phosphorylase (PNP), similarly leads to a buildup of toxic products that are particularly damaging to the neurologic system and T cells. Eventually, all lymphoid tissues—thymus, tonsils, lymph nodes and spleen—are depleted. Paradoxically, even though children with this condition are markedly immunodeficient, autoimmune disease is common in these patients.

RECOMBINASE DEFICIENCIES. Recombination-activating genes *(RAG)* 1 and 2 code for enzymes involved in the rearrangement of the Ig genes in pre-B cells and the T cell receptor genes in pre-T cells (see Chapters 6 and 9). Both enzymes are absolutely required for rearrangement, so mutations in either result in complete absence of T cells, B cells, and Ig. Maturation stops at the pre-T and pre-B cell stages. Typically, NK cell function is intact.

T^+B^- Subgroup

OMENN SYNDROME. Omenn syndrome is a "leaky" SCID with reduced but partial *RAG* activity. A complete understanding of this disease is still lacking. The patients' clinical presentations are similar to individuals with severe graft versus host (GVH) disease (discussed in Chapter 19) rather than to those lacking *RAG* activity. Although severely immunodeficient in that they cannot mount an effective immune response to any pathogen, these patients also demonstrate a dysregulation of the immune system. These patients are $T^+B^-$by peripheral blood analysis and have massive skin and gastrointestinal infiltration by eosinophils and activated T cells, producing T_H2 type cytokines (see Chapters 10 and 11). This results in hyper-IgE syndrome and malnutrition due to protein loss. The success rate of bone marrow transplants in individuals with Omenn syndrome is low compared to other types of SCID patients. The failures are due to graft rejection. Thus, although Omenn syndrome patients are immunodeficient, they still need pretreatment with immunosuppressive therapy.

T^+B^+ Subgroup

BARE LYMPHOCYTE SYNDROME. Bare lymphocyte syndrome (BLS) results from the failure to express HLA (the human MHC) molecules. BLS is divided into three groups, depending on which class of HLA molecules is missing: class I, class II, or both class I and II. Although there are three groups, only those individuals lacking expression of HLA class II molecules, with or without class I expression, consistently show immunodeficiencies. Circulating T and B cell numbers may be normal; however, in the absence of HLA class II molecules, protein antigens cannot be presented to $CD4^+$ T cells (Fig. 17.3). Therefore, collaboration does not occur between antigen-presenting cells (B cells, macrophages/monocytes, dendritic cells) and $CD4^+$ T cells. In consequence, help is not provided to B cells or for the generation of cytotoxic T cells (see Chapter 10). This results in a clinical presentation of combined immunodeficiency. Since MHC class II expression is required on thymic epithelial cells for positive selection of $CD4^+$ T cells, proportionately fewer $CD4^+$ T cells are produced in the thymus (Fig. 17.1, defect 7). Therefore, most patients have a decreased proportion of $CD4^+$to $CD8^+$ T cells, resulting in a reversed CD4:CD8 T cell ratio. The $CD4^+$ T cells present are functional, as demonstrated by their ability to respond when stimulated in vitro. Since GVH disease could occur in these patients, HLA-matched bone marrow donors are required for treatment.

The mutation responsible for BLS is not in the HLA class II genes themselves but in a one of the four genes that codes for regulatory factors required to transcribe the class II

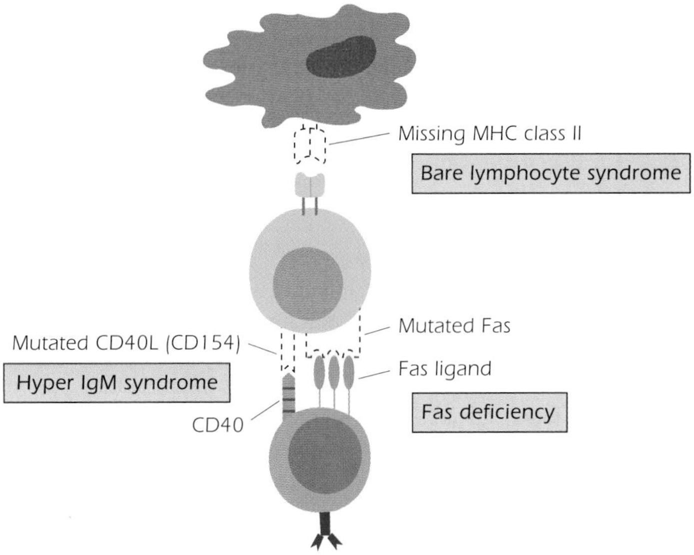

Figure 17.3. Missing cell membrane determinants required for normal T cell–APC interactions result in several primary immunodeficiency syndromes, including bare lymphocyte syndrome, hyper-IgM syndrome and Fas deficiency .

genes. One might speculate that a better understanding of transcription failure in BLS could result in the development of a method to turn off HLA class II expression. This could be applied to prevent graft rejection of transplanted organs (i.e., kidney, liver) in immunocompetent individuals.

Few patients deficient in HLA class I expression have been identified; some were discovered serendipitously. This is undoubtedly due to the fact that not all individuals with deficient HLA class I expression show clinically significant immunodeficiency. As in BLS patients with defective HLA class II expression, patients with HLA class I deficiency do not have a mutation in the HLA class I gene, but rather have a mutated gene for the ***transporter protein*** (TAP). As we described in Chapter 9, the transporter protein transports peptides generated in the cytosol into the endoplasmic reticulum where they interact with and stabilize the structure of the MHC class I molecules. In the absence of the Tap gene product, MHC class I molecule expression on the surface is very low. For reasons that are unclear, when patients with this defect are symptomatic, they have recurrent bacterial pneumonias rather than the expected viral infections.

ZAP-70 MUTATION. Patients with a mutation in the T cell tyrosine kinase ***ZAP-70,*** which transduces the signal transmitted through the T cell receptor, also present with a SCID-like phenotype. This will be described in more detail later in this chapter.

Other Multisystem Disorders. In addition to the combined immunodeficiency diseases we have just discussed, several multisystem inherited disorders result in a SCID-like clinical picture:

WISKOTT-ALDRICH SYNDROME. Wiskott-Aldrich syndrome is an X-linked disease showing a classic triad of symptoms: bleeding diathesis (tendency to bleed) due to thrombocytopenia (low platelet level in blood) and small platelet size, recurrent bacterial infections, and allergic reactions (including eczema, elevated IgE levels, and food allergies). Longer term, patients have increased risk of developing malignancies, particularly of the lymphoid system. The genetic basis of the disease is a mutation in the X-linked gene coding for the Wiskott-Aldrich syndrome protein (***WASP***), which is expressed in all hematopoietic stem cells. Current evidence suggests that WASP interacts with the cytoskeleton and that, in affected cells of patients with this syndrome, the cytoskeleton may not be able to reorganize in response to stimuli.

The immune defects are variable, but both T and B cells are functionally abnormal, with T cell numbers particularly decreased. Characteristically, patients are unable to respond to polysaccharide antigens. Treatment consists of antibiotics and antiviral agents given promptly with each infection. Reconstitution of T and B cells has been reported following bone marrow transplantation. Without treatment, the average life span is approximately 3 years. With extension of survival, the incidence of malignancies would be expected to increase.

ATAXIA TELANGIECTASIA. Ataxia telangiectasia (AT) is another multisystem genetic disorder in which neurologic symptoms (staggering gait or ataxia) and abnormal vascular dilatation (telangiectasia) accompany increased susceptibility to infections; lymphopenia (low lymphocyte numbers in peripheral blood); thymic hypoplasia; and depressed levels of IgA, IgE, and sometimes IgG. The immune defect involves both cellular and humoral (T cell–dependent and T cell–independent) immune responses, severely affecting T-dependent regions of lymphoid tissues. The genetic basis of this syndrome is a mutation in the gene coding for a protein known as ATM, part of a pathway activated when the cell suffers DNA breaks from ionizing radiation and oxidative damage. AT patients have impaired development of their T and B cells. The normal generation of both T and B lineages involves critical phases of extensive cell proliferation, apoptosis, and DNA recombination events, all of which may be dysregulated with a mutated, nonfunctional ATM protein. AT children also have a greatly increased risk of developing malignancy, particularly lymphoid neoplasms. This may be the result of an ATM-dependent defect in DNA repair or cell cycle arrest following chromosomal damage. AT has been grouped with ***Bloom syndrome*** and ***Faconi's anemia,*** both of which show similar variable immune deficiencies and susceptibility to DNA damage.

In summary, the underlying causes resulting in severe defects in both cell-mediated and humoral immunity are varied. They range from mutations in enzymes found in all cells, which should have global effects in the body (deficiencies in ADA and PNP) to mutations involving signaling proteins specifically expressed in T cells (ZAP-70 mutation).

Animal models have been informative, both in understanding the defects observed in human syndromes and in helping delineate steps in normal T and B cell development. The SCID mutant mouse strain, which has a genetic defect in a protein repairing double-stranded DNA breaks, was the first mouse model used for the study of this group of diseases. Since then, knockout mouse models for the majority of these spontaneous human genetic diseases have been produced to aid in their investigation (see Chapter 5). In addition, SCID mice and nude mice (discussed later in this chapter), with diminished ability to reject foreign tissues, can be used as a "living test tube" to study the growth of human hematopoietic stem cells and human tumors.

Immunodeficiency Disorders Associated with T Cells and Cell-Mediated Immunity. As we showed in Table 17.1, patients with T cell–associated deficiency diseases are susceptible to ***viral, fungal,*** and ***protozoal*** infections. Moreover, because T cells are required to help B cells produce antibodies to T-dependent antigens (see Chapter 10), patients with T cell–associated deficiencies also exhibit selective defects in antibody production. Consequently, T cell–deficient patients may be difficult to distinguish clinically from SCID patients.

Congenital Thymic Aplasia (DiGeorge Syndrome). DiGeorge syndrome is a T cell deficiency in which *the thymus, as well as other non-lymphoid organs, develop abnormally.* The syndrome is caused by defective migration of fetal neural crest cells into the third and fourth pharyngeal pouches. This normally takes place during the 12th week of gestation. In DiGeorge syndrome, the heart and face develop abnormally and the thymus and parathyroids fail to form, resulting in ***thymic aplasia*** and ***hypoparathyroidism.*** Thymic aplasia results in an absence of mature T cells and immunodeficiency. The nude mouse is an animal model of DiGeorge syndrome; in these animals, the thymus *and* hair follicles do not develop.

DiGeorge syndrome is not hereditary but occurs sporadically and is generally the result of a deletion in chromosome 22q11. Newborns present with hypocalcemia (low calcium levels), resulting from absence of the parathyroid glands, and congenital cardiac disease. The children suffer from recurrent or chronic infections with viruses, bacteria, fungi, and protozoa. They have either no or very few mature T cells in the periphery (blood, lymph nodes, or spleen) (Fig. 17.1, defect 2). Although B cells, plasma cells, and serum Ig levels may be normal, many patients fail to mount an antibody response after immunization with T-dependent antigens. The lack of helper T cells required for isotype switching results in the absence of IgG and other switched isotypes following immunization. The IgM response to T-independent antigens is intact, however. Since individuals with DiGeorge syndrome lack T cells and fail to generate normal antibody responses, they should never be immunized with live attenuated viral vaccines!

Formerly, children with DiGeorge syndrome were treated with a fetal thymus graft, which resulted in the appearance of host-derived T cells within a week. The fetal thymus used for transplantation needed to be < 14 weeks gestation to avoid GVH reactions, which would occur if mature donor thymocytes were transferred into the immunoincompetent recipient. This donor fetal thymus provided the environment, the thymic epithelial cells, for development of recipient T cells from the patient's normal lymphoid precursors. Although the T cells produced were normal, cell-mediated immunity and help for antibody production were not fully restored. The recipient's T cells learned the MHC of the transplanted thymus as "self" and sometimes collaborated poorly with the body's own antigen-presenting cells (APCs) in the periphery (see Chapters 8 and 9). Since this treatment strategy was not successful, therapy now is mostly in response to symptoms. Some patients have remnants of thymic tissue, allowing delayed though still diminished T cell maturation. The other medical problems associated with the syndrome, such as congenital heart disease, add to the overall poor prognosis.

T-Cell Deficiencies with Normal Peripheral T Cell Numbers. A number of patients have been identified with functional, rather than numerical defects in their T cells. Clinically, they may present with opportunistic infections and a strikingly high incidence of autoimmune disease. Family studies show autosomal recessive patterns of inheritance. Molecular analysis demonstrates that the underlying cause is heterogenous, with deficient expression of ***ZAP-70 tyrosine kinase, CD3ϵ,*** or ***CD3γ*** (Fig. 17.4).

As we described in Chapter 10, ZAP-70 is required for intracellular transduction of the signal after binding to the T cell receptor. For reasons that are not clear, patients defective in ZAP-70 expression present with a SCID-type clinical picture (defective cell-mediated and humoral immunity, as described earlier in the chapter). The absence of T cell activity suggests that ZAP-70 plays a critical role in the function of mature T cells (Fig. 17.1, defect 3), however, the reason for the effect on B cell function is unclear. In addition, although the peripheral blood counts, lymph nodes, and thymus are essentially normal, $CD8^+$ T cells are missing in patients defective in ZAP-70 expression. This suggests that ZAP-70 is also required for $CD8^+$ T cell differentiation in the thymus.

Mutations in the CD3 chains are quite rare and only a handful of patients with such defects have been described.

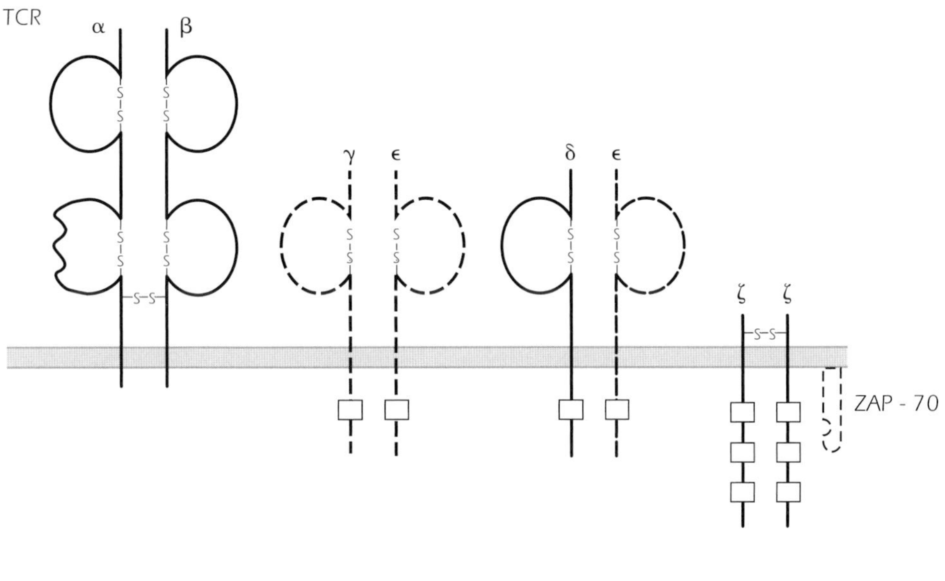

Figure 17.4. Deficiencies of molecules involved in T cell signaling through the antigen-specific receptor (the T cell receptor).

Animal models confirm that all the CD3 peptide chains are required for normal signaling through the T cell receptor. It is not clear, however, that these mice accurately mimic the few patients reported.

Autoimmune Lymphoproliferative Syndrome. Autoimmune lymphoproliferative syndrome (ALPS) is an inherited disease characterized by massive proliferation of lymphoid tissue with early lymphoma development. It may be considered an autoimmune disease since this genetic defect results in systemic autoimmune phenomena and susceptibility to only chronic viral infections. Patients have an increased number of double negative ($CD4^-CD8^-$) T cells and may eventually develop B cell lymphomas. Most ALPS patients have a mutation in the gene coding for the ***Fas protein*** (CD95) (Fig. 17.3). Signaling through this protein normally activates ***apoptosis,*** or programmed cell death (see Chapters 10 and 12). Without activation of apoptosis, cells that should have died live, and immune responses that should have been turned off continue. Most ALPS patients have one normal and one mutated Fas molecule. This suggests that the mutated Fas molecule somehow interferes with the function of the normal molecule. Some ALPS patients have defects in other components of the apoptosis pathway, such as Fas ligand or caspase 10.

Two mouse strains—*lpr* and *gld*—have a phenotype similar to ALPS patients. *lpr* mice have a mutation in their Fas gene and *gld* mice have a mutation in their Fas ligand gene. For many years, *lpr* mice were studied as a model for autoimmune disease, specifically systemic lupus erythematosus (SLE), before their Fas gene defect was discovered.

Chronic Mucocutaneous Candidiasis. Chronic mucocutaneous candidiasis is a poorly defined collection of syndromes characterized by *Candida* infections of skin and mucous membranes. This fungal organism is normally present but nonpathogenic. Patients usually have normal T cell–mediated immunity to microorganisms other than *Candida* and normal B cell–mediated immunity (antibody production) to all microorganisms, including *Candida*. Thus they have only a *selective defect in the functioning of T cells.* This disorder affects both males and females, particularly children, and there is some evidence that it may be inherited.

B Cell–or Immunoglobulin-Associated Immunodeficiency Disorders. B cell– or immunoglobulin-associated immune diseases range from those having defective B cell development with complete absence of all Ig classes to those associated with deficiencies in a single class or subclass of Ig. Patients suffer from recurrent or chronic infections that may start in infancy (Bruton's agammaglobulinemia) or in young adulthood. Evaluation includes analysis of B cell number and function and immunoelectrophoretic and quantitative determinations of Ig class and subclass.

X-Linked Infantile Agammaglobulinemia. First described in 1952 by Bruton, X-Linked Infantile Agammaglobulinemia (XLA) is also called ***Bruton's agammaglobulinemia.*** The disorder is relatively rare (1 in 100,000). It is first noticed at 5–6 months of age, when the infant has lost the maternally derived IgG that had passed through the placenta. At that age, the infant presents with serious and repeated bacterial infections as a result of severe depression or virtual *absence of all Ig classes.*

The major defect lies in the inability of pre-B cells, which are present at normal levels, to develop into mature B cells. The ***BTK gene,*** which is mutated in XLA, normally codes for a tyrosine kinase enzyme residing in the cytosol. *BTK* seems to be essential for signal transduction from the pre-B cell receptor on developing B cells. Without this signal, the cell develops no further (Fig. 17.1, defect 4). All mature B cells from female carriers of the mutant gene have only the nonmutated X chromosome active. XLA is, therefore, one of several inherited immunodeficiency diseases described in which a mutation in a cytoplasmic tyrosine kinase is responsible. The JAK3 form of SCID and the ZAP-70 form of T cell deficiency were described above.

Analysis of the blood, bone marrow, spleen, and lymph nodes of XLA patients reveals near *absence of mature B cells and plasma cells,* explaining the depressed Ig levels. Characteristically, the children have markedly underdeveloped tonsils. The limited number of B cells generated appear normal in their ability to become plasma cells. Infants with XLA have recurrent bacterial otitis media, bronchitis, septicemia, pneumonia, arthritis, meningitis, and dermatitis. The most common microorganisms found are *Hemophilus influenzae* and *Streptococcus pneumoniae*. Frequently, patients also suffer from malabsorption due to infestation of the gastrointestinal tract with *Giardia lamblia*. Unexpectedly, they are also susceptible to infection by viruses which enter through the gastrointestinal tract—for example, echovirus and polio. The infections do not respond well to antibiotics alone. Treatment, therefore, consists of periodic injections of ***intravenous gamma globulin*** (*IVGG*) containing large amounts of IgG (discussed further in Chapter 21). Although this passive immunization has maintained some patients for 20–30 years, the prognosis is guarded, as chronic lung disease due to repeated infections often supervenes.

Transient Hypogammaglobulinemia. At 5–6 months of age, passively transferred maternal IgG disappears and production by the infant begins to rise. Premature infants may have transient IgG deficiency if they are not yet able to synthesize Igs. Occasionally, a full-term infant may also fail to produce appropriate amounts of IgG, even when levels of IgM or IgA are normal. This appears to be due to a deficiency in number and function of helper T cells. Transient hypogammaglobulinemia may persist for a few months to as long as 2 years. It is not sex linked and can be distinguished from the X-linked disease by the presence of normal numbers of B cells in the blood. Although treatment is usually not necessary, infants need to be identified since immunizations should not be given during this period.

Common Variable Immunodeficiency Disease. Patients with common variable immunodeficiency disease (CVID) have markedly decreased serum IgG and IgA levels, with normal or low IgM and normal or low peripheral B cell numbers. The cause of the disease, which affects both males and females, is not entirely clear and is probably not uniform. Onset may occur at any age, with two peaks at 1–5 years and at 15–20 years. Affected individuals suffer from recurrent respiratory and gastrointestinal infections with ***pyogenic bacteria*** and ***autoimmune diseases,*** such as hemolytic anemia, thrombocytopenia, and SLE, that are associated with autoantibodies. Many also have disorders of cell-mediated immunity. Long term, these patients have a high incidence of ***cancer,*** particularly lymphomas and gastric cancers.

CVID is characterized by a *failure of maturation of B cells into antibody-secreting cells* (Fig. 17.1, defect 5). This defect may be due to an inability of the B cells to proliferate in response to antigen, normal proliferation of B cells without secretion of IgM, secretion of IgM without class switching to IgG or IgA (due to an intrinsic B cell or T cell abnormality), or failure of glycosylation of IgG heavy chains. In most cases, the disorder appears to be the result of diminished synthesis and secretion of Igs. The disease is familial or sporadic, with unknown environmental influences triggering onset.

Treatment depends on severity. For severe disease, with many recurrent or chronic infections, IVGG therapy is indicated. Treated patients can have a normal life span. Women with CVID have normal pregnancies but, of course, do not transfer maternal IgG to the fetus.

Selective Immunoglobulin Deficiencies

Several syndromes are associated with selective deficiency of a single class or subclass of Igs. Some are accompanied by compensatory elevated levels of other isotypes, as exemplified by increased IgM levels in cases of IgG or IgA deficiency.

IgA deficiency is the most common immunodeficiency disorder in the Western world, with an incidence of approximately 1 in 800 (Fig. 17.1, defect 6). The cause is unknown but appears to be associated with decreased release of IgA by B lymphocytes. IgA deficiency can also occur transiently as an adverse reaction to drugs. Patients may suffer from recurrent sinopulmonary viral or bacterial infections, celiac disease (defective absorption in the bowel), or may be entirely asymptomatic.

Treatment of symptomatic patients consists of broad-spectrum antibiotics. Therapy with immune serum globulin is not useful because commercial preparations contain only low levels of IgA, and because *injected* IgA does not reach the areas of the secretory immune system, where it is normally the protective antibody. Furthermore, patients may mount antibody responses (usually IgG or IgE) to IgA in the transferred immune serum, causing hypersensitivity reactions. In general however, the prognosis for selective IgA deficiency is good, with many patients surviving normally.

There are selective deficiencies in other Ig isotypes. An example is ***IgM deficiency,*** a rare disorder, in which patients suffer from recurrent and severe infections with polysaccharide-encapsulated organisms, such as pneumococci and *Haemophilus influenzae.* Selective deficiencies in subclasses of IgG have been described but are extremely rare.

Disorders of T–B Interactions. There are at least two diseases in which the T and B lineages appear to mature normally but interactions between the lineages are abnormal. Although both are due to underlying T cell abnormalities, the predominant clinical symptoms are in the B cell or humoral immune response. These diseases are hyper-IgM syndrome and X-linked lymphoproliferative disease.

Hyper-IgM Syndrome. Patients with X-linked hyper-IgM syndrome (XHIM) present with recurrent respiratory infections at 1–2 years of age and very low serum IgG, IgA, and IgE with normal to elevated IgM (Fig. 17.1, defect 8). Their B cells, which are normal in number, are functional in vitro and will isotype switch when appropriately stimulated. Their T cells are also normal in number, subset distribution, and proliferative responses to mitogens. A mutation in the ***CD40L gene*** on the X chromosome results in the absence of CD40 ligand (CD154) on T_H cells (Fig. 17.3). CD40L binds to CD40 expressed on B cells (see Chapter 10). This interaction rescues the B cell from apoptosis and appears important, if not necessary, for isotype switching. In XHIM, recruitment of B cells into follicles also does not occur, resulting in lack of germinal center formation. Boys with this condition also have subtle changes in T cell function and a partial block in neutrophil differentiation and macrophage activation. This may explain their propensity for opportunistic infections, particularly *Pneumocystis carinii* pneumonia (PCP) and their poorer prognosis than XLA patients.

A second group of patients, with similar presentations to XHIM but with an autosomal recessive pattern of inheritance, may have a B cell defect, possibly in CD40. A third group, which has a defect in the interaction of CD40 with a modulator of the transcription factor NF-κB (see Chapter 10), has an X-linked mode of inheritance. As is common in genetic disorders involving such intracellular regulatory molecules, these children also show abnormalities in non-immune system cells, reflecting the use of these molecules in multiple cell types.

X-Linked Lymphoproliferative Disease (Duncan Syndrome) X-linked lymphoproliferative (XLP) disease was originally observed in six maternally related males of the Duncan family, thus its common name. An inability of T cells to regulate B cell growth is considered to be a major part of the underlying defect in this rare disease. Before exposure to ***Epstein-Barr virus*** (EBV), patients are clinically healthy with normal T and B cell numbers. Exposure to EBV, however, results in a severe course of infectious mononucleosis, which may be fatal. Development of malignant lymphoma or dysgammaglobulinemia frequently follows survival from infection. Lymphoma and Ig deficiency may also occur without prior exposure to EBV. The lymphomas are predominantly aggressive B cell lymphomas at extranodal sites, particularly the gastrointestinal tract. Burkitt's lymphoma (described later in the chapter) is the most frequent type. Although the pattern of lymphomas is similar to those in other patients with poorly controlled EBV-induced B cell proliferations due to T cell defects (such as in AIDS or immunosuppressed transplant patients), the lymphoma incidence is much greater in XLP. Prognosis is extremely poor.

Phagocytic Dysfunctions. Phagocytic cells—polymorphonuclear leukocytes and macrophages/monocytes—play a critical role in both innate and acquired immunity to pathogens, acting either alone or in concert with lymphocytes. Inherited deficiencies in phagocytic cells have helped identify many of the molecules required in each step of the phagocyte's action that are required to eliminate the pathogens. These steps and the associated deficiencies are migration and adhesion of phagocytic cells (leukocyte adhesion deficiency), phagocytosis and lysosomal fusion (Chédiak-Higashi syndrome), and respiratory burst for killing (chronic granulomatous disease) (Fig. 17.5). Phagocytic dysfunction may be secondary, caused by ***extrinsic factors,*** such as drugs and systemic diseases (e.g., diabetes mellitus) or by defects in other arms of the immune system.

Leukocyte Adhesion Deficiency. As discussed in Chapter 11, for leukocytes to arrive at sites of infection in tissues, they must first leave the bloodstream. This is accomplished in a series of steps; initially, by the cell's slow rolling along the endothelium through the interaction of ***selectins*** on endothelium and ***selectin ligands*** on leukocytes (see Fig. 11.2). Chemoattractants then cause the cell to stop rolling. The cell adheres more firmly, followed by transendothelial migration. These latter steps involve the interaction of ***integrins*** on leukocytes and their ligands on endothelial cells.

Leukocyte adhesion deficiency (LAD) is a group of disorders in which leukocyte interaction with vascular endothelium is disrupted (Fig. 17.5A). ***LAD I*** is an autosomal recessive disease mapping to chromosome 21. Patients have a defect in the β-subunit of integrin molecules, preventing their expression. The β-subunit is common to three integrins found on granulocytes, monocytes, and lymphocytes; LFA-1 (CD11a/CD18), Mac-1 (CD11b/CD18) and p150,95 (CD11c/CD18). As a result, adhesion and migration of all white blood cells (WBCs) are impaired. LAD I individuals suffer from recurrent soft tissue bacterial infections and have increased WBC counts but without pus formation or effective wound healing. As expected, lymphocyte function is also affected due to the lack of LFA-1 expression. Newborns with LAD I have a characteristically delayed separation of their umbilical cord.

LAD II individuals have a defect in selectin ligands, so cells from these patients cannot roll along the endothelial surface, a preliminary step for migration (Fig. 17.5A). The

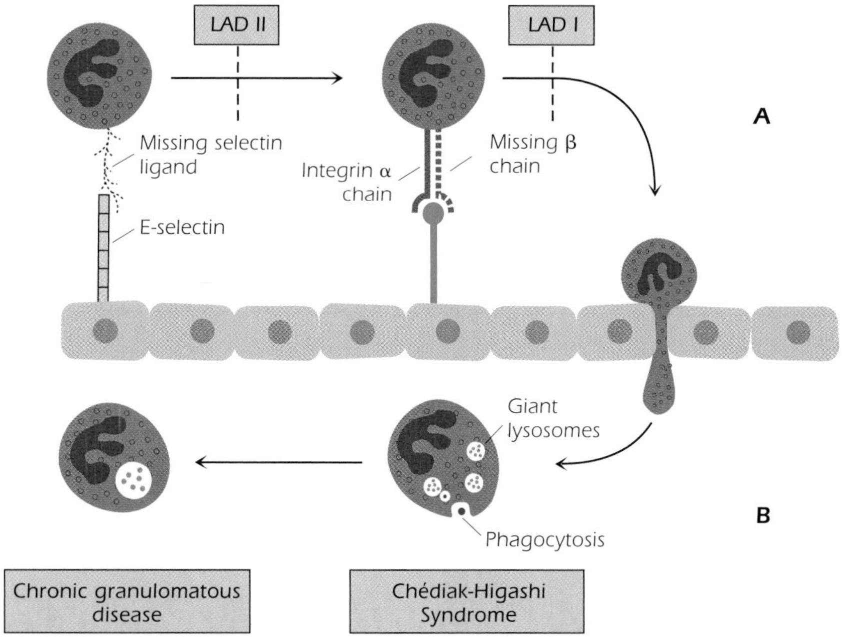

Figure 17.5. **(A)** Defects in cell adhesion disrupt the ability of leukocytes to interact with vascular endothelium, causing impairment of migration of these cells from the blood to sites of infection. **(B)** Impairments in mechanisms required for phagocytosis result in defective intracellular killing of microorganisms.

underlying defect in LAD II is in fucose metabolism, which results in the absence of fucosylated ligands for selectins to bind to. Although the immunodeficiency symptoms are milder, the defect in fucose metabolism results in other developmental abnormalities. As in LAD I, there is little or no pus formation, and the children do not show classical clinical signs of severe infection.

Chédiak-Higashi Syndrome. Chédiak-Higashi syndrome is an autosomal recessive disease characterized by abnormal giant granules and organelles in the cells (Fig. 17.5B). Lysosomes and melanosomes are particularly affected, resulting in defects in pigmentation and neutrophil, NK cell, and platelet function and in neurologic abnormalities. Neutrophils show diminished intracellular killing of organisms, the result of both defective degranulation and impaired fusion of lysosomes with phagosomes. With time, patients develop massive infiltrates of lymphocytes and macrophages in the liver, spleen, and lymph nodes. Pyogenic organisms such as *Streptococcus* and *Staphylococcus* cause recurrent, sometimes fatal infection. Prognosis is poor.

Chronic Granulomatous Disease. In chronic granulomatous disease (CGD), the final step in killing of ingested organisms is defective (Fig. 17.5B) and the continued intracellular survival of the organisms results in granuloma formation. In normal individuals, activated neutrophils and mononuclear phagocytes kill organisms via the ***respiratory burst,*** which consumes oxygen and generates hydrogen peroxide and free superoxide radicals. Mutations in any of the subunits of the enzyme that catalyzes the burst—NADPH oxidase—can result in CGD. The most common form of CGD is due to a mutation in one of the membrane-bound subunits, $gp91^{phox}$, which is coded for by the *CYBB* gene located on the X chromosome. Thus the majority of patients show an X-linked recessive pattern of inheritance. The other subunits of NADPH oxidase are coded for by autosomal genes. CGD patients with mutations in these other subunits show autosomal recessive inheritance. Mostly, these patients have mutations in one of the two cytosolic subunits of the enzyme, $p47^{phox}$ or $p67^{phox}$.

Symptoms appear during the first 2 years of life. Patients have enhanced susceptibility to infection with organisms that are normally of low virulence, such as *Staphylococcus aureus, Serratia marcescens,* and *Aspergillus*. Associated abnormalities include lymphadenopathy (increase in lymph node size) and hepatosplenomegaly (increase in liver and spleen size) due to the chronic and acute infections. Treatment consists of aggressive immunization and therapy with wide-spectrum antibiotics, antifungal agents, and interferon-γ.

In addition to CGD, disorders with reduced or absent levels of phagocyte-associated enzymes, including ***glucose-6-phosphate dehydrogenase, myeloperoxidase,*** and ***alkaline phosphatase,*** result in decreased intracellular killing of organisms.

Interferon-γ Receptor Deficiency. A mutation in the *IFNγR1* gene results in an inability of monocytes to respond to interferon-γ (IFNγ) with secretion of tumor necrosis factor-α (TNFα). Patients with this mutation are selectively susceptible to weakly pathogenic mycobacteria, demonstrating the importance of IFNγ in controlling mycobacterial infections. This also suggests that other effects of IFNγ in these individuals are compensated for. Immunization with live bacillus Calmette-Guérin (BCG), common in some parts of the world, is dangerous for patients with this defect.

Natural-Killer Cell Deficiency. Very little is known about natural-killer (NK) cell deficiency in humans, and only a few such cases have been reported. Animal studies suggest that NK cell deficiency impairs allograft rejection and is linked to higher susceptibility to viral diseases and increased metastases from tumors. NK cell defects are seen in severe combined immunodeficiency disorders, in some T and phagocytic cell disorders, and in X-linked lymphoproliferative syndrome.

Diseases Caused by Abnormalities in the Complement System. As we described in Chapter 13, complement is important in the ***opsonization*** and ***killing*** of bacteria and altered cells, in ***chemotaxis,*** and in ***B cell activation***. Complement components also participate in the elimination of antigen–antibody complexes, preventing ***immune complex deposition*** and subsequent disease. Deficiencies in complement are inherited as autosomal traits, with heterozygous individuals having half the normal level of a given component. For most components, this is sufficient to prevent clinical disease. The half-life of activated complement components is also normally carefully controlled by inhibitors, which break down the products or dissociate the complexes.

Deficiencies of Early Complement Components. The early components of complement are particularly important in generating the opsonin C3b (Fig. 17.6). Patients with ***deficiencies of C1, 4, or 2 from the classical pathway*** or with ***C3 deficiency*** itself have increased infections with encapsulated organisms (*Streptococcus pneumoniae, Streptococcus pyogenes, Haemophilus influenza*) and increased rheumatic diseases due to improper clearance of immune complexes as a consequence of low C3b generation. Often the autoimmune disease is most striking. In fact, SLE is the most common presenting symptom of some complement deficiencies. SLE in these individuals is of earlier onset and more severe than without this association and can occur in the absence of antibodies that are frequently found in other cases of SLE (see Chapter 12). Deficiencies of the mannose-binding lectin, which binds to the surface of microbes without antibody and activates the classical pathway, also results in risk of bacterial infections and lupus-like symptoms. Since all the complement activation pathways—classical,

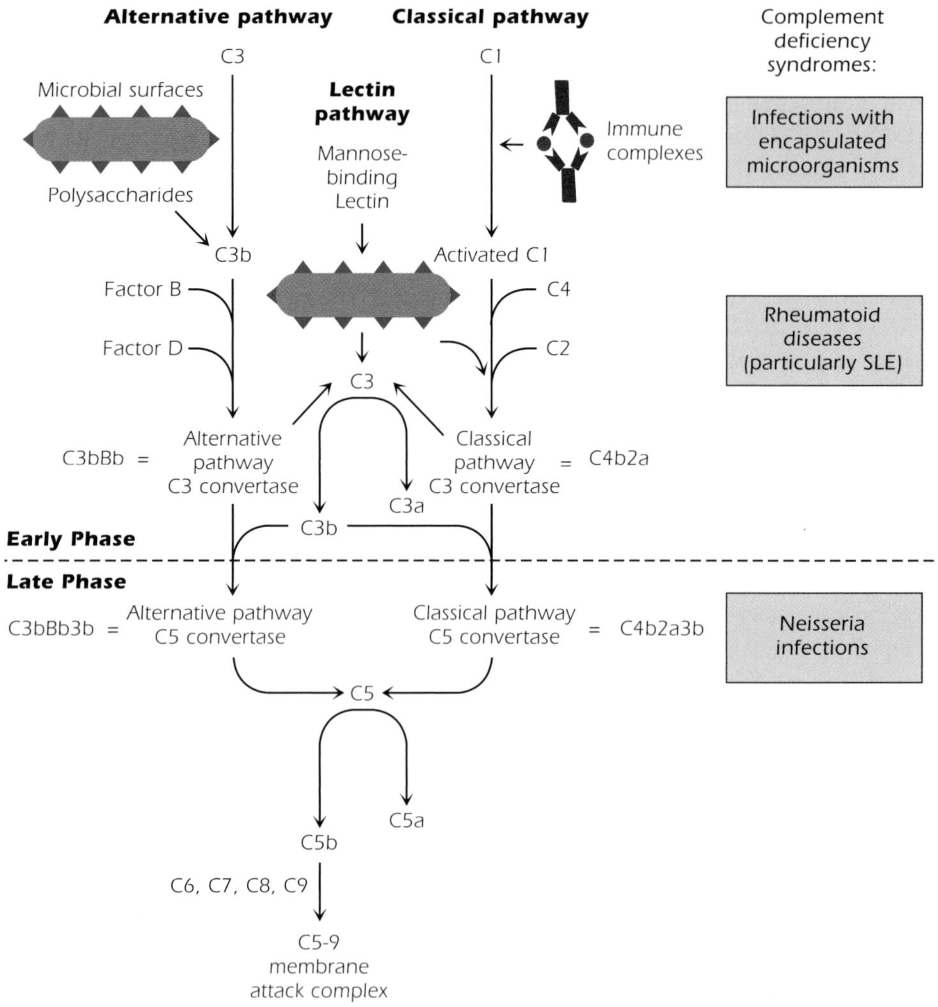

Figure 17.6. Complement cascade showing that deficiencies in early-phase complement components predispose individuals to infections caused by encapsulated microorganisms and rheumatoid syndromes. Late-phase complement deficiencies are associated with *Neisseria* infections.

mannose-binding lectin, and alternative—require C3 activation, deficiencies of C3 itself are associated with the most severe symptoms, particularly infectious complications.

Deficiencies of Late Complement Components.

Deficiencies of the later complement components, **C5–C9**, interfere with the generation of the ***membrane attack complex*** (MAC). The MAC is directly lytic and the primary defense against gram-negative bacteria, particularly *Neisseria meningitidis* (Fig. 17.6).

Defective Control of Complement Components

HEREDITARY ANGIOEDEMA. In hereditary angioedema, patients lack a functional ***C1 esterase inhibitor.*** Without this inhibitor, the action of C1 on C4, C2, and the kallikrein system is uncontrolled, generating large amounts of vasoactive peptides. These peptides cause increased blood vessel permeability. Patients suffer from localized edema, which is life-threatening when it occurs in the larynx, obstructing the airway passage. Treatment includes avoidance of precipitating factors, usually trauma, and infusion of C1 esterase inhibitor.

GLYCOSYL PHOSPHATIDYL INOSITOL PROTEIN DEFICIENCIES. A family of proteins with glycosyl phosphatidyl inositol (GPI) anchors is expressed on the membranes of red blood cells (RBCs), lymphocytes, granulocytes, endothelial cells (blood vessel lining cells) and epithelial cells. These proteins, which include ***decay-accelerating factor*** (DAF, or CD55) and ***CD59,*** protect the cells against spontaneous lysis by complement (see Fig. 13.4). In the absence of these cell surface inhibitors, granulocytes, platelets and, particularly RBCs are susceptible to spontaneous lysis by complement. Rare families exist with inherited mutations in DAF, CD59, or all the GPI proteins. The patients show symptoms of severe anemia, thrombotic events, and chronic infections.

An acquired form of the disease, called ***paroxysmal nocturnal hemoglobinuria*** (PNH), is more common. In PNH, patients have a deficiency in an enzyme required for the production of all the GPI anchored proteins. This is due to an acquired somatic mutation in an early myeloid stem cell. The three nonlymphoid lineages—granulocytes, platelets, and erythrocytes—are affected. In many patients, the stem cells with this mutation eventually acquire additional mutations, dominate the normal cells in the bone marrow, and stop maturing, resulting in acute myelogenous leukemia. During the chronic course of PNH, intravascular hemolysis occurs, more prominently in the kidneys at night where the acidic environment activates the alternative complement pathway. This clinical presentation is reflected in its name, paroxysmal nocturnal hemoglobinuria.

Secondary Immunodeficiency Diseases

Secondary immune deficiency diseases are the consequence of other diseases. By far the most common cause of immunodeficiency disorders worldwide is malnutrition. In developed countries, immunodeficiency is more often iatrogenic—that is, inadvertently caused by medical treatment, particularly from using ***chemotherapeutic agents*** in cancer therapy or deliberate ***immunosuppression*** in cases of organ transplantation or autoimmune disease. Secondary immunodeficiencies are also seen in untreated autoimmunity and with overwhelming infections by bacteria. Malignancies of the immune system also frequently suppress the nonmalignant components, resulting in increased susceptibility of these patients to infection.

ACQUIRED IMMUNODEFICIENCY SYNDROME (AIDS)

Initial Description and Epidemiology

In 1981 several cases of an unusual *Pneumocystis carinii pneumonia (PCP)* were reported in homosexual males in California. This was followed by the recognition of an aggressive form of Kaposi's sarcoma in a similar population in New York City. Since those first recognized cases of AIDS until today, >20 million people have died worldwide and >40 million are currently infected.

AIDS is caused by infection with the human immunodeficiency virus (HIV). The virus is transferred through blood and body fluids. Blood, semen, vaginal secretions, breast milk, and (to a small extent) saliva of an infected individual contain free virus or cells harboring virus. Thus HIV can be transmitted through sexual contact, sharing of needles, transfusion of blood or blood products, placental transfer, passage through the birth canal, and breast feeding.

Although first recognized in sexually active homosexual males in large U.S. cities, the infection and the disease have no sexual preference. Worldwide, heterosexual transmission is most common. In the United States, although homosexual males and intravenous drug abusers still constitute the major infected groups, the greatest increase in rate of AIDS incidence is in heterosexual women and minorities, African-Americans and Hispanics. Transmission of the virus through transfusion of blood and blood products has been virtually eliminated in the United States through screening of donors, testing of collected blood units, and heat inactivation of clotting factor concentrates. A dangerous "window period" still exists in which infection of blood units cannot be detected. The reasons for this will become clear later. Transmission from mother to infant, which accounts for >80% of the pediatric cases, can be greatly diminished by antiviral therapy of the mother and avoidance of vaginal childbirth and breast feeding. These positive statements exist almost as a footnote, however, to an epidemic that continues to spread worldwide without signs of abating, particularly in Africa and Southeast Asia.

Human Immunodeficiency Virus

HIV is an enveloped human retrovirus of the lentivirus family. Two strains of HIV have been described, HIV-1 and HIV-2, the latter found mostly in West Africa. HIV-1 is the more virulent strain. The viral particle contains two identical single strands of genomic RNA and three enzymes: ***integrase, protease,*** and ***reverse transcriptase*** (Fig. 17.7). These are packaged in the ***p24*** and ***p7/9*** capsid proteins and surrounded by the ***p17*** matrix protein. The viral envelope, which is derived from the host cell membrane, displays viral glycoproteins including ***gp120*** and ***gp41,*** which are critical for infection. Gp120 is noncovalently bound to gp41, which is a transmembrane protein. Gp120 has high affinity for CD4. All cells expressing CD4 are potential targets for the virus; in the human, these include macrophages, monocytes, and dendritic cells as well as $CD4^+$ T cells.

After binding to CD4, gp120 undergoes a conformational change and must then also bind a second molecule, a ***coreceptor,*** on the surface of the target cell for HIV to enter the cell. Several ***chemokine receptors*** (see Chapter 11) have been identified that act as coreceptors for HIV. The particular coreceptor used by the virus depends on the variant of the gp120 molecule expressed on its surface. Variation in gp120, therefore, determines what is referred to as the ***tropism*** of the virus, dictating which $CD4^+$ target cell can be infected by that viral particle. ***Macrophage tropic HIV*** uses the chemokine receptor CCR5, and requires only a low level of CD4 expression on the host cell. CCR5 is expressed by macrophages and dendritic cells—both expressing low levels of surface CD4—and $CD4^+$ T cells. ***Lymphotropic HIV*** uses the chemokine receptor CXCR4 expressed on T cells and requires a high density of CD4 on the cell surface. HIV variants using CCR5 are now termed R5, those using CXCR4 are termed X4; variants able to bind both chemokine co-receptors are referred to as R5X4. Both coreceptors are G-coupled proteins with seven transmembrane spanning domains. CCR5 normally binds the chemokines RANTES, macrophage inflammatory protein 1α (MIP-1α), and MIP-1β. CXCR4 binds stromal-derived factor 1.

CCR5 is thought to be the major coreceptor for establishing primary infection, since individuals with mutations in CCR5 appear to be at least partially protected. If an individual is first infected with a macrophage tropic variant via sexual contact, viral infection can be established in the macrophage

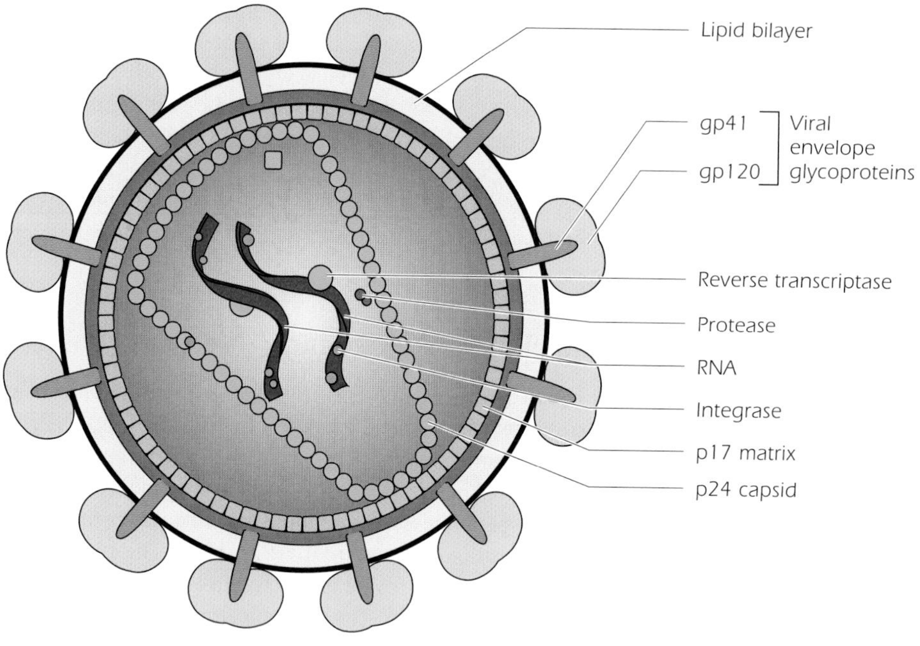

Figure 17.7. Structure of HIV-1 showing two identical RNA strands (the viral genome) and associated enzymes, including reverse transcriptase, integrase, and protease, packaged in a cone-shaped core composed of p24 capsid protein with surrounding p18 protein matrix, all surrounded by a phospholipid membrane envelope derived from the host cell. Virally encoded membrane proteins (gp41 and gp120) are bound to the envelope.

and dendritic cells of the mucosal-associated lymphoid tissue. These infected cells will then provide a ***reservoir*** of virus, since they are not killed by the infection and are capable of migrating throughout the body. Exposure to antigen promotes viral replication in the macrophages in particular, a switch to the lymphotropic form, and further rapid dissemination in the body. Thus the tropism of the virus produced within the infected individual changes over time. This evolution is due to mutations in the gp120 gene, resulting in alterations in its amino acid sequence.

Following binding of gp120 to CD4 and its coreceptor, gp41 penetrates the cell membrane, allowing fusion of the viral envelope with the cell membrane and subsequent viral entry. In the host cell, viral RNA is replicated to a complementary DNA (cDNA) copy by the viral enzyme reverse transcriptase. The cDNA may remain in the cytoplasm or may enter the nucleus where it is integrated into the host genome as a provirus with the help of the viral enzyme integrase. Viral replication continues at a low level, sometimes for several years, so that HIV infection remains in a relatively, but not truly, latent phase.

The HIV genome has a long terminal repeat (LTR) region at each end (Fig. 17.8). The LTR region is required for viral integration and has binding sites for regulatory proteins. When the T cell is activated by antigen, a cascade of reactions leads to activation of the transcription factor NF-κB. NF-κB binds to a promoter region in the LTR area, activating transcription of the provirus by host RNA polymerase.

Transcription of the provirus produces a long mRNA transcript that is spliced at alternative sites for the synthesis of different proteins. The first two proteins made are ***Tat*** and ***Rev.*** Tat enters the nucleus, where it acts as a transcription factor. It binds to the LTR region and increases the rate of viral transcription. Rev also acts in the nucleus, binding to the Rev responsive element in the viral mRNA transcript. Rev binding increases the RNA transport rate to the cytoplasm. When the

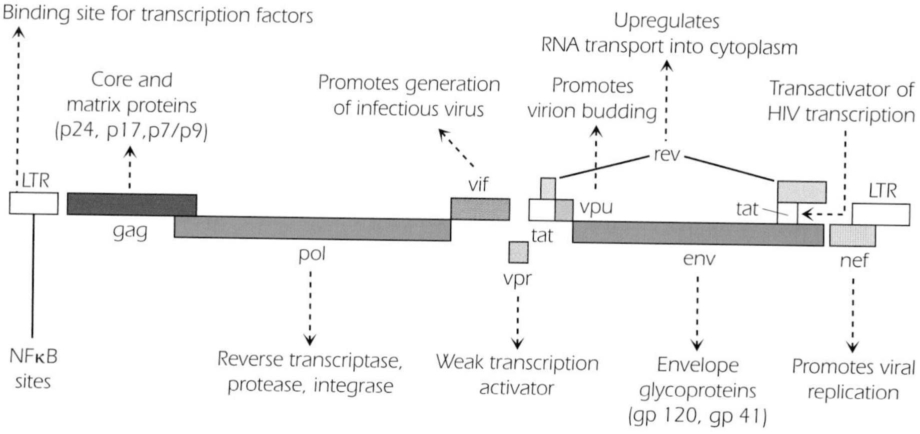

Figure 17.8. The genes and proteins of HIV-1. The HIV-1 RNA genome is flanked by LTR regions required for viral integration and regulation of the viral genome. Several viral genes overlap, resulting in different reading frames, thus allowing the virus to encode many proteins in a small genome. The functions of the gene products are also shown.

mRNA is transported more rapidly into the cytoplasm, less splicing occurs in the nucleus and different proteins can then be made from these mRNA forms. In this second wave of viral protein synthesis, structural components of the viral core and envelope are produced in precursor form. In the third wave, unspliced RNA is transported to the cytoplasm and serves as the RNA for the new viral particles and for the translation of *gag* and *pol*. *Gag* codes for p24, p17, and p7/p9. *Pol* codes for the viral protease, reverse transcriptase, and integrase. The protease cleaves the product of the *env* gene to produce gp120 and gp41.

Release of virus from $CD4^+$ T cells frequently results in lysis of the cell. Macrophages and dendritic cells are generally not killed by HIV but serve as a reservoir, transporting virus to other parts of the body (lymphoid tissue and central nervous system) and producing a small number of particles without cytopathic consequences. Dendritic cells carry the virus mostly on their surface, whereas the macrophages allow a constant low level of viral production. The stimulation of infected macrophages and T cells by cytokines or antigen results in increased viral replication and the productive phase.

Clinical Course

The clinical course can be divided into three phases.

Acute Infection. Upon initial infection with HIV, many patients are asymptomatic. Others show a flu-like illness, characterized by fever, sore throat, and general malaise starting 2–4 weeks after infection and lasting 1–2 weeks. During this time, there is a viremia (virus in peripheral blood) and a precipitous drop in the number of circulating $CD4^+$ T cells. The immune system responds by generating cytotoxic T cells (CTLs) and antibodies specific for the virus. The CTLs are partially responsible for the drop in $CD4^+$ T cells, killing virally infected cells. At this point, the patient has ***seroconverted,*** expressing detectable antibody specific for HIV proteins. The number of $CD4^+$T cells in the peripheral blood then partially recovers. Infected macrophages and dendritic cells disseminate the virus to lymphoid tissue throughout the body.

Chronic Latent Phase. Although the immune response seems standard for a viral infection, it merely contains rather than eradicates the virus. The extremely high rate of mutations of the virus may explain the ineffectiveness of the immune response. A "latent" phase is established, which may last as long as 15 years. During this relatively asymptomatic period, a low level of viral replication continues associated with a gradual decline in $CD4^+$ T cell number. HIV, therefore, never has a true latent phase. In contrast to what might be expected, the number of virus-infected T cells in the peripheral blood is extremely low. Lymph nodes are the predominant location of infected cells. As we described above, macrophages act as a reservoir. Follicular dendritic cells of the germinal center (see Chapter 7) function not only as a reservoir but also to present virus captured on their surface. This results in continuous presentation of virus to T and B cells, culminating in the intense follicular (germinal center) hyperplasia and lymphadenopathy (lymph node enlargement) typical of this phase.

T cells undergo a slow rate of lysis, which eventually results in involution of the lymph node. This T cell death seems to be the result of a combination of factors. First, production of virus in the cells themselves causes lysis. Second, the infected cell seems to be more susceptible to apoptosis. Third, CTLs kill some of the infected cells. Finally, uninfected $CD4^+$ T cells may be killed in a bystander antibody-dependent, cell-mediated cytotoxicity-like mechanism as a result of binding soluble gp120 and anti-gp120 antibody to their surface CD4 molecules.

During this phase, patients have traditionally been followed by their peripheral $CD4^+$T cell counts and CD4:CD8 cell ratio. In healthy people the CD4:CD8 cell ratio is normally approximately 2, but in this phase of HIV infection the ratio is reversed, with CD8 cells outnumbering CD4 cells. A reversed CD4:CD8 cell ratio can be seen in other viral infections, often due to an increase in $CD8^+$ cells. In HIV, however, the number of $CD4^+$ T cells is diminished. As the number of $CD4^+$ cells reaches progressively lower values, the patient becomes symptomatic, entering the final phase, AIDS.

Crisis Phase. AIDS was originally recognized by the clinical appearance of unusual infections and malignancies and these continue to be the hallmarks of full-blown AIDS. The Centers for Disease Control and Prevention (CDC) have identified illnesses that are considered AIDS associated (Table 17.3). They fall into three categories: ***unusual malignancies, opportunistic infections,*** and ***neurologic syndromes,*** reflecting the primary effects of HIV on the immune system and central nervous system (CNS).

Several factors acting concurrently appear to initiate this symptomatic or crisis phase. The gradual drop in $CD4^+$ T cells eventually results in an ***immunodeficient state,*** leaving the individual susceptible to opportunistic infections, as is also seen in patients with primary immunodeficiency or in immunosuppressed transplant patients. ***Activation of virally infected T cells*** by antigen results in stimulation of viral transcription and progeny formation. This leads to accelerated T cell death, exacerbating the immunodeficient state. Rapid viral replication also increases the ***viral mutation*** rate, allowing escape from any immune controls that might remain.

The patterns of infections and malignancies in an individual with full-blown AIDS may partially reflect the mode of transmission of HIV to that patient—that is, sexual transmission versus intravenous drug use. This is suggested by differences between the infections and malignancies seen in

TABLE 17.3. AIDS-Associated Diseases Defined by the CDC[a]

Infections—frequently disseminated		
	Fungal	
		Candidiasis
		Cryptococcosis
		Histoplasmosis
		Coccidioidomycosis
	Parasitic	
		Toxoplasmosis
		Pneumocystis
		Cryptosporidiosis
		Isosporiasis
	Bacterial	
		Mycobacteriosis, including atypical *Salmonella*
	Viral	
		Cytomegalovirus
		Herpes simplex virus
		Progressive multifocal leukoencephalopathy
Neoplasms		
	Sarcoma	
		Kaposi's sarcoma
	Lymphoma	
		Burkitt lymphoma
		Diffuse large B cell lymphoma
		Effusion-based lymphoma
		Primary CNS lymphoma
	Carcinoma	
		Invasive cancer of the uterine cervix
General Conditions		
	HIV encephalopathy and dementia	
	Wasting syndrome	

[a]Selected illnesses are discussed in the text.

AIDS patients versus other immunosuppressed individuals and among AIDS patients with different modes of exposure. This is particularly true for ***malignancies*** associated with viral infections.

Some individuals infected with HIV are also infected with other sexually transmitted diseases. ***Human papillomavirus*** (HPV) is associated with the development of cervical cancer in women. Exposure to HPV, combined with the individual's immunodeficient state, may be responsible for a markedly increased incidence of ***invasive cervical cancer*** in HIV^+ women. The CDC have now included invasive cervical cancer in the AIDS-associated malignancies.

The aggressive form of ***Kaposi's sarcoma*** (KS) is virtually unique to AIDS patients, particularly male homosexuals, in whom it may occur early in the course of the disease. KS is an abnormal proliferation of small blood vessels that normally presents as a slow-growing tumor on the skin of the lower extremities of elderly men. ***Human herpes virus 8*** (HHV-8) has been identified in KS from AIDS patients. Whether these vessels grow in response to the virus or the virus is directly oncogenic is unknown. This virus is also associated with an unusual form of aggressive lymphoma seen in AIDS patients, ***primary effusion lymphoma.*** This malignancy is more common in male homosexual AIDS patients; some have the lymphoma and KS concurrently.

Aggressive ***B-cell lymphomas,*** mostly ***EBV associated,*** are seen at an incidence similar to that observed in immunosuppressed transplant patients. These lymphomas are usually ***Burkitt's*** or ***diffuse large B cell lymphoma*** (see below) and are often found outside the lymph nodes (extranodal). In AIDS patients, the CNS is a frequent site of primary lymphoma.

The ***infectious diseases*** associated with AIDS reflect the inability of the patient's markedly depressed cell-mediated immune system to handle organisms that are normally nonpathogenic (opportunistic infections). As in any T cell immunodeficient patient, ***PCP*** is a major infectious complication. ***Candidiasis*** is also frequently seen. Granuloma formation—a T cell–dependent function—is poor in these patients, leading to uncontrolled ***mycobacterial infections. Mycobacterium avium,*** not normally a human pathogen, can also cause overwhelming infection. ***Cryptosporidia, Mycobacterium avium,*** and ***CMV*** are among the most common organisms infecting the gastrointestinal tract and cause severe diarrhea. The CNS is susceptible to infection by ***cryptococcus, toxoplasma,*** and ***CMV.***

The multiple infections cause continuous cell necrosis (death), a major feature of AIDS. The organisms and cell debris provide chronic antigenic stimulation to a deficient immune system. B cells show evidence of responding to the chronic stimulation: Patients have polyclonal hypergammaglobulinemia (elevated serum Igs), circulating immune complexes, and markedly increased plasma cell production. In spite of this B cell activity, patients are unable to mount an effective antibody response to newly encountered antigens, perhaps due to the T cell defect; however, they also have particular difficulty with T cell–independent responses to encapsulated organisms. In addition, B cells infected with EBV, normally eliminated by T cell responses, are susceptible to additional transforming events, resulting in the B cell malignancies discussed above.

The CNS is infected with HIV, presumably via transport by macrophages. The virus infects microglia (bone-marrow derived cells in the same lineage as the macrophage), oligodendrocytes, and astrocytes. This may start the process resulting in AIDS-related ***dementia*** and progressive ***encephalopathy,*** which have been frequently documented. In total, up to 50% of AIDS patients show CNS symptoms and >70% have CNS changes at autopsy.

Finally, these patients suffer from ***cachexia,*** or wasting syndrome. This wasting syndrome is much more severe than found in other illnesses known to be associated with weight loss and fatigue. It is thought that HIV alters the cytokine profile of macrophages to increase TNF production, leading to the development of cachexia.

Prevention, Control, Diagnosis, and Therapy of HIV Infection

Prevention and control of HIV is best accomplished by avoiding unprotected contact with blood and body fluids from infected individuals. Education and public awareness of both what to avoid and what is safe (casual contact) is required to control the disease and to prevent possible panic.

Starting in 1985, all blood donations in the United States were tested for antibodies to HIV. Because the development of an antibody response after exposure to HIV can take five weeks, this antibody screening approach still left a long window period in which a recently infected person might not be detected. Blood donors were—and still are—screened by an interview process and asked direct questions orally and in writing about high-risk behavior. Testing for viral RNA, which requires a polymerase chain reaction (PCR) amplification step, is very sensitive and is currently being put in place. The viremia following infection precedes the immune response. Detection of the viral RNA will decrease the window period to <2 weeks but will not entirely eliminate it.

HIV^+ pregnant women are placed on anti-viral therapy to decrease viral load and thereby diminish risk of transplacental virus transfer. Caesarean sections are performed to eliminate infection during passage through the birth canal. Finally, exposure through breast milk is avoided. For people who are accidentally exposed to infected products, therapy is administered as soon as possible after exposure to prevent establishment of infection.

Diagnosis of HIV infection is generally made by detection of antibodies to the viral protein p24 by enzyme-linked immunosorbent assay (ELISA) and confirmed by Western blot analysis. Patients were originally monitored by following their absolute $CD4^+$ T cell count in the peripheral blood. Correlations have shown that opportunistic infections generally are not seen with CD4 counts $>500/\mu L$. The CDC have designated CD4 counts $<200/\mu L$ as an indicator of full-blown AIDS.

Therapy Azidothymidine (AZT), also called Zidovudin, is a nucleoside inhibitor of reverse transcriptase and was the first promising drug used for HIV infection. Protease inhibitors form a second class of agents in use and non-nucleoside reverse transcriptase inhibitors, a third class of therapeutic agents. Drug resistance to single agents develops rapidly, however, because HIV is capable of an amazing rate of spontaneous mutation during the course of infection in a single individual. This results from the lack of fidelity of the reverse transcriptase and RNA polymerase.

Individuals who are HIV positive but asymptomatic are now placed on ***triple-agent antiviral therapy*** referred to as ***highly active antiretroviral therapy*** (HAART). HAART combines three drugs from at least two of the inhibitor classes directed against HIV's reverse transcriptase and protease. It is hoped that the triple-agent therapy will delay the appearance of mutant strains. This therapy prevents infection of new cells; previously infected cells remain until they are lysed, however. After initiating therapy the fall in virus titer—currently monitored for viral load by quantitative analysis of viral RNA following PCR—is rapid and dramatic, but a small baseline titer almost always remains. As one would expect, discontinuation of the drugs for a prolonged period results in a resurgence of virus. Unfortunately, mutations allow escape from control by these agents, so there is a great need to develop an extensive armory of drugs to treat the disease. This therapy is not without side effects, particularly suppression of hematopoietic cells. More time is needed to see how successful this approach will be.

Extension of life span and improvement in quality of life were first achieved by aggressive, even prophylactic, treatment of infections, particularly PCP. Infection still remains the major immediate cause of death in AIDS patients.

Many infectious diseases have been controlled by vaccines, with the most effective way of preventing the spread of infection by inducing long-lasting immune response before exposure to the infectious agent (see Chapter 21). Vaccine development for HIV presents serious challenges, however. First, we do not yet know which arm of the immune response—antibody, CTL, etc.—needs to be boosted, to mount a response that would eliminate the virus; HIV escapes eradication despite both antibody and cytotoxic T cell responses in recently infected individuals. Second, the virus's ability to "hide out" in reservoir cells and its high mutation rate are major problems that need to be overcome. In addition, animal models to test candidate vaccines, which have been used extensively in other infectious diseases, are limited. The best model is the monkey, which develops a disease similar to AIDS after infection with simian immunodeficiency virus (SIV). Testing of vaccines in humans is also fraught with ethical problems. Understanding the molecular biology and structure of all components of HIV will be essential for developing a safe vaccine.

NEOPLASMS OF THE LYMPHOID SYSTEM

A common theme throughout this chapter has been the idea that dysregulation of the immune system can result in the emergence of neoplasms, particularly neoplasms of lymphoid cells. This is described in patients with primary immunodeficiency diseases, AIDS, and immunosuppressed transplant patients (also see Chapter 19). In these circumstances, the malignancies that arise are most often aggressive B cell lymphomas, frequently associated with EBV infection. In this section, we first describe general characteristics of lymphoid neoplasms followed by specific examples of important types.

Lymphoid leukemias and lymphomas were originally categorized by cell morphology and clinical outcome. A ***leukemia*** designation implies that the malignant cells are

TABLE 17.4. WHO Classification for Lymphoid Neoplasms

- B cell neoplasms
  - Precursor B cell lymphoblastic leukemia/lymphoma
  - Mature B cell neoplasms
    - Chronic lymphocytic leukemia, small lymphocytic lymphoma, prolymphocytic leukemia
    - Follicular lymphoma
    - Mantle cell lymphoma
    - Marginal zone lymphoma of MALT type
    - Nodal marginal zone lymphoma
    - Splenic marginal zone lymphoma
    - Hairy cell leukemia
    - Diffuse large B cell lymphoma (including mediastinal, primary effusion, intravascular)
    - Burkitt's lymphoma
    - Plasmacytoma
    - Plasma cell myeloma
    - Lymphoplasmacytic lymphoma
- B cell poliferations of uncertain malignant potential
  - Lymphomatoid granulomatosis
  - Posttransplant lymphoproliferative disorders
- T/NK cell neoplasms
  - Precursor T cell lymphoblastic leukemia/lymphoma
  - Mature T/NK cell neoplasms (selected)
    - T cell large granular lymphocytic leukemia
    - NK cell leukemia
    - Peripheral T cell lymphoma (unspecified)
    - Mycosis fungoides
    - Sézary syndrome
    - Primary cutaneous anaplastic large cell lymphoma
    - Systemic anaplastic large cell lymphoma
    - Extranodal NK/T-cell lymphoma, nasal type
    - Intestinal T cell lymphoma
    - Hepatosplenic $\gamma\delta$ T cell lymphoma
    - Adult T cell leukemia/lymphoma
- Hodgkin lymphoma
  - Nodular lymphocyte predominant Hodgkin lymphoma
  - Classical Hodgkin lymphoma
    - Nodular sclerosis
    - Mixed cellularity
    - Classical, lymphocyte rich
    - Lymphocyte depleted

[a] Selected neoplasms are discussed in the text.

predominantly in the circulation and/or bone marrow. A ***lymphoma*** presents as solid masses in the lymph nodes, spleen, thymus, or extranodal organs. Sometimes the same malignant cell type can show either presentation (***leukemia/lymphoma***).

In 1996, the World Health Organization (WHO) recommended a classification system based on cell of origin—B vs. T/NK—and stage of differentiation—immature (precursor) vs. mature (peripheral) (Table 17.4). The tumors are considered outgrowths of a transformed lymphoid cell that appears frozen in development. They have the same surface markers and many of the same properties as the corresponding normal cells at that developmental stage. The malignant cells, however, may not continue to mature, accumulate in large numbers, and all originate from a single clone (i.e., they are monoclonal). They will also occupy the same sites or traffic in the same pattern as their normal counterparts—that is, bone marrow for immature B cells, thymus for immature T cells, etc.

Southern blot analysis of DNA extracted from B and T cell neoplasms shows a single band for the Ig gene and T cell receptor gene, respectively. This demonstrates that all the tumor cells have the same rearrangement of these genes and establishes the monoclonality of that lymphoid growth. PCR may be used before the Southern blot to detect a small population of monoclonal cells. For some lymphoid neoplasms, a unique molecular abnormality, which may contribute to the transformation of that cell, has been identified. These molecular changes are also incorporated into the classification scheme. Since the WHO classification is based on cell of origin rather than clinical presentation, leukemias versus lymphomas are no longer separated if they are derived from the same malignant cell type. The WHO grouping makes practical sense since the treatment is often the same.

B Cell Neoplasms

Precursor B Cell Lymphoblastic Leukemia/ Lymphomas. B cell acute lymphoblastic leukemias (B-ALLs) correspond to the pro-B, pre-B, or immature B cell stages of development, as demonstrated by the expression of surface CD markers and the stage of Ig gene rearrangement in the individual patient's leukemia (Fig. 17.9). The malignant cells may express the blast or stem cell marker CD34 (particularly pro-B cells) and will express CD10 and CD19, early B cell markers. Similar to the normal pro-B or pre-pre-B cell and pre-B cell, corresponding ALLs express terminal deoxynucleotidyl transferase (TdT) in their nucleus. The expression of this enzyme, normally required to rearrange the Ig genes (and T cell receptor genes), reflects the fact that B-ALL cells are in the process of gene rearrangement. The corollary of this is that these cells do not yet express a complete Ig molecule on their surface and have only cytoplasmic μ-chains if at the pre-B cell stage. Chemotherapy has been successful in treating children with these leukemias.

There is also an aggressive immature B-ALL that is the leukemic counterpart of Burkitt's lymphoma and that demonstrates the same characteristic translocation (described below). These cells correspond to immature B cells just entering the periphery from the bone marrow. They express CD20; have turned off TdT, and, having completed their Ig gene rearrangement, now display surface IgM.

Burkitt's Lymphoma/Leukemia. Burkitt's lymphoma may present as a leukemia or a lymphoma, characterized by a translocation that places the ***c-myc oncogene*** next to either the Ig H chain gene or one of the two L chain

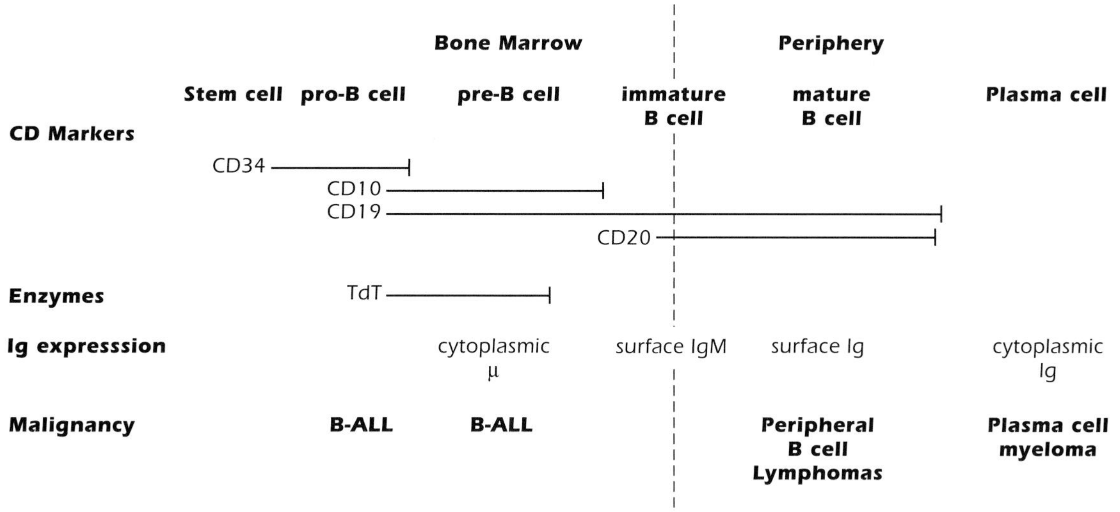

Figure 17.9. Correlation of B cell development with B cell malignancies.

genes—t(8;14), t(8;22), or t(2,8) (Fig. 17.10). The c-*myc* protein is normally involved in activating genes for cell proliferation when a resting cell receives a signal to divide. Translocation to the Ig genes leads to increased expression of c-*myc* and increased cell proliferation. Possibly, antigenic stimulation of the B cell initiates the overexpression of c-*myc,* now under the control of the Ig gene.

In equatorial Africa, this lymphoma is endemic and is associated with EBV infection of the B cells. Burkitt's lymphoma is one of the malignancies seen in immunosuppressed patients (AIDS and medically immunosuppressed) in which the EBV genome is also sometimes found in the lymphoma cells. The other malignancy, diffuse large B cell lymphoma, is discussed later in the chapter.

Follicular Lymphoma. Follicular lymphomas represent transformation of the B cells normally found in lymph node follicles (Fig. 17.11). As we described in Chapter 7, B cells are stimulated by antigen in the follicle, generating a germinal center. The B cells may respond by proliferating and undergoing affinity maturation, by isotype switching, and by differentiating into memory or plasma cells (see Chapter 7). If their antibody is a poor match for that antigen or of low affinity, the cell undergoes ***apoptosis,*** or cell death. In

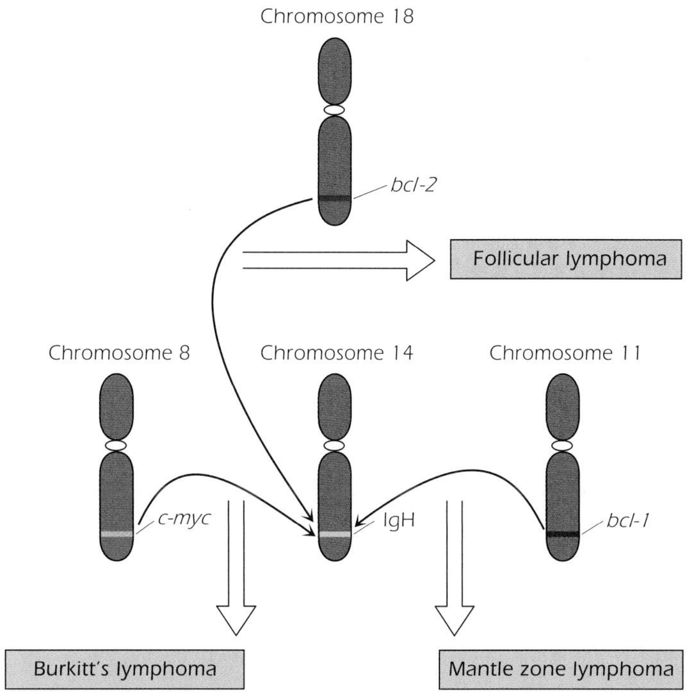

Figure 17.10. Some of the B cell neoplasms associated with translocations of genes to the chromosomal locus encoding the Ig H chain gene on chromosome 14.

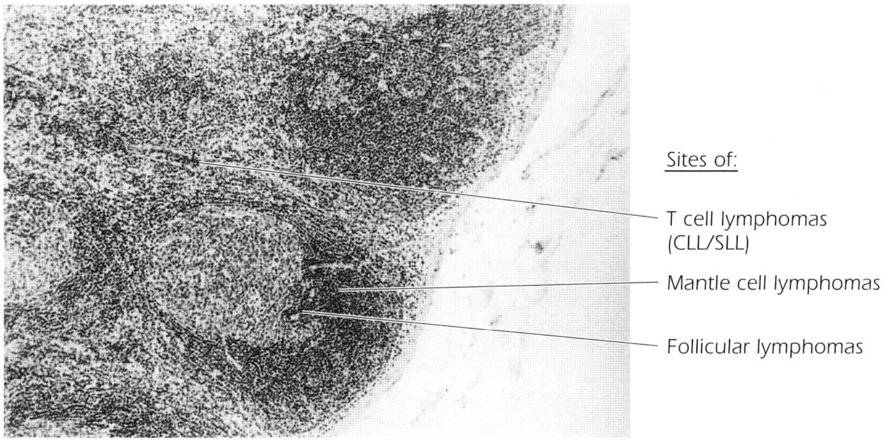

Figure 17.11. A section through a normal lymph node showing sites that become involved by T and B cell lymphomas. CLL/SLL, mantle cell lymphoma, and follicular lymphoma are all B cell derived.

follicular lymphomas, the ***bcl-2 gene,*** which produces a protein that interferes with apoptosis, is translocated to the Ig H chain gene, t(14;18) (Fig. 17.10). This results in continuous expression of bcl-2 protein, preventing death of the cells. In fact, these B cell neoplasms have only a low rate of proliferation and a long chronic clinical course. They display the phenotype (surface CD markers) of normal follicular center B cells: $CD19^+$, $CD20^+$, $CD10^+$, and surface Ig.

Mantle Cell Lymphoma. The normal germinal center is surrounded by a collar of small quiescent B cells that have not responded to antigen (Fig. 17.11). A neoplasm of these mantle zone cells has the same B cell phenotype as their normal counterpart, $CD19^+$, $CD20^+$, $CD5^+$, sIgM. Many mantle cell lymphomas have a translocation of the ***bcl-1 gene*** to the Ig H chain gene—t(11;14)—resulting in overexpression of ***cyclin D1* protein** (Fig. 17.10). Cyclin D1 is normally responsible for promoting cell cycle progression from G_1 to S phase, leading to cell division. This lymphoma has a higher proliferative rate and a more aggressive course than follicular lymphomas.

Marginal Zone Lymphoma. Marginal zone lymphomas most commonly arise in the mucosal-associated lymphoid tissue (MALT) and, interestingly, may be associated with chronic antigenic stimulation or autoimmune disease of that organ. For example, chronic ***Helicobacter pylori*** infection of the stomach may lead to the development of gastric lymphoma and thus may be preventable by antibiotic treatment for the organism. Similarly, patients with autoimmune thyroiditis (***Hashimoto thyroiditis***) and autoimmune disease of the salivary glands (***Sjögren syndrome***) have a high incidence of this B cell lymphoma developing in the affected organ.

The association between these autoimmune diseases or infection and lymphoma suggest two interesting and not mutually exclusive hypotheses. First, that chronic antigenic stimulation provides fertile ground for the development of a B cell lymphoma. B cells, which continue to undergo somatic mutation of their Ig genes, may accumulate transforming mutations with continuous stimulation. The second hypothesis is that a defect in the regulation of the B cells, whether intrinsic or due to lack of T cell downregulation, leads to both autoimmune disease and, eventually, lymphoma.

As we described earlier in this section, the malignant cells of the immune system follow the trafficking pattern of their normal counterpart. Marginal zone lymphomas remain localized for a prolonged period and then follow the circulatory pattern for normal MALT cells, traveling to other MALT sites.

Chronic Lymphocytic Leukemia/Small Lymphocytic Lymphoma. Chronic lymphocytic leukemia (CLL) or small lymphocytic lymphoma (SLL) is thought to be a malignant transformation of the subset of B cells known as B-1 cells (see Chapter 7). In some patients, it presents first with a leukemic picture (blood and bone marrow involvement),whereas in others it presents first in the lymph nodes (Fig. 17.11). Similar to normal B-1 cells, CLL/SLL cells express CD19 and CD20, the mature B cell marker, as well as CD5 and sIgM.

B-CLL is the most common leukemia in North America and western Europe, seen mostly in older individuals. These patients are extremely susceptible to infection, suggesting that their nonmalignant cells are not functioning properly. Autoimmune antibodies are common, particularly against RBCs, resulting in autoimmune hemolytic anemia. The antibodies may be produced by the malignant clone or, more often, by nontransformed B cells. The association of this autoimmune condition with a leukemia/lymphoma again suggests a lymphoid neoplasm arising in the setting of or causing immune dysregulation. CLL has a long clinical course, but eventually there is massive involvement of every organ, peripheral blood, and bone marrow by malignant cells.

Diffuse Large B Cell Lymphoma

The diffuse large B cell lymphomas are a heterogeneous group of lymphomas that may arise de novo at a single site, may be a progression of one of the above-described slow-growing lymphomas (e.g., follicular lymphoma), or may be a consequence of a poorly controlled EBV infection in immunosuppressed individuals (e.g., HIV^{+}, transplant, or immunodeficiency patients). In all cases, the cells express B cell markers, CD19 and CD20, and frequently express surface Ig. A subgroup has a translocation of the *bcl-6* gene. *Bcl-6* is a proto-oncogene gene that normally acts as a transcriptional repressor of several genes required for normal B cell and germinal center development.

The behavior of the de novo diffuse large B cell lymphomas has been historically unpredictable. Recent application of cDNA microarray analysis (see Chapter 5) to a series of these tumors has divided the lymphomas into two major groups, based on patterns of gene expression (mRNA production), and has demonstrated a correlation between these two groups and tumor behavior. This molecular characterization should lead to a better understanding of the biology of these lymphomas, suggesting practical applications for treatment.

The association of EBV infection with diffuse large B cell lymphomas and Burkitt's lymphoma in immunosuppressed patients is an important illustration of the consequences of a breakdown in the immune system's ability to regulate itself. EBV infection of B cells (via the EBV receptor CD21) leads to polyclonal B cell proliferation. In healthy individuals, these expanded EBV-infected B cells are removed by the body's CTLs (see Chapter 10). In situations in which T cell control is lacking, however, the infected B cells continue to expand, and some may acquire additional mutations, such as c-*myc* translocation, that cause transformation and subsequent independent growth. For example, EBV can be used to immortalize B cells in tissue culture, where the B cells are not subject to T cell control. This is also important clinically: for patients on immunosuppressive therapy, there is a point at which it is still possible to prevent the development of B cell lymphomas by withdrawing the immunsuppressive treatment and allowing the body's immune system to handle the abnormal B cell proliferation. Of course, this option is not possible in AIDS patients.

Plasma Cell Neoplasms. Neoplastic growths of plasma cells may occur at a single site, resulting in a ***plasmacytoma,*** or may be at multiple sites, predominantly throughout the bone, and are called ***multiple myeloma*** or ***plasma cell myeloma.*** As for normal plasma cells, interleukin-6 (IL-6) functions as an autocrine growth factor for myeloma cells.

The neoplastic plasma cells may continue to synthesize and secrete their Ig product. In many cases, this secreted monoclonal protein causes more difficulties than the transformed cells for the patient. Light chain deposits called ***amyloid*** can cause organ failure, especially in the kidneys. As we described in Chapter 4, excretion in the urine of free light chains derived from some multiple myeloma patients—***Bence-Jones proteins***—provided early insights into understanding Ig light chain structure. These proteins are monoclonal and detectable in the serum and sometimes in the urine as an M spike in the gamma region of an electrophoretic evaluation (see Fig. 4.1). A spike rather than a broad band forms because all the Igs are identical and migrate to the same place by size and charge (see Chapter 5). Most cases produce monoclonal IgG; IgA is the next most frequent isotype found. The levels of all other normal Igs are severely decreased in these patients, who are immunosuppressed with respect to antibody production and therefore susceptible to infection. Before the appearance of full-blown myeloma, patients may have a small amount of monoclonal Ig for many years. Many individuals remain at this stage, never progressing to disease. Small M spikes may be found in association with other lymphoid neoplasms, such as CLL, and even with nonmalignant conditions.

Lymphoplasmacytic Lymphoma (Waldenström Macroglobulinemia). Lymphoplasmacytic lymphoma/ Waldenström's macroglobulinemia is a neoplasm of a single clone of B cells in which their microscopic appearance is a mixture of lymphocytes, plasma cells, and something in between—lymphoplasmacytoid cells. The neoplastic cells involve the lymph nodes, bone marrow, and spleen. Although uncommon these lymphomas are of interest to immunologists because they overproduce IgM. The large size and high concentration of the IgM in the blood may combine to slow blood flow and clog vessels (hyperviscosity syndrome). In some patients, the IgM has an abnormal structure, causing it to precipitate in the cold (cryoglobulin) and cause circulatory problems in their extremities (fingers and toes).

T-Cell Neoplasms

Precursor T Cell Acute Lymphoblastic Leukemia/ Lymphoma. Precursor T cell acute lymphoblastic leukemia (T-ALL) is a neoplasm of immature T cells and has characteristics identical to those of thymocytes frozen in their immature state. As Figure 17.12 shows, T-ALLs express the pan-T cell markers, CD2, CD5, and CD7, that appear early in T cell development. Some T-ALLs have the characteristics of immature thymocytes, and do not express CD4 or CD8 (i.e., they are *double negative*). The majority of normal thymocytes and the majority of T-ALLs are slightly more mature, expressing both CD4 and CD8 (*double positive*) but little or no CD3 on their surface (referred to as *common thymocytes*). These cells have not yet completed rearrangement of their T cell receptor (TCR) genes and still express TdT. T-ALL presents as a leukemia or as a thymic mass. Treatment has not been as successful as for B-ALL.

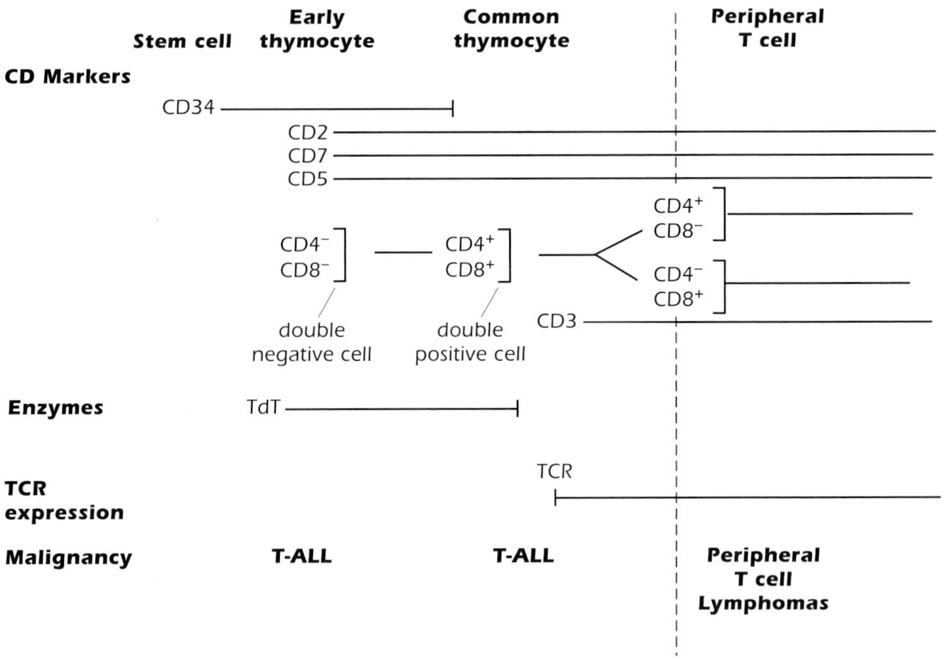

Figure 17.12. Correlation of T cell development with T cell malignancies.

Peripheral T-Cell Neoplasms. Peripheral T cell lymphomas have varied presentations. They are found wherever T cells normally migrate—namely, skin, lung, vessel wall, gastrointestinal tract, and lymph nodes. They also retain some of the functions of normal mature T cells; consequently, cytokine production by the neoplastic cells results in a background of inflammatory cells that includes eosinophils, plasma cells, and macrophages. Peripheral T cell lymphomas usually seem to have a more aggressive course than B cell lymphomas. Two are highlighted here.

Cutaneous T Cell Lymphoma. When confined to the skin, this cutaneous T cell lymphoma is still known by its historical name, ***mycosis fungoides,*** because patients were originally believed to have a chronic fungal infection of the skin that waxed and waned over many years. We now understand that the skin disease is due to infiltration of the epidermis by malignant $CD4^+$ T cells. Eventually, the cells spread to the lymph nodes and even into the blood. The malignant T cells found in the circulation are called Sezary cells and the patient is said to have ***Sezary syndrome.***

Adult T Cell Leukemia/Lymphoma. Adult T cell leukemia/lymphoma (ATLL) is an aggressive T cell neoplasm that was described in the 1970s in a region of Japan, where it is endemic. It is also found in the Caribbean, parts of central Africa, and a small region of the southeast United States. Usually ATLL is a neoplasm of mature $CD4^+$ T cells. IL-2 is an autocrine growth factor for these cells. In early attempts at treatment, the neoplasm was found to respond temporarily—a few months—to administration of an antibody (known as anti-Tac) that was later found to be specific for the α-chain of the IL-2 receptor (CD25).

ATLL is caused by the retrovirus human T cell lymphotropic virus 1 (HTLV-1), which was described and isolated before recognition of AIDS and HIV. The proviral genomic structure is similar to HIV, containing an LTR and coding for structural and regulatory proteins as well as viral enzymes, reverse transcriptase, integrase, and protease. Tax, the viral protein that transactivates HTLV-1 transcription by binding to the LTR region, activates host genes, including those coding for IL-2, IL-2R α-chain, and a parathyroid-like hormone (not normally expressed by T cells). Therefore activation of proviral transcription is associated with activation and proliferation of host T cells. Patients with ATLL frequently have extreme elevations in serum calcium levels as a result of the increased synthesis of the parathyroid-like hormone.

Transmission of HTLV-1 is similar to HIV in that it is transmitted through contact with blood and body fluids, with more efficient transfer through breast milk. Thus many patients are infected with HTLV-1 during infancy. The incubation period of this virus is long, typically 20–40 years. The virus mostly infects $CD4^+$T cells and also infects the nervous system. A subset of patients presents with neurologic disease.

Fortunately, only approximately 1% of infected patients develop ATLL. What initiates its development after so many years is unknown. The $CD4^+$ T cells harbor the virus in a quiescent state. Unlike HIV, the virus is not cytolytic for these cells once activated. To the contrary, HTLV-1 leads to transformation of the T cells. Once diagnosed with ATLL, survival is generally 6–12 months. The blood supplies of the United States and the United Kingdom are screened for HTLV-1 infection.

Hodgkin Lymphoma

Hodgkin lymphoma is characterized by the presence of relatively small numbers of large binucleate malignant cells named Reed-Sternberg cells (described below) in a reactive background of small T cells, eosinophils, plasma cells, macrophages, and fibrosis. This reactive milieu is the result of abundant cytokine production, particularly IL-5, by the tumor cells and/or the background cells. Patients show clinical signs of increased cytokine production with fevers, night sweats, and weight loss. Classically, they also show evidence of depressed cell-mediated immune responses, with no delayed-type hypersensitivity (DTH) reaction to common test antigens, and with increased susceptibility to viral and parasitic infections.

The lineage origin of the Reed-Sternberg cell, which expresses no lineage markers and is characterized by the expression of only CD15 and CD30, has been the subject of much debate. Recent studies using molecular techniques on single malignant cells have shown rearrangements in the Ig genes, supporting a B cell origin. The finding of hypermutation in those Ig genes suggests that the Reed-Sternberg cell derives from a postgerminal center B cell. Although the malignant cell has been identified as a B cell, this lymphoma behaves differently from large B cell lymphomas and, therefore, remains separately classified. Lymphomas are grouped as Hodgkin versus non-Hodgkin lymphomas.

Immunotherapy

The expanding knowledge of lymphoma biology combined with the technical advances in monoclonal antibody and protein production have led to the development of a new generation of treatment options. Currently, chimeric and humanized monoclonal antibodies directed against CD20, in particular, are widely used for the treatment of B cell lymphomas. These antibodies either are used alone ("cold"), causing tumor cell elimination by opsonization of antibody-coated cells, or are conjugated to a toxin that directly kills the cell (see Chapter 20). Additional agents to block cytokines or cytokine receptors required for malignant cell proliferation are being combined with conventional chemotherapy. Conventional chemotherapies, which are largely nonspecific agents, kill all dividing cells. The technology used in developing these new specific therapies is also widely applicable to drug development for the treatment of autoimmune diseases and nonlymphoid cancers, such as breast cancer.

The immune system normally works as a finely regulated network, responding to foreign invaders, causing no harm to itself, and returning to a more quiescent state (but with memory) once the threat is over. Eliminating, chronically stimulating, or allowing uncontrolled growth of any single component perturbs the remaining elements. Thus, if the network is no longer properly regulated, the occurrence of any one of the major categories of disorders—immunodeficiency, autoimmune disease, or lymphoid neoplasm—allows the emergence of one or both of the other two disease types.

SUMMARY

1. Immune deficiency disorders are called primary when the deficiency is the cause of disease and secondary when the deficiency is a result of other diseases or the effects of treatment regimens.
2. Immune deficiency diseases may be due to disorders in the development or function of B cells, T cells, phagocytic cells, or components of complement.
3. Immune deficiency disorders predispose patients to recurrent infections. The type of infection that develops is usually characteristic of the particular arm of the immune system that is deficient: Defects in humoral immunity lead to increased susceptibility to bacterial infections; defects in cell-mediated immunity, to viral and fungal infections; defects in phagocytic cells, to infections with pyogenic organisms; and defects in complement components, to bacterial infections and autoimmunity.
4. Immune deficiencies constitute one type of defect or disorder of the immune system. Other aspects of such disorders are the unregulated proliferation of B or T lymphocytes, the overproduction of lymphocyte or phagocytic cell products, and the unregulated activation of complement components. This may account for the association of immune deficiencies with autoimmune disease and malignancies.
5. HIV, by infecting and killing $CD4^+$ lymphocytes, causes a massive immunosuppressive illness known as AIDS.
6. Lymphoid neoplasms of the immune system are uncontrolled monoclonal proliferations that can be related to their normal cell counterparts and stage of differentiation. Many lymphoid neoplasms have specific chromosomal translocations causing dysregulation of cell proliferation and death. Some are associated with infections with viruses, such as EBV and HTLV-1, acting either as growth promoters or as oncogenic viruses.

REFERENCES

Ammann AJ (1994): Mechanisms of immunodeficiency. In Stites DP, Terr Al, Parslow TG (eds): Basic and Clinical Immunology, 8th ed. East Norwalk, CT: Appleton & Lange.

Anderson DC, Springer TA (1987): Leukocyte adhesion deficiency: an inherited defect in Mac-1, LFA-1, and p150, 95 glycoproteins. *Annu Rev Med* 38:175.

Baltimore D, Feinberg MB (1989): HIV revealed: towards a natural history of the infection. *N Engl J Med* 132:1673.

Berger EA, Murphy PM, Farber JM (1999): Chemokine receptors as HIV-1 coreceptors: roles in viral entry, tropism and disease. *Annu Rev Immunol* 17:657.

Clerici M, Shearer GM (1994): The T_H1-T_H2 hypothesis of HIV infection: new insights. *Immunol Today* 14:107.

Fahey JL (1993): Update on AIDS. *Immunologist* 1:131.

Fauci AS (1993): Multifactorial nature of human immunodeficiency virus disease: implications for therapy. *Science* 262:1011.

Green WC (1993): AIDS and the immune system. *Sci Am* (Sept):99.

Hazenberg MD, Hamann D, Schuitemaker H, Miedema F (2000): T cell depletion in HIV-1 infection: how $CD4^+$ T cells go out of stock. *Nature Immunol* 1:285.

Helbert MR, L'Age-Stehr J, Mitchison NA (1993): Antigen presentation, loss of immunological memory and AIDS. *Immunol Today* 14:340.

Jaffe ES, Harris NL, Stein H, Vardiman JW, eds. (2001): World Health Organization Classification of Tumours. Pathology and Genetics of Tumours of Haematopoietic and Lymphoid Tissues. Lyon, France: IARC Press.

Kohler H, Muller S, Nara P (1994): Deceptive imprinting in the immune response against HIV-1. *Immunol Today* 15:475.

Lusso P, Gallo RC (1995): Human herpes virus 6 in AIDS. *Immunol Today* 16:67.

Ochs HD, Smith CIE, Puck JM (1999) Primary Immunodeficiency Diseases. New York: Oxford University Press.

Orkin SH (1989): Molecular genetics of chronic granulomatous disease. *Annu Rev Immunol* 7:277.

Rosenberg ZF, Fauci AS (1990): Immunopathogenic mechanisms of HIV infection: cytokine induction of HIV expression. *Immunol Today* 11:176.

Snapper SB, Rosen FS (1999): The Wiskott-Aldrich syndrome protein (WASP): roles in signalling and cytoskeletal organization. *Annu Rev Immunol* 17:905.

REVIEW QUESTIONS

For each question, choose the ONE BEST answer or completion.

1. An 8-month-old baby has a history of repeated gram-positive bacterial infections. The most probable cause for this condition is that
   A) the mother did not confer sufficient immunity to the baby in utero.
   B) the baby suffers from erythroblastosis fetalis (hemolytic disease of the newborn).
   C) the baby has a defect in the alternative complement pathway.
   D) the baby is allergic to the mother's milk.
   E) None of the above.

2. A 50-year-old worker at an atomic plant who previously had a sample of his own bone marrow cryopreserved was accidentally exposed to a minimal lethal dose of radiation. He was subsequently transplanted with his own bone marrow. This individual can expect
   A) to have recurrent bacterial infections.
   B) to have serious fungal infections due to deficiency in cell-mediated immunity.
   C) to make antibody responses to thymus-independent antigens only.
   D) All of the above.
   E) None of the above.

3. Which of the following immune deficiency disorders is associated exclusively with an abnormality of the humoral immune response?
   A) X-linked agammaglobulinemia (Bruton's agammaglobulinemia)
   B) DiGeorge syndrome
   C) Wiskott-Aldrich syndrome
   D) chronic mucocutaneous candidiasis
   E) ataxia telangiectasia

4. A sharp increase in levels of IgG with a spike in the IgG region seen in the electrophoretic pattern of serum proteins is an indication of
   A) IgA or IgM deficiency.
   B) multiple myeloma.
   C) macroglobulinemia.
   D) hypogammaglobulinemia.
   E) severe fungal infections.

5. Patients with DiGeorge syndrome may fail to produce IgG in response to immunization with T-dependent antigens because
   A) they have a decreased number of B cells that produce IgG.
   B) they have increased numbers of suppressor T cells.
   C) they have a decreased number of T helper cells.
   D) they have abnormal antigen-presenting cells.
   E) they cannot produce IgM during primary responses.

6. A 2-year-old child has had three episodes of pneumonia and two episodes of otitis media. All the infections were demonstrated to be pneumococcal. Which of the following disorders is most likely to be the cause?
A) an isolated transient T cell deficiency
B) a combined T and B cell deficiency
C) a B cell deficiency
D) transient anemia
E) AIDS

7. A healthy woman gave birth to a baby. The newborn infant was found to be HIV seropositive. This finding is most likely the result of
A) the virus being transferred across the placenta to the baby.
B) the baby's making anti-HIV antibodies.
C) the baby's erythrocyte antigens cross-reacting with the virus.
D) the mother's erythrocyte antigens cross-reacting with the virus.
E) maternal HIV-specific IgG being transferred across the placenta to the baby.

8. Immunodeficiency disease can result from
A) a developmental defect of T lymphocytes.
B) a developmental defect of bone marrow stem cells.
C) a defect in phagocyte function.
D) a defect in complement function.
E) All of the above.

9. A 9-month-old baby was vaccinated against smallpox with attenuated smallpox virus. He developed a progressive necrotic lesion of the skin, muscles, and subcutaneous tissue at the site of inoculation. The vaccination reaction probably resulted from
A) B lymphocyte deficiency.
B) reaction to the adjuvant.
C) complement deficiency.
D) T cell deficiency.
E) B and T lymphocyte deficiency.

10. The most common clinical consequence(s) of C3 deficiency is (are)
A) increased incidence of tumors.
B) increased susceptibility to viral infections.
C) increased susceptibility to fungal infections.
D) increased susceptibility to bacterial infections.
E) All of the above.

CASE STUDY

A senior pediatrician recounts this story: In 1985, a mother who had just moved into town brought her 4-year-old child into my office. She complained about the child's failure to thrive, including loss of appetite, weight loss, and persistent cough. On physical examination, the child appeared pale and sickly, with a low-grade fever but had no other physical signs. His past history was unremarkable except for a fractured leg at 1 year of age that required a blood transfusion during surgery, but the fracture healed without complication. I performed a battery of tests. X-ray examination showed some bilateral pulmonary infiltrates. Blood count was normal, with slightly reduced white cell numbers. An ELISA to detect serum Igs showed elevated IgG, IgM, and IgA. Skin tests performed with mumps, tetanus, and *Candida* antigens were negative. Antibiotic therapy was started, but on the next visit the child was sicker and now had enlarged lymph nodes, spleen, and liver. What diagnosis should I have made and how should I have confirmed it?

ANSWERS TO REVIEW QUESTIONS

1. *E* None of these is likely to be the underlying cause for the history. The baby is probably hypogammaglobulinemic. Hypogammaglobulinemia leads to recurrent bacterial infections. Viral and fungal infections are controlled by cell-mediated immunity, which is normal in hypogammaglobulinemic individuals. Answer A is incorrect because the mother's IgG, which passed through the placenta, would have a half-life of 23 days and would, therefore, not be expected to remain in the baby's circulation for 8 months. At this age, any Ig present in the baby's circulation is synthesized by the baby. Answer B is irrelevant, since erythroblastosis fetalis is caused by the destruction of the newborn's Rh^+ erythrocytes by the Rh^- mother's antibodies to Rh antigen. Answer C is unlikely since the classical complement pathway would still be protective; moreover, a defect in the alternative pathway would not result in the selective inability to protect from only gram-positive bacterial infections. Answer D is incorrect because even if allergic to the mother's milk the baby should not suffer from increased frequency of bacterial infections.

2. *E* The autologous bone marrow cells, which contain stem cells, will replicate, differentiate, and repopulate the hematopoietic-reticuloendothelial system, rendering the individual immunologically normal. Thus the individual is not expected to have bacterial, viral, or fungal infections or to respond to antigens differently from a normal individual.

3. *A* The only immune deficiency disorder that is associated with an abnormality exclusively of the humoral response is X-linked (Bruton's) agammaglobulinemia. DiGeorge syndrome results from thymic aplasia, in which there is a deficiency in T cells that influence IgG responses, which require T helper cells. Wiskott-Aldrich syndrome is associated with several abnormalities. Ataxia telangiectasia is a disease with defects in both cellular and humoral immune responses, with T cell–dependent areas of lymphoid tissues the most severely affected. Chronic mucocutaneous candidiasis is a poorly defined collection of syndromes associated with a selective defect in the functioning of T cells.

4. ***B*** This pattern is characteristic of multiple myeloma (IgG myeloma). Multiple myeloma may be recognized by the synthesis of large amounts of homogeneous antibody of any one isotype. Although patients with multiple myeloma may suffer from a decreased synthesis of other Ig isotypes, the electrophoretic pattern is not necessarily an indication of IgA or IgM deficiency.

5. ***C*** Patients with DiGeorge syndrome have a decreased number of T cells; in particular, T helper cells, which are essential for the IgG response to T-dependent antigens. These patients have normally functioning B cells and are capable of responding to T-independent antigens or with only IgM responses (primary responses) to T-dependent antigens.

6. ***C*** The cause for the described case history is very likely due to B cell deficiency, which is characterized by recurrent bacterial infections leading to otitis media and pneumonia. T cell deficiency would usually result in viral, fungal, and protozoal infections. The same is true for combined T and B cell deficiency. Answer D (transient anemia) is irrelevant in this case; anemia is not generally associated with increased infections. It is unlikely that with a history of only pneumococcal infections the child would have AIDS. The latter syndrome is associated more with characteristic infections such as with *Pneumocystis carinii* and various viral infections.

7. ***E*** The most likely explanation is that the "healthy" mother has been infected with HIV-1 and is making anti-HIV IgG, which is transferred to the fetus and newborn transplacentally. While it is possible that the HIV was transferred to the infant across the placenta, this would not cause the newborn to make antibodies to the virus at this young age. Thus answers A and B are incorrect. Answers C and D are false because this unlikely situation would result in the recognition of the viral antigen as "self"and the individual would not make anti-self antibodies.

8. ***E*** All are correct. Immunodeficiency disorders may result from defects in the development of bone marrow stem cells into lymphocytes and other cells that participate in the immune response. They can also result from defects in phagocyte functions, which are important in phagocytosis and presentation of antigen. Immunodeficiency disorders may also result from defects in complement function and absence or malfunction of one or more of the complement components, activators, or regulators.

9. ***D*** T cell deficiency would result in the absence of the crucial immunological defenses against viral infection—that is, cell-mediated immunity. Cell-mediated immunity plays the major role in immunity to viral infections, much greater than the role of either antibody or complement. In fact, individuals with impaired T cell–mediated immunity should not be vaccinated with live virus, which, even if attenuated, may cause a serious infection.

10. ***D*** Deficiency in C3 is associated with increased susceptibility to bacterial infections, because C3 plays an important role in the opsonization and destruction of bacteria. C3 is a component of all the complement activation pathways: alternative, classical, and mannose-binding lectin pathways. Cell-mediated immunity is generally more important in the resistance of the host to viral and fungal infections. In general, cell-mediated immunity is also considered to be more important than complement in the resistance of the host to tumors.

ANSWER TO CASE STUDY

Most likely, this was a case of childhood AIDS, presumably attributable to the earlier transfusion with blood obtained from a blood bank. Following a long incubation period, the child presented with a slightly lowered white cell count, somewhat elevated Ig levels, but a seriously compromised T cell function. The latter was determined by the absence of skin reactions to mumps, tetanus toxoid, and candida antigens, all of which elicit T cell–mediated DTH reactions in normal individuals. A follow-up test of the levels of circulating $CD4^+$ and $CD8^+$ cells revealed a ratio of 0.4, indicating that $CD4^+$ T cells, the target of the HIV virus, had declined markedly. Further study of the lung infiltrate, which failed to respond to antibiotic therapy, would be done by bronchoscopy and lavage. Microscopic examination of the lung washings would probably have shown an opportunistic organism such as *Pneumocystis carinii,* a common cause of death in patients with AIDS. Final confirmatory evidence of HIV infection would have come from evaluation of the child's serum for the presence of antibody to HIV antigens. Currently, the presence of viral genomes would be confirmed by using an HIV-specific PCR.

Fortunately, cases of HIV transmission by blood transfusion are now very rare in the United States, because of the measures taken to screen the blood supply. This has been a major step forward in preventing the spread of AIDS via blood transfusion.

18

TRANSPLANTATION

INTRODUCTION

The immune system has evolved as a way of discriminating between self and non-self. Once foreignness has been established, the immune response proceeds toward its ultimate goal of destroying the foreign material, be it a microorganism or its product, a substance present in the environment or a tumor cell. The triggering of the immune system in response to such foreign substances is, of course, of great survival value.

The same discriminating power of the immune system between self and non-self is undesirable in instances that are highly artificial, such as the transplantation of cells, tissues, or organs from one individual to another for therapeutic purposes. Indeed, results of transplants were formerly disastrous, culminating in the phenomenon of ***graft rejection,*** with one notable exception—namely, blood transfusions. Blood transfusions represent the earliest and most successful cell-based "transplants" and they continue to be the most common of all transplants. Why are these transplants uniformly successful if preformed properly? The reason is that it is easy to match the red blood cells (RBCs) of the donor and recipient—the population expresses only a limited number of different types of the major RBC antigens, the ABO and Rh blood group antigens (four and two, respectively). Matching prevents rapid antibody-mediated destruction of donor RBCs. By contrast, the antigens expressed on tissues and organs as well as leukocytes (MHC antigens, see Chapter 9), are highly ***polymorphic*** in the population, so matching donor and recipient is extremely difficult.

Our current understanding of cellular and molecular mechanisms associated with graft rejection and the advent of effective immunosuppressive therapies have made transplantation of various cells, tissues, and organs for therapeutic purposes very commonplace (Table 18.1). For example, >10,000 kidneys are transplanted annually worldwide with a high degree of success. Transplantations of heart, lungs, cornea, liver, and bone marrow, considered spectacular and widely publicized as recently as 25 years ago, have now become commonplace. Although rejection episodes have been significantly reduced due to the use of immunosuppressive therapies, they have not been eliminated. Thus transplantation immunology continues to be a major area of research. Later in this chapter, we will briefly describe the experience of one of us (E.B.) who has undergone heart transplantation.

RELATIONSHIP BETWEEN DONOR AND RECIPIENT

Before we discuss the immunologic mechanisms associated with graft rejection, it is important to understand the various gradations in relationships of transplantation from donor to recipient. These are shown in Figure 18.1 and are described below.

- An ***autograft*** is a graft or transplant from one area to another on the same individual, such as would occur in the transplantation of normal skin from one area of

Immunology: A Short Course, Fifth Edition, By Richard Coico, Geoffrey Sunshine, and Eli Benjamini
ISBN 0-471-22689-0

TABLE 18.1. Transplantation of Specific Organs and Tissues

Organ/Tissue	Clinical Uses	Comments
Skin	Burns, chronic wounds, diabetic ulcers, venous ulcers	Commonly autologous grafts; increasing use of artificial skin consisting of stromal elements and cultured cells of allogeneic or xenogeneic origin
Kidney	End-stage renal failure	Graft survival now exceeds 85% at one year even with organs from unrelated donors
Liver	Hepatoma and biliary atresia	Successful in about two-thirds of recipients at 1 year
Heart	Cardiac failure	Survial rates in excess of 80% at 1 year
Lung	Advanced pulmonary or cardiopulmonary diseases	Sometimes performed together with heart transplantation
Bone marrow	Incurable leukemias and lymphomas, congenital immunodeficiency diseases	Risk of GVH disease a unique feature of bone marrow transplantation; increasingly, transplantation of hematopoietic stem cells being used
Cornea	Blindness	HLA matching not advantageous since this is a "privileged" site that normally lacks lymphatic drainage
Pancreas	Diabetes mellitus	Pancreas and kidney transplantation sometimes performed together; success rates approaching that seen with kidney transplants

an individual to a burned area of the same individual. The graft is recognized as autochthonous or ***autologous*** (self), and no immune response is induced against it. Barring technical difficulties in the transplantation process, the graft will survive, or *take,* in its new location.

- An ***isograft*** or ***syngraft*** is a graft or transplant of cells, tissue, or organ from one individual to another individual who is ***syngeneic*** (genetically identical) to the donor. An example of an isograft is the transplantation of a kidney from one identical (homozygotic) twin to the other. As in the case of an autograft, the recipient who is genetically identical in regard to the donor MHC and all other loci, recognizes the donor's tissue as "self" and does not mount an immune response against it. The two individuals (i.e., donor and recipient) are described as histocompatible.
- An ***allograft*** is a graft or transplant from one individual to an MHC-disparate individual of the same species. Because of the high degree of MHC polymorphism within a given outbred species, this ***allogeneic*** transplant will result in rejection of the grafted foreign tissue. The donor and recipient, in this case, are nonhistocompatible or histoincompatible.
- A ***xenograft*** is a graft between a donor and a recipient from different species. The transplant is recognized as foreign, and the immune response mounted against it will destroy or reject the graft. Donor and recipient are again histoincompatible.

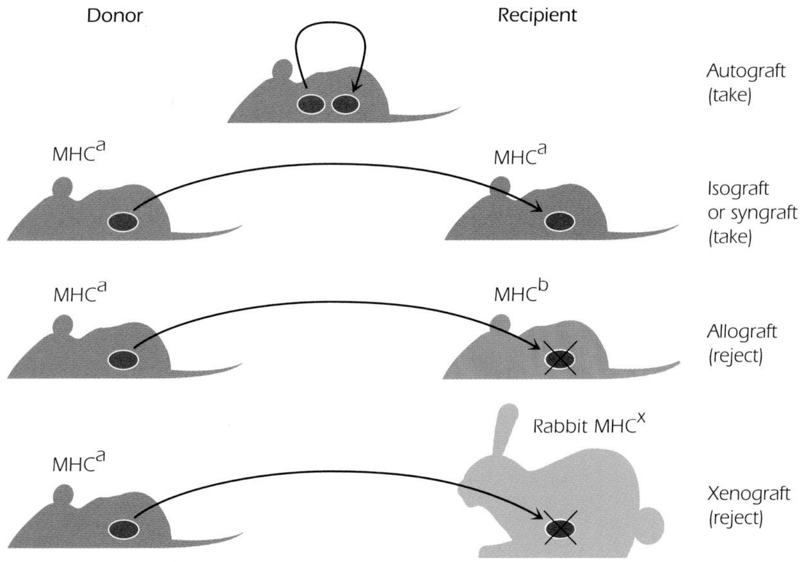

Figure 18.1. Situations of tissue transplantation.

IMMUNE MECHANISMS AND ALLOGRAFT REJECTION

The most direct evidence that an immune response is involved in graft rejection is provided by experiments in which skin is transplanted from one individual to a genetically different individual of the same species—namely, between allogeneic donor and recipient. Skin from a mouse with black hair transplanted onto the back of an MHC-disparate white-haired mouse appears normal for 1 to 2 weeks. However, after approximately 2 weeks, the skin allograft begins to be rejected and is completely sloughed off within a few days. This process is called ***first-set rejection.*** If, after this rejection, the recipient is transplanted with another piece of skin from the same initial donor, the graft is rejected within 6–8 days. This accelerated rejection is termed a ***second-set rejection.*** By contrast, grafting skin from a different MHC-disparate mouse strain will result in rejection at a rate similar to that of the initial graft—with so-called ***first-set kinetics.*** Thus second-set rejection is an expression of specific immunologic memory for antigens expressed by the graft. The participation of $CD4^+$ and $CD8^+$ T cells in the rejection response can be shown by transferring these cells from an individual sensitized to an allograft into a normal syngeneic recipient. If the second recipient is transplanted with the same allograft that was used on the original T cell donor, a second-set rejection ensues. This establishes that T cells primed in the initial grafting mediate the accelerated rejection in the second host. However, antibodies can also contribute to the destruction of grafted tissue in second-set rejection.

Many other lines of evidence establish the immunologic nature of graft rejection. For example, (1) histologic examination of the site of the rejection reveals lymphocytic and monocytic cellular infiltration reminiscent of the delayed-type hypersensitivity (DTH) reaction (see Chapter 16); both $CD4^+$ and $CD8^+$ cells are present at the site, and (as we shall see later) both play a crucial role in graft rejection. (2) Animals that lack T lymphocytes (such as athymic, or *nude,* mice or humans with DiGeorge syndrome; see Chapter 17) do not reject allografts or xenografts. (3) The process of rejection slows down considerably or does not occur at all in immunosuppressed individuals. It has also been demonstrated that in a normal individual, T cells are primed and circulating antibodies are induced to the antigens expressed by an allograft or a xenograft.

RESPONSES TO ALLOANTIGENS AND ALLOGRAFT REJECTION

Clinically, allograft rejections fall into three major categories: ***hyperacute rejection, acute rejection,*** and ***chronic rejection.*** The following are descriptions of the rejection reactions as might be observed, for example, after transplantation of a kidney; they also apply for rejection of other tissues.

Hyperacute Rejection

Hyperacute rejection occurs within a few minutes to a few hours of transplantation. It is a result of destruction of the transplant by so-called ***preformed antibodies*** to incompatible MHC antigens and, in some cases, to carbohydrates expressed on transplanted tissues (e.g., on endothelial cells). Such antibodies have been produced in the recipient before transplant. In some cases, these preformed antibodies are generated as a result of previous transplantations, blood transfusions, or pregnancies. These cytotoxic antibodies activate the complement system, followed by platelet activation and deposition, causing swelling and interstitial hemorrhage in the transplanted tissue, which decrease the flow of blood through the tissue. Thrombosis with endothelial injury and fibrinoid necrosis is often seen in cases of hyperacute rejection. The recipient may have fever and leukocytosis and produce little or no urine. The urine may contain various cellular elements, such as erythrocytes. Cell-mediated immunity is not involved at all in hyperacute rejection.

Acute Rejection

Acute rejection is seen in a recipient who has not previously been sensitized to the transplant. This form of rejection is mediated by T cells, and it is believed that it is the result of their direct recognition of alloantigens expressed by the donor cells (as discussed in more detail later in this chapter). It is the common type of rejection experienced by individuals for whom the transplanted tissue is a mismatch or who receive an allograft and insufficient immunosuppressive treatment to prevent rejection. For example, an acute rejection reaction may begin a few days after transplantation of a kidney, with a complete loss of kidney function within 10–14 days. Acute rejection of a kidney is accompanied by a rapid decrease in renal function. Enlargement and tenderness of the grafted kidney, a rise in serum creatinine level, a fall in urine output, decreased renal blood flow, and presence of blood cells and proteins in the urine are characteristic. Histologically, ***cell-mediated immunity,*** manifested by intense infiltration of lymphocytes and macrophages, is taking place at the rejection site. The acute rejection reaction may be reduced by immunosuppressive therapy, for example, with corticosteroids, cyclosporine, and other drugs, as we shall see later in this chapter.

Chronic Rejection

Chronic rejection caused by both antibody and cell-mediated immunity occurs in allograft transplantation months or years after the transplanted tissue has assumed its normal function. In cases of kidney transplantation, chronic rejection is characterized by slow, progressive renal failure. Histologically, the chronic reaction is accompanied by cell-mediated inflammatory lesions of the small arteries, thickening of the glomerular basement membrane, and interstitial fibrosis. Because the damage caused by immune injury has already taken place, immunosuppressive therapy at this point is useless, and little can be done to save the graft.

While the preceding example is for kidney transplantation, it is important to point out that the rate, extent, and underlying mechanisms of rejection may vary, depending on the transplanted tissue and site of the transplanted graft. The recipient's circulation, lymphatic drainage, expression of MHC antigens on the graft, and several other factors determine the rejection rate. For example, bone marrow and skin grafts are very sensitive to rejection compared to heart, kidney, and liver grafts.

ROLE OF MHC MOLECULES IN ALLOGRAFT REJECTION

Antigens that evoke an immune response associated with graft rejection are sometimes referred to as ***transplantation antigens,*** or ***histocompatibility antigens.*** Indeed, the MHC was so-named because of its central role in graft rejection. Why do these molecules serve as the major antigenic targets for the T cells that are ultimately responsible for graft rejection? There are at least two reasons for this: As discussed in Chapter 9, gene products of the MHC are cell-surface proteins. All nucleated cells express MHC class I molecules whereas class II molecules are normally expressed only on a subset of hematopoietic cells and by thymic stromal cells. Other cell types may also be induced to express MHC class II following their exposure to the proinflammatory cytokine, interferon γ (IFN-γ). In an organ transplantation scenario in which donor and recipient are MHC disparate (allogeneic), the immune response will be directed predominantly against foreign MHC class I antigens expressed on the cells in the grafted tissue. Furthermore, foreign MHC molecules activate an enormous number of T cell clones in the recipient. It is estimated that up to 5% of all T cell clones in the body may be activated in response to alloantigen activation, orders of magnitude higher than the response to a other antigens. The combination of non-self MHC molecule and bound peptides cross-reacts with T cell receptors (TCRs) expressed on many different T cell clones. Other mechanisms, discussed below, also contribute to how alloantigens on the transplant are presented to the recipient's T cells.

Mechanisms of Alloantigen Recognition by T Cells

As we discussed in Chapters 8 and 9, the specificity of T cells is normally restricted by self-MHC, the allelic specificity seen in the thymus during T cell differentiation. Thus the exposure of an individual to non-self MHC molecules expressed on the graft represents an artificial but clinically relevant situation.

There are two mechanisms of alloantigen recognition by T cells: ***direct*** and ***indirect.*** When T cells are exposed to foreign cells expressing non-self MHC (class I or class II), many clones are "tricked" into activation because their TCRs bind to (ligate) the foreign MHC–peptide complex being presented. This direct mechanism is presumably due to the recognition of foreign MHC and bound, donor-derived peptides that produce a structure that has functional cross-reactivity with the self MHC–peptide combination to which these clones would normally respond. Why are these donor cells expressing MHC bound to donor-derived peptides? It is important to recall from our discussion of MHC structure and function in Chapters 9 and 10 that MHC molecules can, and do, normally bind to self-peptides. Self-proteins are routinely digested within cytosolic organelles called proteosomes, and peptides are delivered to the endoplasmic reticulum where they can bind to MHC class I molecules. Such MHC-self peptide complexes are believed to stabilize the structure of the MHC molecules and are of no consequence when expressed on the surface of cells in a normal individual, since there is tolerance to self-peptides. However, when such peptides are presented by donor cells (acting as antigen-presenting cells; APCs) to T cells of the recipient, they are recognized as foreign. Thus these T cells are reacting directly to the donor APCs expressing allogeneic MHC in combination with peptide. In addition, these donor APCs also have co-stimulatory activity needed to generate the second signal required for T cell activation. It is now known that a major source of the donor-derived peptides presented in this fashion are the so-called ***minor histocompatibility antigens*** (minor H antigens).

Minor H antigens are encoded by genes outside the MHC. Differences in the polymorphic minor H antigens evoke less potent immune responses compared to differences in the MHC. Minor H antigens are peptides of donor origin derived from polymorphic cellular proteins presented by MHC class I molecules on the graft. Responses to minor H antigens are generally mediated by $CD8^+$ T cells, because they are presented by MHC class I molecules. As we will discuss later in this chapter, minor H antigens appear to be important in bone marrow transplantation and have been implicated in graft versus host (GVH) disease (discussed later in this chapter) in cases of human leukocyte antigen (HLA)-matched bone marrow transplantations.

The second mechanism of alloantigen recognition by T cells (indirect) involves the APCs of the recipient. When these APCs encounter the graft, they take up the alloantigenic proteins, process these molecules, present the resulting peptides on self (recipient) MHC molecules to allopeptide-specific T cells, and activate them. Thus alloactivation of recipient T cells can be direct, via recognition of foreign MHC antigens expressed by donor cells, or indirect, via recognition of donor-derived cellular peptides (minor H antigens) bound to MHC antigens expressed by these cells (Fig. 18.2).

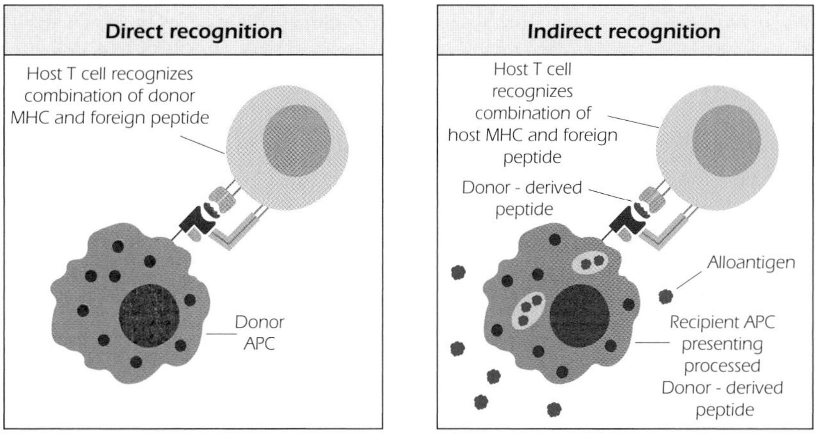

Figure 18.2. Direct and indirect recognition of alloantigens in grafted organs and tissues.

The relative contribution of these two mechanisms to graft rejection is not known. ***Direct alloactivation*** is believed to be of importance in acute rejection of grafts, as discussed earlier in this chapter. The destruction of donor cells, in this case, is therefore directly mediated by T cells. In contrast, ***indirect alloactivation*** of T cells generates a response that also involves activation of macrophages, which cause tissue damage and fibrosis. Moreover, such activation leads to the development of cytotoxic alloantibody responses, which may also play a role in the destruction of the graft.

Role of Cytokines in Allograft Rejection

Alloactivation of T cells activates the immune response by triggering both $CD4^+$ and $CD8^+$ cells. As a result, cytokines are synthesized largely by activated $CD4^+$T cell clones, and alloreactive cytotoxic T cells are activated. The most important cytokines generated are during these responses are interleukin-2 (IL-2), IFN-α, IFN-β, and IFN-γ, tumor necrosis factor-α (TNFα), and TNFβ. IL-2 is important for T cell proliferation, and for differentiation of cytotoxic T lymphocytes (CTLs), and T_H1 cells participating in the delayed-type hypersensitivity (DTH) reactions associated with allograft rejection (see Chapter 16). IFN-γ is important for the activation of macrophages that migrate to the graft area, causing tissue damage, and TNFβ is cytotoxic to the graft. Moreover, IFN-α, IFN-β, as well as TNFβ and TNFα increase the expression of MHC class I molecules, while IFN-γ increases the expression of MHC class II molecules on allograft cells, thus increasing the effectiveness of antigen recognition and enhancing graft rejection.

LABORATORY TESTS USED IN TISSUE TYPING

To minimize the risks of graft rejection, laboratory tests are performed before transplantation to phenotype the MHC of both the donor and the recipient (cross-matching). These tests are often referred to as ***tissue typing.*** Tissue typing consists of the analysis of histocompatibility antigens (HLA in humans) and allows a determination of the degree of foreignness between the two individuals, thus serving to predict the outcome of a transplant procedure. With the advent of more efficacious immunosuppressive drugs and modalities, matching donor and recipient by the similarity of their HLA antigens is becoming less and less essential. Nevertheless in many instances (e.g., bone marrow transplantation), HLA analyses are critical to minimize graft rejection or, in the case of bone marrow transplantation, the chances for development of graft versus host disease (see below).

There are several ways to determine the degree of MHC parity or disparity between donor and recipient. These are discussed below and include serologic and genotyping methods as well as functional assays (mixed leukocyte reactions) to measure the recipient's T cell proliferative responses to donor alloantigens (or, in the case of bone marrow transplants, the response of donor T cells to the recipient's alloantigens).

Serologic Detection of MHC Antigens

A panel of antibodies (HLA-specific antisera or monoclonal antibodies) is often used to determine the phenotype of the MHC antigens expressed on cells. The antisera are sometimes obtained from people who have had multiple transplantations or transfusions and from multiparous (multiple birth) women. These antibodies can be used in a variety of phenotyping assays, including immunofluorescence staining and fluorescene-activated cell sorting (FACS) analysis (see Chapter 5) or the ***lymphocytotoxicity test.*** In this test, MHC-specific antibodies, in the presence of complement, are used as cytotoxic, complement-fixing antibodies to determine their ability to damage the target cells, which are lymphocytes. Thus lymphocytes of the donor and recipient are reacted with a panel of antibodies with specificity for a wide range of MHC class I and class II alleles (e.g., HLA-A1, HLA-DRB1). Complement-mediated killing (lymphocytotoxicity) of such cells indicates that the test antibody has reacted with the cell-surface MHC, thus the cells are positive for that MHC allele.

Serologic tissue typing provides a fairly reliable measure of parity (or disparity) between MHC antigens of the donor and the recipient. However, because the number of antisera available for such tests is finite, there is always the possibility that, although the panel of sera shows a "match," differences would be found if the panel of antisera were enlarged or if polymerase chain reaction (PCR) based genotyping assays were used, as discussed below.

Genotyping of MHC

Molecular approaches to tissue typing are now used routinely in tissue-typing laboratories. DNA segments are amplified by PCR to obtain DNA quantities that afford sequencing oligonucleotides and sequence comparison. Genetic variation in the PCR-amplified DNA can then be detected in a number of ways, including restriction fragment length polymorphism (RFLP), PCR fingerprinting, sequence analysis, allele-specific oligonucleotide typing, and PCR sequence-specific primer typing. These highly sensitive methods are far more accurate than serologic typing, because they can detect differences on the level of a single amino acid. Indeed, typing at the genomic level has shown differences in instances where a *complete* match has been shown by serologic means.

Mixed Leukocyte Reactions

In the ***mixed leukocyte reaction*** (MLR), leukocytes from donor and recipient are cultured together for several days. Donor T cells respond to allo-MHC antigens expressed on the recipient cells and are stimulated to produce cytokines and proliferate in the presence of these antigens (Table 18.2). The same is true for recipient leukocytes, which will proliferate in the presence of alloantigens on the donor cells. The proliferation is usually measured by introducing a radioactively labeled precursor to DNA (e.g. radiolabeled thymidine) into the culture. The greater the extent of proliferation, the more DNA is synthesized by the proliferating cells and the more radioactivity is incorporated into the cells' DNA.

In most cases, it is essential to ascertain whether the recipient lymphocytes will react against the donor histocompatibility antigens (rather than whether the donor lymphocytes will react against the recipient alloantigens). For this purpose, an MLR is set up as a "one-way MLR" in which the donor cells have been treated with mitomycin C or X-irradiation to prevent their proliferation. In this way, the only cells with the ability to proliferate are the recipient T cells. Under these conditions, recipient $CD4^+$ T cells will proliferate when stimulated with foreign MHC class II molecules. This response will lead to the production of cytokines, which help activate alloreactive cytotoxic $CD8^+$ T cells. The functional activity of such cells can subsequently be measured in CTL assay cells (see Chapters 5 and 10).

Although MLR testing for histocompatibility is a highly effective indicator of the degree of parity between donor and recipient, it is a lengthy procedure and requires several days, whereas the serologic and molecular typing methods take less than a day to perform. Thus, while transplantation of cells, tissues, or organs from a living donor can await the results of the MLR test, sufficient time for this test may not be available in cases of organs obtained from recent cadavers. This is one reason why organ banks are set up to select the best-matched recipient when an organ becomes available.

As has been pointed out earlier, tissue or organ transplantation is relying more and more on immunosuppressive agents to prolong graft survival and less and less on tissue typing. In fact, recent results comparing graft survival with immunosuppressive agents show that, depending on the transplanted

TABLE 18.2. Cases of Mixed Lymphocyte Reaction Associated with Different Transplantation Situations

Transplantation Situation	HLA Relationship	Treatment of Reacting Leukocytes	MLR
Tissue between identical twins	HLA identical (syngeneic)	No treatment	(−) No reaction
Tissue between nonrelated donor and recipient	HLA different (allogeneic)	No treatment	(+) Reaction intensity depends on the degree of HLA difference between donor and recipient
Tissue between nonrelated donor and recipient	HLA different (allogeneic)	Donor's cells are treated with a mitotic inhibitor, thus testing reactivity of only recipient cells (performed to test for donor-recipient match)	(+) This is a one-way MLR; reaction intensity depends on the degree of HLA difference between donor and recipient
Bone marrow transplantation, or tissue grafting to an immunoincompetent recipient	HLA different (allogeneic)	Recipient's cells are treated with a mitotic inhibitor, thus testing reactivity of only donor's cells (performed to avoid GVH reaction)	(+) This is a one-way MLR; reaction intensity depends on the degree of HLA difference between donor and recipient

tissue, there is little difference in graft survival regardless of whether tissue typing or cross-matching indicated a match between donor and recipient, as long as an effective immunosuppressive regimen is used.

PROLONGATION OF ALLOGRAFT SURVIVAL

A major clinical issue in transplantation immunology is to determine how the components and regulatory interactions involved in graft rejection might be manipulated to allow allograft (or xenograft) acceptance. Nonspecific approaches using immunosuppressive drugs that reduce the overall immunocompenence of the recipient to all foreign antigens have been used with success to achieve this goal. However, given the need to treat patients chronically with these drugs to maintain the immunosuppressed state, such individuals are predisposed to opportunistic infections as well as malignancies. Accordingly, chemoprophylaxis using antimicrobial drugs is used in patients undergoing nonspecific, generalized immune suppression to help reduce the incidence of infections. The potential malignancy problem is one that cannot be addressed prophylactically.

More recently, experimental strategies that seek to prevent responses only to the antigens of a particular donor have been investigated. The ultimate goal of this approach is to achieve tolerance, which is lasting and ensures donor-specific nonresponsiveness. As discussed in Chapter 12, there are several mechanisms by which T cell and B cell tolerance to self-antigens is achieved. These include clonal deletion, anergy, and suppression. Although clinical trials have begun in which tolerance-inducing strategies are combined with conventional immunosuppressive therapies (discussed below), none of these strategies have been used to replace such chronic therapy in clinical transplantation.

Several of the standard and experimental immunosuppressive agents used in transplantation cases are listed in Table 18.3 and discussed below. Commonly, they are used in various combinations with each other to prevent graft rejection in transplantation of heart, kidney, lungs, liver, and other organs and tissues.

TABLE 18.3. Immunosuppressive Drugs Used in Transplantation

Inhibitors of lymphocyte gene expression	Corticosteroids Cyclosporine (Neoral) FK-506
Inhibitors of cytokine signal transduction	Anti-CD25 Rapamycin Leflunomide
Inhibitors of nucleotide synthesis	Azathioprine (Imuran) Mercaptopurine Chlorambucil Cyclophosphamide

Anti-inflammatory Agents

Corticosteroids, such as ***prednisone, prednisolone,*** and ***methylprednisolone,*** are powerful anti-inflammatory agents. As pharmacologic derivatives of the glucocorticoid family of steroid hormones, their physiologic effects result from their binding to intracellular steroid receptors that are expressed on almost every cell of the body. The immunosuppressive action of corticosteroids is due to several effects, most of which are a consequence of corticosteroid-induced regulation of gene transcription. Corticosteroids downregulate the expression of several genes that code for inflammatory cytokines, including IL-1, IL-2, IL-3, IL-4, IL-5, IL-8, TNFα, and granulocyte-macrophage colony-stimulating factor (GM-CSF). Cortocosteroids also inhibit expression of adhesion molecules, causing inhibition of leukocyte migration to sites of inflammation. Therefore, they inhibit the activity of inflammatory cells. In addition, they promote the release of cellular endonucleases, leading to the induction of apoptosis in lymphocytes and eosinophils. Moreover, they reduce phagocytosis and killing by neutrophils and macrophages and reduce expression of MHC class II molecules. In this way, cortocosteroids inhibit T cell activation and function.

It is important to acknowledge that despite these beneficial anti-inflammatory effects, corticosteroids also have potent toxic effects, including fluid retention, weight gain, diabetes, thinning of the skin, and bone loss. Therefore, the efficacy of corticosteroids in the control of disease involves the judicious use of these agents to strike a careful balance between their beneficial and toxic effects. As will be discussed below, given the growing arsenal of immunosuppressive therapies, corticosteroids are often used in combination with other panimmunosuppressive agents in an effort to keep the dose and toxic side effects to a minimum.

Cytotoxic Drugs

Antimetabolites that suppress immune responses include the purine antagonists ***azathioprine, mercaptopurine,*** and ***mycophenolate mofetil,*** which interfere with the synthesis of RNA and DNA by inhibiting inosinic acid, the precursor for the purines adenylic and guandylic acids. ***Chlorambucil*** and ***cyclophosphamide,*** compounds that alkylate DNA, also interfere with the metabolism of DNA. These agents were originally developed to treat cancer. The observation that they are also cytotoxic to lymphocytes led to their use as immunosuppressive therapeutic agents. As expected, however, they have a range of toxic effects, since they interfere with DNA synthesis in many tissues in the body. Consequently, in addition to their immunosuppressive activity, they can also cause anemia, leukopenia, thrombocytopenia, intestinal damage, and hair loss. Indeed, fatal reactions to these cytotoxic drugs have also been reported. As noted above, the availability of other immunosuppressive agents allows them to be used in combination therapies at lower, less toxic doses.

Agents that Interfere with Cytokine Production and Signaling

Several agents that interfere with cytokine activity (cytokine production or cytokine-mediated signaling) are commonly used as supplements to immunosuppressive antimetabolite and cytotoxic drugs and include ***cyclosporine, FK-506*** (tacrolimus), and ***rapamycin*** (sirolimus). They exert their pharmacologic effects by binding to immunophilins, a family of intracellular proteins involved with lymphocyte signaling pathways. Upon binding to immunophilins, these agents interfere with signal-transduction pathways needed for clonal expansion of lymphocytes.

Cyclosporine A (also referred to as cyclosporine) is a compound that is widely used for immunosuppression during allotransplantation. In many instances, enhancement in survival of an allograft between unmatched donor and recipient was almost as effective in cyclosporine-treated patients as when transplantation was performed between matched individuals. Cyclosporine is a cyclic peptide derived from a soil fungus (*Tolypocladium inflatum*). It enhances graft survival by interfering with cytokine gene transcription in T cells. The complex of cyclosporine and its cytoplasmic receptor cyclophilin binds to and blocks the phosphatase activity of ***calcineurin,*** which is an intracellular signaling protein that is essential for transcriptional activation of the IL-2 gene. It also suppresses production of IL-4, and IFN-γ as well as the synthesis of IL-2 receptors (CD25). In addition, it is known to induce the synthesis of TGFβ, a cytokine that has immunosuppressive activity. Cyclosporine is effective when administered before transplantation but is ineffective in suppressing ongoing rejection. Evidence indicates cyclosporine is nephrotoxic and is also associated with an increased risk of cancer in patients who take this drug long-term. It has been suggested that these and other side effects are largely due to the TGFβ-inducing property of cyclosporine.

FK-506 (tacrolimus) is also widely used to treat transplant patients. It is a macrolide compound obtained from the filamentous bacterium *Streptomyces tsukabaenis.* Macrolides are compounds that have a multimembered lactone ring to which is attached one or more deoxy sugars. Although its structure is considerably different from that of cyclosporine, its biologic and immunosuppressive activities are similar. Like cyclosporine, its affect is on T cell activation by blocking calcineurin activity and the accompanying cytokine production.

Rapamycin (sirolimus) is another macrolide compound and is derived from the bacterium *Streptomyces hygroscopicus.* Like cyclosporin and FK-506, it inhibits T cell activation, but it does so using a different pharmacologic mechanism. Unlike cyclosporin and FK-506, which block calcineurin activity, rapamycin inhibits T cell activation by blocking signal transduction mediated by IL-2 and other cytokines not by inhibiting IL-2 production.

Immunosuppressive Antibody Therapy

Antilymphocyte antibody preparations, such as horse antilymphocyte and rabbit antithymocyte globulin (ATG), have been used as adjuncts to standard immunosuppressive therapy for many years. While this therapeutic approach can effectively remove unwanted lymphocytes, treatment of humans with large amounts of foreign protein has the disadvantage of inducing a serum sickness caused by the formation of immune complexes (see Chapter 15). Nevertheless, ATG is still used today to treat acute graft rejection. Clearly, the challenge for those attempting to develop new antibody-based therapies for transplant patients is to develop less immunogenic antibodies while maintaining their targeted effects. To this end, monoclonal antibodies and engineered mouse–human chimeric antibodies or humanized antibodies are being used (see Chapter 5 for a discussion about these antibodies). The first mouse monoclonal antibody to be used as an immunosuppressive agent in humans was OKT3 which is directed against CD3 expressed on T cells. More recently, two chimeric antibodies (Daclizamab and Basiliximab) with specificity for the IL-2 receptor α-chain (CD25) have been used. Their molecular effect downregulates expression of the IL-2 receptor on activated T cells—a phenomenon that interferes with the ability of T cells to proliferate in response to IL-2. The advent of engineered antibodies holds great promise in reducing the limitations of alloantibody therapy by minimizing the antigenicity of these proteins.

New Immunosuppressive Strategies

The use of antibodies to several other molecules important for T cell adhesion (e.g., anti-intercellular adhesion molecule 1; anti-ICAM-1) and T cell activation are currently under investigation. Among the latter category of T cell determinants, a humanized mouse antibody against human CD154 (also known as CD40 ligand) has recently been shown to prevent acute renal allograft rejection in nonhuman primates. Other target antigens include the co-stimulatory molecules B7.1 (CD80) and B7.2 (CD86). As discussed in Chapter 10, binding of B7.1 or B7.1 to CD28 initiates a cascade of T cell activation events. Conversely, binding of CTLA-4, an alternate ligand for these co-stimulatory molecules, delivers inhibitory signals to the responding T cells. As predicted, blocking CD28 ligation interferes with the transmission of signals needed for gene expression and T cell activation. Thus antibodies that interfere with co-stimulatory molecule-mediated

T cell activation may have efficacy in transplant patients. It should be noted that a related experimental approach uses the inhibitory ligand, CTLA-4, to suppress the function of these co-stimulatory molecules. In animal studies, injection of soluble CTLA-4 has been found to allow the long-term survival of certain grafted tissues. Evidence suggests that the mechanism responsible for the beneficial effect of CTLA-4 involves the blocking of co-stimulation of the T cells that recognize donor antigens, thus inducing a state of unresponsiveness (anergy).

It should be clear from the above that several experimental approaches are being taken with the hope of finding immunosuppressive agents that will be less toxic and will not leave the recipient highly susceptible to opportunistic infections in the absence of a fully competent immune response. However, it should be stated that with all the experimental approaches mentioned above the main agents that are most commonly used for clinical immunosuppression are corticosteroids, cyclosporin, FK506, and azathioprine.

BONE MARROW AND HEMATOPOIETIC STEM CELL TRANSPLANTATION

Attempts to use bone marrow cells of a healthy individual to restore the lost marrow function of an ill patient are at least 60 years old. Early attempts at human marrow transplantation were largely unsuccessful because the scientific basis for success was not yet known. Marrow transplantation as a form of treatment began to be explored scientifically at the end of World War II. Transplantation of bone marrow constitutes a special transplantation situation because it is performed mostly between an immunocompetent donor and an immunocompramised recipient. Usually these immunoincompetent patients have severe combined immunodeficiency (SCID), Wiskott-Aldrich syndrome (see Chapter 17), or advanced leukemia, and they receive bone marrow from identical siblings. Bone marrow transplantation is also being used to treat blood cell diseases such as thalassemia and sickle cell diseases, in which a mutant gene is inherited. The mutant gene expresses itself only in the blood-forming hematopoietic cells. In this sense, transplantation for these patients is a form of genetic therapy: The genetically abnormal blood-forming stem cells are replaced with normally functioning cells.

The ultimate goal of bone marrow transplantation is to restore or reconstitute normal hematopoiesis of the recipient by infusion with a rich source of hematopoietic stem cells—the pluripotential population responsible for production of all blood cells (red cells, phagocytes, and platelets) and immune cells (lymphocytes). Stem cells also circulate in the blood in very small numbers and various cytokines (colony-stimulating factors) are available that increase the numbers of stem cells both in the marrow and blood. Today, sufficient quantities of these stem cells for transplantation are recovered (sometimes following pretreatment of the donor with appropriate CSFs) by circulating large volumes of blood through a *hemapheresis* machine and skimming off a population of cells that contains stem cells. Therefore, peripheral blood is an increasingly frequent source of stem cells for transplantation. Thus *bone marrow transplantation* as a generic term for the procedure has been modified to mean blood or marrow transplantation, permitting the continued use of the familiar acronym, BMT. In many cases, the more specific term ***stem cell transplantation*** is now used. The two most common types of BMT are referred to as ***allogeneic*** and ***autologous*** stem cell transplantation. A more rare BMT scenario is one in which transplantation is performed between identical twins (syngeneic transplantation). Syngeneic stem cell transplantation is associated with a relatively low immunologic risk because of the genetic similarity between donor and recipient.

Autologous stem cell transplantation is an important therapy; although, strictly speaking, it is not transplantation but a technique of obtaining stem cells from blood or marrow and returning them to the same individual. Therefore, immunologic transplantation barriers do not exist. This procedure is commonly used to treat patients with hematologic malignancies such as leukemia, lymphoma, and myeloma. The stem cells are recovered from the bone marrow or blood and stored frozen (cryopreserved) while the patient is intensively treated with chemotherapy and/or irradiation to control the malignancy and to markedly decrease the malignant cells in marrow and blood. Finally, the autologous stem cells are infused into the patient so that blood cell production can be restored.

Allogeneic stem cell transplantation involves the use of donor cells obtained from bone marrow, blood, or from umbilical cord sources and placental blood where the concentration and growth of blood cell–forming stem cells is even greater than in the blood of adults. Unlike autologous stem cell transplantation in which there is no risk of immune reactivity to the infused cells, in allogeneic stem cell transplantation, two potential immune rejection outcomes may result: The donated stem cells may be rejected by the recipient (host versus graft disease) or an immune reaction by the donor's cells to MHC antigens of the recipient (graft versus host [GVH] disease; see below) may occur. When immunocompetent recipients are used, immune rejection by host T cells is usually prevented by intensive treatment of the recipient before the transplant to suppress the immune system. Such treatment is also performed in patients with malignancies to destroy the rapidly dividing cancer cells (induction therapy). Patients with immunodeficiency diseases (e.g., SCID) do not require such induction therapy since there is no risk of rejection by the host. To reduce this risk of GVH disease, T cells are rigorously eliminated from the donor cell population. This removal, which can be achieved by a number of methods (e.g., treatment with monoclonal anti-T cell antibodies and complement), widens the choice of bone marrow donors.

GRAFT VERSUS HOST REACTIONS

As noted above, transplantation of immunocompetent lymphocytes from a donor to a genetically different recipient can result in a reaction mounted by the grafted T cells against the recipient's MHC (and/or minor H) antigens. This ***graft versus host*** (GVH) reaction is particularly important in cases in which immunocompetent lymphoid cells are transplanted into individuals who are immunologically incompetent and, therefore, cannot reject the transplanted cells. This situation is best exemplified in cases where bone marrow cells are transferred into individuals with various immunodeficiency disorders or in cases of bone marrow transplantation into an immunosuppressed recipient. It is interesting that GVH disease may occur in bone marrow transplant recipients even if the donor and recipient are perfectly HLA-matched. This is probably due to differences in minor histocompatibility antigens of the recipient, which are recognized by donor T cells.

In experimental animals, a GVH reaction may lead to a wasting syndrome in the recipient; in humans, GVH reactions may produce splenomegaly (enlarged spleen), hepatomegaly, lymphadenopathy (enlarged lymph nodes), diarrhea, anemia, weight loss, and other disorders in which the underlying causes are inflammation and destruction of tissue. The GVH reaction is initiated by the transferred T lymphocytes from the donor, which recognize the recipient's MHC antigens (and minor H antigens) as foreign. Donor T cells thus become activated as in an allograft response. In GVH disease, however, most of the inflammatory cells that participate in the reaction and that are mainly responsible for destruction of tissue are host cells recruited to the site of the reaction by cytokines released by the donor's lymphocytes.

XENOGENEIC TRANSPLANTATION

It is estimated that >50,000 people who need organ transplants die each year while waiting for a compatible donor. To address the critical shortage of donated human organs for transplantation, studies are underway in the use of nonhuman organs. For ethical and practical reasons, species closely related to the human, such as the chimpanzee, have not been widely used. Attention has focused on the pig, some of whose organs are anatomically similar to the human. Interestingly, the human T cell response to xenogeneic MHC antigens is not as strong as to allogeneic MHC molecules.

The major problem with using pig organs, and organs from other species, in human recipients, however, is the potential for the existence of natural or preformed antibodies to carbohydrate moieties expressed on the graft's endothelial cells. As a consequence, the activation of the complement cascade occurs rapidly and hyperacute rejection ensues. Finally, another concern that has stimulated debate about the safe use of xenografts concerns the possibility that animal organs and tissues may harbor viruses that might infect humans. This fear is underscored by the possibility that the HIV pandemic may have been caused by the transmission of a virus from monkeys to humans. In the United States, the Centers for Disease Control and Prevention (CDC) and other public health agencies have drafted guidelines to monitor patients who receive xenografts using sensitive assays to detect viruses that may be present.

THE FETUS: A TOLERATED ALLOGRAFT

A puzzling phenomenon associated with allograft rejection is that the fetus, which expresses paternal histocompatibility antigens that are not expressed by the mother, is not rejected by the mother as an allograft. It is clear that the mother can mount an antibody response against fetal antigens, as exemplified by anti-Rh antibodies produced by Rh^- mothers. More important, women who experience multiple births have antibodies to the father's MHC. It appears, however, that in most cases the antibodies are harmless to the fetus, and what is important is the mother's ability or, rather, inability to respond with the production of cytotoxic T cells against the fetus. There is evidence that fetal trophoblast cells that constitute the outer layer of the placenta that come in contact with maternal tissue do not express polymorphic MHC class I or class II molecules but express only the nonpolymorphic MHC class Ib molecule, HLA-G. Thus the fetal trophoblast does not prime for a cellular immune response associated with allograft rejection. It has been suggested that the major function of HLA-G is to provide a ligand for the killer cell inhibitory receptors (KIRs) on maternal natural-killer (NK) cells, thus preventing them from killing the fetal cells (see Chapter 2). HLA-G is also expressed in thymic medullary epithelium, where it might ensure T cell tolerance to this molecule. Finally, no cells expressing large amounts of MHC class II molecules (e.g., dendritic cells) have been found in the placenta.

Other factors that affect the immune response and may be involved in the fetal–maternal relationship include cytokines, complement inhibitory proteins, and other as yet unknown factors. Another factor that appears to operate in the survival of the fetus, is α-fetoprotein, a protein synthesized in the yolk sac and fetal liver. α-Fetoprotein has been demonstrated to have immunosuppressive properties. All in all, the fetus and several other tissues in the body that do not initiate an immune response or are not affected by immune components are termed ***immunologically privileged sites.*** Overall, it appears that multiple factors are responsible for one of the most spectacular immunologically privileged sites: the fetus.

Increased knowledge of the immunologic mechanisms responsible for tolerance to the fetus might provide new insights for how we might induce tolerance to grafted cells, tissues, and organs.

HEART TRANSPLANTATION: A PERSONAL STORY

It is strictly coincidental and not associated with any deliberate pedagogic exercise that one of us (E.B.) has undergone a heart transplant, which is briefly described here.

The realization that one requires a heart transplant as a last resort comes as a shock, in spite of years of cardiomyopathy. Before being accepted into the transplant program at the University of California San Diego Medical Center, dozens of tests, some of which are uncomfortable and painful, had to be performed to ensure that a healthy heart would not be transplanted into a "sick" body or a body that may develop malignancies as a result of immunosuppression (e.g., intestinal polyps, which may become malignant).

Having undergone all the necessary tests and having been accepted into the program, the long wait for a suitable heart began. I was kept in the cardiac intensive care unit waiting for a blood group- and Rh-matched donor heart for 2 months. My awareness of time became blurred, and I nearly forgot why I was there and what I was waiting for. While some patients less moribund may wait at home until a suitable heart becomes available, the wait may range from a few days or weeks to many months. Not all patients survive the wait.

Finally, and rather unexpectedly, the transplant coordinator brought the good news: A suitable heart was available. This was one of the most emotional moments of the transplantation process. Despite all the rationalization that the donor did not die for my sake, the realization that the precious gift of the heart of someone who died tragically in a car accident would be transplanted into me was a very emotional experience.

In the hands of a very competent heart transplant surgeon, the surgical procedure is almost routine. Immediately before surgery, I was given a cocktail of immunosuppressive agents (cyclosporin, prednisone, and azathioprine) along with a host of antibiotics, antiviral and antifungal agents, and other medications to help prevent infections due to nonspecific immunosuppression that I, like all other organ allograft recipients, will continue to take for the rest of my life. The immunosuppressive agents have severe side effects, including nephrotoxicity, diabetes, and increased susceptibility to malignancies. The blood level of cyclosporine is routinely monitored and the side effects of other medications are evaluated periodically. The fact that I am capable of writing and retelling my story six years after transplantation testifies to their effectiveness.

It is hoped that in the future, more palatable and effective immunosuppressive agents will become available to make allotransplantation, or even xenotransplantation, less dangerous. We remain confident that with continued research in this arena, the hope for an even higher quality of life for patients following transplantation will become a reality.

SUMMARY

1. Alloreactive T cells (cell-mediated immunity) are principally responsible for allograft (and xenograft) rejection. Alloantigen-specific antibodies are responsible for hyperacute rejection, and they can also participate in other types of rejection.

2. The most important transplantation antigens, which cause rapid rejection of the allograft, are derived from the donor MHC, which is called HLA in humans and H-2 in mice. Genetic differences between donor and host can also result in allogeneic cellular peptides (minor H antigens) being presented by host MHC molecules to T cells. Reactions to these allogeneic proteins can also lead to graft rejection.

3. Two mechanisms for host T cell alloantigen recognition are known to exist: (1) direct recognition, in which donor APCs stimulate alloreactive T cells, and (2) indirect recognition, in which recipient APCs process and present allogeneic peptides derived from the donor organ or tissue.

4. The degree of histocompatibility between donor and recipient can be determined by serologic or, more commonly, molecular tissue typing and by the MLR.

5. Survival of allografts is prolonged using a cocktail of immunosuppressive agents, including antiinflammatory agents, cytotoxic agents, and antimetabolites and by using agents that interfere with IL-2 production and cytokine-mediated signaling. Newer modalities include the use of biologic agents that target costimulatory molecules associated with T cell activation.

6. The fetus is a natural allograft that is tolerated. Multiple factors appear to be involved in this form of tolerance, including the absence of MHC class I and II molecules on fetal trophoblast cells and the "absence" of MHC class II expression on placental cells.

REFERENCES

Armitage JO (1994): Bone marrow transplantation. *N Engl J Med* 330:827. Auchincloss H Jr, Sachs D (1998): Xenogeneic transplantation. *Annu Rev Immunol* 16:433.

Auchincloss H Jr, Sykes M, Sachs D (2003): Transplantation immunology. In Paul WE (ed): Fundamental Immunology, 5th ed. New York: Lippincott-Raven.

Beniaminovitz A, Itescu S, Lietz K, Donovan M, Burk EM, Groff BD, Edward N, Mancini DM: (2000) Prevention of rejection in cardiac transplantation by blockade of the interleukin-2 receptor with a monoclonal antibody. *N Engl J Med* 342:613.

Charenoud L (1998): Tolerogenic antibodies and fusion proteins to prevent graft rejection and treat autoimmunity. *Mol Med Today* 4:25.

Charlton B, Auchincloss H Jr, Fathman CG (1994): Mechanisms of transplantation tolerance. *Annu Rev Immunol* 12:707.

Ferrara JLM, Deeq HJ (1991): Graft versus host disease. *N Engl J Med* 324:667.

Garovoy MR, Stock P, Baumgardner G, Keith F. Linker C (1994): Transplantation. In Stites DP, Terr AI, Parslow TG (eds): Basic and Clinical Immunology, 8th ed. East Norwalk, CT: Appleton & Lange.

Hunt JS (1992): Immunobiology of pregnancy. *Curr Opin Immunol* 4:591.

Kirk, AD (1999): Treatment with humanized monoclonal antibody against CD154 prevents acute renal allograft rejection in nonhuman primates. *Nat Med* 5:686.

Lechler RI, Lombardi G, Batchelor JR, Reinsmoen N, Bach FH (1990): The molecular basis for alloreactivity. *Immunol Today* 11:83.

Roopenian DC (1992): What are the minor histocompatibility loci? A new look at an old question. *Immunol Today* 13:7.

Schreiber SL, Crabtree GR (1992): The mechanism of action of cyclosporin A and FK-506. *Immunol Today* 13:136.

Sherman LA, Chattopadhyay S (1994): The molecular basis of allorecognition. *Annu Rev Immunol* 11:385.

Suthanthiran M, Strom TB (1994): Renal transplantation. *N Engl J Med* 331:365.

Winkelstein A (1994): Immunosuppressive therapy. In Stites DP, Terr AI, Parslow TG (eds): Basic and Clinical Immunology, 8th ed. East Norwalk, CT: Appleton & Lange.

REVIEW QUESTIONS

For each question, choose the ONE BEST answer or completion.

1. Serologic tissue typing before kidney transplantation reveals that the leukocytes of a prospective recipient are killed by the following anti-HLA antibodies in the presence of complement: anti-B27, anti-A1, and anti-A3. Which of the following statements can be concluded from these results?

A) The prospective recipient expresses the B27, A1, and A3 HLA specificities.
B) The prospective recipient does not express the B27, A1, and A3 HLA specificities.
C) The potential donor and the prospective recipient are not siblings.
D) The potential donor and the prospective recipient are not identical twins.
E) The prospective recipient should not receive a kidney graft that expresses these HLA specificities.

2. In clinical transplantation, preformed cytotoxic antibodies reactive against MHC antigens expressed on the grafted tissue cause

A) chronic rejection.
B) hyperacute rejection.
C) acute rejection.
D) delayed-type hypersensitivity.
E) no serious problems.

3. The MHC contains all of the following except which?

A) genes that encode transplantation antigens
B) genes that encode immunoglobulins
C) genes that regulate immune responsiveness
D) genes that encode some components of complement
E) genes that encode class I and class II antigens

4. Which of the following statements regarding GVH disease is incorrect?

A) GVH can result from MHC differences between donor and recipient.
B) GVH requires immunocompetent donor cells.
C) GVH may result from infusion of blood products that contain viable lymphocytes into an immunologically incompetent recipient.
D) GVH requires natural killer cells.
E) GVH may occur in an immunosuppressed individual.

5. Graft rejection may involve

A) cell-mediated immunity.
B) type III (immune complex) hypersensitivity.
C) complement-dependent cytotoxicity.
D) the release of IFN-γ by alloreactive T_H1 cells.
E) All of the above.

6. Which of the following statements concerning the MLR is correct?

A) MLR results in clonal expansion of alloreactive B cells.
B) MLR results in clonal expansion of alloreactive T cells.
C) MLR between unrelated individuals who differ according to HLA serology is usually negative.
D) Stimulation of proliferation is controlled primarily by the HLA-A region alleles.
E) All of the above.

7. A clinical trial investigating the efficacy of a humanized anti-CD28 monoclonal antibody in prolonging kidney allograft survival shows that patients treated with this biologic reagent have significantly fewer episodes of chronic rejection. The probable mechanism responsible for this effect is best explained by
A) the binding of anti-CD28 to B cells, which blocks their interaction with B7.1 and B7.2 expressed on T cells.
B) the formation of circulating CD28-anti-CD28 immune complexes.
C) the binding of anti-CD28 to T cells, which interferes with signal transduction needed for T-cell activation.
D) the binding of anti-CD28 to suppressor T cells, which then become activated.
E) the binding of anti-CD28 to B and T cells, which interferes with signal transduction and activation of both populations.

CASE STUDY

A three-year-old boy is brought to the hospital suffering from an aplastic bone marrow after ingestion of benzene. All blood elements are at low levels, and death is imminent. The child and an older sibling were rapidly typed as both being RBC blood group antigen A^+ Rh^+, HLA-A3,7: B4,8, and bone marrow was transfused from the sibling to the younger brother. Within a few days, the patient's RBC count rose, indicating a successful take. However, 3 weeks later the child began to experience diarrhea and a skin rash on the palms and soles of the feet, spreading to the trunk. This was followed by jaundice and enlarged liver and spleen. Administration of an anti-CD3 monoclonal antibody plus cyclosporine produced some improvement. What went wrong, and why?

ANSWERS TO REVIEW QUESTIONS

1. ***A*** These findings are the results of a lymphocytotoxicity test. Killing of cells following incubation with MHC-specific antibodies and complement indicates the expression of the MHC antigens for which the antibodies are specific, in this case, MHC class I determinants B27, A1 and A3. The results tell us nothing about the relationship between the donor and recipient; therefore, C and D are incorrect. Answer E is incorrect because we have no information about the recipient's MHC antigens to guide such a decision.

2. ***B*** Hyperacute rejection is caused by preformed cytotoxic, complement-fixing antibodies that cause platelet activation and deposition, leading to swelling and hemorrhage in the transplanted tissue. This quickly leads to decrease in the flow of blood through the tissue and ultimate rejection of the graft. Choices A, C, and D are T cell–mediated, therefore, they are incorrect. Choice E is wrong for obvious reasons.

3. ***B*** The MHC complex contains all genes mentioned except genes that encode immunoglobulins. They are on different chromosomes.

4. ***D*** GVH disease is caused by the destruction of cells or tissue of an immunoincompetent recipient by immunocompetent lymphoid cells transferred from a histoincompatible donor. The GVH reaction does not require natural-killer cells.

5. ***E*** All are correct. The important process in the rejection of an allotransplant is cell-mediated immunity. Here, T cells, which recognize the alloantigens, become activated; the T cells release cytokines, one of which is IFN-γ, which recruits and activates phagocytic cells that, together with cytotoxic T cells, destroy the graft. However, the reaction to the allotransplant may also involve antibodies (IgM and IgG), which can cause damage to tissue via activation of complement and the recruitment of polymorphonuclear cells to the site of the reaction. The polymorphonuclear cells would damage the graft by the release of their lysosomal enzymes.

6. ***B*** The MLR results in the proliferation of alloreactive T cells that recognize foreign MHC antigens expressed on recipient cells used in the assay. Although clones of B cells may also expand, the major cellular expansion is that of the T cells. The MLR between unrelated individuals who differ according to HLA serology is usually positive (rather than negative). Thus only choice B is correct.

7. ***C*** Experimental models have demonstrated that injection of allografted mice with anti-CD28 monoclonal antibody does, indeed, prolong survival of the allograft. Blocking CD28 ligation interferes with the transmission of signals needed for gene expression (e.g., IL-2 synthesis) and T cell activation. B7.1 (CD80) and B7.2 (CD86) are costimulatory molecules that ligate CD28 expressed on APCs, leading to T cell activation.

ANSWER TO CASE STUDY

The symptoms are typical of GVH disease. The hasty matching presumably involved serologic typing only and matching for MHC class II molecules by PCR genotyping or by MLR was not done. In addition, care was not taken to deplete the donor bone marrow of mature T cells. Presumably, histoincompatibility between the donor and recipient triggered the donor's T cells to attack the recipient's cells, resulting in the clinical manifestations seen. Therapy aimed at destroying or inhibiting activated donor T cells is not as effective as eliminating them in the first place.

19

TUMOR IMMUNOLOGY

INTRODUCTION

Immune responses against tumor cells occur, in large part, due to expression of surface components of the malignant cell that are not expressed on the cell's normal counterpart and that give rise to structures that are antigenic. In 1943, Gross observed that when tumor cells were injected subcutaneously into syngeneic (histocompatible) mice, the cells formed nodules that grew for a few days and then regressed. When identical tumor cells were reinjected into the mice, they did not produce nodules or grow. These findings were interpreted to mean that the mice that rejected the tumor did so because they had generated an immune response to the tumor. Subsequently, ***tumor-specific transplantation antigens*** (TSTAs) or, as they are more commonly called, ***tumor antigens,*** have been demonstrated for many tumors in a variety of animal species, including humans.

The major focus of this chapter concerns the role of the immune system in tumor cell destruction. It is believed that throughout life, tumor cells are generated in normal individuals and then destroyed by normal immune effector mechanisms, without notice or consequence. Obviously, the immunologic mechanisms that thwart the threat of cancer by destroying the cancer-causing tumor cells are not always successful. The hope is that our growing knowledge of host effector mechanisms associated with immune surveillance will provide new insights into how we might prevent and better treat cancer. Thus the goals of the field of tumor immunology are (1) to elucidate the immunologic relationship between the host and the tumor, and (2) to use the immune response to tumors for the purpose of diagnosis, prophylaxis, and therapy. In this chapter we discuss various approaches to meeting these goals.

TUMOR ANTIGENS

Advances in immunologic and molecular biologic methodology have greatly facilitated the identification of tumor antigens capable of eliciting immune reactions. Before defining the different categories of tumor antigens, it is important to underscore the principle biologic mechanisms that may lead to the appearance of immunogenic tumor antigens, including ***mutation, gene activation,*** and ***clonal amplification.*** Like normal immune responses to foreign antigens, the immunogenic potential of tumor antigens is manifested when expression of these antigens stimulates immune effector mechanisms. The antigenic prerequisites that apply to foreign immunogens also apply to tumor antigens. As discussed in Chapter 3, a substance must possess the following characteristics in order to be immunogenic: (1) foreignness, (2) high molecular weight, (3) chemical complexity, and (4) degradability with the ability to interact with host MHC antigens. Immunogenic tumor antigens fulfill these criteria and thus have the potential to induce effector responses.

Some tumor antigens may consist of structures that are unique to the cancerous cells and are not present on their normal counterparts. Other tumor antigens may represent

Immunology: A Short Course, Fifth Edition, By Richard Coico, Geoffrey Sunshine, and Eli Benjamini
ISBN 0-471-22689-0 © 2003 John Wiley & Sons, Inc.

structures that are common to both malignant and normal cells but are masked on the normal cells and become unmasked on malignant cells. Still other antigens on tumor cells represent structures that are qualitatively not different from those found on normal cells but that are overexpressed—present at significantly increased levels on the cancer cell as products of cellular oncogenes. An example is the high levels of human epidermal growth factor receptor (HER) due to increased expression of the *HER-2/neu-1* oncogene (e.g., in certain breast and ovarian cancers) and the elevated *ras* oncogene products present on some human prostate cancer cells. Still other antigens on malignant cells represent structures that are present on fetal or embryonic cells but absent on normal adult cells. These latter antigens are referred to as ***oncofetal antigens.*** Normal genes that were previously silent may also be activated by carcinogens. It is generally assumed that unique tumor antigens on tumors induced by carcinogens are products of mutated genes with *hot spots* for mutations. There is little or no cross-reactivity among carcinogen-induced tumors. This absence of cross-reactivity is probably due to the random mutations induced by the chemical or physical carcinogens, leading to a large array of different antigens. For example, if the chemical carcinogen methylcholanthrene is applied in an identical manner to the skin of two genetically identical animals or on two similar sites on the same individual, the cells of the developing tumors (sarcomas) will exhibit antigens unique to each tumor, with no immunologic cross-reactivity between the tumors. As with chemically induced tumors, there is little or no cross-reactivity between physically induced tumors, such as those induced by ultraviolet light or by X-irradiation.

Carcinogens can also cause clonal amplification of single cells expressing a particular normal antigen and convert an otherwise nonimmunogenic molecule to an immunogenic antigen. The carcinogen-induced transformation event(s) that cause the emergence of such expanded clones most likely affects the genes that possess mutation-sensitive hot spots while sparing the genes responsible for other normal proteins. When these normal proteins are clonotypic (i.e., expressed only by single clones of cells), their expression is dramatically amplified, making them targets for immune responses, assuming tolerance can be broken. As an example, the idiotypes of antigen-specific receptors expressed by B or T cells may not be sufficient to elicit a response in the normal host but may serve as target antigens for tumor cells bearing the same idiotype.

Tumor antigens are particularly well demonstrated by ***virus-induced tumors*** which tend to show cross-reactivity among tumors induced by the same virus. Several members of the *Herpesvirus* family and retroviruses which infect but do not kill their target cells can stimulate uncontrolled growth of these infected cells. Specific examples of such ***oncogenic viruses*** are discussed later in this chapter.

The following two sections provide examples and overviews of the various categories of tumor antigens and the immune effector mechanisms that play a physiologic role in preventing tumor cell development. Our expanding knowledge of these areas of tumor immunology continues to facilitate the development of clinically useful tumor-specific immonotherapies.

CATEGORIES OF TUMOR ANTIGENS

Tumor antigens may be classified into several major categories (Table 19.1). The categories differ in both the factors that induce the malignancy and the immunochemical properties of the tumor antigens.

Normal Cellular Gene Products

Some tumor antigens are derived from normal genes that, under normal circumstances, are programmed to be expressed

TABLE 19.1. Categories of Tumor Antigens

Category		Type of Antigen	Name of Antigen	Types of Cancer
Normal cellular gene products	Embryonic	Oncofetal antigens	MAGE-1	Several
			MAGE-2	Several
			CEA	Lung, pancrease, breast, colon, stomach
			AFP	Liver, testis
	Differentiation	Normal intracellular enzymes	PSA	Prostate
			Tyrosinase	Melanoma
		Oncoprotein	HER-2/neu	Breast, ovary
		Carbohydrate	Lewis	Lymphoma
	Clonal amplification	Immunoglobulin idiotype	Specific antibody of B cell clone	Lymphoma
Mutant cellular gene products	Point mutations	Oncogene product	Mutant RAS proteins	Several
		Suppressor gene product	Mutant p53	Several
		CDK	Mutant CDK-4	Melanoma
Viral gene products	Transforming viral gene	Nuclear proteins	E6 and E7 proteins of HPV	Cervical

only during embryogenesis—namely, ***oncofetal antigens.*** Examples of these tumor antigens include the ***melanoma-associated antigen*** (MAGE) family of proteins, which are not expressed in any normal adult tissues except for the testes (an immunologically privileged site). MAGE antigens are candidate tumor vaccine antigens, because their expression is shared by many melanomas. Indeed, like many other tumor-associated antigens, the HLA restriction elements of the antigenic epitopes have been identified for MAGE-1. This information is being exploited in experiments aimed at developing immunogenic tumor peptide vaccines that can be presented by MHC class I antigens on antigen-presenting cells (APCs) to activate cytotoxic ($CD8^+$) T cell responses.

Other examples of oncofetal antigens include the ***carcinoembryonic antigen*** (CEA) and ***α-fetoprotein*** (αFP). CEA is found primarily in serum of patients with cancers of the gastrointestinal tract, especially cancer of the colon. Elevated levels of CEA have also been detected in the circulation of patients with some types of lung cancer, pancreatic cancer, and some types of breast and stomach cancer. However, it should be noted that elevated levels of CEA have also been detected in the circulation of patients with nonneoplastic diseases, such as emphysema, ulcerative colitis, and pancreatitis, as well as in the sera of alcoholics and heavy smokers. αFP is normally present at high concentrations in fetal and maternal serum but absent from serum of normal individuals. It is rapidly secreted by cells of a variety of cancers and is found particularly in patients with hepatomas and testicular teratocarcinomas.

Finally, amplified clones of malignant B or T cells that express antigen-specific receptors represent yet another example of how normal cellular gene products can be characterized as tumor antigens. The idiotype of the particular immunoglobulin or T cell receptor (TCR) expressed by the transformed B or T cell, respectively, effectively identifies that clone as a unique population of malignant cells.

Mutant Cellular Gene Products

The genetic origins of several unique tumor antigens that are products of mutated genes have been identified. In every case, the antigen was caused by a somatic mutation (i.e., by a genetic change absent from autologous normal DNA). Often, these mutations occur in genes that code for functionally important parts of the expressed protein. There are several well characterized examples of tumor antigens derived from mutant cellular gene products. ***Chronic myelogenous leukemia*** (CML) is characterized by the ***Philadelphia chromosome,*** a shortened chromosome 22 resulting from a reciprocal translocation between the *bcr* gene on chromosome 22 and the *abl* gene on chromosome 9 [t(9;22)]. The molecular equivalent of t(9;22) can be detected in virtually all cases of CML. It manifests with the expression of a *bcr/abl* fusion gene that encodes chimeric RNAs, which produces copious amounts of the *abl* gene tyrosine kinase activity. This chimeric gene product, at least in part, appears to be responsible for uncontrolled cell proliferation. Recently, clinical trials using a potent inhibitor of the *bcr/abl*-derived tyrosine kinase have shown promise for inducing complete hematologic responses in a sizable portion of patients with CML.

Another example of a mutant cellular gene product is seen in many cases of familial melanoma. This disease is associated with a mutation in ***cycline-dependent kinase 4*** (CDK-4), which reduces binding to its inhibitor (p16INK-4) and happens to be a ***tumor-suppressor protein.*** Yet another example of a tumor antigen that is generated as a result of a mutant cellular gene is the ***mutant p53 protein.*** The p53 mutation generates common conformational changes in p53a protein that normally acts as a suppressor of cellular growth. Mutations in p53 are among the most common seen in tumors of human and experimental animals. They typically occur in evolutionarily conserved regions of the p53 gene and result in overproduction of the protein, which then serves as an antigen for B and T cells. Antibody and T-cell responses are also seen when mutations occur in *ras* oncogene-encoded proteins. Mutant ras proteins, resulting from a glycine substitution at position 12 of ras, represent one of the most common mutations in human cancers.

The potential use of mutated proteins as immunologic targets for therapy is best illustrated by experimental evidence showing that tumor immunity in vivo can be induced by vaccination against mutant p53 peptides if given with interleukin-12 (IL-12). Because p53 is commonly expressed in cancer cells, T cells directed against normal p53 might preferentially destroy tumor cells. Furthermore, p53 knockout mice can be induced to generate cytotoxic T cells specific for normal p53 that, on adoptive transfer into p53 wild-type mice, can eradicate p53-overexpressing tumors without signs of autoimmunity to the host.

Tumor Antigens Encoded by Oncogenes

Although a full discussion of carcinogenesis is beyond the scope of this chapter, it is important to summarize the ***oncogene theory*** in order to better understand the properties of certain oncogene-derived proteins that can be tumor antigens. All retroviral oncogenes are known to have close relatives in the genomes of virtually all normal vertebrate cells called *c-onc* genes or ***proto-oncogenes.*** The gene products of proto-oncogenes have been identified as proteins with known functions in normal cells, including growth factor receptors and signal transducers. The oncogene theory postulates that such proto-oncogenes, when mutated or activated by other aberrant mechanisms, display increased expression or inappropriate expression of mutated forms of their gene products, thereby contributing to neoplastic transformation and the development of cancer. Oncogenes are aberrantly activated in somatic cells in many forms of human cancer, including carcinoma, sarcoma, leukemia, and lymphoma. The chief mechanisms of activation are chromosomal translocation, point mutation,

TABLE 19.2. Activation of Cellular Proto-Oncogenes in Human Cancers

Proto-Oncogene	Activation Mechanism	Chromosomal Change	Associated Cancer
c-*myc*	Genetic rearrangement	Translocation: 8-14. 8-2, or 8-22	Burkitt's lymphoma
c-*abl*	Genetic rearrangement	Translocation, 9-22	CML
c-*H-ras*	Point mutation		Bladder carcinoma
c-*K-ras*	Point mutation		Lung and colon carcinoma
N-*myc*	Gene amplification		Neuroblastoma

and gene amplification. Table 19.2 gives a partial list of the known proto-oncogenes and their associated cancers.

Animal studies have shown that tumors induced by oncogenic viruses exhibit extensive immunologic cross-reactivity. This is because any particular oncogenic virus induces the expression of the same antigens in a tumor, regardless of the tissue of origin or the animal species. For example, in animals, DNA viruses such as polyoma, SV40, and Shope papilloma virus induce tumors that exhibit extensive cross-reactivity within each virus group. Many leukemogenic viruses, such as Rauscher leukemia virus, induce the formation of tumors that exhibit cross-reactivity not only within each virus group but also between some groups. In this connection, there is considerable evidence to suggest that several human cancers are caused by viruses including ***Epstein-Barr virus*** (EBV) (Burkitts lymphoma and nasopharyngeal carcinoma), ***human T cell leukemia virus-1*** (HTLV-1) (adult T cell leukemia), and ***human papilloma virus*** (HPV) (hepatocarcinoma).

As might be expected, the viral proteins, which ultimately serve as unique tumor antigens, are expressed intracellularly as predominantly nuclear proteins. In order for cytotoxic T lymphocytes (CTLs) to recognize these antigens, they must be processed and presented as MHC-associated peptides. Studies using SV40-specific CTLs have confirmed that these cells can recognize processed fragments of proteins that are primarily located intracellularly. The unique tumor antigens of cells transformed by SV40 and several other viruses, including polyoma virus, adenovirus, and HPV, have been studied extensively and, in many cases, shown to be clearly related to the transformed phenotype and the establishment of malignancy. Such viruses have so-called early region genes, designated E1A/E1B and E6/E7, that are transcribed during early stages of viral replication and in transformed cells. Like other categories of tumor antigens, these proteins are candidate targets for therapy.

Immunologic Factors Influencing the Incidence of Cancer

In the late 1950s, a hypothesis emerged to help explain the primary reason for development of T cell–mediated immunity during the evolution of vertebrates. It was proposed that the main function of the T cell–mediated arm of the immune system was to provide specific defense against altered self or neoplastic cells. The term ***immune surveillance*** was coined to describe the concept of immunologic resistance against the development of cancer. We now know that T cell immunity is necessary for resistance to a variety of infections—most notably, viral infections. Animal studies as well as epidemiologic and immunologic studies of patients with various immunodeficiencies (primary, secondary, or acquired) have now provided evidence to support this hypothesis but only in regard to cancers associated with viruses or, in some cases, UV exposure. By contrast, most common forms of cancer are not increased in immunocompromised individuals. However, patients with immunodeficiency diseases are usually susceptible to viral infections and certain malignant neoplasms (Table 19.3). The apparent lack of immune surveillance of spontaneous cancers or those induced by carcinogens does not imply that such tumors are not antigenic. Indeed, there is

TABLE 19.3. Malignant Neoplasms with an Increased Incidence In Immunodeficiency Patients

Type of Immunodeficiency	Cancer	Associated Virus[a]
Primary (congenital)	Hepatocellular carcinoma	HBV
	B cell lymphoma	EBV
Secondary, drug induced	B cell lymphoma	EBV
	Squamous cell carcinoma (skin)	HPV
	Hepatocellular carcinoma	HBV
	Cervical carcinoma	HPV
AIDS	Cellular carcinoma	HBV
	Cloagenic or oral carcinoma	HPV
	B cell lymphoma	EBV

[a] *HBV,* hepatitis B virus; EBV, Epstein-Barr virus; HPV, human papilloma virus.

sufficient evidence to support the conclusion that these tumor cells, like those induced by viruses, are sensitive to immunologic destruction. Nevertheless, the natural development of immunologic responses usually fails to prevent cancer from developing. It is hoped that the successful manipulation of such responses (e.g., vaccination with tumor antigens) will serve as a viable option for the prevention or treatment of cancer in the future.

EFFECTOR MECHANISMS IN TUMOR IMMUNITY

Until recently, most of the information concerning antitumor immune effector mechanisms and their capacity to destroy tumor cells has been derived from experiments with transplantable tumors in animals or from in vitro experiments. There is now ample evidence to suggest that adaptive and innate immune responses play important roles in the relationship between the host and the tumor in humans as well.

Immune effector mechanisms that are potentially capable of destroying tumors in vitro are summarized in Table 19.4. In general, destruction of tumor cells by these mechanisms is more efficient in the case of dispersed tumors (i.e., when the target tumor cells are in single-cell suspension) than in the case of solid tumors, probably because dispersed cells are more accessible to the immune system.

B Cell Responses to Tumors

Both IgM and IgG antibodies have been shown to destroy tumor cells in vitro in the presence of complement. Several studies conducted with mice indicate that, in the presence of complement, antitumor antibodies are effective in vivo in destroying some leukemia and lymphoma cells and in reducing metastases in several other tumor systems. Other studies in vivo and in vitro, however, show that the same antibodies, in the presence of complement, are ineffective in destroying the cells of the same tumor in a solid form.

Destruction of Tumor Cells by Opsonization and Phagocytosis. Destruction of tumor cells by phagocytic cells has been demonstrated in vitro, but only in the presence of antitumor immune serum and complement. The relevance of this finding in vivo is unknown.

Antibody-Mediated Loss of Adhesive Properties of Tumor Cells. It appears that metastatic activity of certain kinds of tumors requires the adhesion of the tumor cells to each other and to the surrounding tissue. Antibodies directed against tumor cell surfaces may interfere with the adhesive properties of the tumor cells. The relevance of this mechanism in vivo is also unknown.

Cell-Mediated Responses: Direct Destruction of Tumor Cells by Cytotoxic T Lymphocytes

Destruction of tumor cells in vitro by specific immune T lymphocytes has been demonstrated numerous times for a variety of tumors, both dispersed and solid. Moreover, from many studies with experimental animals (primarily but not exclusively mice), there is good evidence that tumor-specific CTLs are responsible for destruction of virally induced tumors in vivo. Although $CD4^+$ T helper cells participate in the induction and regulation of cytotoxic T cells, the destruction of the tumor cell is achieved by the $CD8^+$ CTL with specificity for the antigens on the surface of the tumor cell.

Antibody-Dependent Cell-Mediated Cytotoxicity. Antibody-dependent cell-mediated cytotoxicity (ADCC) involves (1) the binding of tumor-specific antibodies to the surface of the tumor cells; (2) the interaction of various cells, such as granulocytes and macrophages, which possess surface receptors for the Fc region of the antibody attached to the tumor cell; and (3) the destruction of the tumor cells by substances that are released from these cells that carry receptors for the Fc region of the antibody. The importance of this mechanism in the destruction of tumor cells in vivo is still not clear.

TABLE 19.4. Effector Mechanisms in Cancer Immunity

Effector Mechanism	Comments
Antibodies and B cells (complement-mediated lysis, opsonization)	Role in tumor immunity poorly understood
T cells (cytolysis, apoptosis)	Critical for rejection of virally and chemically induced tumors
NK cells (cytolysis, ADCC, apoptosis)	Tumor cells not expressing one of the MHC class I alleles are effectively rejected by NK cells
LAK cells (cytolysis, apoptosis)	Antitumor responses seen in certain human cancers following adoptive transfer of LAK cells
Macrophages and neutrophils (cytostasis, cytolysis, phagocytosis)	Can be activated by bacterial products to destroy or inhibit tumor cell growth
Cytokines (apoptosis, recruitment of inflammatory cells)	Growth inhibition can occur using adoptively transferred tumor cells transfected with certain cytokines (e.g., GM-CSF)

Destruction of Tumor by Natural-Killer, Natural-Killer/T, and Lymphokine-Activated Killer Cells. Natural-killer (NK) cells are a distinct subpopulation of lymphocytes that, without prior sensitization and without MHC restriction, can kill certain tumor cells. Tumor cells that fail to express at least one of the MHC class I molecules are targets for NK cells (see Fig. 2.5). These cells can lyse a variety of target cells, such as virally infected cells, antibody-coated cells, undifferentiated cells, and cells from a number of different tumors. NK cells have receptors for the Fc region of IgG (CD16) and, as we saw in Chapter 4, can participate in ADCC. Like activated macrophages, NK cells secrete tumor necrosis factor-α (TNFα), which induces hemorrhage and tumor necrosis; however, the exact mechanism by which NK cells recognize and kill the tumor cells is still not clear. More recently, evidence has been obtained indicating that NK/T cells make up another innate immune cell population essential for tumor elimination in vivo (see Chapter 10).

Lymphokine-activated killer (LAK) cells are tumor-specific killer cells obtained from the patient. The cells are grown in vitro in the presence of IL-2 and then are adoptively transferred back to the same patient. LAK cells constitute a heterogeneous population of lymphocytes, which includes NK cells. However, their activity cannot be attributed solely to NK cells, since they can kill, in vitro, tumor cells that are not killed by NK cells. Although the natural biologic function of LAK cells is still obscure, they are now being tested for efficacy in tumor immunotherapy in humans (a topic discussed later in this chapter). A more recent innovation is the use of T cells isolated from the tumor and expanded and activated with IL-2. These tumor-infiltrating lymphocytes (TILs) show promise of greater specificity.

Destruction of Tumor Cells by Activated Macrophages and Neutrophils. Macrophages and neutrophils are generally not cytotoxic to tumor cells in vitro. They can be activated by bacterial products in vitro to cause selective cytostasis or cytolysis of malignant cells. Macrophages may also become highly cytotoxic (Figs. 19.1 and 19.2) when they are activated by cytokines, most notably interferon-γ (IFNγ) produced by an activated population of T lymphocytes, which, by themselves, are not cytotoxic. These CD4$^+$T cells are tumor-specific: They release IFNγ after activation by tumor antigen. Other cytokines released by these antigen-activated T lymphocytes attract macrophages to the area of the antigen. IFNγ also prevents migration of macrophages away from the antigen. The mechanism of activation of macrophages by T cells specific for tumor antigen, leading to destruction of tumor cells, is similar to mechanisms involved in delayed-type hypersensitivity (DTH) reactions in allograft rejection or in the killing of microorganisms: antigen-specific T cells become activated by antigen, and they release cytokines, which attract and activate macrophages. These activated macrophages are cytotoxic to the microorganism, to tumor cells, and even to "self" cells in the vicinity of the activated macrophages. The damaging and killing activity of activated macrophages is due to several products that they release, notably lysosomal enzymes and TNFα.

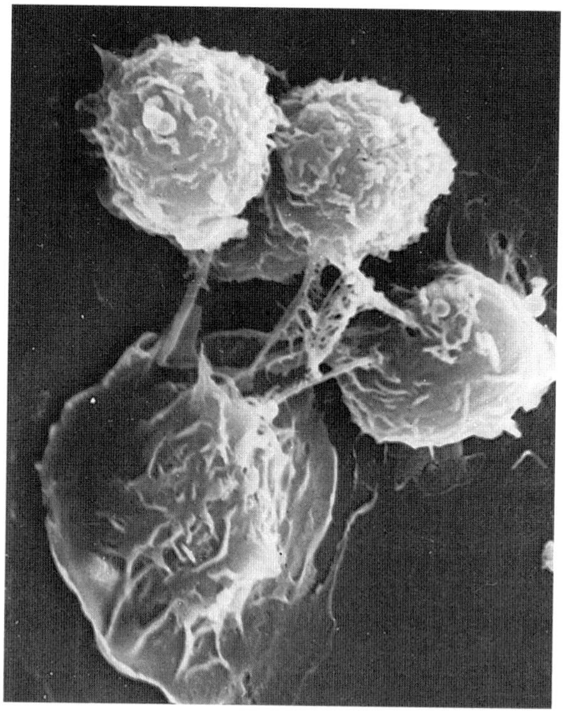

Figure 19.1. A scanning electron micrograph showing an activated macrophage with filopodia extending to the surface of three melanoma cells. $\times$4500. (Courtesy of K.L. Erickson, School of Medicine, University of California, Davis; reproduced with permission of Lippincott/Harper & Row).

Mounting evidence indicates that destruction of tumor cells by activated macrophages occurs in vivo. For example, resistance to a tumor can be abolished by specific depletion of macrophages. In addition, increased resistance to tumors accompanies an increase in the number of activated macrophages. Finally, activated macrophages are frequently found at the site of regression of a tumor. However, the relationship between the tumor and the tumor-associated macrophages is quite complex. On one hand, macrophages can and, indeed, do kill tumor cells. In addition, macrophages and tumor cells have been shown to produce reciprocal growth factors, leading to an almost symbiotic relationship. Thus changes in the delicate balance between macrophages and tumor cells may drastically affect the fate of the tumor.

Cytokines

As discussed above, cytokines can have a variety of ancillary functions that facilitate immune effector mechanisms in cancer immunity. It is important to note that, depending on the cytokines produced, immune effector mechanisms may be stimulated or inhibited. Consequently, the result may either be stimulation or inhibition of the growth of premalignant or malignant cells by acquired and/or innate immunity. The

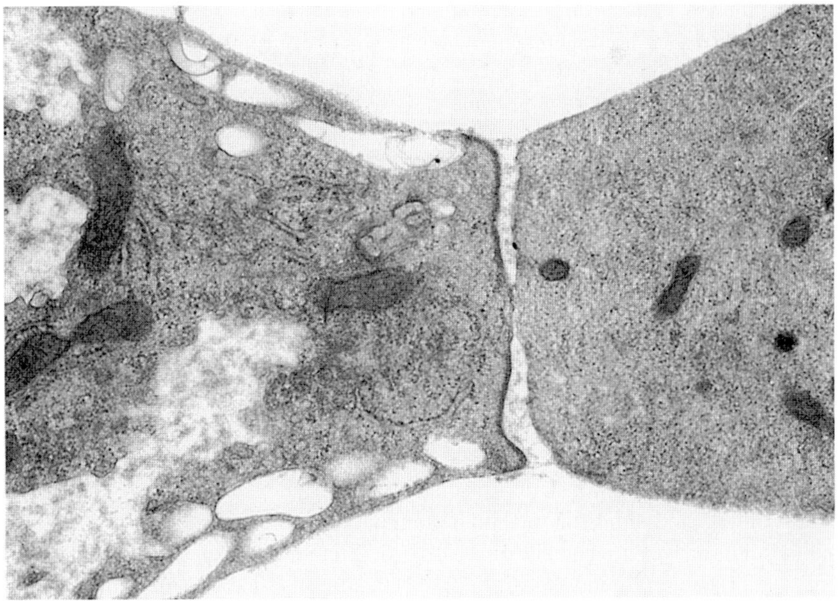

Figure 19.2. "The kiss of death." An electron micrograph showing a contact point between an activated macrophage (*left*) and a melanoma cell after 18 h of co-culture, leading to cytolysis of the melanoma target cell. Flocculent material is found between the cells; a dense plate is associated with the cell membranes of the macrophage process; microtubules also appear in these projections. ×26,000. (Courtesy of K.L. Erickson, School of Medicine, University of California, Davis; reproduced with permission of Lippincott/Harper & Row).

growth-promoting effects of cytokines is seen in the case of certain tumor cells that produce and respond to cytokines in an autocrine fashion. Similarly, production of transforming growth factor-β (TGFβ) by some tumor cells promotes tumor growth due to the angiogenic properties of this cytokine.

Cytokines such as TNF and IFNγ have antitumor effects because, among other functions, they upregulate MHC class I and class II MHC molecules on some tumor cells. Decreased expression of these MHC determinants allows tumor cells to evade the actions of cytotoxic T cells and NK cells. Cytokine upregulation of MHC molecules thereby facilitates important cell-mediated effector mechanisms. The effects of sustained high levels of certain cytokines have been studied using tumor cells transfected with cytokine genes. Transfection with genes coding for cytokines IL-1, IL-7, and IFNγ followed by adoptive transfer of such cells into tumor-bearing mice has been shown to significantly inhibit the growth of tumors.

LIMITATIONS OF THE EFFECTIVENESS OF THE IMMUNE RESPONSE AGAINST TUMORS

There is no question that an immune response can be induced against tumors. Why, then, in spite of the immune response, does the tumor continue to grow in the host? Several possible mechanisms may be operational either alone or in combination with each other. As shown in Table 19.5, tumor-related and host-related factors may influence the escape of tumor cells from destruction by the immune system. Tumor-related factors include those that relate to defective immunosensitivity and range from the lack of an antigenic epitope to resistance of tumor cells to tumoricidal effector pathways. Defective immunogenicity of the tumor may also account

TABLE 19.5. Mechanisms of Tumor Escape from Immunologic Destruction

Tumor-related	*Failure of the tumor to provide a suitable target* • Lack of antigenic epitope (tumor antigen) • Lack of MHC class I molecule • Deficient antigen processing by tumor cell • Antigenic modulation • Antigenic masking of the tumor • Resistance of tumor cell to tumoricidal effector pathway *Failure of the tumor to induce an effective immune response* • Lack of antigenic epitope • Decreased MHC or tumor antigen expression by the tumor • Lack of co-stimulatory signal • Production of inhibitory substances (e.g., cytokines) by the tumor • Shedding of tumor antigen and tolerance induction • Induction of T cell signaling defects by tumor burden
Host-related	*Failure of the host to respond to an antigenic tumor* • Immune suppression or deficiency of host, including apoptosis and signaling defects of T cells due to carcinogen (physical, chemical), infections, or age. • Deficient presentation of tumor antigens by host APCs • Failure of host effectors to reach the tumor (e.g., stromal barrier) • Failure of host to kill variant tumor cells because of immunodominant antigens on parental tumor cells

for a tumor's escape from immunologic destruction. Here, again, the lack of an antigenic epitope heads the list of possible mechanisms. Several other mechanisms, including lack of expression of co-stimulatory molecules by tumor cells and shedding of tumor antigens, and subsequent tolerance induction may also contribute to the failure of such cells to induce immune responses. Finally, the stromal environment is critical for preventing or permitting the immunologic destruction of tumor cells. Under certain circumstances, the stroma is the site for paracrine stimulatory loops that cause rapid malignant growth and thereby impede immunologic destruction.

Host-related mechanisms that promote the evasion of tumors from immunologic destruction are also summarized in Table 19.5. Immune suppression, deficient presentation of tumor antigens by APCs, and failure of host effectors to reach the tumor due to stromal barriers or the possible privileged-site setting of the tumor may facilitate immune evasion. Finally, studies have shown that expression of an immunodominant tumor antigen tends to prevent sensitization to other tumor antigens, thus preventing immune attack on variants.

Nonspecific suppression mediated by tumor cells can also allow tumors to escape from immunologic destruction. Certain types of tumors synthesize various compounds, such as prostaglandins, which reduce many aspects of immune responsiveness. However, the role of this mechanism in the escape of tumors from destruction by the immune response is still unclear.

Finally, the immune response and its various components have a finite capacity for the effective destruction of tumors (or, for that matter, of invading microorganisms). Thus, while immunization may result in effective protection against an otherwise lethal dose of tumor cells, it is ineffective if the dose of tumor cells is sufficiently large. The progression of the growth of a tumor in an immunocompetent host, in the face of an immune response, may be due to a rapid increase in the mass of the tumor, which outstrips the increase in immune responsiveness, until the large mass of the tumor overwhelms any effects of the immune response.

IMMUNODIAGNOSIS

Immunodiagnosis of tumors may be performed to achieve two separate goals: (1) the immunologic detection of antigens specific to tumor cells and (2) the assessment of the host's immune response to the tumor. Immunodiagnosis is predicated on immunologic cross-reactivity, and immunologic methods may be used to detect tumor antigens and other "markers" in cases in which tumor antigens exhibit similarities from individual to individual. In the presence of such immunologic cross-reactivity, antibody or lymphocytes from individuals with the same type of tumor would be expected to react with the cross-reactive tumor antigens, regardless of the individual from which they have been derived. Nevertheless, although useful in monitoring patients for tumor recurrence after therapy, no tumor marker has undisputed specificity or sensitivity for application in early diagnosis or mass cancer screening.

As discussed earlier in this chapter, tumor cells may express cytoplasmic, cell-surface or secreted products that are different in nature and/or quantity from those produced by their normal counterparts. Because of the generally weak antigenicity of the tumor-specific markers, such differences—either qualitative or quantitative—have generally been demonstrated by the use of antibodies produced in xenogeneic animals. The use of mouse monoclonal antibodies has greatly enhanced the specificity of immunodiagnosis of human tumor cells and their products. Monoclonal antibodies are currently gaining use not only in the detection of antigens and products associated with the presence of tumor cells but also for their efficacy in the localization and imaging of tumors. Injection of radiolabeled tumor-specific antibodies (radioimmunoconjugates) into the tumor-bearing individual permits visualization by computerized topography (CT) studies of the radiolabeled antibodies attached to the tumor. This method allows the detection of small metastases as well as the primary tumor mass. Some of the most widely used and reliable immunodiagnostic procedures for the detection of malignancies are described below.

Detection of Myeloma Proteins Produced by Plasma Cell Tumors

Abnormally high concentration in serum of monoclonal immunoglobulins of a certain isotype or the presence of light chains of these immunoglobulins (***Bence-Jones proteins***) in the urine is indicative of plasma cell tumors. The concentration of these myeloma proteins in the blood or urine is a reflection of the mass of the tumor. Consequently, the effectiveness and duration of therapy for these tumors may be monitored by measurement of the concentration of myeloma proteins in the serum and urine.

Detection of Alpha Fetoprotein

Alpha fetoprotein (αFP) is a major protein produced by fetal liver cells and found in fetal serum. After birth, the level of αFP falls to approximately 20 ng/mL. Levels of αFP are elevated in patients with liver cancer (hepatomas), but they are also elevated in ovarian and testicular embryonal carcinoma as well as noncancerous hepatic disorders, such as cirrhosis and hepatitis. Serum αFP concentrations of 500–1000 ng/mL generally indicate the presence of a tumor that is producing αFP, and monitoring αFP levels determines regression or progression of the tumor.

Carcinoembryonic Antigen

Carcinoembryonic antigen (CEA) is a term applied to a glycoprotein produced normally by cells that line the gastrointestinal tract, in particular the colon. If the cells become malignant, their polarity may change, so that CEA is released into the blood instead of the colon. Concentrations in the blood of CEA exceeding 2.5 ng/mL generally indicate malignancy, and monitoring CEA levels is helpful in determining tumor growth or regression. Here again, however, higher than normal levels of CEA in blood may be due to noncancerous diseases, such as cirrhosis of the liver and inflammatory diseases of the intestinal tract and lung.

Detection of Prostate-Specific Antigen

Prostate-specific antigen (PSA) is a glycoprotein located in ductal epithelial cells of the prostate gland. It can be detected in low concentrations in the sera of healthy men. Levels above 8–10 ng/mL blood suggest prostate cancer. Confirmatory tests are required, since prostatitis and benign prostate hypertrophy may also release into the bloodstream PSA derived from glandular prostate epithelium. The test is especially useful for monitoring significant increases or decreases of serum of PSA that correlate with increases or decreases of tumor size.

Cancer Antigen-125

A clinically useful tool for diagnosing and monitoring therapy for ovarian cancer involves the immunodiagnostic measurement of serum ***cancer antigen-125*** (CA-125) levels. Circulating levels of CA-125 also increase during peritoneal inflammatory processes.

Other Markers

B72.3 is a monoclonal antibody that recognizes all carcinomas in humans (***pancarcinoma antigen***). This reagent is being used in tumor localization studies to find occult tumor deposits. Other markers are associated with malignancies, such as enzymes and hormones, that can be detected by immunologic methods. Qualitative and quantitative determinations of all tumor markers are useful in monitoring the extent of malignancy and the effect of therapy on it.

TUMOR IMMUNOPROPHYLAXIS

Immunization against an oncogenic virus would be expected to provide prophylaxis against the virus and, hence, against the subsequent induction of tumor by the virus. Indeed, this approach has been successful in the protection of chickens against Marek disease, and a significant degree of protection against feline leukemia and feline sarcoma has been achieved by immunizing cats with the respective oncogenic viruses. As we have already discussed, immunization against the tumor itself requires that the tumor possess specific tumor antigens and that these antigens cross-react immunologically with any prepared vaccine. There are literally thousands of reports of effective immunization against transplantable animal tumors, using as immunogens (1) sublethal doses of live tumor cells, (2) tumor cells in which replication has been blocked, (3) tumor cells with enzymatically or chemically modified surface membranes, and (4) extracts of antigens from the surface of tumor cells (either unmodified or chemically modified). Despite these reported successes in the protection of experimental animals against transplantable tumors, the efficacy of immunoprophylaxis for protection of humans and animals against spontaneous tumors has not been sufficiently evaluated. This lack of complete study relates to the need for appropriate immunogens and the danger of inducing the production of immunologic elements that may, in fact, enhance metastasis, and thus be detrimental to the host.

IMMUNOTHERAPY

Leonardo da Vinci (1452–1519) wrote that "the supreme misfortune is when theory outstrips performance." Unfortunately, this is a fairly accurate characterization of the current state of cancer immunotherapy. Numerous attempts have been made to treat cancers in animals and humans by immunologic means. Although reports of successful immunotherapy in human cancers are increasing in the literature, to date, immunotherapy has not been proved to be an effective treatment of cancer, either when used as the sole treatment or as an adjunct to other forms of therapy such as chemotherapy, radiotherapy, or surgery.

Currently, a wide range of strategies in experimental immunotherapy of tumors are in use (Fig. 19.3). ***Tumor-specific monoclonal antibodies*** (e.g., anti-CD20 for the treatment of certain lymphomas; anti-Her2/neu-1 for the treatment of certain patients with breast and ovarian cancers) can mediate cytolysis either by engaging NK cells via Fc receptors (ADCC) or by complement activation. Trials of cancer immunotherapy are underway in which toxins, such as ricin, or radioactive isotopes attached to tumor-specific antibodies are delivered specifically to the tumor cells for direct killing. The extent to which these ***immunotoxins*** will prove effective in the treatment of cancer remains to be established. Xenogeneic antibodies (e.g., mouse anti-human monoclonal antibodies) that have been molecularly engineered using recombinant DNA technology to humanize their constant regions (see Chapter 5) are also being tested as candidates for immunotherapy. ***Bispecific antibody*** constructs designed to bring immune effector cells into contact with tumor cells and to simultaneously stimulate the cytotoxic activity of effector cells are also under investigation. Examples include antibodies that recognize unique tumor antigens and IgG Fc receptors (CD16) to activate NK cells. Similarly, bispecific antibodies constructs containing Fabs specific for tumor antigens and CD3 have also been studied.

A relatively new approach involves the creation of recombinant fusion proteins consisting of antitumor antibodies

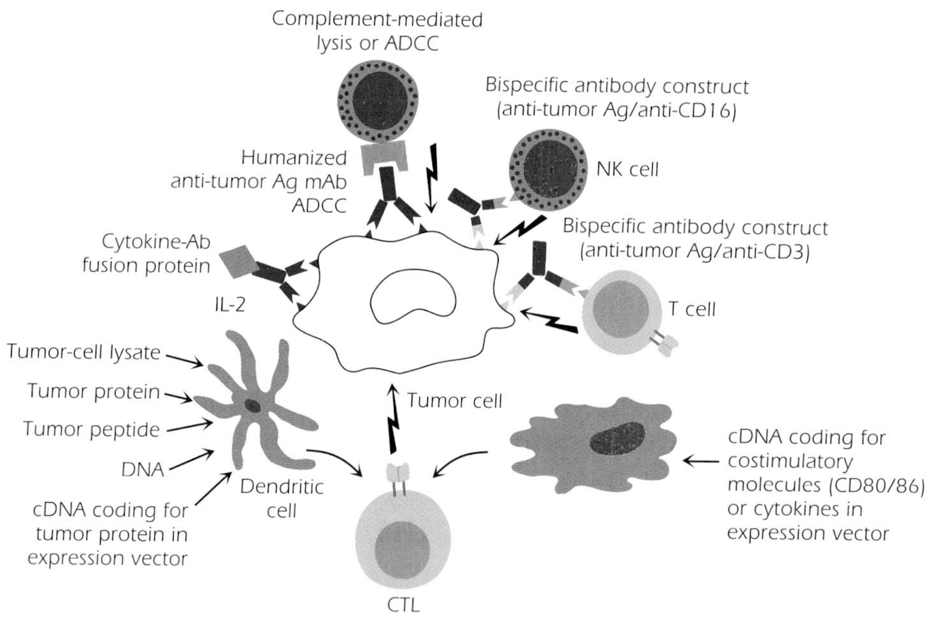

Figure 19.3. Current strategies in experimental immunotherapy. *Ag,* antigen; *mAb,* monoclonal antibody.

and cytokines (***immunocytokines***). Such fusion proteins are designed to concentrate cytokine-mediated immune effector functions at the tumor site. Several approaches are designed to stimulate or bolster the function of tumor-specific CTLs. CTLs can be activated against tumor antigens by tumor cells rendered immunologic by expression of either costimulatory molecules such as CD80/CD86 or cytokines. A highly effective method for stimulating tumor-specific CTLs involves the presentation of MHC class I tumor antigen peptides by ***dendritic cells.*** These highly efficient APCs normally express high levels of cell surface co-stimulatory molecules, therefore enhancing their ability to present tumor antigens to effector T cells (see Chapters 9 and 10). Dendritic cells are either directly loaded with peptides or exposed to tumor cell lysates, tumor proteins, or they are transfected with tumor-derived cDNA in an expression vector. They are then adoptively transferred to the tumor-bearing host in hope of activating cytotoxic T cells to kill the tumor cells.

For tumor antigens that have been molecularly characterized, active vaccination using recombinant vaccines have been developed using vaccinia, *Listeria*, or virus-like particles. Active immunization has also been studied by injection of naked DNA plasmid constructs (***DNA vaccines***) with the goal of having the unique tumor antigen encoded and expressed by muscle cells. In some studies, the genes encoding cytokines (e.g., GM-CSF, IL-2, IL-12) are also introduced to improve the presentation of the tumor antigen by dendritic cells at the site of injection.

Attempts at immunotherapy of animal and human malignancies have also been aimed at the augmentation of specific anticancer immunity, using nonspecific enhancement of the immune response. In particular, stimulation of macrophages, using ***bacille Calmette-Guerin*** (BCG) or *Corynebacterium parvum* has been successfully used in some cases. One example is the use of BCG for treating patients with residual superficial urinary bladder cancer. Repeated instillation of live *Mycobacteria* into the bladder by way of catheter after surgery has become the treatment of choice for superficial bladder cancer.

Trials are also in progress on the effects of ***various cytokines,*** such as IFNα, IFNβ, IFNγ, IL-1, IL-2, IL-4, IL-5, IL-12, TNF, and others—either singly or in combination on tumor regression. To date, these trials are mostly inconclusive. The clinical use of LAK cells and TILs have also been applied to the treatment of cancer with variable results. LAK cells are produced in vitro by cultivation of the patient's own peripheral lymphocytes with IL-2. Upon reinfusion into the patient, dramatic improvement has been reported in a number of cases. A documented success has also been reported using TIL adoptively transferred to patients with melanoma. These lymphocytes, removed from a tumor biopsy, expanded in vitro with IL-2, and given back to the tumor-bearing individual, have an antitumor activity many times higher than LAK cells, thus less is needed for therapy.

Our growing understanding of cancer and of the immune system continues to fuel the development of new immunotherapeutic strategies. In all cases, such strategies must be evaluated in preclinical models for their potential usefulness. The great promise that the immune system can be exploited for the treatment and prevention of cancer must be tempered by the few examples of documented efficacy that have emerged. Nevertheless, given the rapid advances in biotechnology and the molecular identification of human tumor antigens, we are entering a new era of cancer immunotherapy. At the present time, we can say with certainty that tumor immunology has clearly yielded significant improvements in the diagnosis of cancer, and it is likely that immune-based diagnostic methods will continue to offer useful new ways to detect tumor cells and monitor their growth.

SUMMARY

1. Tumor immunology deals with (1) the immunologic aspects of the host–tumor relationship and (2) the use of the immune response for diagnosis, prophylaxis, and treatment of cancer.
2. Tumor antigens induced by carcinogens do not cross-react immunologically. On the other hand, extensive cross-reactivity is exhibited with virally induced tumor antigens. Several types of tumors produce oncofetal substances, which are normally present during embryonic development.
3. The immune response to tumors involves both humoral and cellular immune responses. Destruction of tumor cells may be achieved by (1) antibodies and complement; (2) phagocytes; (3) loss of the adhesive properties of tumor cells caused by antibodies; (4) cytotoxic T lymphocytes; (5) ADCC; and (6) activated macrophages, neutrophils, NK cells, NK/T cells, and LAK cells.
4. The role of immune responses to tumors appears to be important in the host–tumor relationship, as indicated by increased incidence of tumors in immunosuppressed hosts and by the presence of immune components at sites of tumor regression. However, immune responses to a tumor may not be effective in eliminating the tumor because of a variety of tumor- and host-related mechanisms.
5. Immunodiagnosis may be directed toward the detection of tumor antigens or the host's immune response to the tumor.
6. Immunoprophylaxis may be directed against oncogenic viruses or against the tumor itself.
7. Immunotherapy of malignancy employs various preparations for the augmentation of tumor-specific as well as nonspecific immune responses. Approaches include active immunization, passive therapy with antibodies, local application of bacterial vaccines (BCG), use of cytokines, and adoptive transfer of effector cells.

REFERENCES

Alexandroff AB, Robins RA, Murray A, James K (1999): Tumour immunology: false hopes/new horizons? *Immunol Today* 19:247.

Epenetos AA, Spooner RA, George AJT (1994): Application of monoclonal antibodies in clinical oncology. *Immunol Today* 15:559.

Grabbe, GM (2001): Dendritic cells in cancer immunotherapy. *Crit Rev Immunol* 21:133.

Haupt, K, Roggendorf, M, Mann, K. (2002): The potential of DNA vaccination against tumor-associated antigens for antitumor therapy. *Exp Biol Med* 227:227.

Jager E, Chen YT, Drifhout JW (1998): Simultaneous humoral and cellular immune response against cancer-testis antigen NY-ESO-1: definition of human histocompatibility leukocyte antigen (HLA)-A2-binding peptide epitopes. *J Exp Med* 187:265.

Mantovani A, Bottazzi B, Colatta F, Sozzani S, Ruco L (1992): The origin and function of tumor associated macrophages. *Immunol Today* 13:265.

Marshall JL, Hawkins MJ, Tsang KY, Richmond E, Pedicano JE, Zhu MZ, Schlom J (1999): Phase I study in cancer patients of a replication-defective avipox recombinant vaccine that expresses human carcinoembryonic antigen. *J Clin Oncol* 17:332.

Melief CJ, Offringa R, Toes RE, Kast WM (1996): Peptide-based cancer vaccines. *Curr Opin Immunol* 8:651.

Noguchi Y, Richards EC, Chen YT, Old LJ. (1995): Influence of interleukin-12 on p53 peptide vaccination against established Meth A sarcoma. *Proc Natl Acad Sci USA* 92:2219.

Ockert D, Schmitz M, Hampl M, Rieber EP (1999) Advances in cancer immunotherapy. *Immunol Today* 20:63.

Ottmann, OG, Druker, BJ, Sawers, CL, Goldman, JM, et al. (2002): A phase 2 study of imatinib in patients with relapsed or refractory Philadelphia chromosome-positive acute lymphoid leukemias. *Blood* 15:1965.

Rosenberg SA (1999): A new era for cancer immunotherapy based on the genes that encode cancer antigens. *Immunity* 10:281.

Rosenberg, SA, Yang, JC, White, DE, Steinberg, SM (1998): Durability of complete responses in patients with metastatic cancer treated with high-dose interleukin-2: identification of the antigens mediating response. *Ann Surg* 228:307.

Stockert E, Jager E, Chen YT (1998): A survey of the humoral immune response of cancer patients to a panel of human tumor antigens. *J Exp Med* 187:1349.

Vitteta ES, Thorpe PE, Uhr JW (1993): Immunotoxins: magic bullets or misguided missiles? *Immunol Today* 14:252.

Wever, J (2002): Peptide vaccines for cancer. *Cancer Invest* 20:208.

REVIEW QUESTIONS

For each question, choose the ONE BEST answer or completion.

1. The appearance of many primary lymphoreticular tumors in humans is associated with impairments in
- A) humoral immunity.
- B) NK cell activity.
- C) NK/T cell activity.
- D) neutrophil function.
- E) cell-mediated immunity.

2. Tumor antigens have been shown to cross-react immunologically in cases of
- A) tumors induced by chemical carcinogens.
- B) tumors induced by RNA viruses.
- C) all tumors.
- D) tumors induced by irradiation with UV light.
- E) tumors induced by the same chemical carcinogen on two separate sites on the same individual.

3. Which of the following is not considered a mechanism by which cytokines mediate antitumor effects?
- A) They enhance the expression of MHC class I molecules.
- B) They activate LAK and TIL cells.
- C) They have direct antitumor activity.
- D) They induce complement-mediated cytolysis.
- E) They increase activity of cytotoxic T cells, macrophages, and NK cells.

4. Rejection of a tumor may involve which of the following?
- A) T cell–mediated cytotoxicity
- B) ADCC
- C) complement-dependent cytotoxicity
- D) destruction of tumor cells by phagocytic cells
- E) All of the above.

5. Which of the following best defines immunotoxins?
- A) toxic substances released by macrophages
- B) cytokines
- C) toxins completed with the corresponding antitoxins
- D) toxins coupled to antigen-specific immunoglobulins
- E) toxins released by cytotoxic T cells

6. It has been shown that a B cell lymphoma could be eliminated with anti-idiotypic serum. The use of this approach to treat a plasma cell tumor would not be warranted because
- A) plasma cell tumors have no tumor-specific antigens.
- B) plasma cell tumors are not expected to be susceptible to ADCC.
- C) plasma cell tumors can be killed in vivo only by cytotoxic B lymphocytes that bear the same class I MHC antigens.
- D) the plasma cells do not have surface immunoglobulin.
- E) the idiotype on the plasma-cell surface is different from that on the B cell surface.

CASE STUDY

A patient suffering from a rare cancer is treated with a cocktail of cytokines, which includes IL-2 and IL-12 and shows improvement, as measured by a reduced tumor burden, despite various side effects of the therapy. Various functional parameters of the patient's peripheral blood cells were tested before, during, and after therapy. An assay designed to measure macrophage phagocytic activity indicates a significant increase in phagocytosis of antibody-opsonized bacteria one day after injection of the cocktail. Explain what might account for this observed effect. How could you confirm your hypothesis? Discuss how this increased phagocytic activity could be responsible for the patient's improvement.

ANSWERS TO REVIEW QUESTIONS

1. ***E*** There is a nearly 100-fold increase in the incidence of lymphoproliferative tumors in individuals with impaired immunity, in particular with impaired cell-mediated immunity.

2. ***B*** Immunologic cross-reactivity has been demonstrated only in cases of virally induced tumors (caused by either RNA or DNA viruses). Tumors induced by chemical or physical carcinogens do not exhibit cross-reactivity, even if induced by the same carcinogen on separate sites on the same individual.

3. ***D*** INFα, INFβ, and INFγ enhance the expression of MHC class I molecules on tumor cells, which makes them more vulnerable to killing by CTLs. IL-2 activates LAK and TIL cells. TNFα and TNFβ both have direct antitumor activity. IFNγ increases the activity of CTLs, macrophages, and NK cells, each of which plays an important role in tumor cell destruction. Cytokines play no role in the activation of complement; therefore, D is incorrect.

4. ***E*** Destruction of tumor cells may be mediated by T cell–mediated cytotoxicity, by ADCC, by complement-mediated cytotoxicity, and by phagocytic cells, which are attracted to the tumor by T cell lymphokines and/or complement components and which become activated by the cytokines or perform enhanced phagocytosis as a result of the present of opsonins on the target cells.

5. ***D*** Immunotoxins consist of toxic substances (or radioactive atoms) conjugated to immunoglobulin molecules specific for tumor cells or other target cells.

6. ***D*** The only relevant statement is that plasma cells do not have surface immunoglobulins and would, therefore, not be susceptible to treatment with anti-idiotypic antibodies. Plasma cell tumors do have tumor-specific antigens and would be susceptible to ADCC with antibodies to these antigens. Statement C is not correct.

ANSWER TO CASE STUDY

Therapeutic infusion of cytokine cocktails can cause a variety of immunomodulatory effects. IL-12 is known to induce increased IFNγ production by T cells, which, in turn, increases the activity of cytotoxic T lymphocytes, macrophages, and NK cells. Each of these cell populations plays a role in the immune response to tumors. The probable reason why the patient's macrophages showed increased phagocytic activity when exposed to antibody-opsonized bacteria is that IFNγ also increases macrophage Fc receptor expression. Their ability to bind to antibody-coated bacteria would, therefore, be greatly facilitated—thus, phagocytosis would be enhanced. One way to confirm this hypothesis would be to measure IFNγ levels in the patient's peripheral blood after cytokine cocktail infusions. Assuming this mechanism were confirmed, it would help explain the patient's improvement, since increased Fc receptor expression would also be expected to increase ADCC activity directed against tumor antigenes. Thus, if the patient had serum antibody specific for tumor antigens, this antitumor mechanism probably functioned in concert with the cytokine-enhanced tumoricidal activities of macrophages and NK to reduce the tumor burden.

20

RESISTANCE AND IMMUNIZATION TO INFECTIOUS DISEASES

INTRODUCTION

The primary function of the immune system is to defend the body against diseases caused from contact with microorganisms. Historically, infectious diseases have been the leading cause of death for human populations, with most deaths occurring in infancy and childhood. There have been many catastrophic epidemics of infectious diseases in history. For example, the bubonic plague caused by the bacterium *Yersinia pestis* killed one-quarter of the European population in the mid-1300s. Hence infectious diseases have provided tremendous selective pressures for the evolution of the immune system. Host defenses are characterized by a considerable amount of layering and redundancy. Layering refers to defense in depth and includes physical barriers, such as the skin and mucosal membranes, and innate and adaptive immune mechanisms. Redundancy is exemplified by the fact that there are several types of phagocytic cells, antigen-presenting cells, (APCs), cytokine-producing cells, opsonins, and so on, such that for many immune functions, multiple mechanisms are in place to achieve the desired end. The redundancy of the immune system allows some hosts to survive for prolonged times, despite severe immune impairment. For example, some individuals with deficiencies in some immunoglobulin isotypes (e.g., IgA deficiency) are thought to live a normal existence because other immunoglobulin classes are able to compensate for the immune deficit.

Microbes differ in their pathogenicity and virulence. Only a small minority of all microorganisms on earth are pathogens for humans. Pathogens are defined as microbes capable of causing host damage. Host damage can occur at the cellular, tissue, or organ level. When host damage reaches a certain threshold, it can manifest itself as disease. If sufficient damage occurs, the host can die. Host damage can result from a variety of mechanisms and can be mediated by the microbe, the host, or both. Examples of mechanisms of microbe-mediated damage include the production of toxins, cellular apoptosis resulting in depletion of immune cells, and the elaboration of enzymes that cause tissue necrosis. Examples of mechanisms of host-mediated damage include destructive inflammation, fibrosis, and autoimmunity. The realization that host damage is the relevant parameter by which to characterize the outcome of the host–pathogen interaction is the basis of the recently proposed ***damage–response framework*** of microbial pathogenesis. According to this conceptual framework, the term *pathogenicity* is defined as the capacity of a microbe to cause damage in a host, and *virulence* is defined by the relative capacity of a microbe to cause damage in a host. Virulence and pathogenicity are not singular microbial properties, because they can be expressed in only susceptible hosts and reflect complex interactions between hosts; microbes; and myriad environmental, social, and human factors.

Human hosts harbor many species of microbes. When a human host encounters a microbe, the interaction can result

Contributed by Dr. Arturo Casadevall, Department of Microbiology and Immunology, Albert Einstein College of Medicine.

Immunology: A Short Course, Fifth Edition, By Richard Coico, Geoffrey Sunshine, and Eli Benjamini
ISBN 0-471-22689-0

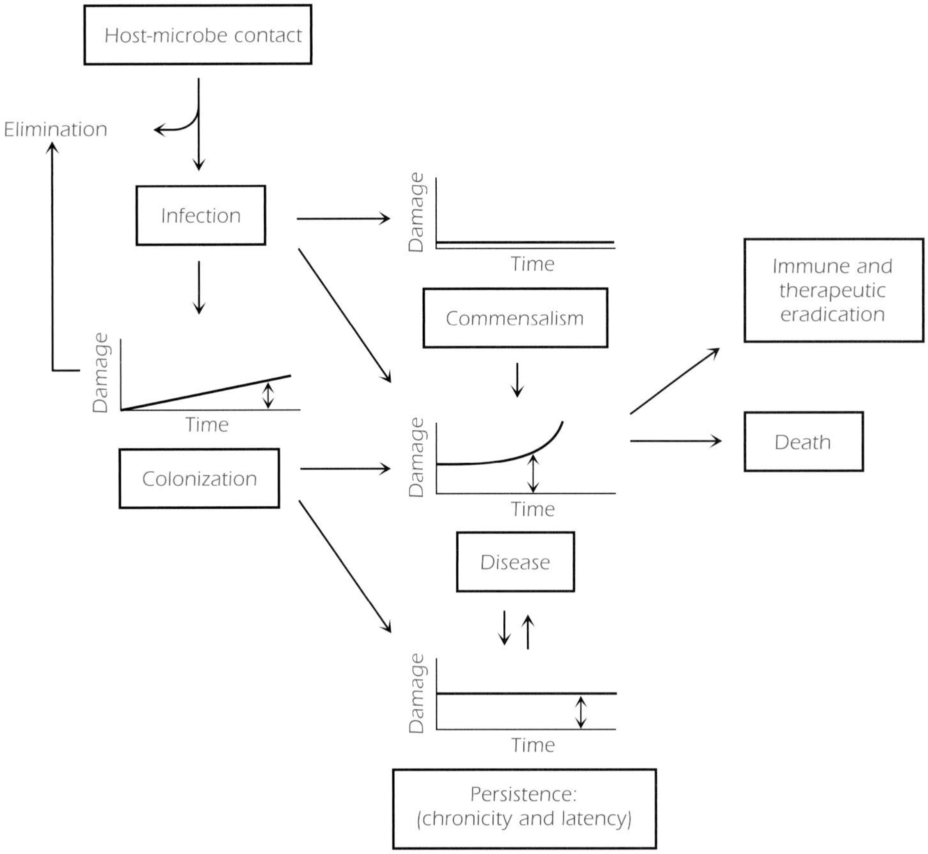

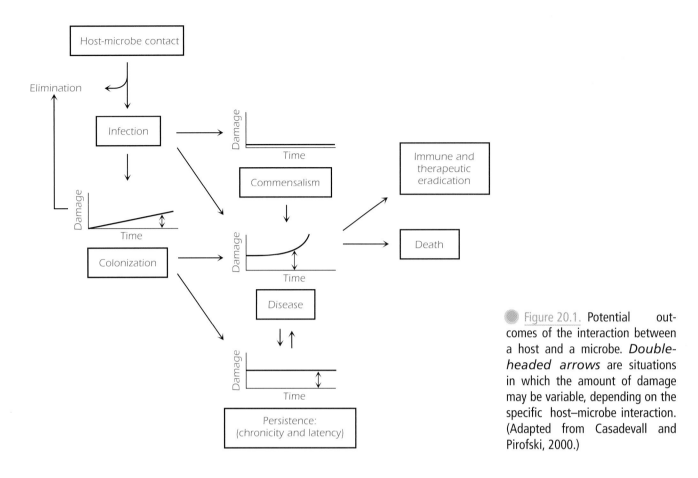

Figure 20.1. Potential outcomes of the interaction between a host and a microbe. *Double-headed arrows* are situations in which the amount of damage may be variable, depending on the specific host–microbe interaction. (Adapted from Casadevall and Pirofski, 2000.)

in one of two outcomes: elimination or infection. Elimination can occur when the host–microbe encounter does not result in the establishment of the microbe in the host. Infection is the acquisition of a microbe by a host. Note that although the term ***infection*** is often used synonymously with the word ***disease,*** the two are not the same. Infection is followed by one of five outcomes: ***elimination, commensalism, colonization, persistence*** (or latency), and ***disease.*** In the latter four outcomes, the relationship between the host and microbe is maintained but the amount of damage sustained by the host differs (Fig. 20.1). Elimination can follow infection as a result of action by host defense mechanisms or therapeutic intervention. Neither commensalism or colonization rarely, if ever, results in symptomatic or clinically evident host damage, but these states can differ in the amount of host damage and in their ability to progress to disease. When there is no host damage commensalism and colonization are essentially indistinguishable states.

Colonization is a term that is usually used for microbes with significant pathogenic potential that establish themselves in the host without causing symptoms. Colonization can lead to elimination, persistence, or disease, depending on the competency of host defenses, the virulence of the microbe, and the effectiveness of the immune response. Many colonizing events are immunizing and prevent future infection and/or disease caused by the relevant microbe. For example, a microbe with high pathogenic potential may establish itself on a mucous membrane, cause a small amount of damage that is insufficient to cause clinical symptoms, and elicit an immune response that eradicates it. In that situation, colonization immunized the host against reacquisition of the microbe.

Persistence (or latency) is a state whereby microbes take up residence in the host and cannot be eradicated, despite causing host damage. For example, in many humans, *Mycobacterium tuberculosis* infection is not symptomatic, even when the microbe has established itself in the host and is able to survive for long periods of time in a granuloma. In this state of persistence, local tissue damage and alterations in normal tissue occur due to granuloma formation, but the damage is not sufficient to produce clinical disease. However, unlike colonization, the host defense mechanisms cannot eradicate the mycobacteria and the infection becomes persistent. In most individuals, this state is maintained with the infection confined to a granuloma. However, in some individuals, this state progresses to tuberculosis, the disease caused by *M. tuberculosis.* In the damage–response framework, disease occurs when the presence of the microbe in the host results in sufficient damage to manifest clinical symptoms.

In patients with intact immune systems, microbes must be sufficiently virulent to establish themselves and cause infection. However, in patients with weakened immune systems, low virulence microbes can cause serious infections. Microbes that are pathogenic in individuals with weakened immune systems are often referred to as ***opportunistic pathogens.*** Hence the microbial properties of pathogenicity and virulence are associated with, and partially depend on, the immune status of the host. In circumstances of normal immune function, commensal microorganisms are not harmful and can serve important roles for the host, such as the production of vitamin K by gut bacteria. However, commensals can become pathogens in circumstances in which the normal host defenses are breached. For example, both *Staphylococcus epidermitis* and *Candida albicans* are part of the normal skin flora but can cause life-threatening infections in patients with intravenous catheters that provide a break in the skin. Some therapies for cancer produce immune suppression, which leaves patients at risk for serious infections with low-virulence microbes, such as commensals.

In this chapter, we will discuss how mammalian hosts protect themselves against various types of pathogens and how the immune system can be primed for antimicrobial defense through active and passive immunization. It is assumed that the reader is now familiar with the principle concepts underlying innate and adaptive immune defenses.

HOST DEFENSE AGAINST THE VARIOUS CLASSES OF MICROBIAL PATHOGENS

The most effective immune response to a particular microbe varies with the type of pathogen and the microbial strategy for pathogenesis. Viruses, bacteria, parasites, and fungi each use different strategies to establish themselves in the host, and, consequently, the effective immune response for each of these classes of microbial pathogens is different. Although each pathogen is different, certain themes emerge when one considers immune responses to the various classes of pathogens.

Immunity to Viruses

All viruses are ***obligate intracellular pathogens*** and many have evolved to have highly sophisticated mechanisms for cellular invasion, replication, and evasion of the immune system. Host defenses against viral infections aim to first slow viral replication and then to eradicate infection. The antiviral response can be complex, with several factors affecting the outcome of the host–pathogen interaction, such as the route of entry, site of attachment, aspects of pathogenesis by the infecting virus, induction of interferon, antibody response, and cell-mediated immunity. An important early defense mechanism consists of the production of various types of interferons including IFNα by leucocytes, IFNβ by fibroblasts, and INFγ by T and natural-killer (NK) cells. Interferons are antiviral proteins, or glycoproteins, produced by several different types of cell in the mammalian host in response to viral infection (or other inducers, such as double-stranded RNA). Interferons serve as an early protective mechanism. IFNα and IFNβ produced by virally infected cells diffuse to adjoining cells and activate genes that interfere with viral replication. These interferons also stimulate production of MHC class I molecules and proteasome proteins that enhance the ability of virally infected cells to present viral peptides to T cells. Furthermore, IFNα and IFNβ activate NK cells that recognize and kill host cells infected with viruses, thus limiting viral production.

NK cells are characterized by their ability to kill certain tumor cells in vitro without prior sensitization and constitute an early cellular defense against viruses. Later in the course of infection, when ***antibodies*** to viral antigens are available, NK cells can eliminate host cells infected with virus through ***antibody-dependent cell-mediated cytotoxicity*** (ADCC). NK cells also produce INFγ, a potent activator of macrophage function that helps prime the immune system for producing an adaptive immune response. ***Complement*** system proteins damage the envelope of some viruses which may provide some, measure of protection against certain viral infections.

While IFNs, NK cells, and possibly complement function to slow and partially contain many viral infections, the infection may progress, with viral replication and damage triggering an immune response. The humoral response results in the production of antibodies to viral proteins. Some antibodies can prevent viruses from invading other cells, and these are called ***neutralizing antibodies.*** IgG appears to be the most active isotype against viruses. Opsonization represents a convergence of humoral and cellular immune mechanisms. IgG, which has combined, through its Fab region, with viral antigens on the surface of infected host cells, links also to Fc receptors on several cell populations, including NK cells, macrophages, and polymorphonuclear (PMN) cells. These cells then can phagocytose and/or damage the virus-infected cell (ADCC).

Antibodies to viral proteins can prevent infection by interfering with the binding of virus to host cells. The production of secretory IgA can protect the host by preventing infection of epithelial cells in mucosal surfaces. Antibodies can also interfere with the progression of viral infection by agglutinating viral particles, activating complement on viral surfaces, and promoting phagocytosis of viral particles by macrophages. The production of an antibody response serves to limit viral spread and facilitates the destruction of infected host cells by ADCC. Hence the effective antibody response to viruses include the production of antibodies that

- Neutralize (or impede) the infectivity of viruses for susceptible host cells.
- Fix complement and promote complement damage to virions.
- Inhibit viral enzymes.
- Promote opsonization of viral particles.
- Promote ADCC of virus-infected cells.

Different types of antibodies may be necessary for the control of specific types of viral infections. Consider the case of influenza and measles virus infections. Infection of the epithelium of the respiratory tract by influenza virus leads to production of virus in epithelial cells and spread of the virus to adjacent epithelial cells. An appropriate and sufficient immune response would involve the action of antibody at the epithelial surface. This action might be effected through locally secreted IgA or local extravasation of IgG or IgM. On the other hand, some viral diseases, such as measles and poliomyelitis, begin by infection at a mucosal epithelium (respiratory and intestinal, respectively) but exhibit their major pathogenic effects after being spread hematogenously to other target tissues. Antibody at the epithelial surface could protect against the virus, but circulating antibody could do likewise.

However, once a virus has attached to a host cell, it is usually not displaced by antibody. Hence an effective antibody response is usually not sufficient to eliminate a viral infection, particularly when the virus has established itself inside host cells. The eradication of an established viral infection usually requires an effective cell-mediated response. The cellular adaptive response results in the production of specific $CD4^+$ and $CD8^+$ T cells that are essential for clearance of viral infections. $CD4^+$ T cells are believed to be intimately involved in the generation of effective antibody responses by facilitating isotype class switching and affinity maturation (Chapter 7). $CD4^+$ T cells also produce important cytokines to stimulate inflammatory responses at sites of viral infection and activate macrophage function. Cytotoxic $CD8^+$ T cells (cytotoxic T lymphocytes; CTLs) are the principal effector T cells against viruses. They are generated early in viral infection and usually appear before neutralizing antibody. $CD8^+$ T cells can recognize viral antigens in the context of MHC class I molecules and can kill host cells harboring viruses. Since MHC class I molecules are expressed by most cell types in the host, $CD8^+$ T cells can recognize many types of infected cells and thus represent a critically important component of the host adaptive response against viral infections. However, for certain noncytopathic viruses, such as hepatitis B, $CD8^+$ T cells can be responsible for tissue injury. Hence, chronic hepatitis B infection results in persistent inflammation and damage to liver cells, resulting in fibrosis and progress to organ failure.

In summary, innate immune mechanisms initially interfere with viral infection through the production of IFNs and the killing of infected cells by NK cells. These early defenses buy time until powerful adaptive immune responses are generated. The adaptive immune responses produce neutralizing antibodies that reduce the number of viral particles and CTCs that kill infected cells. The presence of neutralizing antibody would then protect against subsequent exposure against the same virus.

Immunity to Bacteria

Host protection against bacterial pathogens is achieved through a variety of mechanisms that include both ***humoral*** and ***cellular immunity.*** Antibacterial defenses include bacterial lysis, via ***antibody and complement, opsonization,*** and ***phagocytosis,*** with elimination of phagocytosed bacteria by the liver, spleen, and other components of the reticuloendothelial system. Bacteria and their products are internalized by APCs such as macrophages and dendritic cells and processed; peptides resulting from such processing are presented to T cells on MHC class II molecules (Chapter 9). This process amplifies the host response as T cells produce cytokines that activate macrophages and recruit additional inflammatory cells. The relative efficacy of the various immune mechanisms depends on the type of bacteria and, in particular, the cell surface properties of the bacteria. Bacterial pathogens can be roughly divided into four classes: ***gram-positive, gram-negative, mycobacteria,*** and ***spirochetes,*** depending on their cell wall and membrane composition. Some gram-positive and gram-negative bacteria have polysaccharide capsules. Another crucial distinction between bacterial pathogens is whether they are ***intracellular*** or ***extracellular*** pathogens. Intracellular bacterial pathogens reside in cells and are partially shielded from the full array of host immune defenses, whereas extracellular bacterial pathogens are found outside cells. In general, humoral immunity is very important for protection against extracellular bacteria, whereas cellular immunity tends to be the primary immune mechanism for the control and eradication of intracellular bacteria.

Gram-Positive Bacteria. Gram-positive bacteria have thick electron-dense cell walls composed of complex cross-linked ***peptidoglycan*** that allow them to retain the stain crystal violet (hence gram-positive). In addition to a thick layer of peptidoglycan, the cell wall of gram-positive bacteria contains teichoic acids, carbohydrates, and proteins. ***Teichoic acids*** are immunogenic and constitute major antigenic determinants of gram-positive bacteria. This type of cell wall provides the gram-positive bacteria with a thick layer of protection that makes them ***resistant to lysis by the complement system.*** Defenses against gram-positive bacteria include ***specific antibody*** responses to provide opsonins and phagocytic cells, such as neutrophils and macrophages, to ingest and kill them. ***Opsonization*** and ***phagocytosis*** involve the action of IgG and IgM alone or in concert with C3b. The alternative complement pathway may be triggered directly by the gram-positive bacterial cell wall, resulting in the deposition of complement opsonins in the cell surface and the production of mediators of the inflammatory response. Although the complement system does not lyse gram-positive bacteria directly, it provides opsonins and mediators of inflammation that are critical for host defense.

Gram-Negative Bacteria. Gram-negative bacteria do not retain crystal violet stain and have a layered cell wall structure composed of outer and inner membranes separated by a thin layer of peptidoglycan in the periplasmic space. Hence gram-positive and -negative bacteria have major differences in their cell wall structure. The outer membrane of gram-negative bacteria contains ***lipopolysaccharide*** (LPS), which is also known as ***endotoxin.*** The polysaccharide portion of LPS has antigenic determinants that confer antigenic specificity. Many gram-negative bacterial species include variants with different LPS structure that can be identified serologically as serotypes. LPS is highly toxic to humans and can produce cardiovascular collapse, hypotension, and shock during infection with gram-negative bacteria. The alternative complement pathway may be activated directly by the LPS found in the walls of gram-negative bacteria or by the polysaccharide capsule of gram-negative bacteria acting on C3. Activation of the alternative pathway leads to the generation of the chemotactic molecules C3a and C5a and the opsonin C3b and can result in bacteriolytic action by the C5–C9 membrane attack complex (see Chapter 13). The ability of the complement system to lyse some gram-negative bacteria directly is an important distinction from gram-positive bacteria, which are impervious to complement-mediated lysis because of the thick peptidoglycan layer. Defenses against gram-negative bacteria include the ***complement system, specific antibody,*** and ***phagocytic cells.***

Mycobacteria. Mycobacteria have cell walls distinct from gram-positive and gram-negative bacteria. Mycobacterial cell walls are characterized by a high lipid content, which makes the bacteria difficult to stain. Another property of the mycobacterial cell wall is ***acid fastness,*** which allows them to retain certain dyes after being treated with acid. Mycobacteria grow slowly and have hydrophobic surfaces that make them clump. Mycobacterial cell wall components elicit strong immune responses during infection, including ***delayed-type hypersensitivity*** (DTH) reactions that form the basis for the ***tuberculin test.*** Hypersensitivity reactions to mycobacterial proteins may be involved in the pathogenesis of mycobacterial infections. Mycobacteria elicit strong antibody responses but the role of humoral immunity is uncertain. The primary defense mechanisms against mycobacteria are ***macrophages*** and ***cell-mediated immunity.***

Spirochetes. Spirochetes are thin helical microorganisms and include the etiologic agents of syphilis (*Treponema pallidum*) and Lyme disease (*Borrelia burgdorferi*). Spirochetes lack cell walls such as those found in gram-positive bacteria, gram-negative bacteria, and mycobacteria. Instead they have a thin outer membrane that contains few proteins. Spirochetes are thin, fragile, and require special techniques for visualization in the microscope, such as dark-field microscopy and immunofluorescence. Important host defenses against spirochetes include ***complement, specific antibody,*** and ***cell-mediated immunity.***

Immunity to Parasites

The parasites are a diverse group of complex pathogens that include the single-celled ***protozoa*** and ***helminths.*** Many parasites have a variety of tissue stages that may differ in cellular location and antigenic composition, thus providing a difficult problem for the immune system. The diversity of parasites is such that it is difficult to make generalizations about effective host mechanisms that protect against parasitic diseases. However, it is clear that both ***innate and adaptive defense mechanisms are critically important for protection against parasitic infections.*** Some parasites are protozoa, single-celled eukaryote organisms that may exist in either a metabolically active form called a trophozoite or a dormant tissue form known as a cyst. The protozoal diseases include amebiasis, malaria, leishmaniasis, trypanosomiasis, and toxoplasmosis. Host defenses against protozoa include both innate and adaptive humoral and cellular mechanisms, but their relative importance may vary with the individual pathogen. Some protozoal parasites, such as trypanosomes, are able to activate the complement system through the alternative pathway.

Complement activation combined with ***phagocytosis*** by neutrophils and macrophages of the innate immune system provide an important line of defense again many parasitic pathogens. For some protozoal infections—such as amebiasis, malaria, and trypanosomiasis—humoral immunity in the form of antibody has been shown to mediate protection against infection. However, for other protozoal infections—such as leishmaniasis and toxoplasmosis—cellular immunity is more important.

Other parasites are multicellular worms called helminths. Unlike other pathogenic microorganisms, the helminths are large macroscopic pathogens that can range from 1 cm to 10 m. Their large size poses particular problems for host defenses, and the control of helminth infections requires a complex interplay between tissue and immune responses. The helminths are notorious for causing chronic infections that can elicit intense immune responses to worm antigens. There is general agreement that components of the innate immune system such as ***eosinophils*** and ***mast cells*** are important effector cells against helminths, but many aspects of the host response to worms remain obscure. ***IgE*** specific for helminth antigens is believed to be important for host defense by priming eosinophils for ***ADCC*** (see Fig. 14.8). Worm infections are often accompanied by an increase in blood eosinophils and serum IgE levels.

Immunity to Fungi

Fungal pathogens are eukaryotes that tend to cause serious infections primarily in individuals with impaired immunity. Fungi cause tissue damage by the elaboration of proteolytic enzymes, inducing inflammatory responses. The most common fungal pathogen is *Candida albicans.* This organism is usually a harmless commensal but can cause disease in situations in which the normal defense mechanisms are compromised, such as breaks in skin resulting from intravenous catherters or surgery. Another group at risk for serious *C. albicans*–related diseases are individuals who have transient depletion of neutrophils as a result of chemotherapy.

The fact that most cases of serious *Candida* infection require a break in the skin or a depletion in neutrophils suggests that ***innate defense mechanisms*** are largely responsible for preventing systemic diseases. However, patients with advanced HIV infection suffer from mucosal candidiasis, highlighting the importance of ***cell-mediated immunity*** in protection against this organism at the mucosal surfaces.

Other fungi, such as *Histoplasma capsulatum* and *Cryptococcus neoformans,* are acquired from the environment by inhalation in regions where the organism is found in soils. Prevalence studies of asymptomatic individuals in such regions have shown a high incidence of infection with a very low incidence of disease, as evidenced by antibody responses or positive skin testing. Hence, for these organisms, it is likely that initial acquisition of the microbe results in an adaptive immune response that controls the infection. Some fungi, such as *H. capsulatum,* survive inside macrophages and are intracellular pathogens. One fungal pathogen, *C. neoformans,* has a polysaccharide capsule that is required for virulence.

Fungi differ from bacteria in having a different type of cell wall, composed of cross-linked polysaccharides. Fungal cells are generally impervious to lysis by the complement system. The host response to fungal infections includes both humoral and cellular responses. The primary form of host defense against fungal pathogens is widely acknowledged to be cell-mediated immunity. The need for intact T cell function in resistance to fungi is particularly evident in the predisposition of patients with AIDS to life-threatening infections with such fungi as *H. capsulatum* and *C. neoformans.* Historically, antibody-mediated immunity was not thought to be very important against fungi, but several protective monoclonal antibodies have been described in recent years against *C. albicans* and *C. neoformans.* Hence it is likely that both cellular and humoral immune mechanisms contribute to protection against fungi.

MECHANISMS BY WHICH PATHOGENS EVADE THE IMMUNE RESPONSE

Despite the formidable defenses of the immune system some, microorganisms manage to establish themselves in the host and cause life-threatening infections. Many pathogenic microbes have special adaptations that allow them to evade the immune system. Learning about the mechanisms by which microbial pathogens evade the host immune response is important because it can teach us about the efficacy and limitations of host defense mechanisms. Furthermore, a better understanding of the strategies used by microbes to survive immune attack can be used to design new therapies and vaccines to fight infection.

Encapsulated Bacteria

Polysaccharide capsules are important ***virulence factors*** for several human pathogens, including *Streptococcus pneumoniae* (pneumococcus), *Haemophilus influenzae, Neisseria meningitidis* (meningococcus), and *Cryptococcus neoformans.* These ***capsules are antiphagocytic*** and thus protect the pathogen from ingestion and killing by host phagocytic cells. Some capsules also interfere with the action of the complement system. Polysaccharide molecules are often weakly immunogenic, and infection by encapsulated pathogens may not necessarily elicit high titer antibody responses. Infants and young children are particularly vulnerable to life-threatening infections with encapsulated bacteria because their immature immune systems do not mount adequate antibody responses. Other individuals at high risk are those with inherited or acquired deficiencies in antibody production and those who lack normal spleen function. Because the bacteria are cleared by the reticuloendothelial system in the spleen and liver, these organs are critical for protection against encapsulated pathogens. Individuals with compromised reticuloendothelial function as a result of disease (e.g., sickle cell anemia) or surgical removal of the spleen are particularly vulnerable to encapsulated bacteria. The mechanism of antibody action against encapsulated pathogens involves ***opsonins for phagocytosis*** and killing by neutrophils and macrophages. Antibodies to capsular polysaccharide function by promoting phagocytosis directly through Fc receptors or indirectly by activating complement.

Toxins

For some bacterial infections, the manifestations of disease are caused by ***virulence factors*** called ***toxins.*** Bacterial toxins are proteins that produce their physiologic effects at minute concentrations. Examples of toxin-producing bacteria are *Corynebacterium dipththeriae, Vibrio cholerae,* and *Clostridium tetani,* the causes of diphtheria, cholera and tetanus, respectively. Diphtheria is a condition in which *C. dipththeria* replication and toxin production in the nasopharynx results in the formation of a tenacious membrane in the throat that can asphyxiate the patient. Cholera is a diarrheal illness caused by *V. cholerae,* resulting from toxin-mediated alteration of water resorption in the cells of the intestinal mucosa. Tetanus is a condition in which toxin produced by *C. tetani* produces unchecked excitation of peripheral muscles, resulting in titanic spasms. The relationship of the toxin function to bacterial invasion and evasion of the immune response is variable and may differ for each pathogen. Some toxins, such as tetanus and botulinum toxin, do not appear to injure the immune system directly. Diphtheria toxin may promote bacterial infection by damaging the mucosa. *Bacillus anthracis,* the causative agent of anthrax, produces pathogenic toxins that cause apoptosis in macrophages. The principle mechanism for this immune evasion involves a toxin called

TABLE 20.1. Protection of Humans by Diphtheria Antitoxin Given on Indicated Day of Disease[a]

Day	Number of Cases	Fatality Rate
1	225	9.0
2	1445	4.2
3	1600	11.1
4	1276	17.3
5 (or later)	1645	18.7

[a] From AM Pappenheimer, 1965, with permission.

lethal toxin (LT). LT inhibits a macrophage protein kinase that is required for the transcription of antiapoptotic genes following cell activation.

Most toxins are highly immunogenic and elicit strong humoral and cellular immune responses. Specific antibodies can bind to and neutralize bacterial toxins. Protection against toxins is predominantly associated with IgG, although IgA may also be important in neutralization of certain exotoxins (e.g., secreted toxins) such as cholera enterotoxin. Because the exotoxins bind firmly to their target tissue, they generally cannot be displaced by subsequent administration of ***antitoxin*** (passive immunization using toxin-specific antibody; discussed later in this chapter). Hence in toxin-mediated diseases (e.g., diphtheria) prompt administration of antitoxin is necessary to prevent attachment of (additional) exotoxin and the damage caused by the exotoxin. This can be illustrated by the effectiveness of antitoxin given at varying times as protection against the lethal effects of diphtheria toxin in humans (Table 20.1). As the infection progresses, the effectiveness of administration of diphtheria antitoxin is significantly reduced. Some bacterial toxins are enzymes, such as the lecithinase of the bacterium *Clostridium perfringens* and snake venom. However, antibodies that bind the toxin may not necessarily inhibit the enzymatically active sites of toxin.

Superantigens

The interaction of certain toxins with the immune system can have major immunologic consequences when they are able to bind the T cell receptor (TCR) of large numbers of T cells. These toxins are known as ***superantigens*** and include the staphylococcal ***toxic shock syndrome*** toxin (see Chapter 10). In the early 1980s, many cases of staphylococcal toxic shock syndrome were associated with tampon use in menstruating women. Since then, the frequency of the disease has decreased significantly in response to changes to the manufacture of tampons. Superantigens stimulate large numbers of T cells to proliferate, synthesize cytokines, and then die by apoptosis, resulting in the loss of important immune cells. This phenomenon is associated with ***hypotension, hypolemia,*** and ***organ failure,*** which can lead to death. B cell superantigens that bind to and alter the expression of certain immunoglobulin gene families have also been described.

Antigenic Variation

Pathogens can escape the immune system by generating variants with different antigenic composition. This mechanism for evasion of host defenses is known as ***antigenic variation.*** Classical examples of pathogens that evade the host response by antigenic variation are influenza virus, HIV, *Streptococcus pneumonia,* trypanosomes, and Group A streptococcus. Each of these pathogens provides an illustrative example of a mechanism for antigenic variation. In the case of Group A streptococcus, the M protein is required for virulence and functions by preventing phagocytosis through a mechanism that involves deposition of fibrinogen on the bacterial surface. M proteins elicit protective antibody but are antigenically variable, so that streptococcal infection with one strain does not elicit resistance to other strains.

Influenza virus generates antigenic variation because it has a segmented RNA genome that can be resorted to yield virions expressing new combinations of the two main surface antigens: the hemagglutinin and neuraminidase surface proteins. Antigenic variation for influenza virus occurs through both antigenic drift and antigenic shift. ***Antigenic drift*** is the result of point mutations in the influenza virus genome, which produce antigenic changes in the hemagglutinin and neuraminidase. ***Antigenic shift*** occurs when influenza virus expresses a new allele of hemagglutin or neuraminidase protein that results in a major antigenic change and the emergence of a new viral strain. The result of antigenic drift and shift for the influenza virus is that the virus changes rapidly and one influenza infection does not confer protection against subsequent infection. Furthermore, since each epidemic is antigenically different, a new vaccine against influenza must be reformulated every year.

HIV undergoes rapid antigenic variation in vivo because it has an error-prone reverse transcriptase that produces mutations that translates into antigenic changes in surface proteins. The problem of antigenic variation in HIV has been a major hurdle preventing the development of an effective vaccine. Other pathogens, such as *Streptococcus pneumoniae* (pneumococcus), present the host with antigenic variation because they exist in multiple serotypes, each of which has a different antigenic composition. There are >80 pneumococcal serotypes, and infection with one serotype does not confer protection against infection with a different serotype. Hence the host must deal with infection by each pneumococcal serotype as if it were an infection by a different microbe.

Pathogens may also encode for antigenic variation in their genomes. ***Trypanosomes*** cause chronic infections by the *emergence of new antigenic types during infection* that express different variant surface glycoproteins (VSGs). In a trypanosome infection, the host mounts an antibody response to the VSG being expressed by the majority of parasites, which clears most parasites. However, in every trypanosome infection there are small numbers of organisms that express a different VSG antigen that is not recognized by the antibody response. As the antibody response helps clear the original typanosome population, the remaining organisms expressing a different VSG then proliferate and at the same time generate a new subpopulation of antigenic variants that can survive the new antibody response. The cycle then repeats itself. Since there are many VSG genes, trypanosomes are able to cause persistent infections by producing escape variants that differ in antigenic composition in every generation.

Intracellular Survival

Some microorganisms are taken up by ***phagocytic cells*** but manage to survive in the intracellular environment. These pathogens include the bacteria *Mycobacterium tuberculosis* and *Listeria monocytogenes,* the fungus *Histoplasma capsulatum,* and the protozoa *Toxoplasma gondii. M. tuberculosis* is the cause of tuberculosis, a pulmonary infection. *L. monocytogenes* is a food-borne microbe that can cause meningitis in individuals with immune suppression. *H. capsulatum* is a fungus common in the soil of the Ohio and Mississippi River valleys that usually causes a self-limited pneumonia in normal individuals. However, in individuals with impaired immunity, *H. capsulatum* can cause disseminated infections that are life threatening. *T. gondii* is a parasite that is acquired from eating undercooked food, which usually causes asymptomatic infections. However, in pregnant women *T. gondii* can infect the fetus, causing severe birth defects. Patients with advance HIV infection are particularly vulnerable to toxoplasmosis. These organisms cause very different types of diseases, but each has in common the ability to survive inside host cells.

Intracellular residence has the advantage that it places these microbes in an environment that is nutrient-rich yet outside the reach of humoral factors and neutrophils. In general, protection against intracellular microorganisms is the domain of cell-mediated immunity, although for several pathogens antibody responses also contribute to host defense. This concept is illustrated by the fact *M. tuberculosis, L. monocytogenes, H. capsulatum,* and *T. gondii* cause serious diseases in individuals with impaired T cell function, such as patients with AIDS. Furthermore, NK cells may play an important role during early stages of infection by destroying infected cells before the development of specific resistance. Granulomatous inflammation is a tissue manifestation of cell-mediated immunity associated with containment of several intracellular pathogens.

Although phagocytic cells are generally efficient antimicrobial cells, microbes capable of intracellular survival use any of several strategies to avoid being killed after phagocytosis. *M. tuberculosis* blocks the fusion of lysosomes with the phagocytic vacuole, thus preventing delivery of antimicrobial substances to the phagosome (Chapter 2). *H. capsulatum* interferes with acidification of the phagolysosomal vacuole, a phenomenon that is believed to interfere with killing of yeast cells inside macrophages. *L. monocytogenes* produces bacterial products that allow it to escape from the phagolysosomal vacuole to the cell cytoplasm, a mechanism that presumably provides a more nutritionally favorable niche and defeats intracellular antimicrobial mechanisms. *T. gondii* generates its own vacuole in which it remains insulated from host lysosomes; this avoids triggering recognition of infected cells by the immune system. Other bacteria—such as *Shigella flexneri,* a microbe that causes a diarrhaeal illness—may promote their survival inside phagocytic cells by triggering apoptosis and death of the phagocytic cell.

Suppression of the Immune System

Some pathogens ensure their survival in a mammalian host by actively suppressing the immune response. Many viruses include genes capable of modulating the immune response. For example, Epstein-Barr virus (EBV), which infects B cells, encodes a gene that produces a protein that is a homolog of interleukin-10 (IL-10) and that downregulates the immune response. Other viruses like herpes simplex have virally encoded Fc and complement receptors that interfere with the function of antibody and complement. Herpes simplex virus can also interfere with recognition of infected cells by the immune system through a mechanism that inhibits MHC class I expression on the infected cell thereby thwarting its ability to present virally derived peptides. Adenoviruses encode genes that downregulate the host inflammatory response. The fungus *Cryptococcus neoformans* sheds large amounts of capsular polysaccharide, which interferes with the formation of inflammatory responses in tissue. HIV infects a variety of cells, including $CD4^+$ T cells and hence is able to directly interfere with the cells necessary for an effective immune response. HIV-induced $CD4^+$ T cell depletion produces a spiraling deterioration of immune function that culminates in AIDS and leaves the patient vulnerable to many opportunistic infections.

Extracellular Enzymes

Some bacteria produce enzymes that degrade immune molecules. For example, *Neisseria meningitidis* and *N. gonorrhoeae,* the causes of meningococcal meningitis and gonorrhea, respectively, produce ***IgA proteases*** that destroy IgA in mucosal surfaces. Streptococci, such as Group A streptococcus (which causes ***strep throat***), produce ***hemolysins,*** which are believed to aid the organism in dissemination; some elaborate a ***peptidase*** that cleaves the C5a complement protein.

Expression of Antibody-Binding Proteins

Some bacteria, such as *Staphylococcus aureus,* express cell-surface proteins that can bind immunoglobulins through their Fc region. Examples of these ***Fc-binding proteins*** are ***protein A*** and ***protein G.*** The ability of these proteins to bind immunoglobulin molecules is exploited in immunologic research by using them in affinity chromatography to purify IgG (Chapter 5).

PRINCIPLES OF IMMUNIZATION

Protection against infectious diseases by the use of vaccines represents an immense, if not the greatest, accomplishment of biomedical science. One disease, smallpox, has been totally eliminated by the use of vaccination, and the incidence of other diseases has been significantly reduced—at least in areas of the world where vaccines are available and administered properly.

If a large enough number of individuals can be immunized, ***herd immunity*** is achieved, and the transmission of communicable diseases among people is interrupted. Although deliberate immunization alone can sometimes reduce the incidence of a disease to a very low level, successful immunization programs require the intelligent practice of other measures, both hygienic and sanitary, which contribute to general improvements in public health.

Immunization can be either active or passive. ***Active immunization*** generally refers to the *administration of a vaccine* that can elicit a protective immune response. ***Passive immunization*** refers to the *administration of antibodies or lymphocytes,* which then provide protection in the recipient host (Table 20.2).

OBJECTIVES OF IMMUNIZATION

The objective of active immunization is to provide the individual with long-lasting immunologic protection against exposure to infectious agents. Many vaccines are given in childhood to protect against infections that are usually acquired early in life. The objective of passive immunization is to provide transient protection against a particular infection. For example, an individual bitten by a rabid animal may be given an injection of immune globulin to rabies virus to protect against infection with this virus. Protection against the development of disease can also be conferred by postexposure immunization. For example, an individual exposed to the rabies virus can be protected against this lethal infection by administration of both rabies vaccine and immune globulin against rabies virus. Other examples of postexposure immunization include the use of toxoid and antitoxin against diphtheria, vaccination with tetanus toxoid after trauma, and administration of immune serum globulins against hepatitis A virus (HAV) and hepatitis B virus (HBV) after exposure. Great effort is currently aimed at the development of therapeutic vaccines that will forestall the relentless progression of AIDS in HIV-infected individuals.

The potential for use of vaccines to prevent certain cancers in humans was discussed in Chapter 19. Some cancers may be prevented by vaccines that prevent infections associated with the subsequent development of carcinoma. For example, there is a strong association between primary carcinoma of the liver and infection by HBV. Hence the use of the recombinant HBV vaccine in high-risk groups may provide protection against both hepatitis and the subsequent development of hepatoma.

TABLE 20.2. Examples of Active and Passive Immunization

Type of Immunity	How Acquired
Active	
Natural (unintended)	Infection
Artificial (deliberate)	Vaccination
Passive	
Natural	Transfer of antibody from mother to infant in placental circulation or colostrum
Artificial	Passive antibody therapy (serum therapy, administration of immune human globulin)

ACTIVE IMMUNIZATIONS

As discussed in Chapter 1, the terms *vaccination* and *vaccine* derive from the work of Edward Jenner who, more than 200 years ago, showed that inoculating people with fluid obtained from the skin lesions of cows who were infected with cowpox virus protected them from the highly contagious and frequently fatal disease smallpox. Jenner's process came to be called *vaccination,* after *vacca,* the Latin word for "cow," and the substance used to vaccinate was called a *vaccine.* Cowpox (vaccinia virus) induces protective immune responses to smallpox virus because the two viruses share antigenic epitopes, thus inducing a protective immune response. Table 20.3 lists some of the different kinds of vaccines currently in use. Later in this chapter, we discuss more recent approaches to vaccine development.

Recommended Immunizations

The usual recommended schedule in the United States for active immunization at various ages is given in Table 20.4. It is important to note that in other parts of the world, the immunization schedule may be different. In recent years, a *Haemophilus influenzae* type b polysaccharide diphtheria

TABLE 20.3. Vaccines Used in Active Immunization

Vaccine Type	Vaccine Composition	Examples
Killed whole organisms	Made from the entire organism, killed to make it harmless	Typhoid
Attenuated bacteria	Organism cultured to reduce its pathogenicity but still retains some of the antigens of the virulent form	Bacille Calmette-Guérin, vaccine against *M. tuberculosis* used in many European countries but rarely used in the United States
Toxoids	Bacterial toxins treated (e.g., with formaldehyde) to denature the protein so that it is no longer dangerous but still retains some epitopes that will elicit protective antibodies	Diphtheria, tetanus
Surface molecules	Purified surface molecules isolated from various pathogens (e.g., hemagglutinins from influenza virus)	Influenza, hepatitis B surface antigen, *S. pneumoniae* capsular polysaccharides, and *H. influenzae* type b capsular oligosaccharides (the latter are formulated as protein conjugates)
Inactivated virus	Whole virus particles treated (e.g., with formaldehyde) so that they cannot infect the host's cells but still retain some unaltered epitopes	Salk vaccine for polio
Attenuated virus	Live viruses that are weakened and nonpathogenic	Sabin oral polio vaccine, measles, mumps, rubella vaccines

toxoid conjugate was added to the vaccination schedule of young children (first dose at 2 months of age). *H. influnzae* type b is a major cause of meningitis in nonimmunized children. The use of this vaccine has resulted in a dramatical reduction in *H. influenzae* type b infections in vaccinated children. Recently, a heptavalent pneumococcal conjugate vaccine was approved for use in children for the prevention of invasive disease, including otitis media.

Use of Vaccines in Selected Populations

In addition to the usual schedule of immunizations given in Table 20.4, some individuals receive additional vaccinations (listed in Table 20.5). Influenza virus (inactivated) is given to people older than 60 years of age and to children and adults with cardiorespiratory ailments. Hepatitis B vaccine (viral protein produced by recombinant DNA technology) is given to health-care and emergency workers who are exposed to human blood. Hepatitis A (inactivated virus) has been approved for use in children and adults. Adenovirus vaccines are used to prevent outbreaks of respiratory infections in military recruits. Anthrax vaccine is used in military personnel, given the threat posed by the use of *Bacillus anthracis* spores in biological warfare. Vaccination against smallpox is no longer recommended for civilians but is still given to selected military personnel. However, there is currently a great debate on whether to make greater use of this vaccine given heightened concerns about the use of smallpox as a biological weapon.

TABLE 20.4. Schedule for Active Immunization in Children[a]

Age	Vaccine
Birth	Hepatitis B (Hep B), first dose
1–4 months	Hep B, second dose
2 months	Dipththeria, tetanus toxoids, acellular pertussis vaccine (DTP); *H. influenzae* type b (Hib); inactivated polio vaccine (IPV); and pneumococcal conjugate vaccine (PCV), first doses
4 months	DTP, Hib, IPV, and PCV, second doses
6 months	DTP, Hib, and PCV, third doses
6–18 months	Hep B and IPV, third doses
12–15 months	Measles, mumps, rubella (MNR), first doses varicella vaccine
15–18 months	DTP, fourth dose
4–6 years	DTP, fifth dose; IPV, fourth dose; MMR, second dose
11–12 years	Tetanus toxoid booster

[a] Adapted from Centers for Disease Control and prevention (www.cdc.gov/nip).

TABLE 20.5. Additional Vaccinations[a]

Vaccine	Population(s)
Anthrax	Military personnel; handlers of animal hides, furs, bone meal, wool, and animal bristles; researchers who work with *B. anthracis;* veterinarians likely to be exposed
Bacille Calmette-Guérin	Health-care personnel in close contact with tuberculosis patients
Hepatitis A	Children and adults in high-risk areas
Hepatitis B	All children, susceptible health-care workers, homosexual males, intravenous drug users, individuals exposed to blood products
Japanese B encephalitis	Travelers to high-risk areas
Influenzae	Persons >65 years of age, children at high-risk
Measles, mumps, influenza, varicella, rubella	Susceptible health-care personnel
Meningococcus	Military personnel, young adults living in college dormitories
Plague	Persons in regular contact with rodents, investigators working with *Yersinia pestis*
Rabies	Veterinarians, animal handlers, animal bite victims
Typhoid	Travelers to high-risk areas
Yellow fever	Travelers to high-risk areas

[a] Adapted from the centers for Disease Control and Prevention (www.cdc.gov).

Several vaccines against bacterial infections are also used in specific populations. A polyvalent vaccine consisting of several antigenic types of capsular polysaccharides from *Streptococcus pneumoniae* is given to individuals with cardiorespiratory ailments, to anatomically or functionally asplenic individuals, and to patients with sickle-cell anemia, renal failure, alcoholic cirrhosis, or diabetes mellitus. These individuals have limited capability to mount the antibody/complement/phagocytic activity required against the encapsulated bacteria such as *S. pneumoniae.* Unfortunately, this vaccine may not be as effective in persons at high risk for pneumococcal pneumonia as in normal individuals because the immune defects preclude the generation of strong antibody responses. *Neisseria meningitidis* vaccine (several serogroups of capsular polysaccharide) is given to military recruits and to children in high-risk regions. This vaccine is also recommended for young adults who live in college dormitories who are at high risk for meningococcal meningitis. Both live attenuated and a polysaccharide vaccines are available for protection against *Salmonella typhi,* the cause of typhoid fever. Because of unique needs or limited efficacy, some vaccines are recommended under only limited circumstances. These vaccines and appropriate circumstances are listed in Table 20.5.

BASIC MECHANISMS OF PROTECTION

Significance of the Primary and Secondary Responses

The rapidity of the ***anamnestic response*** to a reencounter with antigen provides the host with potential protection on repeated exposures to an infectious agent. This anamnestic response is relevant in at least two significant ways in the application of ***immunoprophylaxis.*** First, it may be of particular importance in infections with a relatively long incubation period (>7 days), as shown in Figure 20.2. Thus an individual infected by agent A, which causes disease after a 3-day incubation period, would produce a primary immune response some time (e.g., 7–14 days) after onset of the infection. On a second encounter with agent A, the individual may again develop disease, because an anamnestic response may not be sufficiently rapid to inhibit agent A. The individual infected with agent B, which causes disease after a 14-day incubation period, would produce a primary response (e.g., 7–14 days after infection). On a second encounter with agent A, the anamnestic response occurring within 7 days would be sufficient to reduce the severity or prevent the disease with the 14-day incubation period.

The second influence of the anamnestic response concerns the level to which the immune response has been raised. In the example cited above, agent A, which causes disease in 3 days, may be prevented from causing disease after a reexposure if there is a persisting high enough level of antibody. Such a level can be achieved deliberately by a series of immunizations (especially applicable with nonviable antigens). Thus it is customary to give several injections of tetanus toxoid (as DTP) over a period of 6 months in childhood immunizations. Such a primary series of injections generates anamnestic secondary responses that successively raise the concentration of antitoxin to protective levels, which are sustained in the serum for 10–20 years.

Age and Timing of Immunizations

The various mechanisms involved in protection can be affected by several factors, including nutritional status,

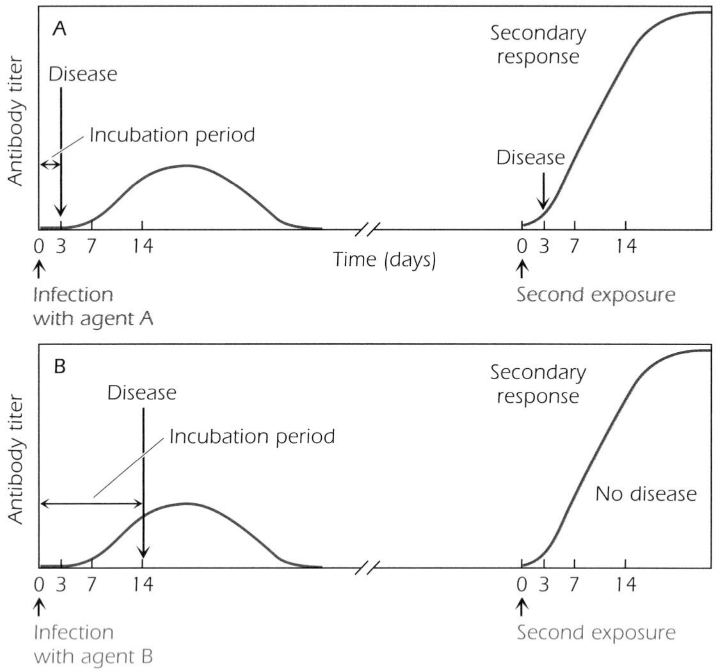

Figure 20.2. The relationship between the primary and secondary immune responses and disease produced by infection with agent A or B. Infection caused by agent A has shorter incubation period than infection caused by agent B.

presence of underlying disease (which affects levels of globulin and cell-mediated immunity), and age. The timing of childhood immunization is driven largely by the fact that the efficacy of certain vaccines depends on the age of the child.

In utero, the human fetus normally appears well insulated from antigens and most infectious agents, although certain pathogens (e.g., rubella virus, *Toxoplasma gondii*) can infect the mother and seriously injure the fetus. The immunity of the mother protects the fetus by permitting interception and removal of infectious agents before they can enter the uterus, or it protects the newborn by virtue of transplacental or mammary gland antibody.

The fetus and neonate have poorly developed lymphoid organs, with the exception of the thymus, which at the time of birth is largest in size relative to the body size at any age. The fetus appears capable of synthesizing mainly IgM, which becomes apparent after 6 months of gestation. Levels of IgM gradually increase to about 10% of the adult level at the time of birth.

IgG becomes detectable in the fetus at about the 2nd month of gestation, but it is IgG of maternal origin. The level of IgG increases significantly at about 4 months of gestation and markedly in the last trimester. At the time of birth, the concentration of IgG slightly exceeds the maternal concentration of IgG. Thus the fetus is provided with maternally synthesized IgG antibodies, which can provide antitoxic, antiviral, and some kinds of antibacterial protection. The levels of these maternal antibodies gradually decline as the infant begins to synthesize its own antibodies, so that total IgG at 23 months of age is <50% of the level at birth. The serum concentrations of immunoglobulins during human development are shown in Figure 20.3.

Some aspects of the immune response of the newborn, for example, against some infectious agents (*Toxoplasma gondii, Listeria monocytogenes,* herpes simplex virus) in which cell-mediated immunity is critical are not well developed. But the newborn can produce antibody to various antigens, such as parenterally administered toxoid, inactivated poliomyelitis virus, hepatitis B antigens, and others. However, administration of pertussis vaccine very soon after birth not only fails to induce a protective response but also creates an impaired response (tolerance?) to the vaccine when it is given again later in infancy. Therefore, with the exception of the hepatitis B vaccine that is given shortly after birth, in most industrialized countries the initial administration of vaccines is deferred until the child is 2 months old. However, the World Health Organization (WHO) recommends earlier commencement of immunization (at 6 weeks) in developing countries.

Maternal antibody, while capable of providing protection to the neonate against a variety of infectious agents or their toxins, may also reduce the response to antigen. For example, a sufficient quantity of maternal measles antibody persists in the 1-year-old infant to interfere with the active response of the infant to the vaccine, so that vaccination is usually delayed until the child is at least 1 year of age.

Children <2 years of age have a general inability to produce adequate levels of antibody in response to injection of bacterial capsular polysaccharides, such as those of *Haemophilus influenzae* type b, various serogroups of *Neisseria meningitidis,* and *Streptococcus pneumoniae* serotypes. It has been suggested that this inability arises because infants do not respond to T-independent antigens, despite their early (in utero) capacity to generate IgM. Chemical linkage of polysaccharide to T-dependent antigens (e.g., diphtheria toxoid) or

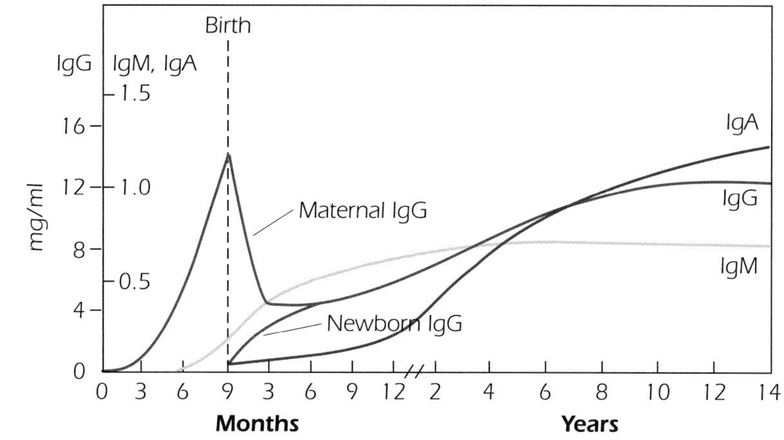

Figure 20.3. Concentration of immunoglobulin in the serum during human development. (After Benich and Johanssen, (1971), with permission.)

to *N. meningitidis* outer membrane protein has improved the immunogenicity so that children younger than 2 years of age respond to polysaccharides. An effective conjugate vaccine is already available against *H. influenzae,* which has virtually eliminated this infection in vaccinated children. For *S. pneumoniae,* a heptavalent vaccine containing polysaccharides of pneumococcal serotypes common in childhood infections is now in routine use.

At the other end of the age spectrum in people older than 60 years of age there also appears to be a reduced capability to mount a primary response to some antigens, such as influenza virus vaccine; but the elderly retain the ability to mount a secondary response to antigens to which they have been previously exposed. The healthy elderly also respond well to bacterial polysaccharides, so that administration of pneumococcal polysaccharide vaccine can usually induce protective levels of antibody. Other groups that are especially susceptible to pneumococcal pneumonia (see earlier in this chapter) should also be immunized. Groups that have enhanced susceptibility to the encapsulated respiratory pathogen *Streptococcus pneumoniae* and those at high risk of exposure (e.g., residents of nursing homes and medical personnel) should also receive influenza virus vaccines.

PRECAUTIONS

Site of Administration of Antigen

The usual site of parenteral (intradermal, subcutaneous, intramuscular) administration of vaccines in adults is the arm, in particular the deltoid muscle. In children, the thigh is routinely used. Studies have shown a suboptimal response to hepatitis B vaccine when given by intragluteal injection than by injection in the arm. The parenteral administration of inactivated polio vaccine may induce a higher antibody response in the serum than the attenuated oral polio vaccine, but the response to the latter, which includes secretory IgA, affords adequate protection. However, use of the attenuated oral polio vaccine has been discontinued because the live virus can in exceptionally rare circumstances cause disease.

Some vaccines may provide a greater antibody response when given by the respiratory route than when given by injection (e.g., attenuated measles vaccine), but administration via the respiratory route remains an investigational method.

Hazards

There are potential hazards associated with the use of some vaccines. Vaccines made from attenuated agents (e.g., measles, mumps, rubella, oral polio, bacille Calmette-Guérin) have the potential for causing progressive disease in the ***immunocompromised patient*** or in the patient on ***immunosuppressive therapy.*** In rare cases, reversion of attenuated poliovirus type III to virulence in the intestine of the vaccinated individual has caused paralytic polio. Concern about vaccine-associated paralytic polio has resulted in a change in recommendations for vaccination against polio virus so that the inactivated poliovirus vaccine is now the recommended vaccine in the United States. This illustrates the need for constant vigilance in monitoring the prevalence of a given infectious disease in a given population and weighing the risks of disease versus the risks of vaccination. Although vaccines are generally associated with very low toxicity, they are administered to large numbers of individuals, and it must be recognized that as the prevalence of an infectious disease is reduced, the risks of vaccination may be magnified. Hence, the paradoxical situation can occur whereby an effective vaccine reduces the prevalence of an infectious disease to such a low level that rare vaccine-related complications are more frequent than the disease in the population. When that happens, public anxiety about vaccination can result in concerns about vaccine use and may reduce its acceptance.

Live attenuated organisms should ordinarily not be given to ***pregnant women*** because of potential damage to the fetus. (The virions in rubella vaccine have been transmitted to the fetus, although without any recognized injurious effect.) Live attenuated vaccines are generally contraindicated for patients with severe immune disorders who may not be able to control the weakened pathogen in the vaccine preparation. Vaccination against smallpox is no longer carried out (except in some military personnel) since the disease has been eradicated. However, as we noted above, concerns about the potential of variola virus as a biological weapon have led to debate as to whether universal vaccination should be reintroduced. At this time, the plan is to vaccinate only individuals who are likely to respond or be exposed to a potential biological attack and reserve the vaccine for use in postexposure prophylaxis. One argument against universal vaccination is that vaccinia virus inoculation carries significant risks, not only in immunocompromised individuals but also in individuals with certain cutaneous lesions. Contact between vaccinated and vulnerable individuals must be avoided until the vaccinia lesions have healed.

Arthritis and arthralgia are common but transient complications following vaccination with attenuated rubella virus, particularly in adult women. Of the inactivated vaccines, the killed *Bordetella pertussis* bacterial vaccine in DTP was associated with some serious side effects, including encephalopathy in the infant. Although serious side effects were relatively rare and the benefits of the pertussis vaccine outweighed any of alleged risks of immunization, the killed bacteria vaccine was replaced by an acellular vaccine containing inactivated pertussis toxin and one or more antigenic components (e.g., filamentous hemagglutinin and fimbriae). The acellular pertussis vaccine has significantly fewer side effects than the earlier vaccine while retaining efficacy.

Tetanus and diphtheria toxoids may provoke local hypersensitivity reactions. Because an adequate initial series of immunizations in childhood appears to give immunity that lasts some 10 years, the use of booster injections of tetanus toxoid should be guided by the nature of an injury and the history of immunization. The increased hypersensitivity to diphtheria toxoid of adolescents and adults necessitates use of a smaller dose of diphtheria toxoid than is used for children. Because influenza virus is cultivated in chick embryos, allergy to egg protein is a contraindication to vaccination against this virus. Whole influenza virus vaccine is used in adults but gives side effects in children, so a split-virus component vaccine is recommended for children younger than 13 years of age. Some vaccines contain preservatives, such as the organomercurial compound thimerosal (Merthiolate), or antibiotics, such as neomycin or streptomycin, to which the vaccinated individual may be allergic.

RECENT APPROACHES TO PRODUCTION OF VACCINES

Advances in recombinant DNA technology and in the technology of rapid, automated synthesis of peptides and other areas of bioengineering (e.g., monoclonal antibodies) hold promise for improvements in available vaccines and new approaches to the production of vaccines.

Vaccines Produced by Recombinant DNA

Recombinant DNA technology provides the means for expressing protein antigens in large amounts for vaccine use. An example of the successful application of recombinant DNA technology to vaccine production is provided by the experience with the hepatitis B vaccine. Hepatitis B is a major cause of liver infection and is associated with a long-term risk of hepatocellular carcinoma. An effective vaccine against hepatitis B was developed in the 1970s by purifying viral antigen from the blood of chronically infected donors. In the 1980s, the HIV epidemic heightened awareness about transmission of blood-borne pathogens, and there were concerns that this vaccine could transmit disease. Although several studies showed the plasma-derived vaccine was safe, an alternative was developed by expressing the hepatitis B antigen in yeast using recombinant DNA technology. This recombinant vaccine simplified the production of antigen by avoiding reliance on human blood plasma and eliminated any potential hazard arising from inadvertent contamination of vaccine antigen with blood-borne pathogens. Recombinant DNA technology has also been used to generate the first effective vaccine against Lyme disease. Other vaccines produced by recombinant DNA technology are in various stages of clinical testing. Some of these molecular approaches may provide practical, safer, and more effective means of immunization than are currently available.

Conjugated Polysaccharides

Conjugated polysaccharide vaccines have revolutionized the approach to vaccination against encapsulated bacterial pathogens. Humoral immunity is critical for protection against encapsulated pathogens, but most microbial polysaccharides are T-independent antigens, which are usually poorly immunogenic. Another problem with polysaccharide vaccines is that young children tend not to mount antibody responses to polysaccharide antigens. Children are at high risk for infection with encapsulated bacteria such as *Streptococcus pneumoniae* and *Haemophilus influenzae*. ***Conjugation of polysaccharide to a protein*** (e.g., ***tetanus*** or ***diphtheria toxoid***) results in a molecule that behaves as a T-dependent antigen and elicits strong antibody responses to the polysaccharide moiety. Conjugation of such (bacterial) polysaccharides or oligosaccharides (e.g., of *H. influenzae*), to proteins such as diphtheria toxoid has provided vaccines that are effective in this age group. Conjugated polysaccharide vaccines are currently available against *H. influenzae* type B and certain serotypes of *S. pneumoniae*. Conjugated polysaccharide vaccines are under development for other pathogens, including meningococci, group B streptococci,

Salmonella typhi and *Shigella* spp. Conjugated polysaccharide vaccines are protective by eliciting strong antibody responses to the polysaccharide portion of the conjugate.

Synthetic Peptide Vaccines

The premise underlying synthetic peptide vaccine development is to use immunogenic peptides to elicit a protective immune response. Synthetic peptide vaccines are designed using the knowledge of the amino acid sequence of the protein antigen that elicits a protective immune response. In theory, synthetic peptide vaccines have the advantage that highly purified peptides may be made in large quantities and their simpler antigenic composition may afford protection with fewer side effects. The general approach is to identify potential epitopes in a protective protein antigen using various algorithms, synthesize a series of peptides corresponding to the amino acid sequence, and test these for immunologic activity. One problem with peptide vaccines is that peptides are poorly immunogenic due to their small size and require conjugation to carrier proteins. Several synthetic peptide vaccines are currently in clinical testing. Peptide vaccines have shown promise against foot and mouth disease virus and malaria.

Anti-Idiotype Vaccines

An antibody (idiotype) induced to a specific epitope of an antigen has a combining site that structurally fits the epitope. If that antibody, in turn, is used as an immunogen to induce an antibody (an anti-idiotype) that reacts with the antigen-combining site of the idiotype, the anti-idiotype may structurally mimic the epitope. This structural mimicry is referred to as an ***internal image.*** Because of the resemblance of the anti-idiotype and the original antigen epitope, its internal image (anti-idiotypic antibody) can be used as an immunogen to induce antibodies against the original epitope (Fig. 20.4). Several anti-idiotypic vaccines are currently being investigated for the effectiveness in treating human cancers.

One example is an immunogen consisting of antibodies made in mice against a monoclonal mouse antibody to hepatitis B surface antigen. Immunization with these anti-idiotypic antibodies that contain the internal image of an epitope on the hepatitis B surface antigen induces antibodies to that epitope. When the toxic effects of certain biologic toxins preclude their use as antigens, anti-idiotypic antibodies can be used to elicit an antitoxic response.

Virus-Carrier Vaccine

It is possible to introduce into a live virus, such as vaccinia, adenovirus, or poliovirus, by means of a vector, a gene from another organism that codes for a desired antigen. The vaccinia virus construct replicates in the host, expresses the foreign gene, and then serves as a vaccine to that particular antigen. This approach is useful provided that the vaccinia virus is not hazardous to the host (as it may be to an immunocompromised individual). This virus-carrier vaccine has the additional advantage in that it can potentially induce both cell-mediated and antibody-mediated immunity to the incorporated antigen.

Bacterium-Carrier Vaccine

Attenuated bacteria such as strains of *Salmonella typhimurium, Escherichia coli,* and bacillus Calmette-Guerin can also serve as carriers for pathogen genes in an effort to elicit pathogen-specific responses. These bacteria are altered by recombinant techniques, which introduce a foreign gene that can express the antigens of pathogenic microbes and induce immune responses. In the future, *Salmonella typhimurium,* an intestinal pathogen, could be used to induce mucosal immunity to the foreign antigens.

DNA Vaccines

Vaccination with a plasmid encoding the DNA sequence for a protective antigen linked to a strong mammalian promoter can elicit an immune response to the protein. DNA vaccines are thought to work by allowing the expression of the microbial antigen inside host cells that take up the plasmid. DNA vaccines function by generating of the desired antigen inside cells and this has the advantage that it may facilitate MHC presentation. Other advantages of DNA vaccines are the absence of infection risk, greater stability relative to protein vaccines, and the possibility of delivering the antigen to cells that are not usually infected by the pathogen for better modulation of the immune response. DNA vaccines could be useful for immunizing young children who still have maternal antibody. The feasibility of DNA immunization has now been demonstrated against several viral, bacterial, and protozoal infections in laboratory animals. Several DNA vaccines are undergoing testing in humans to determine their usefulness in prevention or treatment of HIV, malaria, and hepatitis B infection. However, no DNA vaccines are currently in use in humans. One

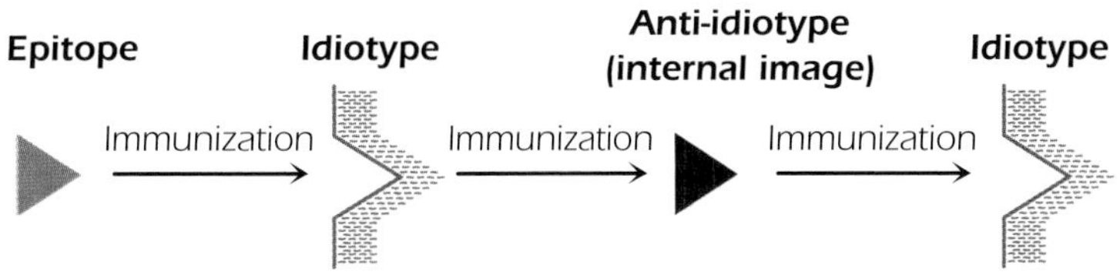

Figure 20.4. An anti-idiotype (internal image) immunogen.

nagging concern with DNA vaccines has been possibility that they could be mutagenic by integrating in host DNA. However, early results in human trials suggest that DNA vaccines are safe. At this time, DNA vaccines continue to be the subject of intense experimental study.

Toxoids

Toxins can be inactivated to produce nonpathogenic toxoids used for vaccination. Toxoids are among the earliest and most successful vaccines. Administration of toxoids prepared from inactivated tetanus, botulism, or diphtheria toxin elicit antibody responses that prevent disease. Toxoids are effective despite the fact that natural infection does not always confer long-lasting immunity, presumably because the amount of toxin produced in infection may not be sufficient to elicit a strong immune response. Hence a bout of tetanus or diphtheria does not confer immunity to recurrent infection but vaccination with a toxoid provides full protection.

PASSIVE IMMUNIZATION

Passive immunization results from the ***transfer of antibody or immune cells*** to an individual from another individual who has already responded to direct stimulation by antigen. Passive immunization differs from active immunization in that it does not rely on the ability of the host's immune system to make the appropriate response. Hence passive immunization with antibodies results in the immediate availability of antibodies that can mediate protection against pathogens. Passive immunization can occur naturally as is the case during transfer of antibodies through the placenta or colostrum or therapeutically when preformed antibody is administered for the prophylaxis or therapy of infectious diseases.

Passive Immunization through Placental Antibody Transfer

The developing fetus is passively immunized with maternal IgG as a result of placental transfer of antibody. Such antibodies are present at birth and protect the infant against infections for which IgG is sufficient and for which the mother had immunity. For example, transfer of antibody to toxins (tetanus, diphtheria), viruses (measles, poliovirus, mumps, etc.) and certain bacteria (*Haemophilus influenzae* or *Streptococcus agalactiae* group B) can provide protection to the child in the first months of life. Hence adequate active immunization of the mother is a simple and effective means of providing passive protection to the fetus and infant. (However, some premature infants may not acquire the maternal antibodies to the extent that full-term infants do.) Toxoid vaccination can elicit IgG responses that cross the placenta to provide protection to the fetus and newborn. This protection is extremely important in areas of the world where an unclean obstetric environment can lead to *tetanus neonatorum* (of the newborn).

Passive Immunization via Colostrum

Human milk contains a variety of factors that may influence the response of the nursing infant to infectious agents. Some of these factors are natural selective factors that can affect the intestinal microflora—namely, by enhancement of growth of desirable bacteria and by nonspecific inhibitors of some microbes, by the action of lysozyme, lactoferrin, interferon, and leukocytes (macrophages, T cells, B cells, and granulocytes). Antibodies (IgA) are found in breast milk, the concentration being higher in the colostrum (first milk) immediately postpartum (Table 20.6). The production of antibody is the result of B cells that are stimulated by intestinal antigens and migrate to the breast where they produce immunoglobulin (the enteromammary system). Thus organisms colonizing or infecting the alimentary tract of the mother may lead to production of colostral antibody, which affords mucosal protection to the nursing infant against pathogens that enter via the intestinal tract. Antibody to the enteropathogens *Escherichia coli, Salmonella typhi, Shigella spp.,* poliomyelitis virus, coxsackievirus, and echovirus have been demonstrated. Feeding a mixture of IgA (73%) and IgG (26%) derived from human serum to low birth weight infants who did not have access to mothers' breast milk protected them against necrotizing enterocolitis. Antibodies to nonalimentary pathogens have also been demonstrated in colostrums—for example, tetanus and diphtheria antitoxins and antistreptococcal hemolysin.

TABLE 20.6. Levels of Immunoglobulin in Colostrum[a]

	Day Postpartum				
Class	1	2	3	4	Approximate Normal Adult Serum Levels
IgA[b]	600	260	200	80	200
IgG[c]	80	45	30	16	1000
IgM	125	65	58	30	120

[a] After Michael, Ringenback, and Hottenstein, 1971; Values given are mg/100 mL.
[b] Approximately 80% is secretory IgA.
[c] IgG_4 represents 15% of colostral IgG and 3.5% of serum IgG.

Tuberculin-sensitive T lymphocytes are also transmitted to the infant through the colostrum, but the role of such cells in passive transfer of cell-mediated immunity is uncertain.

Passive Antibody Therapy and Serum Therapy

The administration of specific antibody preparations was one of the first effective antimicrobial therapies. Antibody against particular pathogens could be raised in animals, such as horses and rabbits (heterologous antibody), and administered to humans for treatment of various infections as serum therapy. Serum from individuals recovering from infection is rich in antibodies and can also be used for passive antibody therapy (homologous antibody). In recent years, some monoclonal antibodies made in the laboratory have been used for passive antibody therapy of infectious diseases. This is an area of great research activity, and it is likely that more antimicrobial therapies based on antibody administration will be developed in the future.

The active agent in serum therapy is specific antibody. In the preantibiotic era (before 1935), serum therapy was often the only therapy available for the treatment of infection. Serum therapy was used for the treatment of diphtheria, tetanus, pneumococcal pneumonia, meningococcal meningitis, scarlet fever, and other serious infections. For example, in World War I, tetanus antitoxin produced in horses injected with tetanus toxoid was used to treat the wounded British troops and resulted in prompt reduction in cases of tetanus. This experience allowed the determination of the minimum concentration of antitoxin needed to provide protection and showed that the period of protection in the human was brief. The basis for the latter is shown in Figures 20.5 and 20.6. The heterologous equine antibody in the human undergoes dilution, catabolism, immune complex formation, and immune elimination. By contrast, the homologous human antibody, which reaches a peak level in the serum about 2 days after subcutaneous injection, undergoes dilution and catabolism with a reduction to half the maximal concentration in about 23 days (the half-life of human IgG_1, IgG_2, and IgG_4 is 23 days; that of IgG_3 is 7 days). The protective level of the human antibody is thus sustained considerably longer than that of the equine antibody. Heterologous antibody, such as that from the horse, can cause at least two kinds of hypersensitivity reaction: type I (immediate, anaphylaxis—see Chapter 14) or type III (serum sickness from immune complexes—see Chapter 15). If no other treatment is available, it is possible to use the heterologous antiserum in an individual with type I sensitivity by administration of gradually increasing but minute amounts of the foreign serum, given repeatedly over several hours. Some preparations of heterologous antibody (e.g., equine diphtheria antitoxin and antilymphocyte serum [ALS]) are still used in humans. In recent years, advances in hybridoma and recombinant DNA technology provided the means to synthesize human immunoglobulins for therapy, and we no longer depend on animal sources for therapeutic antibodies. Human antibodies have significantly longer half-life and reduced toxicity in humans.

Monoclonal and Polyclonal Preparations

Hybridoma technology that allows the production of monoclonal antibodies was discovered in 1975 (see Chapter 5). Polyclonal preparations result from the antibody response to immunization or recovery from infection in a host. In general, antibody to a specific agent is only a small fraction of the total antibody in a polyclonal preparation. Furthermore, polyclonal preparations usually contain antibodies to multiple antigens and include antibodies of various isotypes. Monoclonal antibody preparations differ from polyclonal antibody preparations in that a monoclonal antibody has one specificity and one isotype. As a result, the activity of monoclonal antibody preparations is considerably greater for the amount of protein present than polyclonal preparations. Another advantage of monoclonal preparations is that they are invariant and do not have the lot-to-lot variability associated with polyclonal preparations that depend on quantitative and qualitative aspects of the immune response for their potency. However, polyclonal preparations have the advantage, by

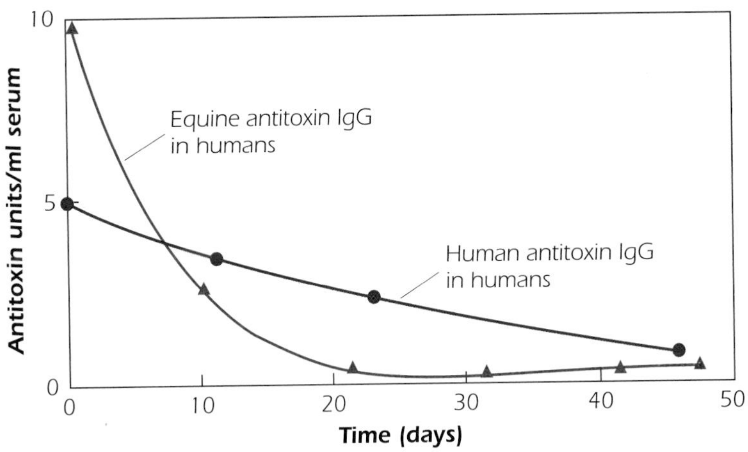

Figure 20.5. Serum concentration of human and equine IgG antitoxin following administration into humans.

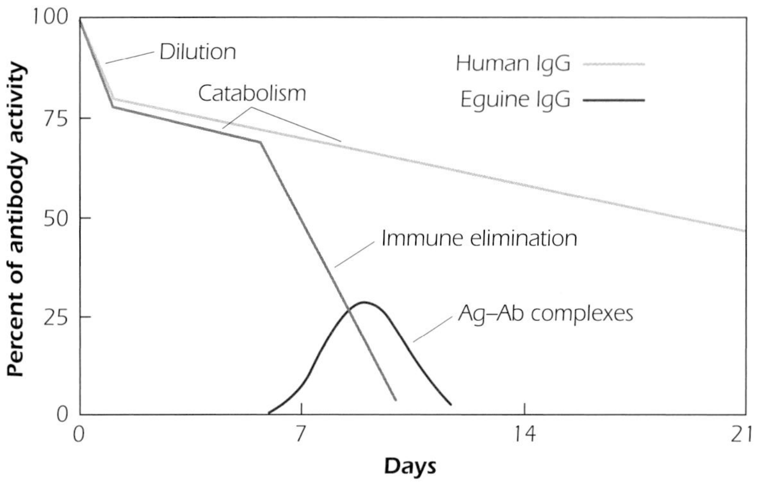

Figure 20.6. The fate of human and equine IgG following administration into humans.

including antibodies with multiple specificities and isotypes, of encompassing a higher biologic diversity. In the past 5 years at least a dozen monoclonal antibodies have been licensed for clinical use. Most of them have been developed for therapy of cancer, although one is now licensed for the prevention of respiratory syncytial virus infections in young children. Several monoclonal and polyclonal antibody preparations are currently used for human therapy.

Preparation and Properties of Human Immune Serum Globulin

The use of immune globulin from human serum began in the early 1900s, when serum of patients convalescing from measles was given to children who had been exposed to measles but had not yet developed symptoms. Additional attempts in 1916 and later showed that early administration of serum obtained from individuals who had recovered from infection with measles virus, could protect against the emergence of clinically apparent measles. In 1933, human placentae were also recognized as a source of measles antibody. A problem with using serum for passive therapy is that it contains relatively little antibody in a large volume. In the early 1940s, Cohn and co-workers devised a method for the separation of the ***gammaglobulin*** (γ-globulin) fraction from human serum by precipitation with cold ethanol. This so-called ***Cohn fractionation*** represented a practical and safe method for production of homologous human antibody for clinical use.

Plasma is collected from healthy donors or placentae. The plasma or serum from several donors is pooled, and the preparation is termed immune serum globulin (ISG) or human normal immunoglobulin (HNI). If the plasma or serum is from donors who are specially selected after an immunizing or booster dose of antigen or after convalescence from a specific infection, the specific immune globulin preparation is designated accordingly: tetanus immune globulin (TIG), hepatitis B immune globulin (HBIG), varicella-zoster immune globulin (VZIG), and rabies immune globulin (RIG). Large quantities can be obtained by plasmapheresis removal of the plasma while returning the blood cells to the donor. The fraction containing antibody globulin(s) is precipitated by cold ethanol. The resultant preparation (1) is theoretically free of viruses such as hepatitis virus and HIV, (2) concentrates many of the IgG antibodies about 25-fold, (3) is stable for years, and (4) can provide peak levels in blood approximately 2 days after intramuscular injection. Preparations that are safe when administered intravenously (called IVIG or IVGG) involve cold alcohol precipitation followed by various other treatments, including fractionation using polyethylene glycol or ion exchangers; acidification to pH 4–4.5; exposure to pepsin or trypsin; and stabilization with maltose, sucrose, glucose, or glycine. Such stabilization reduces aggregation of the globulins that can trigger anaphylactoid reactions (see below). In these newer intravenous preparations, IgG is present in one third to one fourth its concentration in the intramuscular immune globulin preparations and there is only a trace of IgA and IgM (Table 20.7).

Indications for the Use of Immune Globulin

Antibody to RhD antigen (***Rhogam***) is given to Rh^- mothers within a 72-h perinatal period to prevent their immunization by fetal Rh^+ erythrocytes that could affect future pregnancies. As discussed in Chapter 15, Rhogam administration protects by promoting the removal of Rh^+ fetal cells to which the mother is exposed during parturition and thus avoids the sensitizing of the Rh^- mother by Rh^+ antigens. TIG (antitoxin) is used to provide passive protection after certain wounds and in the absence of adequate active immunization with tetanus toxoid. VZIG is given to patients with leukemia who are highly vulnerable to the varicella-zoster (chickenpox) virus and to pregnant women and their infants exposed to or infected with varicella virus. Cytomegalovirus human immune globulin (CMV-IGIV) is used prophylactically for recipients

TABLE 20.7. Comparison of Human Immune Serum Globulin

	Immunoglobulin (mg/100 mL)		
Source	IgG	IgA	IgM
Whole serum	1,200	180	200
Immune serum globulin	16,500	100–500	25–200
Intravenous immunoglobulin	3,000–5,000	trace	trace
Placental immune serum globulin	16,500	200–700	150–400

of bone marrow or renal transplants. RIG is given together with active immunization with human diploid cell rabies vaccine to individuals bitten by potentially rabid animals (human RIG is not universally available, so equine antibody may be necessary in some areas). HBIG may be given to a newborn child of a mother who has evidence of hepatitis B infection, to medical personnel after an accidental stick with a hypodermic needle, or after sexual contact with an individual with hepatitis B. (ISG may also be used against hepatitis B; see below.) Vaccinia immune globulin is given to eczematous or immunocompromised individuals with intimate exposure to others who have been vaccinated against smallpox by live attenuated vaccinia vaccine. Such compromised individuals can develop destructive progressive disease from the attenuated vaccine.

IVIG has been used in certain circumstances for its antimicrobial properties and has had significant success against group B streptococcal infections in premature neonates, echovirus-induced chronic meningoencephalitis, and Kawasaki disease (a condition of unknown cause). Intravenous administration of immune globulin can reduce bacterial infections in patients with hematopoietic malignancies, such as chronic B cell lymphocytic leukemia and multiple myeloma. Chronic IVIG administration has been useful in children who have immunosuppressive conditions and in premature infants; in hypogammaglobulinemia and primary immune deficiency disease, repeated injections of ISG are required. IVIG also has therapeutic value in a variety of autoimmune conditions. For example, in immune idiopathic thrombocytopenic purpura (ITP), IVIG presumably blocks the Fc receptors on phagocytic cells and prevents them from phagocytosing and destroying platelets coated with autoantibodies. IVIG has also been used with varying success in other immune cytopenias.

Precautions on the Use of ImmuneTherapy

The preparations of globulin other than IVIG have to be given by the intramuscular route; intravenous administration is contraindicated because of possible anaphylactoid reactions. These are probably due to aggregates of immunoglobulin formed during the fractionation by ethanol precipitation. These aggregates activate complement to yield anaphylatoxins (IgG_1, IgG_2, IgG_3, and IgM by the classical pathway; IgG_4 and IgA, by the alternative pathway) or cross-link Fc receptors directly, leading to the release of inflammatory mediators. The IVIG that is safe for intravenous administration has been increasingly used, particularly when repeated administration is required, as in agammaglobulinemia.

One unique contraindication to the use of the usual immune globulin preparations is in cases of congenital deficiency of IgA. Since these patients lack IgA, they recognize it as a foreign protein and respond by making antibodies against it, including IgE antibodies, which can lead to a subsequent anaphylactic reaction. The IVIG preparations with only a trace of IgA may pose less of a problem.

Colony-Stimulating Factors

Colony-stimulating factors (CSFs), as discussed in Chapter 11, are cytokines that stimulate the development and maturation of white blood cells (WBCs). Granulocyte colony-stimulating factor (G-CSF), granulocyte-macrophage colony-stimulating factor (GM-CSF), and macrophage colony-stimulating factor (M-CSF) have been cloned by recombinant DNA technology and are now available for clinical use. CSFs have proven to be useful in accelerating the recovery of bone marrow cells in patients who have undergone myelosuppressive therapy for cancer or organ transplantation. In these patients, neutrophil depletion (neutropenia) is a major predisposing factor for severe infection. By shortening the period of neutropenia, CSFs can reduce the incidence of serious infections in patients receiving myelosuppressive therapy. CSFs also enhance leukocyte function, and there is encouraging preliminary information, suggesting that these proteins may be useful as immunotherapy for enhancing host defenses against various pathogens.

Several other cytokines are powerful activators of the immune system, and there is great interest in learning how to use them as adjunctive therapy against infectious diseases. IFNγ is a powerful activator of macrophage function, which has been shown to reduce the incidence of severe infections in patients with chronic granulomatous disease. IFNγ has shown encouraging results as adjunctive therapy for some infections, including drug-resistant *Mycobacterium tuberculosis* infection and several unusual fungal infections.

SUMMARY

1. To cause disease, microbes must cause damage to the host.
2. The effective host defenses against individual pathogens depend on the type of pathogen. In general, successful protection against most pathogens involves both humoral and cellular components of the innate and adaptive immune systems.
3. Pathogens use a variety of strategies to escape host defenses, including polysaccharide capsules, antigenic variation, intracellular survival, proteolytic enzymes, and active suppression of the immune response.
4. In general, an effective host response to a pathogen uses components of both humoral and cellular immunity. However, for some pathogens, one arm of the immune system may provide the primary protection.
5. Protection against infectious diseases may be achieved by active as well as passive immunization.
6. Active immunization may result from previous infection or from vaccination, while passive immunization may occur by natural means (such as the transfer of antibodies from mother to fetus via the placenta or to an infant via the colostrum) or by artificial means (such as by the administration of immune globulins).
7. Active immunization may be achieved by administration of one immunogen or a combination of immunogens.
8. The incubation period of a disease and the rapidity with which protective antibody titers develop influence both the efficacy of vaccination and the anamnestic effect of a booster injection.
9. The site of administration of a vaccine may be of great importance; many routes of immunization lead to the synthesis predominantly of serum IgM and IgG; oral administration of some vaccines leads to the induction of secretory IgA in the digestive tract.
10. Immunoprophylaxis has had striking success against subsequent infection; immunotherapy has had limited success in infectious diseases.

REFERENCES

Allen JE, Maizels RM (1997): Th1Th2: reliable paradigm or dangerous dogma. *Immunol Today* 18:387.

Casadevall A, Pirofski L (2000): Host-pathogen interactions: basic concepts of microbial commensalism, colonization, infection, and disease. *Infect Immun* 68:6511.

Casadevall A, Scharff MD (1994): "Serum therapy" revisited: animal models of infection and the development of passive antibody therapy. *Antimicrob Agents Chemother* 38:1695.

Centers of Disease Control and Prevention (2002): Recommended childhood immunization schedule—United States, 2002. *J Am Med Assoc* 287: 707.

Deitsch KW, Moxon ER, Wellems TE (1997): Shared themes of antigenic variation and virulence in bacterial, protozoal, and fungal infections. *Microbiol Molec Biol Rev* 61:283.

Hemming VG (2001): Use of intravenous immunoglobulins for prophylaxis and treatment of infectious diseases. *Clin Diagn Lab Immunol* 8:859–63.

Hubel K, Dale DC, Liles WC (2002): Therapeutic uses of cytokines to modulate cytokine function for the treatment of infectious diseases: current status of granulocyte colony-stimulating factor, granulocyte-macrophage colony-stimulating factor, macrophage colony-stimulating factor, and interferon-gamma. *J Infect Dis* 185:1490.

Ismail N, Olano JP, Feng H., Walker DH. (2002): Current status of immune mechanisms of killing of intracellular microorganisms. *FEMS Microbiol Lett* 207:111.

Lai WC, Bennett M (1998): DNA vaccines. *Crit Rev Immunol* 18:449.

Negrao-Correa D (2001): Importance of immunoglobulin E (IgE) in the protective mechanism against gastrointestinal nematode infection: looking at the intestinal mucosae. Rev Inst Med trop *S Paulo* 43:291.

Park JM, Greten FR, Li ZW, Karin M (2002): Macrophage apoptosis by anthrax lethal factor through p38 MAP kinase inhibition. *Science* 297:2048.

Pirofski L, Casadevall A (1998): The use of licenced vaccines for active immunization of the immunocompromised host. *Clin Microbiol Rev* 11:1.

Reichert JM (2001): Monoclonal antibodies and the clinic. *Nat Biotech* 19:819.

Tsuji M, Zavala F (2001): Peptide-based subunit vaccines against pre-erythrocytic stages of malaria parasites. *Molec Immunol* 38:433.

REVIEW QUESTIONS

For each question, choose the ONE BEST answer or completion.

1. The usual sequence of events in the development of an effective immune response to a viral infection is
   A) interferon secretion, antibody synthesis, cellular immune response, NK cell ADCC.
   B) antibody synthesis, interferon secretion, NK cell ADCC, cellular immune response.
   C) NK cell ADCC, interferon secretion, antibody synthesis, cellular immune response
   D) interferon secretion, cellular immune response, antibody synthesis, NK cell ADCC.
   E) cellular immune response, interferon secretion, antibody synthesis, NK cell ADCC.

2. Differences between gram-positive and gram-negative bacteria include
   A) staining with crystal violet.
   B) ability of complement to lyse cells.
   C) thickness of the peptidoglycan layer.
   D) endotoxin in the cell walls of gram-negative bacteria.
   E) All of the above.

3. Antigenic variation is a mechanism of immune evasion that results in
   A) interference with attachment to host receptors.
   B) induction of immune suppression.
   C) alterations in important surface antigens so that escape variants arise as a result of immune selection.
   D) mutations in surface antigens.
   E) destruction of antigens by proteolytic enzymes

4. The best way to provide immunologic protection against tetanus neonatorum (of the newborn) is to
   A) inject the infant with human tetanus antitoxin.
   B) inject the newborn with tetanus toxoid.
   C) inject the mother with toxoid within 72 h of the birth of her child.
   D) immunize the mother with tetanus toxoid before or early in pregnancy.
   E) give the child antitoxin and toxoid for both passive and active immunization.

5. Active, durable immunization against poliomyelitis can be accomplished by oral administration of attenuated vaccine (Sabin) or by parenteral injection of inactivated (Salk) vaccine. These vaccines are equally effective in preventing disease because
   A) both induce adequate IgA at the intestinal mucosa, the site of entry of the virus.
   B) antibody in the serum protects against the viremia that leads to disease.
   C) viral antigen attaches to the anterior horn cells in the spinal cord, preventing attachment of virulent virus.
   D) both vaccines induce formation of interferon.
   E) both vaccines establish a mild infection that can lead to formation of antibody.

6. The administration of vaccines is not without hazard. Of the following, which is least likely to adversely affect an immunocompromised host?
   A) measles vaccine
   B) pneumococcal vaccine
   C) bacille Calmette-Guérin
   D) mumps vaccine
   E) Sabin poliomyelitis vaccine

7. The administration of foreign (e.g., equine) antitoxin for passive protection in humans can lead to serum sickness, which is characterized by all of the following except which?
   A) production by host of antibody to foreign antibody
   B) onset in 24–48 h
   C) use of homologous antitoxin
   D) deposition of antigen-antibody complexes at various sites in the host
   E) Although delayed, the reaction is not a cell-mediated delayed, type IV immune response.

8. The pneumococcal polysaccharide vaccine should be administered to all except which group?
   A) individuals with chronic cardiorespiratory disease
   B) the elderly (>60 years of age)
   C) children (<2 years of age)
   D) persons with chronic renal failure
   E) individuals with sickle cell disease

9. The following statements about human immune serum globulin are true except which one?
   A) The source is human placenta.
   B) The globulins are obtained by precipitation with cold ethanol.
   C) The concentration of IgG is more than 10-fold greater than in plasma.
   D) IgA and IgM are present in concentrations slightly lower than in plasma.
   E) The ethanol precipitation does not render preparation of globulin free of hepatitis virus.

ANSWERS TO REVIEW QUESTIONS

1. ***D*** The usual sequence of events in the host immune response to a viral infection is interferon secretion, cellular immune response, antibody synthesis, NK cell ADCC. Interferon is produced early in the course of viral infection and serves to slow the infection of adjoining cells. Cellular immune responses in the form of cytotoxic $CD8^+$ T cells occur early in viral infection and usually precede the appearance of serum-neutralizing antibody or NK cell–mediated ADCC (which requires specific antibody).

2. ***E*** Differences between gram-positive and gram-negative bacteria include staining with crystal violet. Gram-negative cells can be lysed by complement, but gram-positive cells are complement resistant because of a thick peptidoglycan layer. Gram-negative bacteria have endotoxin in their cell walls that can cause hemodynamic compromise and septic shock in patients with gram-negative sepsis. Gram-positive bacteria lack endotoxin but have teichoic acids that are immunogenic.

3. ***C*** Antigenic variation is common to many pathogens and is a mechanism by which they are able to escape the immune system. Antigenic variation can be the result of various mechanisms including mutation, changes in surface protein expression, and natural variation among strains such as occurs in the pneumococci. The potential of a microorganism for antigenic variation is a major consideration in vaccine design.

4. ***D*** The simplest and most effective way to protect the newborn infant against exotoxic disease, such as tetanus and diphtheria, is to induce antibody in the mother. The antitoxic IgG passing through the placenta will provide the necessary protection. While tetanus antitoxin could be used to provide short-term passive protection, it would be more costly and require an otherwise unnecessary and painful injection. Injection of toxoid in the mother within 72 h of delivery of the child would not allow time for induction of antibody. While antitoxin and toxoid could provide immediate passive and future active protection, the latter would have to be accompanied by future injections of toxoid and the former is expensive; both would require undesirable injections.

5. ***B*** Both attenuated and inactivated vaccines lead to formation of circulating antibody, which would provide protection by intercepting the infecting virus before it reaches the target tissue in the central nervous system. While the Sabin vaccine induces mucosal gut IgA that may intercept virus at the portal of entry, the parenterally injected Salk vaccine is not effective in inducing mucosal IgA. Viral antigen in the vaccine might attach to the anterior horn cells in the nervous system, but it probably would not provide durable immunity. Induction of interferon would represent potentially only brief protection. Only the Sabin vaccine, being attenuated and live, would induce a mild infection.

6. ***B*** The pneumococcal vaccine consists of capsular polysaccharides from *Streptococcus pneumoniae* and represents a nonviable vaccine that cannot lead to infection. Measles, mumps, and Sabin polio vaccines contain attenuated viruses, and bacille Calmette-Guerin is an attenuated bacterium. These attenuated organisms are capable of proliferating in the human host. The normal host limits their replication, but the immunocompromised host may not be able to do so, and progressive infection may occur.

7. ***B*** The reactions that constitute serum sickness follow administration of the foreign substance within 6–12 days. During this time, the host produces antibody that reacts with the foreign substance(s), which persists in the host and leads to antigen-antibody complexes that can be deposited in joints, lymph nodes, skin, and elsewhere. The manifestation of the immune reaction, although appearing later, nevertheless are classified as type III rather than cell-mediated delayed (type IV) hypersensitivity because they involve antibodies rather than T cells.

8. ***C*** Children younger than 2 years of age do not respond adequately to immunization with pure bacterial capsule polysaccharide vaccine. Therefore, vaccinating them may be useless. The various other individuals listed are particularly vulnerable to infection with *Streptococcus pneumoniae.* While some of them may mount a suboptimal response to the vaccine, they should nevertheless be vaccinated.

9. ***E*** The potential hazard of hepatitis viruses in human plasma is overcome by the separation of ethanol-precipitated globulins. The concentration of IgG is about 16,500 mg/dL, compared to 1200 mg/dL in plasma. Whereas the IgG thus becomes highly concentrated in immune serum globulin, IgA and IgM are relatively depleted, and their concentration in the ethanol-precipitated immune serum globulin is close to their original concentration in the plasma.

GLOSSARY

ABO blood group system Antigens expressed on red blood cells used for typing human blood for transfusion.

accessory cell A cell required to initiate immune responses, often used to describe antigen-presenting cell (see also antigen-presenting cell).

accessory molecules Molecules other than the antigen receptor and major histocompatability complex that participate in cognitive activation and effector functions of T lymphocyte responsiveness.

acquired immune response The response of antigen-specific lymphocytes to antigen, including the development of immunological memory; also known as acquired immune response.

activation-induced cell death The death by apoptosis of activated B and T cells at the end of an immune response when antigen has been removed.

acute-phase proteins A series of proteins, found in the blood after the onset of an infection, that participate in the early phases of host defense against infection.

acute-phase response (APR) The release of acute phase proteins such as C-reactive protein into the blood within a few hours of exposure to an infectious agent. Acute-phase proteins participate in the early phase of host defense. Inflammation, tissue injury, and, very infrequently, neoplasm may also be associated with the APR.

adapter proteins Key linkers between receptors and downstream members of signaling pathways. All use a similar domain, known as the SH2 domain

adaptive immune response See acquired immune response.

ADCC See antibody-dependent, cell-mediated cytotoxity

adenosine deaminase (ADA) deficiency A form of severe combined immunodeficiency disease (SCID) in which affected individuals lack the ADA enzyme, which catalyzes the deamination of adenosine and deoxyadenosine to produce inosine and deoxyinosine, respectively.

adhesion molecules Mediate the binding of one cell to other cells or to extracellular matrix proteins, integrins, selectins, and members of the Ig gene superfamily.

adjuvant A substance, given with antigen that enhances the response to the injected antigen.

adoptive transfer The transfer of the capacity to make an immune response by transplantation of immunocompetent cells.

affinity A measure of the binding constant of a single antigen-combining site with a monovalent antigenic determinant.

affinity chromatography The purification of a substance by means of its affinity for another substance immobilized on a solid support—for example, an antigen can be purified by affinity chromatography on a column of antigen-specific antibody molecules covalently linked to beads.

affinity maturation The sustained increase in affinity of antibodies for an antigen with time following immunization. The genes encoding the antibody variable regions undergo somatic hypermutation with the selection of B lymphocytes whose receptors express high affinity for the antigen.

agammaglobulinemia See X-linked agammaglobulinemia.

agglutination The aggregation of particulate antigen by antibodies.

agonist peptides Peptide antigens that activate their specific T cells, inducing them to make cytokines and to proliferate.

alleles Two or more alternate forms of a gene that occupy the same position, or locus, on a specific chromosome.

allelic exclusion The ability of heterozygous lymphoid cells to produce only one allelic form of antigen-specific receptor (Ig or T cell receptor) when they have the genetic endowment to produce both. Genes other than those for the antigen-specific receptors are usually expressed codominantly.

allergen An antigen responsible for producing allergic reactions by inducing IgE synthesis.

allergic asthma A clinical phenomenon caused by constriction of the bronchial tree due to an allergic reaction to inhaled antigen.

allergic reaction A response to environmental antigens (allergens) due to preexisting antibody or antigen-primed T cells.

allergic rhinitis An allergic reaction in the nasal mucosa, also known as "hay fever," that causes runny nose, sneezing, and watery eyes.

allergy A term covering immune reactions to nonpathogenic antigens, that lead to inflammation and deleterious effects in the host.

alloantigen A cell-surface-expressed antigen that stimulates a graft response in a genetically different member of the same species.

allogeneic Describes genetic variations or differences among members or strains of the same species; refers to organ or tissue grafts between genetically dissimilar humans or between unrelated members of the same species.

allograft A tissue transplant (graft) between two genetically nonidentical members of a species.

allotypes Antigenic determinants that are present in allelic (alternate) forms. When used in association with Ig, allotypes describe allelic variants of Ig detected by antibodies raised between members of the same species.

alternative complement pathway The mechanism of complement activation that begins with the activation of C3 and the deposition of C3b on the surface of cells.

alveolar macrophage Found in the lung alveoli that may remove inhaled particulate matter.

anamnestic Describes immunological memory, which leads to a rapid increase in response after reexposure to antigen.

anaphylatoxin Substance such as C5a, C3a capable of releasing histamine from mast cells and basophils.

anaphylaxis Immediate hypersensitivity response to antigenic challenge, mediated by IgE and mast cells. It is a life-threatening allergic reaction, caused by the release of pharmacologically active agents.

anergy A state of antigen-specific nonresponsiveness in which a T or B cell is present but functionally unable to respond to antigen.

ankylosing spondylitis A chronic inflammatory disease affecting the spine, sacroiliac joints, and large peripheral joints. There is a major genetic predisposition, as revealed by increased incidence in selected families. Approximately 90% of patients with ankylosing spondylitis are positive for HLA-B27, compared to 8% among individuals who are negative for this HLA determinant in the United States.

antibody Serum protein formed in response to immunization, which is generally defined in terms of its specific binding to the immunizing antigen.

antibody-dependent, cell-mediated cytotoxicity (ADCC) A phenomenon in which target cells, coated with antibody, are destroyed by specialized killer cells (natural-killer cells and macrophages), that bear receptors for the Fc region of the coating antibody (Fc receptors). These receptors allow the killer cells to bind to the antibody-coated target.

antigen Any foreign material that is specifically bound by antibody or lymphocytes; also used loosely to describe materials used for immunization.

antigen presentation The display of antigen as peptide fragments bound to MHC molecules on the surface of a cell; T cells recognize antigen only when it is presented in this way.

antigen processing The degradation of proteins into peptides that can bind to MHC molecules for presentation to T cells.

antigen receptor The specific antigen-binding receptor on T or B lymphocytes, which is transcribed and translated from rearrangements and translocation of V, D, and J genes.

antigen-binding site The location on an antibody molecule where an antigenic determinant or epitope combines with it. It is located in a cleft bordered by the N-terminal variable regions of H and L chain parts of the Fab region.

antigen-capture assay Antigen binds to a specific antibody, and its presence is detected using a second antibody that binds to a different epitope.

antigenic determinant A single antigenic site or epitope on a complex antigenic molecule or particle.

antigenic drift Variations in antigenicity of microorganisms (e.g., viruses, parasites) resulting from point mutations of genes that cause small differences in surface antigen expression.

antigenic shift Mixing (Reassortment) of one influenza virus genome with another, creating radically new surface antigens.

antigen-presenting cell (APC) A specialized type of cell, bearing cell-surface MHC class II molecules, involved in presentation of antigen to T cells.

anti-Ig antibodies Antibodies against Ig constant domains that are useful for detecting bound antibody molecules in immunoassays and other applications.

antiserum (pl., antisera) The fluid component of clotted blood from an immune individual that contains a heterogeneous collection of antibodies against the molecule used for immunization. Such antibodies bind the antigen used for immunization. Each has its own structure, its own epitope on the antigen, and its own set of cross-reactions. This heterogeneity makes each antiserum unique.

antitoxin Antibody specific for exotoxins produced by certain microorganisms, such as the causative agents of diphtheria and tetanus.

APC See antigen-presenting cell

apoptosis A form of programmed cell death caused by activation of endogenous molecules leading to the fragmentation of DNA.

appendix A gut-associated lymphoid tissue located at the beginning of the colon.

Arthus reaction A hypersensitivity reaction produced by local formation of antigen–antibody aggregates that activate the complement cascade and cause thrombosis, hemorrhage, and acute inflammation.

asthma A disease of the lungs characterized by reversible airway obstruction (in most cases), inflammation of the airway with prominent eosinophil participation, and increased responsiveness by the airway to various stimuli. Some cases of asthma are allergic (see allergic asthma) and are mediated, in part, by IgE antibody to environmental allergens. Other cases are provoked by no allergic factors.

ataxia telangiectasia A multisystem disorder characterized by lack of muscle coordination (ataxia), permanent dilation of blood vessels (telangiectasis) in the eyes and skin, and a variable immunodeficiency that affects the function of both T and B lymphocytes.

atopic allergy or atopy Describes IgE-mediated allergic responses in humans, usually showing a genetic predisposition.

autochthonous Pertaining to self.

autograft A tissue transplant from one area to another on a single individual.

autoimmunity An immune response to self tissues or components. Such an immune response may have pathologic consequences, leading to autoimmune diseases.

autologous Derived from the same individual, self.

avidity The summation of multiple affinities—for example, when a polyvalent antibody binds to a polyvalent antigen.

azathioprine A potent immunosuppresive drug that is converted to its active form in vivo and then kills rapidly proliferating cells, including lymphocytes responding to grafted tissues.

B cell The precursors of antibody-forming plasma cell; expresses Ig on its surface. Also known as B lymphocyte

B cell receptor (BCR) The cell-surface receptor of B cells for a specific antigen composed of a transmembrane Ig molecule associated with the invariant Igα and Igβ chains in a noncovalent complex.

B7 A costimulatory homodimeric Ig superfamily protein whose expression is restricted to the surface of accessory cells (e.g., B cells, macrophages) that interact with T lymphocytes. The ligands for B7 include CD28 and CD152.

BALT See bronchus-associated lymphoid tissue

bare lymphocyte syndrome An immunodeficiency disease resulting from the failure to express either MHC class I and class II molecules.

basophils White blood cells containing granules that stain with basic dyes and are thought to have a function similar to mast cells.

bacille Calmette-Guerin (BCG) A *Mycobacterium bovis* strain that has long been used in Europe as a vaccine against tuberculosis, although it never gained popularity in the United States.

BCR See B cell receptor.

Bence-Jones proteins Dimers of Ig L chains in the urine of patients with multiple myeloma.

Blk See tyrosine kinases.

blocking antibody An antibody molecule capable of blocking the interaction of antigen with other antibodies or with cells.

Bloom syndrome A disease caused by mutations in DNA helicase that is characterized by low T cell numbers; reduced antibody levels; and increased susceptibility to respiratory infections, cancer, and radiation damage.

bone marrow The site of hematopoiesis, in which stem cells give rise to the cellular elements of blood, including red blood cells, monocytes, polymorphonuclear leukocytes, platelets, and lymphocytes.

bone marrow transplantation A procedure used to treat both immunodeficiency and neoplastic conditions not amenable to other forms of therapy. It has been especially used in cases of aplastic anemia, acute lymphocytic leukemia, and acute nonlymphocytic leukemia.

bradykinin A vasoactive peptide that is produced as a result of tissue damage and acts as an inflammatory mediator.

bronchus-associated lymphoid tissue (BALT) Secondary lymphoid organs connected to the bronchial tree.

Bruton agammaglobulinemia See X-linked agammaglobulinemia

bursa of Fabricius Site of development of B cells in birds; an outpouching of the cloaca.

calcineurin Cytosolic serine–threonine phosphatase that plays a crucial role in signaling via the T cell receptor. The immunosuppressive drugs cyclosporin A and tacrolimus (FK506) form complexes with cellular proteins (called immunophilins) that inactivate calcineurin, suppressing T cell responses.

calnexin An endoplasmic reticulum protein that binds partly folded proteins of the Ig-superfamily and returns them to the endoplasmic reticulum until folding is completed.

calreticulin The molecular chaperone that binds initially to MHC class I and class II moleculas and other proteins containing Ig-like domains (e.g., T and B cell receptors).

CAM Cell-surface adhesion molecule. See adhesion molecules

carcinoembryonic antigen (CEA) A membrane glycoprotein epitope that is present in the fetal gastrointestinal tract in normal conditions. CEA levels are elevated in almost one third of patients with colorectal, liver, pancreatic, lung, breast, head and neck, cervical, bladder, medullarythyroid, and prostatic carcinoma.

carrier A large immunogenic molecule or particle to which a hapten or other nonimmunogenic, epitope-bearing molecule may attach, allowing it to become immunogenic.

caspases A family of closely related cysteine proteases that cleave proteins at aspartic acid residues and have important roles in apoptosis.

CD See cluster of differentiation

CDR See complementarity-determining regions

CEA See carcinoembryonic antigen

C8 deficiency A very uncommon genetic disorder with an autosomal recessive mode of inheritance. Affected individuals are missing C8 α or β chains; associated with a defective ability to form a membrane attack complex and an increased propensity to develop disseminated infections caused by *Neisseria* microorganisms such as meningococci.

cell-mediated cytotoxicity Killing (lysis) of a target cell by an effector lymphocyte.

cell-mediated immunity (CMI) Also referred to as delayed-type hypersensitivity. Immune reaction mediated by T cells, in contrast to humoral immunity, which is antibody mediated.

central lymphoid organs Early sites of lymphocyte development, in which antigen-specific receptors are acquired. In humans, B lymphocytes develop in bone marrow, whereas T lymphocytes develop with the thymus from bone-marrow derived progenitors.

centroblasts Large, rapidly dividing cells found in germinal centers that undergo somatic hyperrmutation and give rise to antibody-secreting and memory B cells.

C5b The principal molecular product that remains after C5a has been split off by the action of C5 convertase on C5; has a binding site for complement component C6 and complexes with it to begin generation of the membrane attack complex.

C5 convertase A molecular complex that splits C5 into C5a and C5b in both the classical and the alternative pathways of complement activation.

C5 deficiency A very uncommon genetic disorder that has an autosomal recessive mode of inheritance. Individuals with this deficiency have a defective ability to form the membrane attack complex, which is necessary for the efficient lysis of invading microorganisms. They have an increased susceptibility to disseminated infections by *Neisseria* microorganisms.

CFU See colony-forming unit.

Chediak-Higashi syndrome A childhood disorder with an autosomal recessive mode of inheritance that is identified by the presence of large lysosomal granules in leukocytes that are very stable and undergo slow degranulation.

chemokines Small cytokines of relatively low molecular weight released by a variety of cells and involved in inflammatory responses and the migration and activation of primarily phagocytic cells and lymphocytes.

chemotaxis Migration of cells along a concentration gradient of an attractant.

CH50 unit The amount of complement (serum dilution) that induces lysis of 50% of erythrocytes coated with specific antibody.

chimera A mythical animal possessing the head of a lion, the body of a goat, and the tail of a snake. Refers to an individual containing cellular components derived from another genetically distinct individual.

chronic granulomatous disease (CGD) A disorder characterized by an enzyme defect associated with NADPH oxidase, which causes neutrophils and monocytes to have decreased consumption of oxygen and diminished glucose use by the hexose monophosphate shunt. It is inherited as an X-linked trait in two thirds of the cases and as an autosomal recessive trait in the remaining third.

chronic lymphocytic leukemia (CLL) A B cell leukemia in which long-lived small lymphocytes continually collect in the spleen, lymph nodes, bone marrow, and blood. CLL cells express a monoclonal Ig on their surface.

class II-associated invariant chain peptide (CLIP) A peptide of variable length cleaved from the invariant chain by proteases. It remains associated with the MHC class II molecules in an unstable form until it is removed by the HLA-DM protein.

class switch See isotype switch

classical complement pathway The mechanism of complement activation initiated by antigen–antibody aggregates and proceeding by way of C1 to C9.

clonal anergy The interaction of a B or T lymphocyte with an antigen leading to its functional inactivation. Can result when the lymphocyte interacts with antigen in the absence of the second signals usually required for cell activation.

clonal deletion The loss of lymphocytes of a particular specificity due to contact with antigen.

clonal selection theory The prevalent concept that specificity and diversity of an immune response are the result of selection by antigen of specifically reactive clones from a large repertoire of preformed lymphocytes, each with individual specificities.

cluster of differentiation (CD) Cluster of antigens with which antibodies react that characterize cell-surface molecules.

C9 A complement component made up of a single-chain protein that binds to the C5b678 complex on the cell surface. The interaction of 12–15 C9 molecules with one C5b678 complex produces the membrane attack complex.

C9 deficiency A very uncommon genetic disorder with an autosomal recessive mode of inheritance in which only trace amounts of C9 are present in the plasma of affected persons. There is a defective ability to form the membrane attack complex.

cold agglutinin An antibody that agglutinates particulate antigens such as bacteria or red cells, optimally at temperatures $<37°C$. In clinical medicine, usually refers to antibodies against red blood cell antigens, as in the cold agglutinin syndrome.

colony-forming unit (CFU) The hematopoietic stem cell and the progeny cells that derive from it. Mature hematopoietic cells in the blood are considered to develop from one CFU.

colony-stimulating factors (CSF) Glycoproteins that govern the formation, differentiation and function of hematopoietic progenitor cells. They promote the growth, maturation, and differentiation of stem cells to produce progenitor cell colonies in vitro.

combinatorial joining The joining of segments of DNA to generate essentially new genetic information, as occurs with Ig and T cell receptor genes during the development of B and T cells. Allows multiple opportunities for sets of genes to combine in different ways.

common lymphoid progenitors Stem cells that give rise to all lymphocytes.

common variable immunodeficiency (CVID) Failure of B cells to mature into antibody-secreting cells. Hypogammaglobulinemia is common to all of these patients and usually affects all classes of Ig, but in some cases only IgG is affected. A relatively common congenital or acquired immunodeficiency that may be either familial or sporadic. The familial form may have a variable mode of inheritance.

complement A series of serum and cell-associated proteins involved in the effector arm of the immune response to pathogens; can be activated either by antigen–antibody complexes (classical pathway) or by complement components binding directly to the foreign substance (alternative and lectin pathways).

complement receptors (CRs) Cell-surface proteins on various cells that recognize and bind complement proteins that have bound pathogens or other antigens. CR on phagocytes allow them to identify pathogens coated with complement proteins for uptake and destruction. Examples are CR1, the receptor for C1q; CR2; CR3; and CR4.

complementarity-determining regions (CDRs) Parts of Ig and T cell receptors that determine their specificity and make contact with specific ligand. CDRs are the most variable part of the molecule and contribute to the diversity of these molecules. There are three such regions (CDR1, CDR2, and CDR3) in each V domain.

complete Freund's adjuvant (CFA) See Freund's complete adjuvant

concanavalin A (con A) A jack bean (*Canavalia ensiformis*) lectin that induces erythrocyte agglutination and stimulates T lymphocytes to undergo mitosis and proliferate.

C1 esterase inhibitor (C1 INH) A serum protein that inhibits the function of activated C1.

C1 deficiencies Disorders that may manifest as systemic lupus erythematosus, glomerulonephritis, or pyogenic infections as well as an increased incidence of type III (immune complex) hypersensitivity diseases. Only a few cases of C1q, C1r, or C1r and C1s deficiencies have been reported.

C1 inhibitor (C1 INH) deficiency The most frequently found deficiency of the classic complement pathway; may be seen in patients with hereditary angioneurotic edema.

C1q An 18-polypeptide chain component of C1, the first component of the classical complement pathway.

C1q deficiency May be found in association with lupus-like syndromes.

C1r A subcomponent of C1, the first component of complement in the classical activation pathway and a serine esterase.

C1s A serine esterase that is a subcomponent of C1, the first component of complement in the classical activation pathway. It binds two C1s molecules to the C1q stalk

conformational epitopes Discontinuous epitopes on a protein antigen that are formed from several separate regions in the primary sequence of a protein when brought together by protein folding. Antibodies that bind conformational epitopes bind only native-folded proteins.

congenic (also coisogenic) Describes two individuals who differ only in the genes at a particular locus and are identical at all other loci.

constant region (C region) The invariant carboxyl-terminal portion of an Ig or T cell receptor molecule, as distinct from the variable region at the amino terminus of the chain.

contact dermatitis A type IV, T lymphocyte–mediated hypersensitivity reaction of the delayed type that develops in response to an allergen applied to the skin.

contact hypersensitivity A form of delayed-type hypersensitivity in which T cells respond to antigens introduced by contact with the skin. An example is poison ivy hypersensitivity, due to T cell responses to the chemical antigen pentadecacatechol contained in oils on the leaves.

convertase An enzyme component in the complement cascade that converts the inactive form of the next component in the pathway into an active form by cleaving it.

Coombs test A test named for its originator used to detect antibodies by addition of an anti-Ig antibody.

coreceptor A cell-surface protein that increases the sensitivity of the antigen receptor to antigen by binding to associated ligands and participating in signaling for activation.

corticosteroids Steroid hormones that are lympholytic and are derived from the adrenal cortex. Glucocorticoids (e.g., prednisone, dexamethasone) can diminish the size and lymphocyte content of lymph nodes and spleen, while sparing proliferating myeloid or erythroid stem cells of the bone marrow.

costimulatory molecules Membrane-bound or secreted products of accessory cells that activate signal transduction events in addition to those induced by MHC–T cell receptor interactions. They are required for full activation of T cells.

cowpox The common name for the disease in cows caused by vaccinia virus; used by Edward Jenner in the successful vaccination against smallpox.

CR See complement receptors

C-reactive protein Found in serum; produced by hepatocytes as part of the acute phase response. Inflammation induced by bacterial infection, necrosis of tissue, trauma, or malignant tumors may cause an increase in the serum concentration within 48 hours of the inducing condition.

C region See constant region

cromolyn sodium A drug that blocks the release of pharmacological mediators from mast cells and diminishes the symptoms and tissue reactions of type I hypersensitivity (i.e., anaphylaxis) mediated by IgE.

cross-reactivity The ability of an antibody, specific for one antigen, to react with a second antigen; a measure of relatedness between two different antigenic substances.

C7 deficiency Very uncommon genetic disorder with an autosomal recessive mode of inheritance. Serum of affected persons contains only trace amounts of C7 associated with a defective ability to form a membrane attack complex and increased incidence of disseminated infections caused by *Neisseria* microorganisms.

C6 A complement component that participates in the membrane attack complex.

C6 deficiency Very uncommon genetic defect with an autosomal recessive mode of inheritance. Affected individuals have only trace amounts of C6 in their plasma and have defective ability to form a membrane attack complex and an increased susceptibility to disseminated infections by *Neisseria* microorganisms.

C3 The fourth complement component of the classical pathway; also starts the alternative complement pathway; has an internal thioester bond that when broken allows the molecule to link covalently with surfaces of cells and proteins.

C3a A low molecular weight (9 kDa) peptide fragment of complement component C3.

C3b The principal fragment produced when complement component C3 is split by either classical or alternative pathway convertases—C4b2a or C3bBb, respectively.

C3 convertase An enzyme that splits C3 into C3b and C3a. The classical pathway C3 convertase is C4b2a and the alternative pathway C3 convertase is C3bBb.

C3 tickover Phenomenon in which the alternative pathway C3 convertase continually generates a small amount of C3b by hydrolysing the C3 internal thioester bond.

CTLA-4 (CD152) Expressed on activated T cells and binds to the co-stimulatory molecule B7 on antigen-presenting cells; delivers an inhibitory signal.

C2 The third complonent of the classical complement pathway activation; a single polypeptide chain that complexes with C4b molecules on the cell surface in the presence of Mg^{++}.

C2 deficiency Rare condition; it may be symptomless, but autoimmune-like manifestations that resemble features of certain collagen-vascular diseases, such as systemic lupus erythematosus, may appear. It has an autosomal recessive mode of inheritance.

cutaneous lymphocyte antigen (CLA) A cell-surface molecule that is involved in lymphocyte homing to the skin in humans.

cyclophosphamide An immunosuppressive drug that is more toxic for B than for T lymphocytes. Consequently, it is a more effective suppressor of humoral antibody synthesis than of cell-mediated immune reactions.

cyclosporin A An immunosuppressive drug that inhibits signaling in T cells thus preventing T cell activation and effector function. It acts by binding to cyclophilin to create a complex that binds to and inactivates the serine–threonine phosphatase calcineurin.

cytokine receptors Cellular receptors for cytokines. Binding of the cytokine to the cytokine receptor stimulates signal transduction, resulting in new activities in the cell, such as growth, differentiation, or death.

cytokines Soluble substances secreted by cells that have a variety of effects on other cells.

cytophilic antibody Attaches to a cell surface through its Fc region, binding to Fc receptors. For example, IgE molecules bind to the surface of mast cells and basophils in this manner.

cytotoxic T cells T cells that can kill other cells. Most cytotoxic T cells are MHC class I-restricted $CD8^+$ T cells, but $CD4^+$ T cells can also kill target cells in some cases.

cytotoxins Proteins made by cytotoxic T cells that participate in the destruction of target cells. Perforins and granzymes are the major defined cytotoxins.

death domain Originally defined in proteins encoded by genes involved in programmed cell death but now known to be involved in protein–protein interactions.

decay-accelerating factor (DAF, CD55) A membrane glycoprotein of normal human erythrocytes, leukocytes, and platelets, but absent from the red blood cells of paroxysmal nocturnal hemaglobulinuria patients. It facilitates dissociation of the classical complement pathway C3 convertase (C4b2a) into C4b and C2a. It also dissociates the alternative complement pathway C3 convertase, C3bBb, into C3b and Bb.

D gene A small segment of Ig H-chain and T cell receptor DNA, coding for the third hypervariable region of most receptors.

degranulation A mechanism whereby cytoplasmic granules in cells fuse with the cell membrane to discharge the contents from the cell. A classic example is degranulation of the mast cell or basophil in immediate (type I) hypersensitivity

delayed-type hypersensitivity A form of cell-mediated immunity elicited by antigen present in the skin. Reaction is mediated by $CD4^+$ T_{H1} cells and involves release of cytokines and recruitment of monocytes and macrophages. The reaction appears hours to days after antigen is injected.

dendritic cells Interdigitating reticular cells, derived from bone-marrow precursors that are found in T cell areas of lymphoid tissues. They have a branched or dendritic morphology and are the most potent stimulators of T cell responses. In nonlymphoid tissues, they do not appear to stimulate T cell responses until they are activated and migrate to lymphoid tissues.

desensitization A procedure in which an allergic individual is exposed to increasing doses of allergen with the goal of inhibiting their allergic reactions. When successful, the mechanism probably involves shifting the response from $CD4^+$ T_H2 to T_H1 cells and thus changing the antibody produced from IgE to IgG.

determinant Part of the antigen molecule that binds to an antibody-combining site or to a receptor on T cells; also termed epitope (see epitope; hapten).

diapedesis The movement of blood cells, particularly leukocytes, from the blood across blood vessel walls into tissues.

differentiation antigen A cell-surface antigenic determinant found only on cells of a certain lineage and at a particular developmental stage; used as an immunological marker.

DiGeorge syndrome A recessive genetic immunodeficiency disease in which there is a failure to develop thymic epithelium; also associated with absent parathyroid glands and large vessel anomalies. It seems to be due to a developmental defect in neural crest cells.

diphtheria toxoid An immunizing preparation generated by formalin inactivation of *Corynebacterium diphtheriae* exotoxins. Used in the immunization of children against diphtheria; usually administered as a triple vaccine, together with pertussis microorganisms and tetanus toxoid (DPT).

diversity gene segments see D gene

DNA vaccination A vaccination procedure in which plasmid DNA is used to initiate an adaptive immune response to the encoded protein.

domain A compact segment of an Ig or T cell receptor chain made up of amino acids around an S-S bond.

double-negative thymocytes Immature T cells within the thymus that lack expression of the coreceptors CD4 and CD8.

double-positive thymocyte An intermediate stage in T-cell development in the thymus characterized by expression of both the CD4 and the CD8 coreceptor proteins.

DP, DQ, and DR molecules MHC class II molecules of humans expressed constitutively on B cells and antigen-presenting cells.

draining lymph node Any lymph node downstream of an infection or site of antigen injection that receives microbes, antigens, and antigen-presenting cells from the site via the lymphatic system. Often enlarges during an immune response and can be palpated (a phenomenon originally called "swollen glands").

DTH See delayed-type hypersensitivity

ECAM Endothelial cell adhesion molecule. See adhesion molecules

effector cells Lymphocytes that can mediate the removal of pathogens or antigens from the body without the need for further differentiation. Distinct from naive lymphocytes, which must proliferate and differentiate before they can mediate effector functions.

ELISA See enzyme-linked immunosorbent assay

elispot assay An adaptation of ELISA in which cells are placed over antibodies or antigens attached to a surface. The antigen or antibody traps the cells' secreted products, which can then be detected by using an enzyme-coupled antibody that cleaves a substrate to make a localized colored spot.

encapsulated bacteria Bacteria with thick carbohydrate coats that protect them from phagocytosis and can cause extracellular infections; are effectively engulfed and destroyed by phagocytes only if they are first coated with antibody and/or complement.

endocytosis A mechanism whereby substances are taken into a cell from the extracellular fluid through plasma membrane vesicles. This is accomplished by either pinocytosis or receptor-facilitated endocytosis.

endogenous pyrogens Cytokines (e.g., interleukin-1, Tumor necrosis factor α) that can induce a rise in body temperature; exogenous substances such as endotoxin from gram-negative bacteria induce fever by triggering endogenous pyrogen synthesis.

endotoxins Bacterial toxins that are released when bacterial cells are damaged or destroyed. The most important endotoxin is the lipopolysaccharide of gram-negative bacteria, which induces cytokine synthesis.

enzyme-linked immunosorbent assay (ELISA) An assay in which an enzyme is linked to an antibody and a colored substrate is used to measure the activity of bound enzyme and hence the amount of bound antibody.

eosinophils White blood cells that play an important role in allergic responses and are thought to be important in defense against parasitic infections.

epitope An alternative term for antigenic determinant.

erythroblastosis fetalis A human fetal disease induced by IgG antibodies passed across the placenta from mother to fetus that bind to fetal red blood cells, leading to their destruction.

erythropoietin A glycoprotein produced by the kidney, based on the presence of substances such as heme in the kidneys, which are oxygen sensitive. It stimulates bone marrow red blood cell production.

exocytosis The release of intracellular vesicle content to the exterior of the cell. The vesicles make their way to the plasma membrane, with which they fuse to permit the contents to be released to the external environment.

exon The region of DNA coding for a protein or a segment of a protein.

experimental allergic encephalomyelitis (EAE) An experimental inflammatory disease of the central nervous system induced in rodents by immunizing with neural antigens and an adjuvant; it models the human disease multiple sclerosis.

Fab Fragment of antibody containing one antigen-binding site; generated by cleavage of the antibody with the enzyme papain, which cuts at the hinge region N-terminally to the inter-heavy-chain disulfide bond and generates two Fab fragments from one antibody molecule.

F(ab′)$_2$ A fragment of an antibody containing two antigen-binding sites; generated by cleavage of the antibody molecule with the enzyme pepsin, which cuts at the hinge region C-terminally to the inter-heavy-chain disulfide bond.

FACS see fluorescence-activated cell sorter

factor B An alternative complement pathway component that combines with C3b and is cleaved by factor D to produce alternative pathway C3 convertase.

factor H A regulator of complement in the blood that unites with C3b and facilitates dissociation of alternative complement pathway C3 convertase (designated C3bBb) into C3b and Bb.

factor I A regulator of complement pathway activation. In the alternative pathway, it splits C3b initially to iC3b, and then to two additional fragments (C3c, and C3d); in the classical pathway, it cleaves C4b into C4c and C4d.

factor P See properdin.

farmer's lung A hypersensitivity disease caused by the interaction of IgG antibodies with large amounts of an inhaled allergen in the alveolar wall of the lung, causing alveolar wall inflammation and compromising gas exchange.

Fas (CD95) A member of the tumor necrosis factor receptor family that is expressed on certain cells, making them susceptible to killing by cells expressing Fas ligand. Binding of Fas ligand to Fas triggers apoptosis in the Fas-bearing cells.

Fas ligand (Fas-L, CD178) A cell-surface member of the tumor necrosis factor family of proteins. Binding of Fas ligand to Fas triggers apoptosis in the Fas-bearing cell.

Fc Fragment of antibody without antigen-binding sites, generated by cleavage with papain; contains the C-terminal domains of the domains of the Ig H chains.

Fc receptor (FcR) A receptor on a cell surface with specific binding affinity for the Fc portion of an antibody molecule; found on many types of cells.

FITC See fluorescein isothiocyanate

FK506 See tacrolimus.

fluorescein isothiocyanate (FITC) A fluorescent dye, which emits a yellow-green color and can be conjugated to antibody or other proteins.

fluorescence microscopy A microscope method that uses UV light to illuminate a tissue or cell stained with a fluorochrome-labeled substance, such as an antibody against an antigen of interest in the tissue.

fluorescence-activated cell sorter (FACS) An instrument that uses a laser to differentially deflect cells bound to fluorochrome-linked antibodies, thus sorting the cells into fluorescent-positive and -negative populations.

fluorescent antibody An antibody coupled with a fluorescent dye used to detect antigen on cells, tissues, or microorganisms.

follicle Circular or oval areas of lymphocytes in lymphoid tissues rich in B cells that are present in the cortex of lymph nodes and in the splenic white pulp. Primary follicles contain B lymphocytes that are small and medium size. Antigen stimulation causes development of secondary follicles, which contain large B lymphocytes in the germinal centers where tingible body macrophages (those phagocytizing nuclear particles) and follicular dendritic cells are present.

follicular dendritic cells Cells within lymphoid follicles that are crucial in selecting antigen-binding B cells during antibody responses. They have Fc receptors that are not internalized by receptor-mediated endocytosis, thus holding antigen–antibody complexes on their surface for long periods.

Freund's complete adjuvant An oil containing killed mycobacteria that, when emulsified with an immunogen in aqueous solution, enhances the immune response to that immunogen after injection. Termed *incomplete Freund's adjuvant* if mycobacteria are not included.

FYN see tyrosine kinases.

GALT See gut-associated lymphoid tissue

gene knockout Gene disruption by homologous recombination.

gene therapy Correction of a genetic defect by the introduction of a normal gene into bone marrow or other cell types. Also known as somatic gene therapy because it does not affect the germline genes of the individual.

genetic immunization A novel technique for inducing adaptive immune responses in which a plasmid DNA encoding a protein of interest is injected, usually into muscle; the protein is then expressed in vivo and elicits antibody and T cell responses to the protein encoded by the DNA.

genotype All the genes possessed by an individual; in practice, refers to the particular alleles present at the loci in question.

germ line Refers to genes in germ cells as opposed to somatic cells; in immunology, refers to genes in their unrearranged state rather than those rearranged for production of Ig or T cell receptor molecules.

germinal centers Secondary lymphoid structures that are sites of intense B cell proliferation, selection, maturation, and death during antibody responses. They form around follicular dendritic cell networks after migration of B cells into lymphoid follicles.

glomerulonephritis Group of diseases characterized by glomerular injury. Immune mechanisms responsible for most cases of primary and many of the secondary glomerulonephritis group. Patients usually have glomerular deposits of Ig, frequently with complement components.

Goodpasture's syndrome An autoimmune disease in which autoantibodies against basement membrane or type IV collagen are produced and cause extensive vasculitis. It is rapidly fatal.

G proteins Proteins that bind GTP and convert it to GDP in the process of cell-signal transduction.

graft versus host (GVH) disease The pathologic consequences of a response generally initiated by transplanted immunocompetent T lymphocytes into an allogeneic, immunologically incompetent host. The host is unable to reject the grafted T cells and becomes their target.

granulocyte see polymorphonuclear leukocytes.

granulocyte-macrophage colony-stimulating factor (CM-CSF) A cytokine involved in the growth and differentiation of myeloid and monocytic lineage cells, including dendritic cells, monocytes, and tissue macrophages and cells of the granulocyte lineage.

granuloma A structure in the form of a mass of mononuclear cells at the site of a persisting inflammation; the cells are mostly macrophages with some T lymphocytes at the periphery. A typical delayed hypersensitivity reaction associated with continuous presence of a foreign body or infection.

Graves' disease An autoimmune disease in which antibodies against the thyroid-stimulating hormone receptor cause overproduction of thyroid hormone and thus hyperthyroidism.

Guillain-Barre syndrome A type of idiopathic polyneuritis in which autoimmunity to peripheral nerve myelin leads to a condition characterized by chronic demyelination of the spinal cord and peripheral nerves.

gut-associated lymphoid tissue (GALT) Lymphoid tissue situated in the gastrointestinal mucosa and submucosa, which constitutes the gastrointestinal immune system. Present in Peyer's patches, the appendix, and the tonsils.

GVH See graft versus host disease

haplotype A linked set of genes associated with one haploid genome; used mainly in connection with the linked genes of the MHC, which are usually inherited as one haplotype from each parent.

hapten A compound, usually of low molecular weight that is not itself immunogenic but that, after conjugation to a carrier protein or cells, becomes immunogenic and induces antibody, which can bind the hapten alone in the absence of carrier.

Hashimoto's thyroiditis An autoimmune disease characterized by persistent high levels of antibody against thyroid-specific antigens. These antibodies recruit natural-killer cells to the tissue, leading to damage and inflammation.

HAT Hypoxanthine-aminopterin-thymidine, commonly used as a selective media cocktail in cell cultures when generating hybridomas.

H chain See heavy chain

heavy chain (H chain) The larger of the two types of chains that make up a normal Ig or antibody molecule.

helper T cells A class of T cells that helps trigger B cells to make antibody against thymus-dependent antigens. Helper T cells also help in the differentiation of other T cells, such as cytotoxic T cells.

hemagglutinin Any substance that causes red blood cells to agglutinate. The hemagglutinins in human blood are antibodies that recognize the ABO blood group antigens. Influenza and some other viruses have hemagglutinins that bind to glycoproteins on host cells to initiate the infectious process.

hematopoiesis The generation of the cellular elements of blood, including the red blood cells, leukocytes, and platelets.

hematopoietic stem cell A bone marrow cell that is undifferentiated and serves as a precursor for multiple cell lineages. These cells are also demonstrable in the yolk sac and later in the liver in the fetus.

hemolytic disease of the newborn Also called erythroblastosis fetalis; caused by a maternal IgG antibody response to paternal antigens expressed on fetal red blood cells. The usual target of this response is the Rh blood group antigen. The maternal anti-Rh IgG antibodies cross the placenta to attack the fetal red blood cells.

herd immunity Nonspecific and specific immunity that may have a significant role in resistance of a group (herd) of humans or other animals against infection. Also means that an epidemic will not follow if a single member of the herd is infected provided other members are immune to that particular infectious agent.

hereditary angioedema A disorder in which recurrent attacks of edema occur in the skin and gastrointestinal and respiratory tracts. It is due to decreased or absent C1 inhibitor (C1 INH). The most serious consequence of this disorder is epiglottal swelling leading to suffocation.

heterodimer A molecule composed of two components that are different but closely joined structures, such as a protein made up of two separate chains. Examples include the T cell receptor made up of either α and β chains or of γ and δ chains, and MHC class I and class II molecules.

heterophile antigen A cross-reacting antigen that appears in widely ranging species, such as humans and bacteria.

heterozygous Describes individuals who have two different alleles for a particular gene.

HEV See high endothelial venules

high endothelial venules (HEVs) Specialized venules found in lymphoid tissues. Lymphocytes migrate from blood into lymphoid tissues by attaching to and migrating across the high endothelial cells of these vessels.

hinge region A flexible, open segment of an antibody molecule that allows bending of the molecule. The hinge region is located between Fab and Fc and is susceptible to enzymatic cleavage.

histamine A vasoactive amine stored in mast cell granules that is released by antigen binding to IgE molecules on mast cells, causing dilation of local blood vessels and smooth muscle contraction. Histamine release produces some of the symptoms of immediate hypersensitivity reactions.

histocompatibility Literally, the ability of tissues to get along; in immunology, it means identity in all transplantation antigens. These antigens, in turn, are collectively referred to as histocompatibility antigens.

HIV See human immunodeficiency virus

HLA See human leukocyte antigen

Hodgkin disease A malignant disease in which antigen-presenting cells that resemble dendritic cells seem to be the transformed cell type. Hodgkin lymphoma is a form of the disease in which lymphocytes predominate.

homodimer A protein composed of two peptide chains that are identical.

H-2 The MHC of the mouse situated on chromosome 17. Haplotypes are designated by a lower-case superscript, as in H-2^b. It contains the polymorphic regions K, I, D, and L, and other non-polymorphic genes.

human immunodeficiency virus (HIV) Retrovirus that infects human $CD4^+$ T cells and causes AIDS.

human leukocyte antigen (HLA) The human MHC; contains the genes coding for the polymorphic MHC class I and II class molecules and many other important non-polymorphic genes.

humanization Describes the genetic engineering of mouse hypervariable loops of a desired specificity into otherwise human antibodies. The DNA encoding hypervariable loops of mouse monoclonal antibodies or V regions selected in phage display libraries is inserted into the framework regions of human Ig genes. This allows the production of antibodies of a desired specificity that do not cause an immune response in humans treated with them.

humoral immunity refers to immune responses that involve antibody (contrast with cell-mediated immunity: T cell responses in the absence of antibody). Can be transferred to another individual by using antibody-containing serum.

hybridoma An immortalized hybrid cell resulting from the in vitro fusion of an antibody-secreting B cell with a myeloma; it secretes antibody without stimulation and proliferates continuously, both in vivo and in vitro. Also refers to a hybrid T cell resulting from the fusion of a T lymphocyte with a thymoma (a malignant T cell); the T cell hybridoma proliferates continuously and secretes cytokines upon activation by antigen and antigen-presenting cells.

hyperacute graft rejection An rapid reaction caused by natural preformed antibodies that react against antigens on an allogenic tissue graft. The antibodies bind to endothelium and trigger the blood clotting cascade, leading to an engorged, ischemic graft and rapid loss of the organ.

hypergammaglobulinemia Elevated serum Ig levels. A polyclonal increase in Ig in the serum occurs in any condition in which there is continuous stimulation of the immune system, such as chronic infection, autoimmune disease, or systemic lupus erythematosus. May also result from a monoclonal increase in Ig production, as in multiple myeloma. Waldenstrom macroglobulinemia and other conditions associated with the formation of monoclonal Ig.

hyperimmune Describes an animal with a high level of immunity that is induced by repeated immunization to generate large amounts of functionally effective antibodies, in comparison to animals subjected to routine immunization protocols, perhaps with fewer boosters.

hypersensitivity State of reactivity to antigen that is greater than normal; denotes a deleterious rather than a protective outcome. Four types (I–IV) are defined.

hypervariable regions Portions of the L and H Ig chains that are highly variable in amino acid sequence from one Ig molecule to another and that together constitute the antigen-binding site of an antibody molecule. Also, portions of the T cell receptor that constitute the antigen-binding site. (see complementarity-determining regions).

Ia (I region-associated) An older term for mouse MHC class II genes and molecules; comprise I-A and I-E.

IDC See interdigitating dendritic cells

idiotype The combined antigenic determinants (idiotopes) expressed in the variable region of antibodies of an individual that are directed at a particular antigen.

Ig See Ig

Igα See B cell receptor

IgA The class of Ig characterized by α H chains; antibodies are mainly secreted by mucosal lymphoid tissues.

Igβ See B cell receptor

IgD The class of Ig characterized by δ H chains; a cell surface Ig co-expressed on naive B cells together with IgM; may function as a coreceptor that binds to IgD receptors expressed on T cells.

IgE The class of Ig characterized by ϵ H chains; involved in allergic reactions.

IgG The class of Ig characterized by γ H chains; the most abundant class of Ig found in plasma.

IgM The class of Ig characterized by μ H chains. IgM is the first Ig to appear on the surface of B cells and the first to be secreted following B cell stimulation with antigen.

IL See interleukins

immature B cell IgM-positive, IgD-negative cell in the B cell lineage; easily tolerized by exposure to antigen.

immediate-type hypersensitivity Reaction (type I) occurring within minutes after the interaction of antigen and IgE antibody.

immune adherence The adherence of particulate antigen coated with C3b to cells expressing C3b receptors; results in enhanced phagocytosis of bacteria by macrophages.

immune complex Molecules formed by the interaction of a soluble (i.e., nonparticulate) antigen with antibody molecules. Large immune complexes are cleared rapidly, but smaller complexes formed in antigen excess may deposit in tissues resulting in tissue damage.

immune modulators Substances that control the level of the immune response.

immunity General term for resistance to a pathogen.

immunodeficiency Decrease in immune response that results from absence or defect of some component of the immune system.

immunodiffusion Identifies antigen or antibody by the formation of antigen–antibody complexes in a gel.

immunogen A substance capable of inducing an immune response (as well as reacting with the products of an immune response). Compare with antigen.

immunoglobulin (Ig) A general term for all antibody molecules: IgM, IgD, IgG, IgA, IgE; each unit is made up of two H chains and two L chains and has two antigen-binding sites.

immunoglobulin A See IgA

immunoglobulin D See IgD

immunoglobulin E See IgE

immunoglobulin G See IgG

immunoglobulin M See IgM

immunoglobulin superfamily Proteins involved in cellular recognition and interaction that are structurally and genetically related to Ig.

immunoreceptor tyrosine-based activation motif (ITAM) A pattern of amino acids in the cytoplasmic tail of many transmembrane receptor molecules, including Igα and Igβ and CD3 chains, which are phosphorylated and then associate with intracellular molecules as an early consequence of cell activation.

immunoreceptor tyrosine-based inhibitory motif (ITIM) Motifs with opposing effects to immunoreceptor tyrosine-based activation motifs. They recruit phosphatases to the receptor site that remove the phosphate groups added by the tyrosine kinases.

immunotoxins Antibodies that are chemically coupled to toxic proteins usually derived from plants or microorganisms. They are being tested as anticancer agents and as immunosuppressive drugs.

inflammation An acute or chronic response to tissue injury or infection involving accumulation of leukocytes, plasma proteins, and fluid.

innate immunity The antigen-nonspecific mechanisms involved in the early phase of the response to a pathogen; include phagocytic cells, cytokines, and complement; not expanded by repeat stimulation with the pathogen.

inducible NO synthase (INOS) Produced by macrophages and many other cell types. Induced by many stimuli to activate NO synthesis, thereby playing a major role in host resistance to intracellular infection.

integrins A family of two-chain cell-surface adhesion molecules found on leukocytes; important in the adhesion of antigen-presenting cells and lymphocytes and in leukocyte migration into tissues.

intercellular adhesion molecules (ICAMs) 1, 2, and 3 Adhesion molecules on the surface of several cell types, including antigen-presenting cells and T cells that interact with integrins; members of the Ig superfamily.

interdigitating dendritic cells (IDCs) Thymic bone marrow-derived cells that play a critical role in negative selection of developing thymocytes.

interferons (IFNs) A group of proteins having antiviral activity and capable of enhancing and modifying the immune response.

interleukins (ILs) Glycoproteins secreted by a variety of leukocytes that have effects on other leukocytes.

intron A segment of DNA that is transcribed but removed by splicing and thus not present in mRNA. Contrast **exon**.

ISCOMs Immune stimulatory complexes of antigen held within a lipid matrix that act as adjuvants and enable the antigen to be taken up into the cytoplasm after fusion with the cytoplasmic membrane.

isoelectric focusing Protein identification technique; proteins migrate in an electric field under a pH gradient to the pH at which their net charge is zero (their isoelectric point).

isograft Tissue transplanted between two genetically identical individuals (same as syngraft).

isohemagglutinins Naturally occurring IgM antibodies specific for the red blood cell antigens of the ABO blood groups; thought to result from immunization by bacteria in the gastrointestinal and respiratory tracts.

isotype switch The switch, which occurs when a B cell stops secreting antibody of one isotype or class and starts producing antibody of a different isotype but with same antigenic specificity; involves joining rearranged V(D)J gene unit to a different H-chain constant region gene.

isotypes Also known as antibody classes; antibodies that differ in the H chain constant regions: IgM, IgG, IgD, IgA and IgE. These differences result in distinct biologic activities of the antibodies; distinguishable also on the basis of reaction with antisera raised in another species.

ITAM See immunoreceptor tyrosine-based activation motif

ITIM See immunoreceptor tyrosine-based inhibition motif

J chain (joining chain) A polypeptide involved in the polymerization of Ig molecules IgM and IgA.

J gene A gene segment coding for the J or joining segment in Ig or T cell receptor

JAK See Janus kinases

Janus kinases (JAKs) Tyrosine kinases activated by cytokines binding to their cellular receptors.

killer activatory receptor (KAR) A receptor expressed on natural killer or cytotoxic cells that can activate killing by these cells.

killer inhibitory receptor (KIR) A receptor expressed on natural killer cells that binds to MHC class I molecules on target cells; ligation of MHC class I inhibits the signaling that would otherwise lead to target cell killing.

killer T cell A T cell that kills a target cell expressing foreign antigen bound to MHC molecules on the surface of the target cell; also called cytotoxic T cell.

KIR See killer inhibitory receptor

L chain See light chain

LAK cells See lymphokine-activated killer cells

Langerhans cell Cell of the monocyte/dendritic cell family that takes up and processes antigens in the epidermal layer of the skin; migrates through lymphatics to lymph nodes draining the site of exposure to antigen, where it differentiates into a mature dendritic cell.

leukemia Uncontrolled proliferation of a malignant leukocyte.

leukocytes White blood cells; comprise monocytes/macrophages, lymphocytes, and polymorphonuclear cells.

leukocyte common antigen (LCA, CD45) An antigen shared in common by both T and B lymphocytes.

ligand A molecule or part of a molecule that binds to a receptor.

ligation The binding of a molecule or a part of a molecule to a receptor.

light chain (L chain) The smaller chain of the Ig molecule; occurs in two forms: κ and λ.

linked recognition The requirement for the T helper and B cell involved in the antibody response to a thymus-dependent antigen to interact with different epitopes physically linked in the same antigen.

lipopolysaccharide (LPS) Components of gram-negative bacteria cell walls; also known as endotoxin.

LPS See lipopolysaccharide

Lyme disease A chronic infection with *Borellia burgdorfii,* a spirochete that can evade the immune response.

lymph Extracellular fluid that bathes tissues; contains tissue products, antigens, antibodies, and cells (predominantly lymphocytes).

lymph nodes Secondary lymphoid organs, in which mature B and T lymphocytes respond to free antigen and antigen associated with antigen-presenting cells, respectively, brought in via lymphatic vessels.

lymphatic system System of vessels through which lymph travels and that includes organized structures, with lymph nodes at the intersection of vessels. It has three major functions: to concentrate antigen from all parts of the body into a few lymphoid organs, to circulate lymphocytes through lymphoid organs so that antigen can interact with rare antigen-specific cells, and to carry products of the immune response (antibody and effector cells) to the bloodstream and tissues.

lymphoblast A lymphocyte that has enlarged and increased its rate of RNA and protein synthesis.

lymphocytes Express antigen-specific receptors. Small leukocyte with virtually no cytoplasm; found in blood, tissues, and lymphoid organs, such as lymph nodes, spleen, and Peyer's patches. Responsible for specificity, diversity, memory, and self–nonself discrimination.

lymphokine A cytokine secreted by lymphocytes.

lymphokine-activated killer (LAK) cells Heterogeneous population of lymphocytes, including natural killer cells, derived from the in vitro cytokine-driven activation of peripheral blood lymphocytes from a tumor-bearing patient.

lymphoma Lymphocyte tumors in lymphoid or other tissues; not generally found in the blood.

macrophages Large phagocytic leukocytes found in tissues; derived from blood monocytes.

major histocompatibility complex (MHC) A cluster of genes encoding polymorphic cell-surface molecules (class I and class II) that are involved in interactions with T cells. Also plays a major role in transplantation rejection. Several other nonpolymorphic proteins are encoded in this region.

MALT See mucosal-associated lymphoid tissue

mast cell Bone-marrow derived granule-containing cell found in connective tissues; releases mediators such as histamine and cytokines following cell activation; plays a major role in allergic responses.

mature B cell B cells with IgM and IgD on their surface.

membrane attack complex Terminal components of the complement cascade (C7–C9) that form a pore on the surface of a target cell, resulting in cell damage or death.

memory In the immune system, denotes that a second interaction with antigen leads to a more effective and more rapid response than the first interaction (primary response).

MHC See major histocompatibility complex

MHC class I molecule A molecule encoded by genes of the MHC that participates in antigen presentation to $CD8^+$ (cytotoxic) T cells.

MHC class II molecule A molecule encoded by genes of the MHC that participates in antigen presentation to $CD4^+$ T cells.

MHC class III molecules Proteins—including complement components C2 and C4 and factor B—that are encoded by genes of the MHC. Molecules coded for by MHC class III genes are not involved in cellular interactions.

MHC restriction The property of T lymphocytes to respond only when they are presented with the appropriate antigen in association with either self MHC class I or class II molecules.

minor histocompatibility antigens Antigens encoded outside the MHC, which stimulate graft rejection but not as rapidly as MHC molecules.

mitogen A substance that stimulates the proliferation of many different clones of lymphocytes.

mixed lymphocyte reaction (MLR) Proliferative response occurring when leukocytes from two individuals are mixed in vitro; T cells from one individual (the responder) are activated by MHC antigens expressed by antigen-presenting cells of the other individual (the stimulator).

MLR See mixed lymphocyte reaction

molecular mimicry Identity or similarity of epitopes expressed by a pathogen and by a self molecule; may explain how autoimmune responses develop.

monoclonal Derived from a single clone; the progeny of a single cell. Generally refers to a population of T cells, B cells, or antibody that is homogeneous and reactive with the same specificity toward an epitope.

monocyte Phagocytic leukocyte found in the blood; precursor to tissue macrophage.

motif A pattern of amino acids in the sequence of a molecule critical for the binding of a ligand.

mucins Highly glycosylated cell-surface proteins. Mucin-like molecules are bound by L-selectin in lymphoid organs.

mucosal-associated lymphoid tissue (MALT) System that connects lymphoid structures found in the gastrointestinal and respiratory tracts; includes tonsils, appendix, and Peyer's patches of the small intestine.

multiple sclerosis Disease of the central nervous system, believed to be autoimmune in nature, in which an inflammatory response results in demyelination and loss of neurologic function.

myasthenia gravis Autoimmune disease in which antibody specific for the acetylcholine receptor expressed in muscle blocks function at the neuromuscular junction.

myeloma A tumor of plasma cells, generally secreting a single monoclonal Ig.

naive lymphocytes Lymphocytes that have not previously encountered their specific antigen and therefore have never responded to it. All lymphocytes leaving the central lymphoid organs.

natural-killer (NK) cells Large granular lymphocyte-like cells that kill various tumor cells in vitro and may play a role in resistance to tumors in vivo; also participate in antibody-dependent, cell-mediated cytotoxicity.

negative selection Step in development of B and T cells at which cells with potential reactivity to self molecules are functionally inactivated.

neutralization The ability of an antibody to block or inhibit the effects of a virus.

neutropenia A situation in which there are fewer neutrophils in the blood than normal.

NK cells See natural-killer cells

NK1.1 T cells A small subset of T cells that express the NK1.1 marker, a molecule normally found on natural-killer cells; express α and β T cell receptors of limited diversity and either the coreceptor CD4 or no coreceptor.

Nuclear factor of activated T cells (NFAT) A complex of a protein (NFATc) that is held in the cytosol by serine–threonine phosphorylation and the Fos–Jun dimer known as AP-1. Moves from the cytosol to the nucleus on cleavage of the phosphate residues by calcineurin.

oncogenes Genes involved in regulating cell growth that, when defective in structure or expression, can cause cells to grow continuously to form a tumor.

opsonization The coating of a particle, such as a bacterium, with antibody and/or a complement component (an opsonin) that leads to enhanced phagocytosis by phagocytic cells.

paracortical area (or paracortex) The T cell area of the lymph node.

passive cutaneous anaphylaxis (PCA) The passive transfer of anaphylactic sensitivity by intradermal injection of serum from a sensitive donor.

passive hemagglutination Technique for measuring antibody, in which antigen-coated red blood cells are agglutinated by adding antibody specific for the antigen.

passive immunization Immunization of an individual by the transfer of antibody synthesized in another individual.

pathogen An agent that causes disease.

PCA See passive cutaneous anaphylaxis

PCR See polymerase chain reaction

perforin A molecule synthesized by cytotoxic T cells and natural-killer cells that polymerizes on the surface of a target cell and creates a pore in the membrane, resulting in target cell death.

periartiolar lymphoid sheath (PALS) Part of the inner region of the white pulp of the spleen and mainly contains T cells.

peripheral lymphoid organs Lymphoid organs other than the thymus, including spleen, lymph nodes, and mucosal associated lymphoid tissue.

peripheral tolerance Tolerance induced in mature lymphocytes outside the thymus.

Peyer's patches Clusters of lymphocytes distributed in the lining of the small intestine.

PHA See phytohemagglutinin

phagocytosis The engulfment of a particle or a microorganism by leukocytes such as macrophages and neutrophils.

phenotype The physical expression of an individual's genotype.

phosphatase Enzyme that removes phosphate groups from proteins.

phospholipase C γ (PLCγ) Enzyme involved in T and B cell activation pathways; splits phosphatidylinositol bisphosphate into diacylglycerol and inositol triphosphate, leading to the activation of two major signaling pathways

phytohemagglutinin (PHA) A mitogen that polyclonally activates T cells.

pinocytosis Ingestion of liquid or very small particles by vesicle formation in a cell.

plasma Fluid component of unclotted blood.

plasma cell The antibody-producing end stage of B cell differentiation.

platelets Bone marrow–derived cells crucial in blood clotting.

pokeweed mitogen A mitogen that polyclonally activates T and B lymphocytes.

polyclonal activator A substance that induces activation of many different clones of either T or B cells. See mitogen

poly-Ig receptor Binds to IgA at one surface of an epithelial cell, transports it through the cell, and releases it at the opposite lumenal surface; the IgA can then participate in protecting the mucosal system.

polymerase chain reaction (PCR) Produces large amounts of DNA from a sequence by repeated cycles of synthesis.

polymorphism Literally, having many shapes; in genetics, the existence of multiple alleles at a particular genetic locus resulting in variants of the gene and product among different members of the species.

polymorphonuclear leukocytes (PMN) Leukocytes containing cytoplasmic granules with characteristic multilobed nucleus; three major types: neutrophils, eosinophils, and basophils.

positive selection The process by which developing B and T cells receive signals in the primary lymphoid organ in which they are developing to continue their differentiation; in the absence of these signals the cells die.

pre-B cell Cell in the B cell lineage that has rearranged heavy but not light chain genes; expresses surrogate L chains and μ heavy chain at its surface in conjunction with the signal transduction molecules Igα and Igβ; all these molecules make up the pre-B cell receptor.

pre-B cell receptor (pre-BCR) A complex of at least five proteins that, when expressed in pre-B cells, causes them to enter cell cycle and turn off *RAG* genes. Once this process is completed, the pre-B cells are ready to rearrange their light chains.

precipitin reaction The mixing of soluble antigen and antibody in different proportions that can result in the precipitation of insoluble antigen–antibody complexes.

prednisone A synthetic steroid with potent anti-inflammatory and immunosuppressive activity used to treat acute graft rejection, autoimmune disease, and lymphoid tumors.

pre-T cell Cell in T lymphocyte differentiation in the thymus that has rearranged T cell receptor β genes and expresses a T cell receptor β polypeptide on the surface with the molecule pre-T_α (gp33). These molecules, in conjunction with CD3 and ζ form the pre-T cell receptor.

pre-T cell receptor (pre-TCR) The set of molecules expressed on the surface of the pre-T cell, comprising TCR β and pre-T_α associated with CD3 and ζ.

primary follicle Region of a secondary lymphoid organ containing predominantly unstimulated B lymphocytes; develops into a germinal center following antigen stimulation.

primary lymphoid organs Organs in which the early stages of T and B lymphocyte differentiation take place and antigen-specific receptors are first expressed.

primary response The immune response resulting from first encounter with antigen; generally small, with a long induction phase or lag period; generates immunological memory. In the primary B cell response, mainly IgM antibodies are made.

priming The activation of naive lymphocytes by exposure to antigen.

pro-B cell Earliest stage of B cell differentiation in which a H chain D gene segment rearranges to a J gene segment.

programmed cell death See apoptosis

properdin (factor P) A positive regulator of the alternative pathway of complement activation; stabilizes C3bBb.

prophylaxis Protection.

proteasome Multiprotein cytoplasmic complex that catabolizes proteins to peptides.

protein A A membrane component of *Staphylococcus aureus* that binds to the Fc region of IgG and is thought to protect the bacteria from IgG antibodies by inhibiting their interactions with complement and Fc receptors. Useful in purifying IgG.

protein kinase C Enzyme activated by calcium and diacylglycerol during T and B lymphocyte activation.

prostaglandins Lipid products of metabolism of arachidonic acid, which like leukotrienes, have a variety of effects (e.g., inflammatory mediators) on a variety of tissues.

protooncogenes Cellular genes regulating growth control; mutation or aberrant expression can lead to malignant transformation of the cell.

provirus DNA form of a retrovirus integrated into the host DNA.

pseudogene Sequence of DNA resembling a gene but containing codons that prevent transcription into full-length RNA species.

pus A mixture of cell debris and dead neutrophils that is present in wounds and abscesses infected with extracellular encapsulated bacteria.

pyogenic Refers to the generation of pus at the sites of response to bacteria with large capsules.

pyrogen A substance that causes fever.

radioallergosorbent test (RAST) A solid-phase radioimmunoassay for detecting IgE antibody specific for a particular allergen.

radioimmunoassay (RIA) A technique for measuring the level of a biologic substance in a sample, by measuring the binding of antigen to radioactively labeled antibody (or vice versa).

RAG-1* and *RAG-2 Recombination activating genes; their products are critically involved in V(D)J recombination in B and T cells.

rapamycin An immunosuppressive agent used to prevent transplantation rejection; blocks cytokine production.

receptor Generally, a transmembrane molecule that binds to a ligand on the exterior surface of the cell, leading to biochemical changes inside the cell.

receptor editing Process by which the rearranged genes of a cell in the B cell lineage may undergo a secondary rearrangement, generating a different antigenic specificity.

recombination See V(D)J recombination

recombination activating genes See *RAG-1* and *RAG-2*.

Reed-Sternberg cells Large malignant B cells that are found in patients with Hodgkin disease.

repertoire The complete library of antigenic specificities generated by either B or T lymphocytes to respond to foreign antigen.

RES See reticuloendothelial system

reticuloendothelial system (RES) A general term for the network of phagocytic cells.

reverse transcriptase Enzyme that transcribes the RNA genome of a retrovirus into DNA; used in molecular biology to convert RNA into complementary DNA.

rheumatic fever Caused by antibodies elicited by infection with some *Streptococcus species*. Some of these antibodies cross-react with kidney, joint, and heart antigens.

rheumatoid arthritis Autoimmune, inflammatory disease of the joints.

rheumatoid factor An autoantibody (usually IgM) that reacts with the individual's own IgG; present in patients with rheumatoid arthritis.

ring vaccination A public health strategy for immunizing a select group of individuals, usually within a relatively small geographic location, who have either been exposed to or potentially exposed to an infectious microorganism that poses a public health threat, such as a biologic weapon.

SCID See severe combined immunodeficiency disease

second set rejection Accelerated rejection of an allograft in a primed recipient.

secondary lymphoid organs Organs in which mature B and T lymphocytes proliferate and differentiate following antigen recognition.

secretory component Cleaved component of the poly-Ig receptor that attaches to dimeric IgA and protects it from proteolytic cleavage as it is transported through an epithelial cell.

selectins A family of cell-surface adhesion molecules found on leukocytes and endothelial cells; bind to sugars on glycoproteins.

sensitization Prior immunization by antigen; generally used for first encounter with allergen.

sepsis Infection of the bloodstream.

serology Use of antibodies to detect antigens.

serum Residual fluid derived from clotted blood; contains antibodies.

serum sickness A type III hypersensitivity reaction resulting from deposition of circulating, soluble, antigen–antibody complexes and leading to complement and neutrophil activation in tissues such as the kidney; typically induced following therapy with large doses of antibody from a foreign source, such as monoclonal antibodies made in mice (originally, by treating patients with horse serum).

severe combined immunodeficiency disease (SCID) Results from early block in differentiation pathways of both B and T lymphocytes.

signal transducers and activators of transcription (STATs) Intracellular proteins phosphorylated by Janus kinases as a consequence of cytokine–cytokine receptor engagement.

signal transduction Process involved in transmitting the signal received on the outer surface of the cell (e.g., by antigen binding to its receptor) into the nucleus of the cell, which leads to altered gene expression.

SLE See systemic lupus erythematosus

slow-reacting substance of anaphylaxis (SRS-A) A group of leukotrienes released by mast cells during anaphylaxis that induces a prolonged contraction of smooth muscle.

smallpox An infectious disease caused by the virus variola.

somatic gene conversion Nonreciprocal exchange of sequences between genes: part of the donor gene or genes is copied into an acceptor gene, but only the acceptor gene is altered; mechanism for generating diverse Ig repertoire in many nonhuman species.

somatic hypermutation Change in the variable region sequence of an antibody produced by a B cell following antigenic stimulation, resulting in increased antibody affinity for antigen.

spleen Largest of the secondary lymphoid organs; traps and concentrates foreign substances carried in the blood; composed of white pulp (rich in lymphoid cells) and red pulp (containing many erythrocytes and macrophages).

STATs See signal transducers and activators of transcription.

strain Set of animals (particularly mice and rats) in which every animal is bred to be genetically identical.

superantigen A molecule that activates all T cells with a particular V_β gene segment, irrespective of their V_α expression.

suppression A mechanism for producing a state of immunological unresponsiveness by which one cell or its products inhibit the function of another.

surrogate light chains Nonrearranging chains ($V_{\lambda 5}$ and V pre-B) expressed in conjunction with the μ chain in the pre-B cell; form part of the pre-B cell receptor.

switch region Region of B cell H chain DNA at which recombination occurs in an antigen-stimulated cell; allows isotype switch (e.g., IgM to IgE).

syngeneic Literally, genetically identical—for example, monozygotic twins or mice of the same strain.

syngraft Same as isograft.

systemic lupus erythematosus (SLE) An autoimmune disease that affects many organs of the body and causes fever and joint pain. Patients produce high levels of antibodies against the components of cell nuclei, particularly DNA, and form circulating soluble antigen–antibody complexes. These complexes deposit in tissues such as the kidney, activate the complement cascade, and result in tissue damage.

T cells The set of lymphocytes whose differentiation requires the thymus.

T_H1 A subset of $CD4^+$ T cells that synthesizes the cytokines interleukin 2, interferon γ, and tumor necrosis factor β; these cytokines activate the effector cells of cell-mediated immunity: natural killer cells, macrophages, and $CD8^+$ T cells.

T_H2 A subset of $CD4^+$ T cells that synthesizes the cytokines interleukin 4, 5, 10, and 13; these cytokines predominate in the response to allergens and parasites (B cell class switching to IgE and eosinophil activation).

tacrolimus An immunosuppressive polypeptide drug (also called FK506) that inactivates T cells by inhibiting signal transduction from the T cell receptor.

TAP-1 and TAP-2 Molecules that selectively transport peptides from the cytoplasm to the endoplasmic reticulum of cells for binding to MHC class I molecules.

target A cell killed by one of the body's killer cells, such as a cytotoxic T lymphocyte or natural-killer cell.

tapasin A TAP-associated protein that is a key molecule for the assembly of MHC class I molecules. Cells deficient in this protein are unable to express MHC class I molecules on their surface.

Tc cell T cytotoxic cell.

T cell receptor (TCR) A two-chain structure on T cells that binds antigen: α and β on the major set of T cells, γ and δ on the minor set of T cells. The TCR complex makes up the antigen-binding chains associated at the cell surface with signal transduction molecules CD3 plus ζ.

TCR See T cell receptor

T-dependent (TD) antigen An immunogen that requires T helper cells to interact with B cells to induce antibody synthesis.

terminal deoxynucleotidyl transferase (TdT) Enzyme that inserts nontemplated nucleotides at the junctions of V, D, and J gene segments of Ig and T cell receptor locus DNA; these N-nucleotides increase the diversity of antigen-specific receptors.

thymocytes T cells differentiating in the thymus.

thymus The primary lymphoid organ for T cell differentiation, made up of an outer cortex and inner medulla; developing thymocytes interact with epithelial cells and bone marrow–derived macrophages and interdigitating dendritic cells in the thymus.

TIL See tumor infiltrating lymphocyte

T-independent (TI) antigen An immunogen that induces antibody synthesis in the absence of T cells or their products; antibodies synthesized generally only of the IgM isotype, with no memory response.

titer Generally, an empirical measure of the avidity of an antibody; the reciprocal of the last dilution of a titration giving a measurable effect—for example, if the last dilution of an antibody giving significant agglutination is 1:128, the titer is 128.

TNF See tumor necrosis factor

tolerance Antigen-specific unresponsiveness of B or T cells.

Toll pathway An ancient signaling pathway that activates transcription factor $NF_{\kappa}B$ by degrading its inhibitor $I_{\kappa}B$.

Toll-like receptors (TLRs) A family of pattern-recognition receptors expressed on cells of the innate immune system, such as macrophages and dendritic cells, that bind to microorganisms. Interaction results in the production of inflammatory cytokines and the expression of costimulatory molecules that enhance the adaptive immune response.

toxic shock syndrome Systemic reaction produced by the toxin derived from the bacterium *Staphylococcus aureus;* the toxin acts as a superantigen that activates a high proportion of $CD4^+$ T cells to produce cytokines.

toxoid A nontoxic derivative of a toxin used as an immunogen for the induction of antibodies capable of cross-reacting with the toxin.

transplantation Grafting solid tissue (such as a kidney or heart) or cells (particularly bone marrow) from one individual to another. See allograft; xenograft

tuberculin test Antigens derived from the organism causing tuberculosis are injected subcutaneously; individuals who have been exposed to the organism and those who have been previously vaccinated with bacille Calmette-Guerin develop a delayed hypersensitivity response at the injection site 24–48 hours later.

tumor infiltrating lymphocyte (TIL) Mononuclear cell derived from the inflammatory infiltrate of solid tumors.

tumor-specific transplantation antigen (TSTA) Antigens uniquely expressed by certain tumor cells.

TUNEL assay Identifies apoptotic cells in situ by the characteristic fragmentation of their DNA. It uses TdT-dependent dUTP-biotin nick end labeling assay.

type I hypersensitivity Immediate hypersensitivity reactions involving IgE responses and the triggering of mast cells.

type II hypersensitivity Involves destruction of cells mediated by antibody (predominantly IgG) binding to cell-associated antigens.

type III hypersensitivity Involves damage to tissue mediated by the deposition of antigen–antibody complexes, resulting in complement activation.

type IV hypersensitivity T-cell mediated, delayed hypersensitivity reactions.

tyrosine kinases A family of enzymes that phosphorylates proteins on tyrosine residues, a critical step in lymphocyte activation. The key tyrosine kinases in T cell activation are Lck, Fyn, and ZAP-70; those in B cell activation are Blk, Fyn, Lyn, and Syk.

unresponsiveness Inability to respond to antigenic stimulus. Unresponsiveness may be specific for a particular antigen (see tolerance) or broadly nonspecific as a result of damage to the entire immune system— for example, after whole-body irradiation.

V regions See variable regions

V(D)J recombination Mechanism for generating antigen-specific receptors of T and B cells; it involves the joining of V, D, and J gene segments mediated by the enzyme complex V(D)J recombinase, and products of the *RAG-1* and *RAG-2* genes.

vaccination Any protective immunization against a pathogen. Originally referred to immunization against smallpox with the less-virulent cowpox (vaccinia) virus.

variable (V) regions The N-terminal portion of an Ig or T cell receptor that contains the antigen-binding region of the molecule; V regions are formed by the recombination of V(D) and J gene segments.

virion A complete virus particle.

virus An organism made up of a protein coat and DNA or RNA genome; it requires a host cell for replication.

Western blot A technique to identify a specific protein in a mixture; proteins separated by gel electrophoresis are blotted onto a nitrocellulose membrane, and the protein of interest is detected by adding radiolabeled antibody specific for the protein.

wheal and flare Itchy reaction at skin site where antigen is injected into an allergic individual; characterized by erythema (redness due to dilation of blood vessels) and edema (swelling produced by release of serum into tissue).

xenogeneic Originating from a foreign species.

xenograft A tissue transplantation between individuals belonging to two different species.

X-linked agammaglobulinemia A disease in boys (also known as Bruton's agammaglobulinemia) manifesting as absence of mature B cells; B cell differentiation does not progress beyond the pre-B cell due to defective tyrosine kinase BTK.

X-linked hyper-IgM syndrome Disease in boys manifesting as inability to synthesize Ig isotypes other than IgM; result of defect in either CD40 or CD154.

ZAP-70 A T cell specific tyrosine kinase involved in T cell activation.

APPENDIX

Partial List of CD Antigens

CD Antigen	Other Name(s)	Cellular Expression	Function/Comments	Ligand
CD1		Langerhans cells, dendritic cells, B cells, thymocytes	MHC class I–like molecule, presents lipids and glycolipids to T cells	Lipids, glycolipids
CD2	T11, LFA-2	T cells, NK cells	T cell adhesion molecule	CD58
CD3	T3	T cells	TCR signal transduction	
CD4	T4	Thymocytes, major set of mature T cells (MHC class II restricted), monocytes, macrophages	TCR coreceptor, signal transduction	MHC class II, HIV-1 and HIV-2, gp120
CD5	T1, Tp67	B cell subset, T cells	B cell expression associated with polyreactive IgM production	
CD8	T8	Thymocytes, major set of mature T cells (MHC class I restricted) = cytotoxic T cells	TCR coreceptor, signal transduction	MHC class I
CD11a	LFA-1 chain	Leukocytes	Subunit of adhesion molecule CD11a/CD18 (LFA-1)	ICAM-1, -2, -3
CD18		Leukocytes	Integrin chain that associates with CD11a, b, c, or d	
CD19		B cells	B cell signal transduction	
CD20		B cells	Ca^{2+} channel in B cell activation	
CD21	CR2	B cells, follicular dendritic cells	Involved in B cell activation	Complement component C3d and EBV
CD25	TAC	Activated T cells, B cells	IL-2 receptor α chain	IL-2
CD28	Tp44	T cell subsets	T cell costimulator molecule	B7 (CD80 and CD86)
CD32	FcγRII	Monocytes, granulocytes, B cells, eosinophils	Low-affinity receptor for IgG	Aggregated IgG and antigen–antibody complexes
CD34		Endothelial cells, hematopoietic precursors	Marker for early stem cells	L-Selectin (CD62L)
CD40		B cells, macrophages, dendritic cells	Involved in T cell interactions with APCs and class switching; receptor for costimulatory signals	CD154 (CD40L)
CD44	Pgp-1, H-CAM	Leukocytes, erythrocytes	Lymphocyte adhesion to HEV	Hyaluronic acid

CD Antigen	Other Name(s)	Cellular Expression	Function/Comments	Ligand
CD50	ICAM-3	Broad (not on endothelial cells)	Adhesion molecule	LFA-1
CD54	ICAM-1	Broad	Adhesion molecule	CD11a/CD18, rhinovirus
CD55	DAF	Broad	Dissociates C3 convertases of complement cascades	C3b, C4b, CD97
CD58	LFA-3	Leukocytes, endothelial cells, epithelial cells, fibroblasts	Adhesion molecule	CD2
CD62L	L-Selectin, MEL-14	B cells, T cells, monocytes, NK cells	T cell adhesion to HEV	CD34
CD74	Invariant chain	B cells, macrophages, monocytes, activated T cells	Associated with MHC class II in endoplasmic reticulum	
CD79a, CD79b	Igα, Igβ	B cells, pre-B cells	Signal transduction molecules, components of B cell receptor	
CD80	B7.1	B cells, macrophages, dendritic cells	Costimulatory molecule on APC	CD28, CD152 (CTLA-4)
CD81	Target of antiproliferative antibody (TAPA-1)	Broad	Associates with CD19 and CD21 on B cells to form B cell coreceptor	
CD86	B7.2	Activated B cells, macrophages, dendritic cells	Costimulatory molecule on APC	CD28, CD152 (CTLA-4)
CD95	Fas, Apo-1	Activated T and B cells, NK cells	Induces apoptosis following ligation with Fas ligand (CD178, CD95L)	CD178 (Fas ligand, CD95L)
CD97	GR1	Granulocytes, macrophages, activated T and B cells	Counterreceptor for CD55	CD55
CD102	ICAM-2	Endothelial cells, resting lymphocytes, platelets	Adhesion molecule	CD11a (LFA-1)
CD152	CTLA-4	Activated T cells	Negative regulator for T cell activation	CD80 (B7.1) and CD86 (B7.2)
CD154	CD40L	Activated T cells	Ligation with CD40 on B cells induces B cell proliferation and class switching	CD40
CD178	FAS ligand, CD95 ligand	T cells and NK cells	Induces apoptosis in cells expressing CD95; humans and KO mice with CD178 mutation show severe autoimmune disease	CD95 (Fas)
CD210	IL-10 receptor	T and B cells, NK cells, monocytes, macrophages	Receptor for IL-10; ligation with IL-10 inhibits macrophage, monocyte, and dendritic cell cytokine production	IL-10

CD Antigen	Other Name(s)	Cellular Expression	Function/Comments	Ligand
CD212	IL-12 receptor β chain	Majority of T cells, NK cells, some B cell lines	Dimerizes and associates with an unknown chain to form the IL-12 receptor; IL-12 directs immune responses preferentially toward T_H1-type responses.	IL-12
CD213	IL-13 receptor	Broadly expressed in hematopoetic tissue, nervous system, and other tissues	Upon binding to IL-13, mediates signals to suppress inflammatory cytokine production by monocytes and macrophages; IL-13 induces B cell proliferation and Ig production	IL-13
CD217	IL-17 receptor	Broad tissue distribution; cord blood lymphocytes, peripheral blood lymphocytes, thymocytes	Binds IL-17 with low affinity; IL-17 induces pro-inflammatory cytokine secretion	IL-17
CD220	Insulin receptor	Ubiquitous, including erythrocytes, liver, muscle, adipose tissue	Cellular receptor for insulin; mutation in CD220 leads to insulin-resistant diabetes mellitus	Insulin
CD247	T cell receptor ζ chain, CD3 ζ	All T cells	Part of CD3 complex; couples antigen recognition to intracellular signal transduction pathways	Not applicable

INDEX

Note: Page numbers followed by *f* or *t* indicate figures and tables, respectively.